GEORGE ELIOT MUSEUM.
J BURTON

International Congress and Symposium Series

Editor-in-Chief: Hugh L'Etang

The history of anaesthesia
Proceedings of the Second International Symposium on the History of Anaesthesia held in London 20–23 July 1987

The organizers would like to thank the following for their support:

Abbott Laboratories Ltd
Ambu International
Blease Medical Equipment
Cardiac Recorders
Dragerwerk (Lubek) AG
DuPont Ltd
Ferraris Medical
H. K. Lewis & Son Ltd
Hoechst UK Ltd
Imperial Chemical Industries Ltd
Life Support Engineering
Mallinckrodt
May & Baker Ltd
Mediplast
Ohmeda
Penlon Ltd
Portex Ltd
Reckitt & Colman
Rimmer Bros
Schwarz
Tricomed

Paperback edition
Published by Royal Society of Medicine Services Limited
1 Wimpole Street   London W1M 8AE
7 East 60th Street   New York   NY 10022
ISBN 0-905958-69-1

Hardback edition
Published in UK and Europe by
The Parthenon Publishing Group Limited
Casterton Hall, Carnforth, Lancs.
ISBN 0-85070-263-2

Published in USA and Canada by
The Parthenon Publishing Group Inc.
ISBN 0-929858-18-2

These proceedings are published by Royal Society of Medicine Services Ltd with financial support from the sponsor. The contributors are responsible for the scientific content and for the views expressed, which are not necessarily those of the sponsor, of the editor of the series or of the volume, of the Royal Society of Medicine or of Royal Society of Medicine Services Ltd.

British Library Cataloguing in Publication Data

International Symposium on the History of
  Anaesthesia (2nd: 1987: London, England).
  The history of anaesthesia
  1. Medicine. Anaesthesia, to 1975
  I. Title   II. Atkinson, R. S. (Richard
  Stuart)   III. Boulton, Thomas B.
  IV. Series
  617'.96'09

  ISBN 0-905958-69-1

Library of Congress Cataloging in Publication Data

The History of anaesthesia.
  (International congress and symposium series; no. 134)
  Proceedings of the Second International Symposium on
  the History of Anaesthesia, London, July 1987.
  Includes bibliographies and index.
  1. Anesthesia – History – Congresses.
  I. Atkinson, R. S. (Richard Stuart)
  II. Boulton, T. B.   III. International Symposium on
  the History of Anaesthesia (2nd; 1987; London, England)
  IV. Series. [DNLM: 1. Anesthesia – history – congresses.
  W3 IN207 no. 134/WO 11.1 H673 1987]
  RD79.H57   1988   617.9'6'09   89–3300

  ISBN 0-929858-18-2 (Parthenon)

Phototypeset by Dobbie Typesetting Limited, Plymouth, Devon
Printed in Great Britain at the Alden Press, Oxford

The History of Anaesthesia

Edited by

Richard S. Atkinson
Thomas B. Boulton

Royal Society of Medicine Services
London   New York

AND

The Parthenon Publishing Group
International Publishers in Science & Technology

Casterton Hall, Carnforth,
Lancs, LA6 2LA, U.K.

120 Mill Road, Park Ridge
New Jersey, U.S.A.

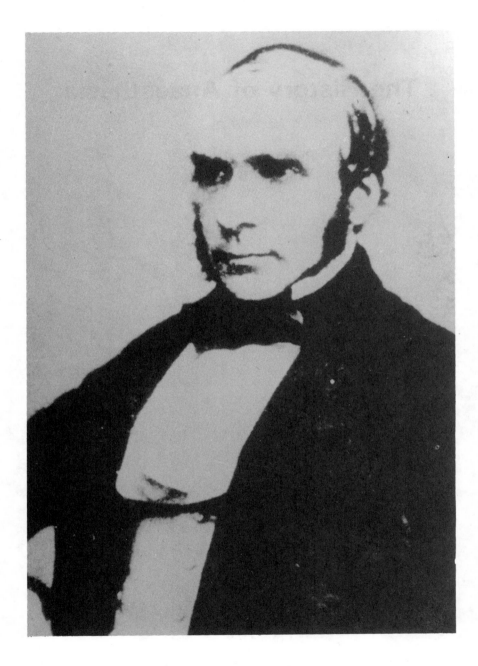

John Snow, MD (1813–1858)

Contributors

R. E. Abdel-Halim
(ch. 3.7, p. 46)

University Hospital, Jeddah, Saudi Arabia

A. K. Adams
(ch. 26.1, p. 619)

Faculty of Anaesthetists, Royal College of Surgeons, London, UK

A. P. Adams
(ch. 26.7, p. 619)

Guy's Hospital, London, UK

C. N. Adams
(ch. 8.8, p. 186)

West Suffolk Hospital, Bury St Edmunds, Suffolk, UK

M. Adt
(ch. 3.6, p. 40)

Deutsches Herzzentrum, Berlin, GFR

M. S. Albin
(ch. 24.1; 25.3; 25.4; 26.3, pp. 495, 533, 539, 619)

University of Texas Health Science Center, San Antonio, Texas, USA

L. G. Allan
(ch. 18.6, p. 368)

Northwick Park Hospital, Harrow, Middlesex, UK

A. A. Al-Mazrooa
(ch. 3.7, p. 46)

University Hospital, Jeddah, Saudi Arabia

R. S. Atkinson
(ch. 8.2; 24.3; 26.1; pp. 162, 500, 619)

Faculty of Anaesthetists, Royal College of Surgeons, London, UK

K. W. Ayisi
(ch. 20.1, p. 386)

University Hospital, Hamburg, GFR

N. Azzopardi
(ch. 5.7, p. 101)

Consultant Anaesthetist, Malta

R. J. Bailey
(ch. 22.6, p. 472)

Royal Alexandra Hospital for Children, Camperdown, NSW, Australia

A. B. Baker
(ch. 8.5, p. 176)

Otago University, Dunedin, NZ

C. Ball
(ch. 16.2; 25.8, pp. 323, 558)

Alfred Hospital, Prahan, Victoria, Australia

P. J. F. Baskett
(p. xxvi)

Bristol Royal Infirmary, Bristol, UK

G. S. Bause
(ch. 23.4, p. 488)

Yale University School of Medicine, New Haven, Connecticut, USA

v

H. Beakers
(ch. 14, p. 287)

State University, Leiden, The Netherlands

H. Beck
(ch. 25.7, p. 551)

University Hospital Hamburg, GFR

J. Beinart
(p. xxviii)

Wellcome Unit for the History of Medicine, University of Oxford, UK

N. A. Bergman
(ch. 23.1, p. 477)

Oregon Health Services University, Portland, Oregon, USA

C. Bernard-Dickstein
(ch. 21.1, p. 433)

Musée, Centre Public d'Aide Sociale, Brussels, Belgium

A. M. Betcher
(ch. 10.7, p. 223)

Mount Sinai School of Medicine, New York, USA

C. E. Blogg
(ch. 12.2, p. 268)

Nuffield Department of Anaesthetics, Oxford University, UK

R. Bodman
(ch. 10.5, p. 216)

Dartmouth, Nova Scotia, Canada

T. B. Boulton
(ch. 8.1, p. 159)

Royal Berkshire Hospital, Reading, UK

J. B. Bowes
(ch. 3.2, p. 26)

Bristol Royal Infirmary, UK

L. Brandt
(ch. 19.2; 19.3; 22.4; 22.5; pp. 375, 382, 464, 468)

Johannes Gutenberg University, Mainz, GFR

S. Calmes
(ch. 3.3; 6.4; 25.6; pp. 29, 129, 547)

Kern Medical Center, Bakersfield, California, USA

R. K. Calverley
(ch. 17.2, p. 333)

University of California, San Diego, USA

D. P. Coates
(ch. 23.3, p. 485)

Sir Humphry Davy Department of Anaesthesia, Bristol University, Bristol, UK

P. Coe
(ch. 23.2; 25.9; 26.7, pp. 481, 559, 619)

Guy's Hospital, London, UK

I. D. Conacher
(ch. 25.2, p. 528)

Freeman Hospital, Newcastle upon Tyne, UK

J. L. Couper
(ch. 3.4; 7.2; 7.3, pp. 34, 147, 149)

Medical University of South Africa, Republic of South Africa

T. F. Dagi
(ch. 18.5, p. 359)

US Navy, Washington, DC, USA

O. P. Dinnick
(ch. 24.5, p. 505)

The Middlesex Hospital, London, UK

D. Duda
(ch. 19.2; 19.3; 22.4; 22.5,
pp. 375, 382, 464, 468)

Johannes Gutenberg University, Mainz, GFR

B. M. Duncum
(ch. 4.3, p. 76)

26 St Edmunds Terrace, London, UK

A. Eccles
(ch. 26.2, p. 619)

St Bartholomew's Hospital, London, UK

M. El Gindi
(ch. 19.2; 19.3; 22.4; 22.5,
pp. 375, 382, 464, 468)

Johannes Gutenberg University, Mainz, GFR

R. H. Ellis
(ch. 1.1; 4.2, pp. 1, 69)

St Bartholomew's Hospital, London, UK

S. Ellmauer
(ch. 19.3, p. 382)

Johannes Gutenberg University, Mainz, GFR

L. W. Fabian
(ch. 10.6, p. 221)

Washington University School of Medicine,
St Louis, Missouri, USA

K. Filos
(ch. 20.1; 25.7, p. 386, 551)

University Hospital, Hamburg, GFR

B. R. Fink
(ch. 3.9, p. 52)

University of Washington, School of Medicine,
Seattle, Washington, USA

E. A. M. Frost
(ch. 25.2, p. 528)

Albert Einstein College of Medicine, New York,
USA

P. Frost
(ch. 26.8, p. 619)

Glan Clwyd Hospital, North Wales, UK

D. M. M. Gillies
(ch. 25.21, p. 614)

Queen Elizabeth Hospital of Montreal, Quebec,
Canada

M. Goerig
(ch. 20.1; 25.7, pp. 386, 551)

University Hospital, Hamburg, GFR

T. Gordh
(ch. 21.2, p. 441)

Karolinska Syukhuset, Stockholm, Sweden

R. A. Gordon
(ch. 8.3, p. 164)

University of Ontario, Toronto, USA

T. C. Gray
(ch. 2.5; 24.8, pp. 16, 518)

University of Liverpool, UK

U. von Hintzenstern
(ch. 3.5; 24.4, pp. 38, 502)

University of Erlangen, GFR

A. J. C. Holland
(ch. 6.3; 24.6, pp. 126, 510)

McGill University, Montreal, Quebec, Canada

D. D. C. Howat
(ch. 4.4, p. 79)

St George's Hospital, London W1, UK

R. Hughes *(ch. 12.1, p. 259)*	*Wellcome Research Laboratories, Beckenham, Kent, UK*
R. M. Humble *(ch. 10.4, p. 214)*	*University of Alberta, Edmonton, Alberta, Canada*
G. Huston *(ch. 18.4, p. 352)*	*Glendale Adventist Medical Center, Glendale, California, USA*
A. I. Hyman *(ch. 11.2, p. 233)*	*College of Physicians and Surgeons, Columbia University, New York, USA*
M. T. Jasser *(ch. 3.8, p. 48)*	*University of Aleppo, Syria*
P. Jones *(ch. 16.3, p. 325)*	*University Hospital of Wales, Cardiff, UK*
J. R. Jude *(ch. 22.3, p. 452)*	*University of Miami, Florida, USA*
W. Jurczck *(ch. 5.8, p. 105)*	*Medical Academy, Poznan, Poland*
L. Kaufman *(ch. 18.1, p. 343)*	*University College Hospital, London, UK*
J. W. van Kleef *(ch. 5.4, p. 92)*	*University Hospital, Leiden, The Netherlands*
S. Kurimoto *(ch. 8.7, p. 184)*	*Osaka Medical School, Takatui, Osaka, Japan*
M. Kuś *(ch. 5.8, p. 105)*	*Medical Academy, Krakow, Poland*
J. J. de Lange *(ch. 5.4, p. 92)*	*Free University Hospital, Amsterdam, The Netherlands*
J. A. Lee *(ch. 2.3, p. 12)*	*Southend Hospital, Southend on Sea, Essex, UK*
K. G. Lee *(ch. 25.18, p. 601)*	*Westminster Hospital, London, UK*
Z. Lett *(ch. 7.4, p. 153)*	*University of Hong Kong, Hong Kong*
J. A. MacDougall *(ch. 6.2, p. 119)*	*St John Regional Hospital, New Brunswick, Canada*
Sir Robert Macintoch *(ch. 2.1, p. 8)*	*Nuffield Department of Anaesthesia, University of Oxford, UK*
J. R. Maltby *(ch. 6.1; 8.6, pp. 112, 178)*	*University of Calgary, Alberta, Canada*
R. Mansfield *(ch. 2.1, p. 8)*	*Brompton Hospital, London, UK*

A. Matsuki   *University of Hirosaki, Hirosaki, Japan*
(ch. 24.2; 26.5, pp. 498, 619)

M. Mauve   *Laren, The Netherlands*
(ch. 5.5, p. 95)

C. A. B. McLaren   *Princess Alexandra RAF Hospital, Wroughton, UK*
(ch. 9.2, p. 195)

I. McLellan   *University of Leicester, UK*
(ch. 10.2, p. 205)

L. E. Morris   *Seattle, Washington, USA*
(ch. 25.11; 25.13; 25.14; 25.15;
26.6, pp. 571, 575, 579, 580, 619)

I. Muller   *Ludwig-Maximilians Universität, München, GFR*
(ch. 3.6, p. 40)

W. W. Mushin   *Welsh National School of Medicine, Cardiff,*
(ch. 2.4, p. 14)   *Wales, UK*

J. F. Nunn   *Clinical Research Centre, Harrow, Middlesex, UK*
(ch. 3.1, p. 21)

Y. V. O'Neill   *Medical Center, University of California at*
(ch. 3.3, p. 29)   *Los Angeles, USA*

B. Owen   *Glan Clwyd Hospital, Bodelwyddan, Clwyd,*
(ch. 22.2, p. 447)   *Wales, UK*

W. K. Pallister   *The Middlesex Hospital, London, UK*
(ch. 25.19, p. 605)

G. R. Park   *Addenbrookes Hospital, University of Cambridge,*
(ch. 13.2, p. 283)   *UK*

C. Parsloe   *Hospital Samaritano, São Paulo, Brazil*
(ch. 25.16, p. 590)

R. W. Patterson   *University of California at Los Angeles, USA*
(ch. 11.1, p. 230)

A. Patwari   *ESI Hospital, Sanathnagar, Hyderabad, India*
(ch. 11.3, p. 236)

J. L. Pettis   *Loma Linda University, California, USA*
(ch. 20.3, p. 402)

K. Quinn   *Addenbrookes Hospital, University of*
(ch. 13.2, p. 283)   *Cambridge, UK*

A. Ramachari   *ESI Hospital, Anathnagar, Hyderabad, India*
(ch. 11.3, p. 236)

J. Ray   *University of San Antonio Health Center, San*
(ch. 24.1, p. 495)   *Antonio, Texas, USA*

L. Rendell-Baker
*(ch. 15.1; 17.1; 20.3, pp. 301,
328, 402)*
Loma Linda University, California, USA

J. Restall
(ch. 9.1, p. 192)
Cambridge Military Hospital, Aldershot, Hants

H. Rheinhold
(ch. 21, p. 433)
Université Libre de Bruxelles, Brussels, Belgium

D. Robinson
(ch. 25.4, p. 539)
*University of Texas Health Sciences Center,
San Antonio, Texas, USA*

Z. Rondio
(ch. 5.8; 11.4, pp. 105, 240)
Institute of Mother and Child, Warsaw, Poland

W. Röse
(ch. 25.5, p. 543)
*Medical Academy, Magdeburg, German
Democratic Republic*

J. Rupreht
*(ch. 5.1; 5.2; Foreword, pp. 82,
86, xxiii)*
Erasmus University, Rotterdam, The Netherlands

T. M. Savege
(ch. 13.3, p. 286)
The London Hospital, UK

P. Schmucker
(ch. 3.6, p. 40)
Deutsches Herzzentrum, Berlin, FDR

W. Schwarz
(ch. 8.4, p. 170)
University of Erlangen-Nurmberg, Erlangen, GFR

C. F. Scurr
(ch. 2.2, p. 9)
Westminster Hospital, London, UK

O. Secher
*(ch. 11.5; 20.4; 24.7, pp. 242,
425, 513)*
University Hospital, Atlanta, Georgia, USA

J. Severinghaus
(ch. 22.7, p. 475)
University of California, San Francisco, USA

W. D. A Smith
(ch. 10.1, p. 199)
University of Leeds, Yorks, UK

S. Smith

(ch. 24.1, p. 495)
*University of Texas Health Center, San Antonio,
USA*

D. Soban
(ch. 5.10, p. 109)
University Hospital, Ljubljana, Jugoslavia

D. H. Soucek
(ch. 17.1, p. 328)
Parma, Ohio, USA

J. E. Steinhaus
(ch. 13.1, p. 278)
Emory University, Atlanta, Georgia, USA

C. R. Stephen
(ch. 10.6, p. 221)
*Washington University School of Medicine,
St Louis, Missouri, USA*

J. B. Stetson
*(ch. 25.10; 25.17; 25.20,
pp. 564, 595, 609)*

Rush Presbyterian—St Luke's Medical Center,
Chicago, Illinois, USA

M. Sych
(ch. 5.8, p. 105)

Medical Academy, Krakow, Poland

M. S. M. Takrouri
(ch. 5.9, p. 107)

Jordan University, Amman, Jordan

T. A. Thomas
(ch. 14.2, p. 295)

Bristol Maternity Hospital, Bristol, UK

P. W. Thompson
(ch. 14.3; 18.2, pp. 298, 346)

University of Wales, Cardiff, Wales, UK

S. Tirer
(ch. 3.10, p. 56)

University of Pennsylvania, Philadelphia, USA

M. Tverskoy
(ch. 6.5; 26.4, pp. 133, 619)

Safed Government Hospital, Israel

M. B. Tyers
(ch. 12.2, p. 268)

Glaxo Group Research, Ware, Herts, UK

L. D. Vandam
(ch. 4.1, p. 64)

Harvard Medical School, Boston, Mass, USA

D. M. E. Vermeulen-Cranch
(ch. 5.6, p. 97)

University of Amsterdam, The Netherlands

R. Westhorpe
*(ch. 15.2; 16.2; 25.12, pp. 319,
323, 574)*

Geoffrey Kaye Museum of Anaesthesia History,
Royal Australian College of Surgeons, Melbourne,
Australia

M. van Wijhe
(ch. 14.1, p. 287)

Streekziekenhuis, Midden Twente, Hengelo,
Netherlands

D. J. Wilkinson
(ch. 18.3; 26.2, pp. 348, 619)

St Bartholomew's Hospital, London, UK

G. Wilson
(ch. 7.1; 25.15, pp. 134, 580)

Australian Society of Anaesthetists, Edgecliff,
NSW, Australia

J. D. P. Wolff
(ch. 16.1, p. 322)

Bloemendaal, The Netherlands

C. H. M. Woollam
(ch. 20.2, p. 393)

Norfolk and Norwich Hospital, Norwich, UK

J. E. Wynands
(ch. 25.21, p. 614)

Queen Elizabeth Hospital of Montreal, Quebec,
Canada

D. Zuck
(ch. 10.3, p. 207)

Chase Farm Hospital, Enfield, Middlesex, UK

Contents

PART VII SPECIAL PRESENTATIONS, 2.

Chapter 26 Posters

Chapter 27 Video and film presentation

The number of anaesthetists studying the history of their profession has increased unexpectedly rapidly, within a very few years. The 'Anaesthesia: Essays on Its History' (Springer-Verlag, 1985) recorded most of presentations from the First International Symposium on the History of Modern Anaesthesia at the Erasmus University Rotterdam in 1982 and, since that meeting was held two enthusiastic groups of historically minded anaesthetists have been established— the North American Anesthesia History Association and its counterpart in Europe based in Great Britain, The History of Anaesthesia Society. Both have attracted more members than might have been reasonably expected.

The great activity and happy enthusiasm of anaesthetist-historians were probably the most remarkable features of the 1987 Second International Symposium on the History of Anaesthesia held at the Royal College of Surgeons of England in London in July 1987. The variety of papers presented was quite astonishing. The excellent scientific part of the meeting was equalled by the non-scientific events. This book of Proceedings is not only an almost complete record of the presentations, but it is also a welcome souvenir of a most stimulating meeting.

The subdivision of these Proceedings into separate parts and chapters was certainly a major challenge but it has been crowned with success. The papers are grouped logically and naturally. The two editors, both prolific medical writers, deserve great credit for their efforts. It is most fortunate that all contributions to the Symposium are included in the volume as this increases their value as a rich source of information for future studies.

Each part of the book is interesting and important but Part I is remarkable. It includes the British pioneers' presentations. It is quite clear that the pioneers, whom we were privileged to have with us at the symposium, have much more to tell which should be recorded. Their contributions to this volume will hopefully encourage the organizers of future meetings to ask pioneers for more information.

It was recorded in the proceedings of the 1982 symposium 'Anaesthesia: Essays on Its History' that reports of studies of anaesthesia history from some very populous regions of this Earth of ours, had been scant. It seems that the situation has not changed in five years. Travelling anaesthetists know that much of historical importance to our profession could be written in areas such as Africa, Latin America, the Socialist Bloc countries and the Far East. One should not underestimate financial and political problems that fellow anaesthesia historians face in such places however. It is worth suggesting that for future symposia on the history of anaesthesia that the reading of papers in the absence of authors who are unable to travel to a meeting in person should be allowed and, indeed, one such paper appears in this proceedings volume.

With the exception of personal reminiscences, most of the authors of papers in these Proceedings are amateur historians. This is remarkable and worthy of admiration but one hopes that more professional medical historians will study the history of our specialty. There are signs that this is happening and at least two such contributions are included in this volume. It is hoped that many more will be stimulated to attend future meetings on the history of medicine and anaesthesia.

These Proceedings appropriately underline the success of the Second International Symposium on the History of Anaesthesia, London, 1987. They form another link in the line of important events in the story of professional anaesthesia. Rich in reminiscences and scientific information they will not fail to be enjoyed by numerous cultivated confreres. The Proceedings testify to and strengthen the universal bond among anaesthesiologists through space and time. They are a landscape through which we walked and a signpost to follow into the future.

Academisch Ziekenhuis,
Rotterdam,
The Netherlands

Joseph Rupreht
Secretary General
First International Symposium on
the History of Anaesthesia 1982

The Second International Symposium on the History of Anaesthesia was both an important conclave for the study of this very interesting subject and a pleasurable and harmonious occasion. We have endeavoured to record both these facets faithfully in this volume of *Proceedings*.

The main headings under which the Scientific Symposia programme was conducted have been echoed in the various Parts of the book, but suitably related Free Papers have been added to the Chapters of each Part, however, thus broadening the treatment of each subject. Part VI contains important biographical material derived from other free papers. Posters and other special presentations have been recorded in Part VII.

We would like to thank the speakers for their ready cooperation and skilled presentations of material suitable for publication—very few papers have escaped the net. We hope contributors will accept our decision to omit medical and academic titles and degrees in the interest of international uniformity. A list of Symposium Registrants and an index is included at the end of the volume.

We are also indebted to Hugh L'Etang, the Editor-in-Chief of the International Congress and Symposium Series and Mr Howard Croft of the Publications Department of the Royal Society of Medicine Services for their advice and ready cooperation.

We hope that our readers will have as much pleasure in reading these pages as we have had in compiling them.

Association of Anaesthetists   *Richard S. Atkinson*
of Great Britain and Ireland,   *Thomas B. Boulton*
9 Bedford Square,   *January 1988*
London W1, UK

Chairman:	Thomas B. Boulton
Deputy:	Richard S. Atkinson
Secretary General:	Peter F. Baskett
Deputy:	Ian R. Verner
Honorary Treasurer:	Michael Rosen
Deputy:	John N. Horton
Scientific Programme:	Peter W. Thompson, Ian McLellan, David J. Wilkinson
Social Programme:	Richard H. Ellis, Nickolas I. Newton
Technical Exhibition:	Ralph S. Vaughan
Audiovisual Presentation:	Colin A. B. McLaren, Trevor A. Thomas

The Officers of the	*President*:	Michael Rosen
Association of Anaesthetists	*Hon. Treasurers*:	Maurice M. Burrows
of Great Britain and Ireland.		William R. MacRae
(ex-officio)	*Hon. Secretaries*:	Michael T. Inman
		Peter Morris
	Editor:	John N. Lunn
	Chairman, Junior	G. William Hamlin
	Anaesthetists Group	

Administrative Secretariat — Barbara Burgess, Ann Muir, Pat Plant, and Una J. Spanner

Liaison with the 50th Anniversary Celebrations of the Nuffield Department of Anaesthetics, Oxford: Gordon M. C. Paterson

International Advisers

Australia:	Gwen Wilson	*Brazil*:	C. Parsloe
Canada:	J. R. Maltby	*Denmark*:	O. Secher
German Democratic Republic:	W. Röse	*Japan*:	A. Matsuki
The Netherlands:	J. Rupreht	*South Africa*:	J. Couper
United States of America:	R. Calverley		

Retrospect of the Second International Symposium on the History of Anaesthesia

The Second International Symposium on the History of Anaesthesia was held at the Royal College of Surgeons at Lincoln's Inn Fields on 20–23 July 1987.

The Royal College proved to be an excellent venue for the 300 delegates from 25 countries. The Symposium was under the Patronage of Her Royal Highness Princess Alexandra who displayed her legendary charm when she opened the Symposium and attended the Reception in the Great Hall of Lincoln's Inn which followed.

The Opening Ceremony was held in the Edward Lumley Hall of the Royal College of Surgeons under the Chairmanship of the Dean of the Faculty of Anaesthetists, Dr Aileen Adams. It was conducted with all the dignity of collegiate ceremonial.

Her Royal Highness referred in her speech to the international comradeship of our specialty and of its immense contribution to the development and improvement of surgical and other treatment of today's patients. In an informal moment she expressed the hope that anaesthetists of the future would find more time for pre- and post-operative visits so that they could become better known as personalities to the patient.

Princess Alexandra found time to visit every stand in the highly successful Pharmaceutical and Technical Exhibition and then went on to mingle informally with delegates and their guests at the Reception. Every person to whom she spoke came away savouring a moment of great pleasure in meeting such a charming and perspicacious lady.

The standard of the papers presented at the scientific session was uniformly high. One hundred and twenty-five papers were presented over the three days in two lecture theatres. The only complaint from the delegates being that they had to make a choice of which lecture theatre to attend at any one time.

Plenary Symposia were held on The Origins and Development of Anaesthesia in Various Countries, the History of Agents and Apparatus, and the History of Resuscitation and Intensive Care. Over 100 free papers were presented ranging from references to anaesthesia in early civilizations to the rise and fall of fazadinium a decade ago. New light was cast also on the work and characters of many famous figures in the development of anaesthesia and others who are not so famous but whose contributions were of great importance.

A highlight of the Scientific Programme was the daily presentation of personal reminiscences by British pioneers, Sir Robert Macintosh, Professor Cecil Gray, Dr Alfred Lee, Professor William Mushin and Dr Cyril Scurr. Each spoke brilliantly to a packed auditorium and made us appreciate the skill, innovation and fortitude of those anaesthetists of former times and all provided guidance and perspective for anaesthetists in the future.

The entire proceedings of the Symposium were recorded on audiotape and a package of slides and descriptive material providing for a self conducted tour of historic sites associates with anaesthesia in London, was available.* The Charles King Collection of historic apparatus was displayed at the headquarters of the Association of Anaesthetists of Great Britain and Ireland, 9 Bedford Square and there was a special complimentary exhibition at the Wellcome Institute. No meeting of anaesthetists would be worth its salt without an exacting social programme and this one was no exception. There was a reception and private view of the Summer Exhibition at the Royal Academy, a magnificent banquet at the Banqueting House in Whitehall, and an informal Riverboat Supper which was distinguished by a splendid display of conjuring tricks by an ever youthful Torsten Gordh.

*The audio tapes, the travel package and slides of the Charles King Collection can be obtained by writing to the Administrative Secretary, Association of Anaesthetists of Great Britain and Ireland, 9 Bedford Square, London W1B 3RA, England.

Daytime visits were organized to places of historical interest in the City of London for delegates and accompanying guests. The itineraries included the nineteenth century operating theatre of St Thomas' Hospital, the Chelsea Physic Garden and the National Theatre.

Thanks are due to many individuals and organizations for supporting this very successful Symposium and particularly to the Association of Anaesthetists of Great Britain and Ireland and its President, Professor Michael Rosen, for underwriting the meeting and to the Dean of the Faculty and the Royal College of Surgeons of England for acting as host at the College and smoothing the way for the ceremonial opening.

One of the hallmarks of many British Anaesthetists' meetings is that registration and organization on the day is in the hands of friendly amateurs, rather than professional congress organizers. On this occasion an excellent team, coordinated by Mrs Barbara Burgess, was composed of the wives of the members of the Organizing Committee and junior anaesthetists who acted as stewards. This cheerful band were well matched by the courteous, benign and charming delegates who attended the Symposium.

We now look forward in anticipation to the Third International Symposium on the History of Anaesthesia at Atlanta, Georgia, USA, in 1992—the 150th anniversary of the first administration of ether for a surgical operation by Dr Crawford W. Long in Jefferson, Georgia.

Bristol Royal Infirmary,
Bristol, UK

Peter J. F. Baskett,
Secretary General,
Second International Symposium on the
History of Anaesthesia. 1987

Problems and sources in the history of anaesthesia

JENNIFER BEINART

Wellcome Unit for the History of Medicine, University of Oxford, UK

When a historian offers to talk about the historiography of anaesthesia to people who are not only practitioners of the subject but practising historians themselves, I imagine there are a few inward groans among the audience. Some of the ground covered by this paper will be familiar to all of you, but I hope to raise one or two questions for leisurely debate. These are to do with the issues that constantly tax the ingenuity of all of us who attempt to research and write history. What are the important problems in this field at various points in time? And what use can we make of different sources to increase our understanding of these problems?

Earlier works on the history of anaesthesia

With the notable exception of Fueloep-Miller's 1938 work (1), the first wave of writing about the history of anaesthesia occurred around the centenary of the introduction of anaesthesia in 1946. Victor Robinson's *Victory over Pain* (2) and E. S. Ellis's *Ancient Anodynes* (3) were published that year, Thomas Keys' book the year before (4), and Barbara Duncum's (5) and Chauncey D. Leake's the following year (6). A major theme of most of these, and of several later contributions, was the question of primacy—who really deserved the credit for the innovation of anaesthesia? Although the story is a dramatic one, it does not warrant the amount of attention it has received. Some writers have attempted to deal with historically more interesting problems, such as why anaesthesia was introduced and accepted at that particular time, and its impact on surgery. Barbara Duncum, in a book of unrivalled scope, traced the development of apparatus and techniques through the second half of the nineteenth century. Two of the issues that give shape to her narrative are the rivalry between ether and chloroform, and the development of anaesthesia as a physician specialty in the United Kingdom. Her sources were almost entirely published books and articles, but she had undertaken a more wide-ranging search than many authors.

Later contributions

It would be misleading to talk about a second wave of writing on the history of anaesthesia. Rather, there has been a variable stream of books with titles like *The Conquest of Pain*, *The Control of Pain*, *The Battle for Oblivion* and *Pain and its Conquest*, again mainly dealing with the controversies surrounding the introduction of anaesthesia and largely dependent on published sources.* Three volumes of *Essays on the First Hundred Years of Anaesthesia* (7) and W. D. A. Smith's *Under the Influence* (8) are more original and innovative. The authors use more varied sources including letters, song sheets and so on, and consider a variety of problems.

---

*These are actual titles—the first having been used by two different authors. Other examples and full references can be found in the catalogue of the Wellcome Institute Library, London.

More recent work

Less well known among anaesthetists in this country is a recently published book by Martin Pernick of the History Department at the University of Michigan, called *A Calculus of Suffering: Pain, Professionalism and Anesthesia in Nineteenth Century America* (9). This deals with many aspects of one central problem; that is, the ideology of medical practitioners in relation to their selective use of anaesthesia for surgery. Pernick found that many American doctors made differential use of anaesthesia, depending on their judgment of a patient's ability to bear pain. For the same surgical procedures young children were more likely to receive anaesthesia than adults, women than men, educated than uneducated, white than black, patients. This analysis has not been universally accepted but, nevertheless the book provides a fascinating account of doctors' views, discussions in the literature, and the evidence of actual practice based on a rich array of sources. These include manuscript patient records from hospitals and individual doctors, manuscript MD theses, collected papers of practitioners, and an enormous range of periodicals, journals, and books. Both the method and the result are extremely impressive.

The history of the Nuffield Department of Anaesthesia, Oxford

My own work has been much more modest, both in scope and execution. However, on the basis of three years spent researching and writing up the history of the Nuffield Department of Anaesthetics at Oxford, I have definite views about problems and sources (10). Although we cannot all be concerned with the same problems, I feel that we should all attempt to set our research into a wider context. It is rather as though each of us was digging away, to uncover our own piece of mosaic; we need to step back in order to see the whole pattern. Beyond the merely local issues thrown up by the history of the Oxford department, I was struck by several interrelated problems. I will list these, without elaborating: firstly, professionalization and training, and their relation to the status of anaesthesia within medicine and, after 1948, within the National Health Service; secondly, the development of sub-specialties of anaesthesia, such as pain relief, intensive care and obstetric anaesthesia; thirdly, the use of regional versus general anaesthesia; fourthly, changes in mortality associated with anaesthesia; and finally, the relation of research to clinical practice.

The motley of sources I had to search out for this relatively recent history included personal papers, proceedings of committees, archives of the department, of the University, of the Regional Health Authority and so on—as well as the usual published sources.

The most interesting and also original type of source however was one that is only available for recent history: that is, the living custodians of history, the victims of my tape recorder. A number of people have asked me how much the interviews contributed to the book when I finally came to write it. I would say that I used direct quotes from them relatively little, and regarded them as a source of evidence that always had to be cross-checked on matters of fact such as dates and names. On the other hand, for evidence of what it felt like to be there at the time, and for a wealth of detail that has not found its way into the documentary sources, the oral account is invaluable. Let me take two examples from quite different periods in the history of the Oxford department to illustrate what I mean.

Right at the start, in 1937, Professor Macintosh spent time giving anaesthetics in Spain, and he has described in his own written accounts how that experience led to his determination to devise anaesthetic equipment that could be used in the difficult conditions of wartime. Speaking to him about this added new dimensions and this was further expanded by interviewing a colleague, Dr Kenneth Boston, who made the same expedition under the aegis of Mac and the Department in 1938.* It emerged that there was a slight disagreement between the two, lasting to this day, as to whether the use of the Flagg's Can type of apparatus in Spain in the winter led to a higher incidence of postoperative chest complications. Macintosh has always maintained that the purpose of warming the ether in the Oxford Vaporizer was simply to achieve a constant vapour pressure, and that there would be no difference in recovery rates whether

*The Author's interviews on audiotape now in the archives of the Nuffield Department of Anaesthetics. Dr Kenneth Boston (16/1/84)—units 110–130 Side B, and Sir Robert Macintosh (18/1/84) Side A.

the ether was warmed or not. When we go out for a walk on a frosty day, he says, do we not breathe in freezing cold air—and do we end up with pneumonia? This is partly a didactic position, taken to ensure that the real point of theory behind the vaporizer's ability to deliver a known concentration of vapour is understood. What the interview achieves here is both an angle of the story which would not be recoverable from written records, and also a taste of Macintosh's teaching techniques.

The second example I have chosen touches on a more controversial issue, and illustrates one of the pitfalls of oral evidence. That is, people may tell you things in interviews that they would not wish to become public knowledge. Whereas a historian feels free, within the terms set by the archivists, to use material in archives to the best of his or her ability to make a truthful interpretation, this is not the case with the oral record. To some extent the interviewee has a right of veto over the use of evidence given in an interview—and makes this clear by saying that they are giving a particular piece of information 'off the record'. Thus, I had heard from various sources that there had been attempt to abolish the Nuffield Chair of Anaesthetics in Oxford when the first Professor retired. This was not entirely surprising, since there had been great controversy over its establishment in the first place. However, it was important for me to discover how serious this attempt to abolish the Chair had been, and why it had come to nothing. I accumulated much evidence, the most revealing of which was oral evidence which was 'off the record'. In the end, because of the sensitive nature of these relatively recent events, virtually all I could say in my book was that the continuation of the Chair was ensured by its excellent record up to that date. Although this part of my research was, in a way, frustrating, it offered further confirmation of one of the key themes of the whole project: that is, the continuing low status of anaesthetics compared with several other branches of medicine, well into the postwar period, and its gradual elevation.

Conclusion

The historiography of anaesthesia, which really began forty years ago, has developed enormously in the past few years as evidenced by the 1982 and 1987 symposia on the history of anaesthesia (11). I hope anaesthetists and others will continue to work on it with the same enthusiasm, but with an increasingly critical eye.

References

(1) Fueloep-Miller R. *Triumph over pain*. New York: Literary Guild of America, 1938.
(2) Robinson V. *Victory over pain*. New York: Schuman, 1946.
(3) Ellis ES. *Ancient anodynes*. London: Heinemann, 1946.
(4) Keys TE. *The history of surgical anesthesia*. New York: Schuman, 1945.
(5) Duncum BM. *The development of inhalation anaesthesia*. London: Oxford University Press for Wellcome History of Medicine Museum, 1947.
(6) Leake CD. *Letheon: the cadenced story of anesthesia*. Austin: University of Texas Press, 1947.
(7) Sykes, WS. *Essays on the first hundred years of anaesthesia*. Vols 1, 2 and 3. Edinburgh: Livingstone, 1960, 1961 and 1982.
(8) Smith WDA. *Under the influence*. London: Macmillan, 1982.
(9) Pernick MS. *A calculus of suffering: pain, professionalism and anesthesia in nineteenth century America*. New York: Columbia University Press, 1985.
(10) Beinart JM. *A history of the Nuffield Department of Anaesthetics, Oxford, 1937–1987*. Oxford University Press, 1987.
(11) Rupreht J, van Leiburg MJ, Lee JA, Erdmann W. *Anaesthesia: essays on its history*. Berlin: Springer-Verlag, 1985.

PART I

SPECIAL PRESENTATIONS

Chapter 1
PRESENTATION DURING THE OPENING CEREMONY

1.1 Dr John Snow. His London residences,
and the site for a commemorative plaque in London

RICHARD H. ELLIS
St Bartholomew's Hospital, London, UK

John Snow achieved his most remarkable successes in the years between 1847 and 1858. These years were amongst those which were perceived by the Victorians as ones of confident and perpetual advance. The highlight of this period was the Great Exhibition of 1851 which was staged at the Crystal Palace in Hyde Park (1). It was full of the inventions and works of some 14 000 exhibitors from all over the world (2). Clearly, the Victorian era was not short of great men and women, and—of these—not a few were doctors.

John Snow's contributions to medicine

In many ways the unassuming John Snow was one of the most remarkable of those great Victorian physicians, for he achieved greatness, and an enduring reputation, in a unique way. Most of his distinguished medical contemporaries earned their reputations having made a lasting contribution to one important aspect of medical science. Snow's special claim is that he made lasting contributions to not one but two, completely unrelated aspects of medicine. These were the promotion of early anaesthesia and the discovery of the mode of spread of epidemic cholera. In each of these fields Snow's achievements were both enduring and of enormous humanitarian value.

In achieving this undoubted distinction in two such different subjects Snow had little if any precedent to follow. He had to guide his own inquisitiveness of mind, to initiate his own experiments, to answer his own questions, and to design his own tests, his own trials and his own apparatus. The conclusions he came to were entirely his own. The benefits of Snow's thinking were not confined to Britain alone. As far as cholera is concerned it was Snow who—for all time—solved the enigma of its mode of spread. The results of his work continue to benefit the entire human race, for it was Snow who showed how the dread disease could be controlled or eliminated.

Similarly, the results of Snow's work on anaesthesia—of which we should be particularly mindful—were to be felt worldwide. His earliest work on ether both complemented and catalysed the introduction of anaesthesia in Britain, and—by reinforcing its earlier but somewhat hesitant start in the United States—led to its rapid adoption throughout Europe and the rest of the developed world. His later work with ether and then with chloroform laid the scientific foundations of the speciality for years to come.

A commemorative plaque

Arguably, the debt still owed to John Snow is owed by people all over the world. It is fitting, therefore, that this unique medical meeting in London should begin by commemorating

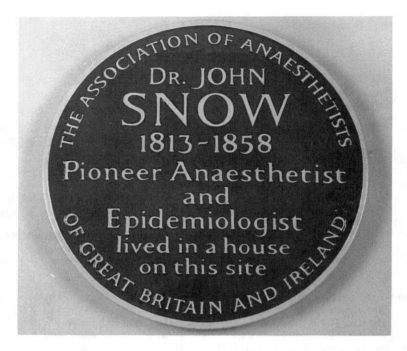

Figure 1   The commemorative plaque, now in place on the site of John Snow's former residence in Frith Street, Soho, London.

Dr John Snow's life in this city by unveiling a plaque (Fig. 1) which, tomorrow (21 July 1987), will be placed at the site of one of his residences here. This project has been sponsored by the Association of Anaesthetists of Great Britain and Ireland, and it is a pleasure to note the interest in it of several of John Snow's descendants. The whole project is made all the more meaningful and memorable by the presence of Her Royal Highness, Princess Alexandra.

John Snow's early life and his achievements and residences in London

John Snow's principal—if not only—biographer was his friend and distinguished Victorian physician Sir Benjamin Ward Richardson (3) who wrote at least two different but very similar accounts of Snow's life. One appeared as a preface to Snow's famous textbook *On Chloroform and other Anaesthetics* (4) and the other was published in *The Asclepiad* (5) and later appeared as a preface to the reprinting of Snow's two original papers on cholera (6).

John Snow was born in York, in 1813. From 1827 to 1833 he worked with a surgeon in Newcastle-upon-Tyne. Then he spent the next 3 years (until 1836) in general practices near Newcastle and York. In 1836, he travelled to London to study medicine more formally. For the remaining 22 years of his life (from 1836 to 1858) Snow lived and worked in London, and it was certainly in London that he accomplished those achievements for which he is now so well known.

During this time he had just three residences. All were in Central London, in what is now known as the West End. From 1836 until 1838 he lived at Bateman's Buildings, in Soho. From late 1838 until sometime in 1853 he lived at nearby Frith Street, also in Soho. In 1853 he moved once more, this time to an address in Sackville Street, Piccadilly, and there he remained until his death in 1858.

I should firstly explain which of these three addresses is the most suitable site at which to commemorate John Snow's life and work in London. The site should be that at which he lived during the most fruitful and productive period of his medical life. With the perspective of history, we can see that Snow's reputation, influence and attainments were more or less different during each of the times he spent at these three different places. At Bateman's Buildings Snow did little more than settle himself in London, and obtain his first medical qualifications. At Frith Street Snow established himself as a doctor, and pioneered his particular subjects of anaesthesia and the epidemiology of cholera. At Sackville Street Snow consolidated, or rounded off, his earlier work, and—to some extent—attained the eminence and public recognition which he so richly deserved.

It would be useful to consider this progression in more detail.

While living at Bateman's Buildings Snow was a medical student and was, virtually, unknown. In 1838 he qualified as a Member of the Royal College of Surgeons of England, and also became a Licentiate of the Society of Apothecaries. These successes seem to have been the signal for him to move to a more congenial address. Although this period of Snow's life was extremely important to him, I do not think that we need to consider Bateman's Buildings as a suitable site for the commemoration of Snow's great achievements in London.

During the time when he was at Frith Street Snow became well established as a doctor. In 1843 he qualified at the new University of London, and a year later he obtained his Doctorate. Gradually he began to develop his reputation in London, principally by working at several London hospitals, and by speaking on a variety of subjects at medical meetings. Most importantly of all he began his pioneering work on the epidemiology of cholera and on anaesthesia.

Cholera

Snow had treated cases of cholera during his time as a family doctor in the North of England, but his real interest—particularly in its mode of spread—did not begin until 1848. In that year he studied a serious outbreak of the disease in London, which caused no less than 7500 fatal cases (7).

In 1848 the cause of cholera was not at all understood, but the generally-held view was that it occurred because of the inhalation of impure or foul, contaminated air—especially that found in overcrowded and insanitary slums (8). This view was supported by most of the medical profession, and also by the Water Companies who had a vested interest in its promotion. Snow, however, thought differently. He believed that some unknown contaminant in drinking water was to blame. Bacteria were at the time virtually unknown, and so Snow had to prove his point by epidemiology, that is by making a careful study of the factors to which the spread of the disease could be related. In 1849 (within a year of beginning his detailed study), he published the first edition of his later-to-be-famous work *On the mode of communication of cholera* (7).

It was Snow's first publication on the subject, and makes it quite clear that by this time—1849—he had convincingly demonstrated that cholera was spread by contaminated drinking water. He wrote 'It remains evident that the only special and peculiar cause connected with the great calamity was the state of the water, which was followed by the cholera in almost every house to which it extended, whilst all the surrounding houses were quite free from it.' However, the medical profession continued to believe, and the Water Companies continued to hope that Snow was wrong, and that the breathing of foul air was, indeed, the cause of cholera. As a result yet another great epidemic occurred (in 1854 in Soho) before the correctness of Snow's views was at last acknowledged.

Anaesthesia

As far as anaesthesia is concerned it is virtually certain that it was on the 28 December, 1846, that Snow had his first experience of the subject (9). On that day Snow saw a demonstration by James Robinson, the Gower Street dentist who had been the very first to use ether in England (10). The 28 December, 1846, was just nine days after ether anaesthesia had first been used in Britain. Undoubtedly, the greatly-overlooked James Robinson was the most important figure in the very earliest weeks of British anaesthesia, but his approach was necessarily empirical.

It was left to the alert and medically-trained John Snow to establish a scientific approach to the subject, and—quite properly—within a matter of 4 to 6 weeks the pioneering mantle passed from Robinson to him.

Snow, alone amongst his contemporaries, explored and deduced the physical principles on which the anaesthetic use of ether depended. He then designed his own inhaler and developed his own, clinically-sound methods. He began to publicize his results, and became a much sought-after and acknowledged expert in the field. For most of 1847 he was ether's champion and logical defender. In the autumn of that year he published his famous textbook on ether (11). Soon after this he began to prefer and promote chloroform rather than ether (12). Again he developed his own clinically-sound method, and lost no time in publicizing his results. He quickly became Britain's leading authority on the use of chloroform, and nurtured and encouraged its safe use in the United Kingdom and abroad.

By 1 May, 1850—within three and a half years of anaesthesia's invention—Snow's reputation as an anaesthetist was such that he had been consulted by Queen Victoria's doctors about the possibility of giving chloroform analgesia to Her Majesty for pain relief during the imminent birth of Prince Arthur (4). This particular occasion was less than two and a half years after chloroform was first introduced and so it is hardly surprising that Snow, although he was consulted, was not actually called in to give Her Majesty the chloroform. But three years later he was asked to go to the old Buckingham Palace and did give chloroform to Queen Victoria for childbirth. This was for the birth of Prince Leopold (13). Snow's use of chloroform on that occasion excited both amazement and criticism in the medical press. The Editor of *The Lancet*, in particular, was outraged (14).

However, Queen Victoria, herself, was unreservedly enthusiastic. She wrote, 'Dr Snow gave that blessed chloroform, and the effect was soothing, quieting and delightful beyond measure' (15). This was in April, 1853, and was Snow's first administration of what became known as 'Chloroform à la Reine'.

It was at about this time that Snow left his home in Frith Street and moved to Sackville Street. It is not possible to be sure precisely when in the spring of 1853 Snow actually made this move. However, what is clear is that during the 5 years from 1853 to 1858 which Snow spent at Sackville Street he attained an increasing degree of public recognition and eminence. In 1855 he was honoured by being elected President of the Medical Society of London. In 1857 he was, again, called in to administer chloroform to Queen Victoria—for the birth of Princess Beatrice (16). On that occasion his critics were silent. He also worked on his famous textbook *On Chloroform and other Anaesthetics* (4), but died in 1858 just as he was completing the manuscript.

The Broad Street pump

It was while at Sackville Street that the celebrated episode of the Broad Street pump-handle took place (17). In September, 1854, a terrible epidemic of cholera raged through Soho. Towards its end, Snow successfully urged the local authorities to remove the handle of the Broad Street water pump from which he was convinced infected water was being drawn. Soon afterwards the epidemic subsided completely, and the medical profession did take notice of Snow's views. The facts surrounding this episode have, over the years, been subjected to enormous distortion, but, nonetheless, it is judged by many to have been Snow's most famous epidemiological achievement.

The site for the commemorative plaque

At this point it is clear which of the sites of Snow's former London residences, in Frith Street or in Sackville Street, is the most suitable for his commemoration with a plaque. The choice must fall on Frith Street, for it was here that Snow spent most of his working life in London, and it was here that the diligent and ascetic Snow conceived his ideas, developed his theories, and honed them into what, for that time, was perfection. Here he was at his most original and progressive, and it was here that he laid the secure foundations for all that came after.

It was while living at Frith Street that, as an anaesthetist, Snow had pioneered and promoted the scientific basis and safe clinical applications of the subject. It was while at Frith Street that he worked to attain such acclamation for anaesthesia, and such eminence for himself, that he was asked (within just three and a half years of anaesthesia's invention) to consider the awesome duty of giving chloroform to Queen Victoria for childbirth.

As far as the epidemiology of cholera is concerned it is true to say that Snow's carefully researched, original ideas were only forced into general acceptance by the action he advised as the 1854 Soho epidemic subsided. Epidemiologically this was indeed his great moment, and he certainly had, by then, moved on from Frith Street. However, viewed with the perspective of history, it is clear that the 1854 epidemic merely provided Snow with the opportunity to prove once again that his previously held views were undoubtedly correct, and could no longer be ignored. These views, of course, he had expounded from his Frith Street home 5 years earlier in 1849 (7).

From Sackville Street Snow continued to dominate British anaesthesia, and to champion his views on the epidemiology of cholera. While at Sackville Street he, deservedly, acquired many outward and visible signs of his success as a doctor, but it is clear that these acquisitions only came because of his reputation previously assured by the work he had already done during his 15 years at Frith Street.

The present-day site of Snow's Frith Street home

As far as his precise address in Frith Street is concerned, there are several records which show that Snow lived at number 54 Frith Street. The relevant Kelly's Postal Directories for London (18), and The Medical Directories (19) all give Snow's address as 54 Frith Street. In addition Snow, when his textbook on ether was published in 1847 (11), was careful to add this address which is also recorded in two of his biographies (4,5). Proof positive of the address can be obtained from the 1841 and 1851 Census Reports (20,21) both of which show Snow as a resident at 54 Frith Street. The Local Authority Rate Books (22) do not help since Snow was never the owner of the house, but, seemingly, merely a lodger.

The house itself was demolished many years ago, but it is still possible to identify its present day site. It is clear from a study of a number of disparate sources that the house which was Snow's Frith Street home stood on precisely the same site as we might expect from the present numbering system of the street. From 1856 onwards to the present-day there have been no changes in this numbering system. 1856 was the year in which the Local Authorities first began to formally record all such alterations, and no relevant changes are to be found (23). That there were no earlier changes in the numbering system (that is during the years from the late 1830s to 1856) can be deduced from records showing the locality 'house by house' and 'street by street'. Over the period of Snow's residence at Frith Street consecutive entries in the Kelly's Street Directories for London (18) and the Local Authority Rate Books (22) show consistency with their later editions, and with still-surviving maps of the area (24–26). These consistently show that the house immediately on the south-west corner of the intersection of Frith Street and Bateman Street is number 55 Frith Street. Number 54 (the house in which Snow lived) was immediately next to number 55, that is, it was the second house down from the south-west corner of that intersection.

The Ordnance Survey Map of 1984 (27) shows the positions of the buildings which occupy the neighbourhood today. There is still a single building on the corner at number 55, but the site of the old 54 Frith Street is now incorporated into a larger development extending from numbers 51 to 54.

A picture of Snow's Frith Street home

An interesting, but hitherto unobserved nineteenth century painting (28) shows what part at least of the house must have looked like during the time of Snow's residence there. The water-colour was painted in 1891 by a London artist named John Emslie (29). It was designed to show the house then on the corner at number 55 Frith Street. Intriguingly, it also shows us on

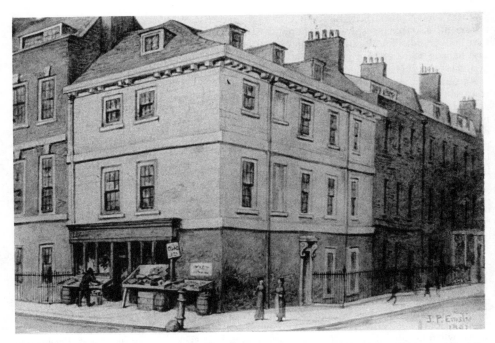

Figure 2   The painting by J. P. Emslie (28) which shows—on the left of the picture—part of the frontage of John Snow's Frith Street residence. Snow lived there from 1838 until 1853.

the left of the illustration (Fig. 2) just about half of the frontage of John Snow's former residence next door at number 54. This is the only illustration which now exists showing even part of the original house in which Snow lived during his most inventive years, and it is probably the only glimpse we can ever have of that important building.

The Association of Anaesthetists' plaque on its site will serve as an appropriate and permanent memorial to John Snow in London. I hope that it will also serve to remind us now, and countless others in the years to come, of the continuing debt which people throughout the world owe to John Snow and his brilliant career.

References

(1) Babbage C. *The Exposition of 1851*. London: Murray, 1851.
(2) ffrench Y. *The Great Exhibition: 1851*. London: Hanvill Press, 1951.
(3) McNalty AS. *A biography of Sir Benjamin Ward Richardson*. London: Harvey and Blythe, 1950.
(4) Snow J. *On chloroform and other anaesthetics*. London: Churchill, 1858.
(5) Richardson BW. John Snow, M.D. *The Asclepiad* 1887; **4**: 274–300.
(6) Snow J. *Snow on cholera*. New York: The Commonwealth Fund, 1936.
(7) Snow J. *On the mode of communication of cholera*. London: Churchill, 1849.
(8) Mackintosh JM. Snow—the man and his times. *Proc Roy Soc Med* 1955; **48**: 1004–7.
(9) Robinson J. Correspondence. *Med Times* 1847; **15**: 274.
(10) Boott F. Surgical operations performed during insensibility. *Lancet* 1847; **1**: 5–8.
(11) Snow J. *On the inhalation of the vapour of ether in surgical operations*. London: Churchill, 1847.
(12) Snow J. On the inhalation of chloroform and ether. *Lancet* 1847; **i**: 177–180.
(13) Anonymous. Birth of a Prince. *The Times* 1853 April 8: page 5, col 5.
(14) Anonymous. Editorial. *Lancet* 1853; **i**, 453.

(15) The Royal Archives, Windsor. *Queen Victoria's Journal*, 1853 April 22.

(16) Anonymous. Birth of a Princess. *The Times* 1857 April 15 page 7, col 1.

(17) Bradford Hill, A. Snow—an appreciation. *Proc Roy Soc Med* 1955; **48**: 1008–12.

(18) Kelly's Post Office Directories. London: Kelly, 1838–1853.

(19) Medical Directories. London: Churchill, 1838–1853.

(20) Census, 1841. London: Public Record Office. HO 107/730, book 2, folio 18, page 27.

(21) Census 1851. London: Westminster City Library (Victoria). Reel 18, Ref. 1510/28.

(22) Poor Rate, St Anne's Westminster, 1838–1853. Westminster City Library (Victoria).

(23) Anonymous. *Names of Streets and Places in the Administrative County of London*. 4th ed. London: London County Council, 1955.

(24) Ordnance Survey, 1894–1896. London: Sheet VII, 63.

(25) Ordnance Survey, 1875. London: Sheet XXXIV.

(26) Insurance Plan of the city of London, 1886–1897. The British Library, reference 145.b.22, (1–12).

(27) Ordnance Survey (SIM), 1984. London: Plan TQ2981SE.

(28) Copy of Watercolour by J. P. Emslie. The premises at 55 Frith Street, Soho; London (1891). Greater London Council Record Office and History Library. London. Reference Westminster CA 26.

(29) Phillips JFC. John Philipps Emslie (1839–1913) and his topographical drawings of the London area. *Guildhall Studies in London History* 1976; **2**: 69–76.

Chapter 2
BRITISH PIONEER PRESENTATIONS

2.1	Saved by the Flagg

SIR ROBERT MACINTOSH
Nuffield Department of Anaesthetics, University of Oxford, UK

I first met Eastman Sheehan, the well-known American Plastic Surgeon, in 1930, when I was working in London. He was quite a wealthy man who crossed the Atlantic every year, spending a good deal of time in our operating theatres to see what was going on in his line of business. The tragic Spanish Civil War broke out in 1936, and facial wounds accumulated because they had no plastic surgeons to deal with them. Sheehan, who was not averse to reasonable publicity, offered his services to the Franco side and these were, of course, accepted.

His first case must have been quite a party. There were language difficulties, but that was nothing. As would be expected, he was allotted their best anaesthetist—a nun who had been trained by nuns. He suggested tracheal intubation but they just did not understand what he was talking about. The anaesthetist insisted on keeping the face-mask firmly applied to the very bit of anatomy which Sheehan intended to repair. The impasse was immediate. Sheehan got in touch with me in Oxford, where I had just started my new job as Professor. He painted the picture as he saw it, and had no doubt that all difficulties would be resolved if I could appear on the scene armed with a laryngoscope and some endotracheal tubes.

Anaesthesia in the Spanish Civil War 1936

When I arrived in Spain laden with 'scopes and tubes, I encountered problems all my own. No Boyle's apparatus which all of us in England just took for granted. No cylinders of gas or oxygen. During the whole of the time I was in Spain, I did not see a cylinder of any description. The only vaporizer known to them was Ombrédanne's a French modification of Clover's portable inhaler. The latter had been described in 1877 (1) and forty years later the French equivalent was described by Ombrédanne (2). In both of these, the face-piece has to be kept in position throughout the operation, so clearly neither would be of the slightest use for the purpose of anaesthetizing for facial surgery. It could have been a very embarrassing position for me.

Flagg's Can

Let me go back a few years. On trips to America, I visited as many anaesthetists as I could manage. One of these was Paluel Flagg of New York, who, despite the fact that he had written several books, was little known in England. On his own territory, however, he was much discussed, being regarded as a Quixotic individual with quite a number of eccentricities, one of which was to prove of great value to me. At that time, ether was sold, not in bottles, but in tin cans. Flagg took out the cork, decanted the ether, and, for some reason or other, punctured additional holes nearby—and a Flagg can resulted. Air enters the holes and passes over the surface of the ether on its way to the patient. The mechanism could not be simpler, but as a scientific inhaler, it leaves room for improvement. In this variant, taken from Flagg's book: *The Art of Anaesthesia*, the leading role is played by a tin of Squibb's ether (3).

The smile on Flagg's face showed quite clearly the satisfaction he derived from demonstrating this tin can in action. Why he ever thought of the idea passed my comprehension, and, in fact, it still does. He was Consulting Anaesthetist to important New York Hospitals, so that any apparatus was at his beck and call, and yet he chose this manifestly primitive vaporizer

8

using ambient air as the source of oxygen. I can only think that he saw merit in it just because it was his own baby. One thing did favour him. He was a great protagonist of ether so that cardiac output and respiration were not impaired.

When faced with anaesthetizing for head and neck surgery, in Spain, I was thankful I had seen Flagg's demonstrations. I cannot think what I would have done without them. I settled for an empty tin of Lyles' Golden Syrup—a strange find in the circumstances, and well it worked.

The development of draw-over anaesthesia at Oxford

When I returned to Oxford a few weeks' later, war against Germany was very much in the air, and if it did materialize, I had no doubt it would be widespread. A greatly improved Flagg's can would be needed, and I sought someone with the requisite knowledge to master-mind the project. My search led me to H. G. Epstein, a D.Phil. graduate of Berlin, *summa cum laude*, or, in the vernacular, 'with first class honours' and he proved to be just the man. He was the one most responsible for the development of the Oxford Vaporizer used extensively by British Military anaesthetists during World War II (4).

After the War, Epstein turned his attention to the E.M.O. which will be more familiar to the present generation. The lineage of this inhaler can be traced back directly to Flagg's can.

The E.M.O. has been described as 'a glorified Flagg's can'—and I would not quarrel with that.

References

(1) Clover J. Portable regulating ether inhaler. *Br Med J* 1877; i: 656.
(2) Ombrédanne L. Appareil pour l'anesthésie par l'éther. *Gaz des Hôpitaux* 1908; **81**: S1095.
(3) Flagg P. *The art of anaesthesia*. Philadelphia: Lippincott 1939: 164.
(4) Epstein HG, Macintosh RR. The Oxford Vaporiser No 1. *Lancet* 1941; ii: 62.
(5) Macintosh RR. A plea for simplicity. *Br Med J* 1955; ii: 1054.

2.2	The introduction of depolarizing muscle-relaxants into clinical practice

C. F. SCURR
Westminster Hospital, London, UK

The relationship between the quaternary ammonium groups of curare and its neuromuscular activity was recognized by Crum-Brown and Fraser in 1868 (1), and we are told that the first attempt at the production of synthetic neuromuscular blocking agents was the production by them of quaternary methyl-strychnine and methyl-brucine derivatives.

More recent efforts in this direction centred around the importance of optimally placed quaternary ammonium groups and in 1948 there appeared in the journal *Nature* the simultaneous publication of letters headed 'Curare-like action of polymethylene bisquaternary ammonium salts,' from Barlow and Ing in Oxford (2) and from Paton and Zaimis (3) working at the Medical Research Council (MRC) in London. Study of a series of bisquaternary compounds with a methylene chain varying in length from two to 20 groups had shown that the lower members of the series (around five or six) were mainly active as ganglion-blockers, at around 10 groups there was significant neuromuscular blocking effect, and the higher members proved to have anti-cholinesterase activity.

Decamethonium

My senior colleague, Geoffrey Organe was at that time in 1948 the Secretary of the MRC anaesthetics committee and it was proposed that he should collaborate with Paton and Zaimis in the first human and clinical trials of decamethonium (C10). As the Senior Registrar at Westminster Hospital I was delegated to the happy position of being the administrator (and if need be the resuscitator) for the first human volunteers who were Organe, Paton and Zaimis (4). The trials took place in the urology theatre at Westminster which had been unused during and since the war. It had a pleasant view from the 7th floor over St John's Gardens, and was equipped with an operating table and full anaesthetic apparatus.

Paton was the first to lie on the table, his blood pressure and pulse were monitored and his ventilation was observed. Muscle power was measured by squeezing an inflated blood pressure cuff held in the subject's hand and noting the rise of the mercury column. I gave him an intravenous dose of 3 m^2 of decamethonium iodide. At the onset of action of the drug Paton said he felt a twinge of pain in his back muscles which he attributed to the initial depolarization—perhaps this was the first herald of suxamethorium fasciculation and after-pains. As paralysis came on over a period of a minute or two speech became slurred and then ineffective, there was ptosis and inability to move the limbs. Fortunately at the chosen dose ventilation remained adequate and the colour was good. Presumably the vital capacity had not fallen below the tidal volume requirement. Paralysis reached a maximum in about four minutes, recovery beginning in about 10 minutes—ability to stand unaided took about 30 minutes.

It was hoped initially that C10 would have a selective effect with respiratory muscle sparing—a feature much sought after at the time—I was never very convinced of this and in any case such an effect was not required once it was appreciated that controlled ventilation was mandatory whenever fully effective doses of relaxants were used.

It had been shown in earlier experimental work on animals that pentamethonium (C5) was an effective antagonist to the neuromuscular blocking action of C10. Accordingly C5 was administered to three volunteers in doses of 20 to 40 mg intravenously at the peak of paralysis by C10. It was possible to show accelerated recovery of hand strength. When the subjects stood up however, postural hypotension was obvious, severe enough in one subject to require administration of methedrine. Appreciation of this hypotensive effect of C5 led us directly to use it for induced hypotension during anaesthesia for lumbo-dorsal sympathectomy for which we had been using total spinal block with procaine.

An investigation into the use of decamethonium in anaesthesia was undertaken following these preliminary trials in volunteers. For several weeks I went down to the Maudsley Hospital to participate in a clinical study comparing decamethonium with d-tubocurarine in the modification of electroconvulsive therapy (ECT). The drugs were given to a series of patients alternating from one ECT administration to the next. We used abdominal and thoracic stethographs and later, a recording spirometer to observe the ventilatory changes. At the conclusion of this work Davies and Lewis wrote a paper for the *Lancet* (5) without acknowledgement of the anaesthetists' role. The next week I published a letter (6) pointing out the fact that during the series it was evident that the effect of d-tubocurarine was abbreviated by the ECT, but that the duration of decamethonium paralysis was unaffected.

Organe was able to report in the *Lancet* (7) in May, 1949, that decamethonium had been used at Westminster Hospital in 150 operations and that it proved a satisfactory substitute for d-tubocurarine. It was soon obvious however that in abdominal surgery or other prolonged operations tachyphylaxis was a serious problem and that repeated doses needed to increase in size. At the end of any procedure in which several doses were given the emergence from the paralysis was incomplete. C5 was not a suitable antidote because of its hypotensive effect, but there was a definite but incomplete reversal if neostigmine was given—we had run into dual block.

I myself found the main value of C10 to be in single doses for ECT and for intubation extending to peroral endoscopy. I therefore wrote a paper on this application and so there evolved, in my thinking, the whole idea of the so-called 'crash' or 'rapid sequence' induction (8).

Suxamethonium and suxethonium

We still hoped for a drug with a quicker action time and a more flexible agent and, consequently, research into other synthetic relaxants was going on in a number of centres.

My war service in Italy had given me a good working knowledge of the language and so I was able to read the monograph by Daniel Bovet (9), who working at the Instituto Superiore di Sanita in Rome had screened a large number of synthetic curarizing agents. Amongst these were the very brief acting compounds—suxamethonium and suxethonium. I noted that suxamethonium by its initial stimulant action on the ganglia could produce severe hypertension in animals and for this reason I first chose to use suxethonium. Some other workers, apparently unaware of this hazard (fortunately rare in man), plunged straight into the use of suxamethonium.

I was next greatly indebted to the chemist, Dr Morrison, who synthesized suxethonium for me at the Roche laboratories in Welwyn and gave me a small sample of 4 g for clinical use.

I had this made up in 60 mg of cation doses in ampoules and this material formed the basis of my first paper in the *British Medical Journal* extolling the value of suxethonium in ECT (10), in intubation and possibly for peritoneal closure.

When plentiful supplies of suxamethonium became available we found it could be used as a drip of 1 g in 500 ml or intramuscularly at the rate of 2 mg per pound (4 mg/kg) for intubation in infants and children; it was effective by this route in 90 seconds and passed off in 12 minutes.

We soon appreciated the drawbacks of bradycardia from repeat doses, and the sequel of muscular after-pains, but it was 15 years before I encountered my own first case of prolonged apnoea and then I had 2 cases in the same week.

The next investigation was focused on the use of suxamethonium in ECT and was undertaken in collaboration with Tony Edridge who volunteered to undergo a series of injections of relaxant and thiopentone in varying sequences and dosage. The purpose of these experiments was to determine the optimal clinical routine from a subjective experience point of view. This aim was achieved and we got some very nice spirometric tracings. The results were presented by Edridge at the Royal Society of Medicine in 1952 (11).

Conclusion

It has been well said that if all the potential complications of suxamethonium had been anticipated, it would perhaps never have been introduced, but on top of this I would say if decamethonium were still available it might be greatly favoured as one of the best agents for atraumatic intubation and I believe it is still in use at East Grinstead for this purpose.

References

(1) Crum-Brown A, Fraser TR. On the connection between chemical constitution and physiological action. *Trans Roy Soc Edin* 1868; **25**: 151.
(2) Barlow BB, Ing HR. Curare-like action of polymethylene bisquaternary ammonium salts. *Nature* 1948; **161**: 718.
(3) Paton WDM, Zaimis EJ. Curare-like action of polymethylene bisquaternary ammonium salts. *Nature* 1948; **161**: 719.
(4) Organe G, Paton WDM, Zaimis EJ. Preliminary trials of bistrimethyl ammonium decane and pentane di-iodide (C10 and C5) in man. *Lancet* 1949; **i**: 21.
(5) Davies DL, Lewis A. Effects of decamethonium iodide (C10) on respiration and on induced convulsions in man. *Lancet* 1949; **i**: 775.
(6) Scurr CF. Decamethonium iodide. *Lancet* 1949; **i**: 842.
(7) Organe G. Decamethonium iodide (bistrimethylammonium decane di-iodide) in anaesthesia. *Lancet* 1949; **i**: 773.
(8) Scurr CF. Use of suxamethonium iodide in anaesthesia for peroral endoscopy. *Br Med J* 1950; **ii**: 1311.
(9) Bovet D. L'utilizzazione del polmone d'acciaio nello studio della tolleranza di dosi elevate di sostanze curarizzantio. *Rendic Instituto Superiore di Sanita* 1949; **12**: 180.

(10) Scurr CF. A relaxant of very brief action. *Br Med J* 1951; **ii**: 831.
(11) Edridge A. Discussion on new muscle relaxants in electric convulsion therapy. *Proc Roy Soc Med* 1952; **45**: 869.

2.3	Anaesthesia in a teaching hospital sixty years ago

J. ALFRED LEE
Southend Hospital, Southend-on-Sea, Essex, UK

When does history begin? Perhaps the 50 year rule is sound. I would like to describe some of the practical details of clinical anaesthesia which I experienced more than 60 years ago at the teaching hospitals of Newcastle-upon-Tyne where I qualified in 1927; but, first, as a matter of historical interest I must mention that, as a surgical dresser to the senior surgeon in the hospital, I saw Lister's antiseptic methods of sterilization employed routinely in his surgical service, although of course all his younger colleagues had adopted the aseptic system many years previously. Gloves, towels, instruments, ligature and swabs were all sterilized by immersion in either 1:20 carbolic acid solution, or in 1:1000 perchloride of mercury. This particular surgeon was the great local expert on the removal of torn semilunar cartilages from the knee-joints of the large number of injured coal miners in the area. The results of these arthrotomies were just as good as those of his younger colleagues who relied on the aseptic system of heat sterilization.

Teaching hospital anaesthetists in the nineteen twenties

The staff anaesthetists at this large teaching hospital were known as 'honoraries' because they were unpaid. This was because the so-called voluntary hospitals at that time, and indeed up until 1948, were paid for by voluntary contributions and local charitable efforts. Two or three of these individuals were whole-time anaesthetists depending for an income on private anaesthetic fees, the remainder combined anaesthetics with general practice in order to make a living. Each anaesthetist attended the hospital two or three mornings each week and always worked with the same surgeon—a tradition still observed, with its advantages and disadvantages, in most British hospitals today. The holders of the post of honorary anaesthetist were not highly respected in the hospital. Though, of course, medically qualified, few anaesthetists possessed postgraduate degrees or diplomas. It was not until 1935 that the first examination to test the candidate's knowledge of the subject was held, the Diploma in Anaesthetics (D.A.) the first such diploma in the world.

The surgeon to whom I acted as house-surgeon, employed, and paid a salary to his anaesthetist who was expected to anaesthetize for all his operating work, both hospital and private. He was little more than a helot but was an engaging personality who had two memorable characteristics. The first was that he required constant urging by the surgeon to get the patient deep enough so that the abdomen would renounce its tone. The second was a morbid fear of germs. He acted as if he knew the cause of AIDS, 60 years before the HIV became a clinical problem, and would never administer an anaesthetic without first donning two pairs of rubber gloves. It was said of him that on a bitterly cold day in the middle of winter, his ever-loving wife asked him to look at her sore throat. He suggested that she should go outside into the garden, stand by the window and open her mouth.

The honorary anaesthetist in charge of the morning list of operations expected to be relieved at 1.30 pm. His duties were taken over by a house surgeon or house physician until the list was finished, and this might be well into the afternoon. We were of course completely inexperienced and sometimes the problems we had to face were serious ones. We learnt as we went along. The clinical teaching we received from our seniors was minimal. How the surgeons and their registrars must have suffered at our hands. All the anaesthetics were however given by qualified doctors, even if very recently qualified, and not by nurses. I will venture no opinion whether it is better to let ignorant young doctors or experienced nurses undertake such duties.

Techniques

How did we set about the task of administering the anaesthetic? Preoperative visiting of the patient, still less preoperative investigation were unknown. Premedication was not routine although some anaesthetists used atropine to reduce the amount of saliva so readily caused by ether.

The surgeon usually told the anaesthetist what anaesthetic to give. It was most important that a porter should be present during the induction in order to contain the restlessness and compulsive movements as the patient passed through the second stage of anaesthesia. The porter was the forerunner of today's skilled Operating Department Assistant (O.D.A.).

Intravenous induction, tracheal intubation, muscle relaxants suction and intravenous drips were not employed, although occasionally saline solution was injected into the outer side of the thigh or beneath the breast, using a Higginson's syringe. Blood transfusion was confined to patients with acute trauma and in medical cases for the temporary relief of pernicious anaemia, and required both donor and recipient to be lying side by side on trolleys. Blood banks were unknown until the 1930s.

The agents used for induction included ethyl chloride, chloroform, ether and a mixture of the last two with ethyl alcohol (ACE). These liquids were dropped on to gauze supported by a wire frame such as a Schimmelbusch mask, the so-called 'open drop' method. Occasionally, nitrous oxide was given from an early and primitive Boyle's machine or via a Clover or Hewitt ether inhaler, but the gas was seldom employed in the operating theatres; its main use was in the Casualty Department for short administrations.

Some skill was required to get a smooth changeover from the stertor of ethyl chloride to ether without interruption of respiration, and we had the constant problem of knowing how deeply anaesthetized the patient was.

Two main difficulties presented themselves; the maintenance of a free airway and the provision of muscular relaxation. Each of these could tax the skills of even experienced anaesthetists. The ability to maintain a free airway by holding the jaw forward is surely even today the one basic skill which should separate the anaesthetist from other doctors, a skill unfortunately not always possessed because of the reliance on and the too frequent practice of tracheal intubation. Dissatisfaction with the tight belly was often expressed by the surgeon and all too frequently made the relationship between surgeon and anaesthetist, somewhat edgy. We had to wait until Harold Griffith introduced curare in 1942 for the too too solid flesh of the abdominal wall to melt in the hands of anaesthetists. If the patient was considered to be too ill to undergo general anaesthesia, he was given a spinal, but always by the surgeon.

Conclusions

May I emphasize three simple lessons born out of experience?
(1) When recalled today our methods may appear to have been unsatisfactory, but were not so regarded at the time. Anaesthetists managed to give reasonable anaesthetics for the operations then in vogue, including thyroidectomies, submucous resections of the nasal septum, caesarean sections, colectomies, hysterectomies and cholecystectomies, but of course the cranial cavity and the chest were seldom opened.
(2) History teaches us that our successors 60 years hence will be just as horrified when they reflect on the methods used today as we are, looking back at the 1920s from the vantage point of the 1980s. Methods extolled today will be despised tomorrow.
(3) History also teaches that the full paraphenalia involved in the application of aseptic methods

in surgery and the use of sophisticated apparatus for the administration of general anaesthesia are both admirable, but that good work can be performed by adopting antiseptic methods of sterilization and the open drop method of general anaesthesia, using a volatile agent. Let us hope that conditions beyond our control never make the use of such outmoded but practical and useful techniques again necessary.

2.4   Anaesthetic books which influenced me in my early days

WILLIAM W. MUSHIN, CBE
Welsh National School of Medicine, Cardiff, UK

Since boyhood I have been a lover of books. Of all the influences that have shaped my professional career, I must place books at the head of the list. To quote from *The Philobiblion* written by Richard de Bury in the 14th century

> *'Since books are the aptest teachers, it is fitting to bestow on them the honour and the affection that we owe to our teachers.'*

I graduated in Medicine in 1933, a time when there were no organized courses in anaesthesia, and when the main books on the subject were simple clinical technical ones. Very few were attractive to one who felt strongly drawn towards mathematics and physics.

By the time the 1939–1945 World War came, I had already read most of the writings of such British authors as Hewitt, Buxton, Blomfield, Minnitt, Boyle, Evans, Rowbotham, Magill, and Nosworthy, as well as those from the United States, such as, Gwathmey, Rovenstine, Guedel, Waters and Lundy.

However, of these, there were a few which influenced me greatly in my thinking and outlook on anaesthesia, and these I will list in chronological order of publication.

1. *Anaesthetics and their Administration* by *Sir Frederick Hewitt*, first published in 1893 and again in 1901, was undoubtedly the first of the truly scientific books on anaesthesia, with perhaps the single exception of John Snow's *On Chloroform and Other Anaesthetics*. Hewitt's book is full of experimental data and should be consulted by any researcher before he appends the adjective 'new' to his own particular theories or discoveries.

2. *Anaesthesia* by *James Taylor Gwathmey* published in 1914 was one of the best. Of the several books on anaesthesia, mostly good, that came from the United States before the war. Gwathmey was the first President of the American Association of Anesthetists and his book is a literary and scientific gem. Many of the contributors were surgeons, indicating how few practitioners of anaesthesia, capable of contributing to such a book, there were in the United States at that time. Even so, this book is still worth reading today, if only as an indication of how far back the roots of modern scientific anaesthesia go.

Its scope is remarkable. Electrical anaesthesia, hypnosis, sequestration anaesthesia, and the effects of such substances as magnesium salts, are just a few examples of material that would be difficult to find elsewhere. The American authorship naturally emphasizes American practice, but the detail and scholarship is of a very high order, especially the very complete and accurate references to source material.

This book is of the same genre as Hewitt's, and both are books I constantly refer to even now. I can recommend them to anyone making a collection of important books in the field of anaesthesia.

3. *Local Anaesthesia* by *H. Braun* first published in 1905 soon after the discovery of procaine, is a model of clarity, although the illustrations are not up to modern standards. It has been the source of most books on regional analgesia since then. The methods described have changed remarkably little since Braun's day!

4. *Recent Advances in Anaesthesia* by *Langton Hewer*. I bought and studied every edition since the first one in 1932, and I still refer to each of them, because with each edition items were omitted from the previous one, often of considerable historic interest.

5. *Biomathematics* by *W. M. Feldman* (1935). This remarkable volume opened my eyes to the place of numeracy in medicine in general, and of the statistical approach to clinical and experimental observations. The lessons of this book have never left me. If a copy can be found, this is a well-worth addition to anyone's collection, even though it now appears a little old fashioned in some of its mathematical presentations.

6. *The Physiology of Anesthesia* by *Henry K. Beecher* (1938). This was a unique book, years ahead of its time, and it really decided me to adopt anaesthesia as a life work. At the time it appeared, I was already lecturing in the short courses on anaesthesia organized by what was then known as the British Medical Postgraduate Federation. Then I bought Beecher's book on the *Physiology of Anesthesia* which had just been published in 1938. Overnight I became an ardent student of the Science as well as of the Art of anaesthesia. There is still much to be learnt from Beecher's account of the early days of scientific investigation of anaesthesia.

There is a curious error in Beecher's book. In discussing soda lime and carbon dioxide absorption, he implies that acapnia may result (during spontaneous breathing!) due to what he refers to as 'too great absorption of the CO_2 in a closed system'.

7. *Spinal Anesthesia* by *L. H. Maxson* (1938). This book was written with great clarity and with good illustrations. It appeared at a time when spinal analgesia was very popular. There was no equivalent book at the time apart from translations of continental authors.

8. *The Art of Resuscitation* and *The Art of Anesthesia* (both in the 1944 editions) by *Paluel Flagg* two books that I found both interesting and somewhat curious. He exposed the unbelievable situation at the time in the United States, regarding the practice of resuscitation, when, even in University Hospitals, the local Fire or Police Force would be called into the Operating Room to resuscitate patients! He brought this deplorable state of affairs to the notice of a wide section of American Medicine. In 1933 he formed SPAD (the Society for the Prevention of Asphyxial Deaths) and this no doubt helped to make resuscitation a serious subject for study and practice by physicians rather than laymen.

9. *The Mode of Action of Anaesthetics* by *T. A. B. Harris* (1951). Although appearing after the War, this too was a book that was years ahead of its time. From this book I began to understand, and to take a keen interest in, the mechanisms of pharmaco-kinetics (the word had hardly been invented then). My interest in this field has never faded.

There were of course many other books, to say nothing of journals, in the English language, all of which one read, with varying degrees of benefit, but the books I have listed come to mind as outstanding.

2.5	Luck was a lady

T. CECIL GRAY, CBE, KCSG
University of Liverpool, UK

I justify my title under two heads: nostalgia and professional. Nostalgia in that I wish to recall the heady and exciting days of the late forties and early fifties. The war was over and anaesthesia was beginning its great efflorescence from an art based on empyricism and craftsmanship to one of the most scientific disciplines in medicine. In 1946, I found myself, still very wet behind the ears in anaesthesia, on the Foundation Board of the Faculty of Anaesthetists of the Royal College of Surgeons of England and in 1948 on the Council of the Association of Anaesthetists of Great Britain and Ireland, with all that such appointments meant in terms of new friends and expanding ambitions.

Professional meetings and social pleasures in London

Meetings were not infrequent—but were much fewer than today when one wonders how anyone who is similarly involved ever manages to do any anaesthesia. The steam trains of those days would not comfortably get one from the North of England to London and back in a day, so there were many chances in the evenings to go on the town in this wonderful city.

I spent quite a few such evenings with John Gillies (Fig. 1), who introduced the concept of 'physiological trespass' exemplified by controlled hypotension, and what good company he was! His base was Edinburgh, but he knew his London better than many indigents. A walk with him in the West End was a great experience. He was a man of the theatre and stage and he knew exactly where the stars of those days lived. He would give a little chuckle, point to a window or apartment and say 'that's where Noel Coward lives', or Jack Buchanan, one of his favourites, or Elsie Randolph, Jessie Mathews and so on and often he would give little spicy insights into their private lives. One evening he took me to see the first London production of that wonderful musical 'Guys and Dolls'. One of Sky Masterson's Damon Runyon type friends was the living image—indeed could have been the twin—of Ivan Magill! Every time he appeared on the stage John laughed as I had never seen him laugh before. It was a night to remember also for another reason: he introduced me for the first time to scampies, claiming it as a Scots dish—which it isn't. A great hit of 'Guys and Dolls' was 'Luck Be A Lady Tonight.' To me she was on such nights.

Liverpool and the early use of curare

My title is redolent of nostalgia for the friends and fun of those times, but it is also an acknowledgement, that to me, professionally, luck has indeed been a real lady. I have been lucky to have lived all my life in so exciting and colourful a town as Liverpool, inhabited by a unique brand of individuals, called scousers—a town still with a collection of the best of Victorian architecture, with two fine Cathedrals, a University founded and financed by the wealthy philanthropists of the early days of the industrial revolution, a waterfront, now refurbished so as to be second only to Boston, and most importantly, with an anaesthetic school of long tradition.

This tradition was maintained in the days before World War 2 by two remarkable men—my teacher R. J. Minnitt and my colleague and friend John Halton, Minnitt's contributions are well known and documented. His gas and air method administered by the patient herself for the relief of pain during child birth was, in its day, an outstanding advance as it was available for use in domiciliary practice by midwives: a foundation member of the Council of our Association of Anaesthetists his greatest contribution, I believe, was his insistence on a very high standard of clinical practice, research and teaching.

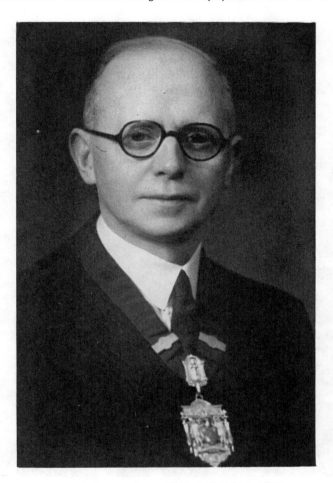

Figure 1   John Gillies, CVO, MC (1895–1976).

Halton's contributions are less recognized and on this historical occasion I would like to say a few words about him. By 1939, when war broke out, Halton (Fig. 2) had established himself as an anaesthetist of quite outstanding ability and ingenuity, so recognized by such men as Nosworthy and Magill who like him were advancing anaesthesia for thoracic surgery. Halton was anaesthetist to the embryonic Thoracic Unit which H. Morriston Davies had established at Clatterbridge Hospital in the Wirral and was developing a method of blind intrabronchial intubation and blockage, when, at the outbreak of the war, as a reservist, he was called to the Royal Air Force.

It was probably Morriston Davies who saw to it that he was appointed medical officer to the Merseyside Balloon Barrage with leave to anaesthetize at the Chest Unit for two half days a week. He made friends with the American medical officers attached to the US Bomber Squadron stationed at Burtonwood, Warrington and became a frequent visitor to their mess. There he heard of the use of curare in the form of Intocostrin in Canada and the USA. Halton persuaded one of his American friends on one of his transatlantic flights to bring back for him some of those precious little bottles of Intocostrin; as his anaesthetic work was limited to thoracic work on two half days a week, he generously gave me some of the precious material to try in general work. We both found Intocostrin to be a little disappointing. We agreed that the real advance offered by curare should be the end of the road for deep or even moderately deep anaesthesia and for this, in our hands, Intocostrin seemed neither sufficiently reliable

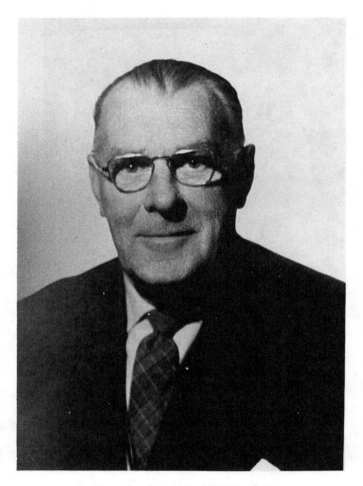

Figure 2   John Halton (1903–1969).

nor potent. Our supply was quickly exhausted and dependence on an unofficially imported drug in those difficult times would certainly have delayed any full exploration of this exciting advance, at least as far as this country was concerned.

We then remembered the 'curare' with which we had experimented on frog muscle in physiology practical classes. Through the good offices of the lecturer in physiology (later Professor) Rod Gregory, we obtained the entire physiology department's stock of those little 6 cm long and 3 mm in diameter vials which contained 100 mg of white powder, labelled 'curarine'. After autoclaving them, one day in 1944 we tipped one vial of 100 mg into a bottle of normal saline, shook it up and dripped it slowly into a lady undergoing, I think, a cholecystectomy, who was very lightly anaesthetized and so far from relaxed. The result of the administration of our curarine seemed miraculous and we recognized at once that the new material was a considerable improvement on Intocostrin. The certainty of effect and controllability of dosage transformed the situation.

The white powder was in fact the alkaloid d-tubocurarine chloride which had been crystallized six years previously by Harold King (1) working in Sir Henry Dale's laboratories at the Wellcome Institute. Dr Ranyard West (2) an Edinburgh physician, reported its intramuscular administration in the treatment of a lady suffering from a spastic condition to the Royal Society of Medicine on January 6th 1935. This was the first time tubocurarine chloride was used clinically. Wintersteiner and Dutcher in the Squibb Laboratories did not report their isolation of the crystalline alkaloid until May 1943 (3). I have enquired from the archives department of Squibb Laboratories in the States whether any of their tubocurarine was used clinically before November 1944. But it seems that they had continued to pin their faith on Intocostrin. Some tubocurarine was issued to a Dr Kay, a psychiatrist, to try in electroconvulsive therapy but no report exists of any trial he may have made. It seems, therefore, for what it is worth, that our administration was the first clinical use of tubocurarine in anaesthesia (4).

The triad of anaesthesia

Luck has been ladylike in providing those with whom I have had the privilege of working. It is invidious to select names, but I don't think anyone is going to be put out if I mention that of Jackson Rees, the first member of my Department—unpaid because he was on a demobilization grant from the RAF. Many thousands of infants will vouch for that having been a good investment! When you collaborate with a colleague with whom you are in complete empathy, a symbiosis occurs, ideas generate and concepts and discoveries evolve with no one individual being responsible.

One such was that a triad of narcosis, analgesia (or reflex depression) and relaxation should replace the established stages and planes of anaesthesia which had become meaningless in the curare era (5). Another was the finding that when relaxants were used and ventilation controlled, the narcotic element of the triad was supplemented. Interestingly enough, this has found support, fairly recently, in work by Forbes, Cohen and Eger which showed that the minimum alveolar concentration (MAC) for halothane is reduced by 25% when pancuronium is used and patients are ventilated (6).

Conclusion

Above all, I have been lucky in practising anaesthesia during four of the most exciting decades in the history of our subject and, resulting from that, in the number of students from far and wide with whom one has formed firm friendships lasting until now, and hopefully for a few years to come.

References

(1) King H. Curare. *Nature* 1935; **135**: 469.
(2) West R. The pharmacology and therapeutics of curare and its constituents. *Proc Roy Soc Med* 1935; **28**: 565.
(3) Wintersteiner O, Dutcher JD. Curare alkaloids from Chodendron tomentosum. *Science* 1943; **97**: 467.
(4) Gray TC, Halton JA. Milestone in anaesthesia? (d-tubocurarine chloride). *Proc Roy Soc Med* 1946; **39**: 400.
(5) Gray TC, Rees GJ. The role of apnoea in anaesthesia for major surgery. *Br Med J* 1952; **ii**: 891.
(6) Forbes AR, Cohen NH, Eger EI. Pancuronium reduces halothane requirement in man. *Anesth Analg* 1979; **54**: 497.

PART II

THE EARLY DEVELOPMENT AND ORGANIZATION OF THE SPECIALTY OF ANAESTHESIA

Chapter 3
THE ORIGINS OF ANAESTHESIA

3.1	Anaesthesia in ancient times—fact and fable

J. F. NUNN

Clinical Research Centre, Harrow, Middlesex, UK

Genesis (chapter 2) says: 'The Lord God caused a deep sleep to fall upon Adam, and he slept'. The phrase 'deep sleep' is translated from the original Hebrew word 'Tardamah', which is the word now used for anaesthesia in Israel and is etymologically more correct (1).

With this exception, one searches the literature and artefacts of pre-Christian times in vain for evidence of the application of anaesthesia to surgical practice as we know it today. Nevertheless, there has developed a considerable mythology attributable to authors with limited knowledge of ancient languages, who have accepted fanciful translations that accord with their own expectations. These have often been copied from book to book without a criticial return to original source material. The plan of this communication is to examine in turn, firstly the evidence for the type of surgery undertaken in classical times, secondly to review the means which were available for rendering the patient free of pain during surgery and finally, and most difficult of all, to consider what use was actually made of such means in classical times.

Surgery

Pharaonic Egypt

The earliest representation of an operation is the circumcision depicted in relief on the wall of the tomb of Ankh-ma-hor, vizier to the pharaoh Teti I, which may be dated to about 2300 BC (Fig. 1).

The inscription above the operator in the left hand scene reads: 'the hem-ka priest is circumcising', the word for circumcising (sb) being very similar to (sebbe) in Coptic, which is the only living language derived from ancient Egyptian. It is far from clear why a hem-ka (or funerary) priest should be circumcising or why Ankh-ma-hor should have wished to have this scene in his tomb. A similar but incomplete scene is depicted in the precinct of Mut in Karnak and there is ample collateral evidence (including Herodotus (2), Book 2, 37) that circumcision was widely practised by the ancient Egyptians.

The original of the Edwin Smith surgical papyrus (3) dates from about 2500 BC in the Old Kingdom. It is largely concerned with trauma but provides clear evidence for the setting of fractures and many references to the suturing of wounds. The word generally accepted to mean 'suture' is 'ider', but is unknown outside the Edwin Smith papyrus and a single mention in the Ebers papyrus no 875 (4). No other ancient Egyptian word is known to mean sew or stitch. Although the Edwin Smith papyrus deals with the head, there is no mention of trephining, and evidence for this procedure in mummies is very uncertain. Apparent laparotomy incisions in mummies were a part of the procedure for mummification.

21

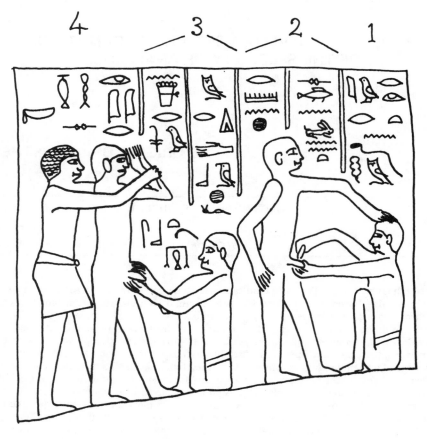

Figure 1   Representation of a circumcision from the tomb of Ankh-ma-hor in Saqqara (approx 2300 BC). The words in front of the seated figure on the left read 'The hem-ka priest is circumcising'. Literal translations of the other inscriptions are: 1. 'I will make it comfortable'. 2. 'Rub it well that it may be effective'. 3. 'Hold him fast. Do not let him fall.' 4. 'I am acting for your praise.' (Reproduced with permission of the Royal College of Surgeons from the Vicary Lecture of 1983 by the author.)

The Ebers papyrus (4) is predominantly medical and dates from about 1550 BC. It contains nine references to the use of 'djwa' which is best translated as 'the knife treatment' and the determinative of the word is a representation of a knife. Amongst the indications for the knife treatment are:

1. A fatty swelling in front of the neck.
2. A 'pus-swelling' with raised head in any part of the body.
3. A painful 'pus-swelling' in the axilla.
4. A swelling of the blood vessels (or nerves).

It is recommended for the last procedure that the knife be heated to prevent bleeding.

Babylonian

The Code of Hammurabi (1792–1750 BC) carefully defines the rewards for success and the punishments for failure of a surgeon (5), and this gives some idea of the scope of contemporary surgical practice.

> *'215: If a physician performed a major operation on a seignior with a bronze lancet and has saved the seignior's life, or he opened up the eye-socket of a seignior with a bronze lancet and has saved the seignor's eye, he shall receive ten shekels of silver.'*

'218: If a physician performed a major operation on a seignior with a bronze lancet and has caused the seignior's death, or he opened the eye-socket of a seignior and has destroyed the seignior's eye, they shall cut off his hand.'

Greek

The Hippocratic writings are sparse in details of surgical procedures although aphorisms 44 and 45 in section 7, for example, refer to the opening of an empyema and liver abscess (6). The rarity of references to surgery is probably because the Hippocratic Oath specifically forbad the practice of surgery, including 'cutting even for the stone', leaving it to 'the practitioners of that craft'. Such practitioners did not commit their procedures to manuscripts which have survived. Nevertheless, the Greek literature contains ample references to the opening of abscesses, the use of cautery, the setting of fractures and the reduction of dislocations.

Roman

Galen, physician to the Emperor Marcus Aurelius (161–192 AD), left a legacy of medical writings which was to dominate the practice of medicine throughout the Middle Ages. Amongst copious references to surgery, he gave detailed accounts of excision of tumours with both knife and cautery. The following excerpt from Retsas (7) makes the intention of the surgeon very clear:

'. . . The purpose of all surgery removing an abnormal growth, is the total resection in a circle of the entire tumour, approaching the normal tissues.'

These brief reviews provide firm evidence that surgery was undertaken in classical times. It ranged from simple procedures such as the opening of abscesses and removal of simple tumours in the third millenium BC to more complex procedures in the 2nd century AD.

Available methods for the relief of pain during surgery

Alcohol

Most ancient civilizations discovered alcohol before writing. In Pharaonic Egypt, the word for wine ('irep') first appeared in the 3rd Dynasty (2686–2613 BC) and beer ('henket') in the 4th Dynasty (2613–2494 BC). Alcoholic beverages were very familiar to the Greeks and Romans.

Opium

The opium poppy was not originally native to Egypt, but opium was imported from Cyprus in the early part of the 18th Dynasty (1551–1436 BC). It was imported in special flasks known as base ring ware which resemble the seed capsule of *Papaver somniferum* when inverted. Opium has been reported in the residue found in four of these jars (8). After the time of Tuthmosis III (1504–1450 BC), *Papaver somniferum* was introduced into Egypt from Palestine and intact burials have featured seed capsules of the opium poppy. From the time of Tuthmosis III, it is unlikely that knowledge of opium was ever lost in the Mediterranean basin.

The Ebers papyrus (4)—no. 782, contains a striking reference to the use of 'shepnen' for the treatment of a crying child, and it is suggested in the authoritative *Worterbuch der ägyptischen Sprache* (9) that this may mean opium. However, the meaning of the word 'shepnen' has never been proven and it seems likely it was translated as opium only because it seemed a logical drug to use for a crying child. This interpretation is not accepted by Von Dienes *et al* (4).

Hyoscine

In the ancient world the most important source of hyoscine was the mandrake (*Mandragora officianarum*) which contains l-hyoscyamine, l-hyoscine and minute quantities of the alkaloid mandragorine. Ingestion of a sufficient quantity of the extract of the root would produce unconsciousness and this was well known in Greco-Roman times. Mandrake fruits modelled in glazed composition feature in a floral collar of the Amarna Period of the Egyptian New Kingdom (1373–1360 BC) (10). Tutankhamen died shortly after the Amarna Period in 1352 BC and eleven mandrake fruits were present in the floral collarette from the third coffin (11). They may have been present for their presumed aphrodisiac properties.

Subsequent references to the magical and medical properties of the mandrake are so numerous that it is unlikely that knowledge of it was lost.

Cannabis

There are few references to the use of cannabis in classical times but Herodotus (2)—Book 4, 76, in his account of the customs of the Scythians reported the following:

> '*Then they take some hemp seed, creep into the tent, and throw the seed on to the hot stones. At once it begins to smoke, giving off a vapour . . . and the Scythians enjoy it so much they howl with pleasure.*'

Herodotus does not refer to any medical application but at least it appears that the Scythians were familiar with the pharmacological effects of cannabis.

Other methods

Apart from those mentioned above, it is difficult to conceive of any drugs available in the ancient world which would relieve the pain of surgery. Alternative techniques might include carotid compression or a blow on the head to induce temporary loss of consciousness. Regional anaesthesia might have been achieved by hypothermia or nerve compression. The author has been unable to trace references to use of such techniques in relation to surgery in classical times.

The use of pain relief for surgery

Regional anaesthesia

By far the earliest indication of any attempt to obtain regional anaesthesia is shown in the right hand panel of Fig. 1. The standing figure is saying: 'Rub it well that it may be effective.', while the squatting figure is saying: 'I will make it comfortable'. Since this is in relation to a circumcision, it seems likely to represent some form of regional anaesthesia. The means employed are by no means obvious. The usual explanation of Egyptologists is that the solid object held by the squatting figure is the 'stone of Memphis', a limestone, which has been dipped in vinegar to release carbon dioxide. Although the inhalation of 30% carbon dioxide induces general anaesthesia, it is clearly ludicrous to suggest that a lump of limestone dipped in vinegar could do anything to relieve the pain of circumcision. Ice would be a possibility but the circumcision was represented in the Old Kingdom and ice was only introduced to Egypt (from Lebanon) in the New Kingdom. Cocaine was only available in the New World.

General anaesthesia

There is no doubt that painful surgery was undertaken since at least the third millenium BC and that suitable drugs were available for producing major pain relief, if not true surgical anaesthesia, in the second millenium BC. It now remains to examine the evidence for their use. The Egyptian medical papyri and the Hippocratic writings do not consider pain relief at all when they refer to operative intervention. This need not surprise us because detailed instructions to naval surgeons for amputations in 1770 AD (12) contain no word on the avoidance of pain during the operation, although in the Stuart period it was suggested that the patient for amputation should receive 'a spoonful of cordial (alcohol) to cherish him' (13). This would hardly rate as anaesthesia!

There are however three classical sources which specifically mention the relief of pain during surgery, but only one of these was by a surgeon. Gaius Plinius Secundus (the elder Pliny) in his monumental Natural History (dedicated to the future Emperor Titus in 77 AD) referring to mandragora says:

> *'administered in doses proportional to the strength of the patient, this juice has a narcotic effect, a middling dose being one cyathus. It is given, too, for injuries inflicted by serpents and before incisions or punctures are made in the body, in order to ensure insensibility to the pain. Indeed for this last purpose, with some persons, the odour of it is quite sufficient to induce sleep.'* (14)

The Greek physician Dioscorides also writing about mandragora in about 100 AD wrote:

> *'Using a cyathus of it for such as cannot sleep, or are grievously pained, and upon whom being cut, or cauterized, they wish to make a non-feeling pain (sic).' and later '. . . and that there be given of it 3 cyathi to such as shall be cut, or cauterized, as is aforesaid. For they do not apprehend the pain, because they are overborn with deep sleep . . .'* (15)

Finally, Apuleius (variously known as Barbarus or Platonicus and sometimes as Pseudo-Apuleius because of the lack of details of his life) wrote a Herbarium probably towards the end of the first century AD. Under the heading of mandragora he wrote:

> *'He who eats this, falls into such a deep sleep, that one can remove a limb without him feeling pain.'* (16)

How far knowledge of the use of mandragora, opium or alcohol was applied for the relief of pain of surgery in classical times can never be known with certainty. We can only say that the means were there and some had recommended their use. It may be that two of the authors copied the first without much reference to what actually happened in contemporary surgical practice. Their comments are suspiciously similar. The novel is often the best indication of customary practice and it is perhaps fitting to close with an excerpt from the Decameron (17), in which Giovanni Boccaccio gives clear evidence of the desire of a surgeon to relieve the sufferings of his patient. This episode must be dated to the time of the Black Death (1348 AD) and, although well outside classical times, is still long before the introduction of the modern concept of true surgical anaesthesia:

> *'The leech saw what was amiss with him, and told his kinsfolk, that unless a gangrened bone that he had in his leg was taken out, he must die, . . . deeming that by reason of the pain 'twas not possible for him to endure the treatment without an opiate, . . . whereby the patient, drinking it, might be ensured sleep during such time as he deemed the operation, . . . might occupy.'*

Acknowledgments

I gratefully acknowledge the valued help which has been given to me by many friends and colleagues in the preparation of this material and translation from other languages. I am particularly indebted, and not for the first time, to Cyril Spaull, Carol Andrews, Maria Arnold, Robert Mahler, Francesca Cook, Joseph Zanelli, Lynette Peat, Michael Denman and to the Library of the Wellcome Institute.

References

(1) Authorised version of the Bible (1611), Genesis II, 21–22.

(2) de Selincourt A. *Translation of Herodotus—the histories.* Harmondsworth, Middlesex, UK: Penguin Books, 1954: 143, 295.

(3) Breasted JH. *The Edwin Smith Surgical Papyrus.* Vols 1 and 2. Chicago: University of Chicago Press, 1930.

(4) von Dienes H, Grapow H and Westendorf W. *Grundriss der medizin der alter Ägyypter. IV 1. Übersetzung der medizinischen Texte.* Berlin: Akademie-Verlag, 1958: 224–228, 292.

(5) Pritchard JB. *The ancient near east.* Volume 1. Princeton, New Jersey: Princeton University Press, 1958: 162.

(6) Lloyd GER. *Hippocratic writings.* Oxford: Blackwell, 1950: 2ֶ33.

(7) Retsas S. On the antiquity of cancer. In: Retsas S, ed. *Paleo-oncology.* London: Ferrand Press, 1986: 49.

(8) Borriau J. *Pottery from the Nile valley before the Arab conquest.* Cambridge: Cambridge University Press, 1981: 126.

(9) Erman A, Grapow H. *Worterbuch der ägyptischen Sprache.* Volume 4. Leipzig: JC Hinrichs'sche, 1930: 445.

(10) *Jewellery through 7000 years.* Catalogue no. 53. London: British Museum Publications, 1976.

(11) Newberry PE. Report on the floral wreaths found in the coffins of Tutankamen. In: Carter H. *The tomb of Tutankhamen.* Vol 3, Appendix 3. London: Cassells, 1933.

(12) Lloyd C, Coulter JLS. *Medicine and the Navy 1200–1900.* Vol 3. Edinburgh: E & S Livingstone, 1961: 367.

(13) Keevil JJ. *Medicine and the Navy 1200–1900.* Vol 2. Edinburgh: E & S Livingstone, 1958: 159.

(14) Bostock J, Riley HT. *Translation of Gaius Plinius Secundus—Natural History.* Volume 5. London: Henry G Bohn, 1861: 139–40.

(15) Gunther RT. *The Greek Herbal of Dioscorides, englished by John Goodyer AD 1655* Oxford: University Press, 1934: 474.

(16) Translated by Joseph Zanelli from the Latin Text of de Herbis by Apuleius, taken from *Herbarum Apulei 1481, Herbolario volgare 1522.* Edizioni il Polifilo.

(17) Rigg JM. *Translation of Boccaccio G—The Decameron.* Volume 1. London: Everyman's Library (no. 845), 1930: 285.

3.2   Mandrake in the history of anaesthesia

J. B. BOWES
Bristol Royal Infirmary, Bristol, UK

The tie of the English Anaesthetic Research Society has a motif which has been variously described as a triffid, against a background of several colours (1). The motif represents the mandrake which is considered to be one of the earliest plants to have what we would now describe as 'anaesthetic significance'.

Mandrake refers to the plant *Mandragora officinarum*. There is the possibility of confusion here for 'mandrake' in America refers to a totally different plant (*Podophyllum peltatum*) which produces resins (2). The mandrake which is part of the history of anaesthesia is a plant with broad fleshy leaves which are close to the ground. The flowers rise from the centre and are a delicate purple colour (3). The normal distribution of the mandrake is in the Mediterranean and coincides with the Olive (3). It is particularly prolific in the eastern part of the Mediterranean. The Greek Islands are covered with its golden yellow berries which are considered a culinary delicacy (3).

The word 'mandrake' is alleged to have come from Sumerian times when 'nam-tar-agar' meant 'demon or fate plants of the fields' (4). In the Old Testament there are several references to the mandrake (5,6). These references consider the mandrake from the point of view of being an aphrodisiac and a drug to improve fertility. This usage arises from the appearance of the root of the mandrake, which resembles the human form. The mandrakes were even split into 'mandrakes' and 'women drakes'. This sort of resemblance leads via sympathetic magic to the 'doctrine of signatories'—that is that when something resembles something it will act in the same way (7). As the mandrake in these conditions was obviously fertile so it could engender fertility in humans. Along with this fertility cult was the idea that, because the plant looked like a homunculus it was 'alive': and therefore pulling it out of the soil would be akin to murder, which would be accompanied by shrieks. By Roman times the mythology was established that these shrieks of a mandrake being pulled from the soil were lethal to either human or animal. So arose the notion of tying a dog to the mandrake to pull it out, and the idea of drowning the sound of these shrieks by blowing a trumpet (8). Also during Roman times there is the possibility that the drink which was given before crucifixion contained mandrake (9), though in such a situation the efficacy of long term sedation mattered more than survival.

In the middle ages there was an interest in the mandrake as a hypnotic as is shown by the quotation:

> *'The rind thereof medled with wine . . . gene to them to drink that shall be cut in the body for they should sleep and not feel the sore knitting.'* (10)

This passage comes from the seventeenth Book of *De Proprietatibus Rerum*, which was written in Latin by Bartholomaeus Anglicus. He not only ranked as a thinker alongside Roger Bacon and Thomas Aquinas but was also one of the few original herbalists of the 13th century. This book became very popular after it was translated into English in 1938 by John of Trevisa.

As the middle ages changed into the Renaissance so the discovery of printing encouraged the production of the Herbals. The first is by Turner, printed between 1551 and 1568. In this herbal Turner states in words which are reminiscent of John de Trevisa's

> *'It [the mandrake] is given to those who must be burned or cut in some place that they should not feel the burning or the cuttying'* (10)

Gerrard set up his herbalist garden in Fetters lane. This is close to the Royal College of Surgeons of England and means that Gerrard was a close neighbour of Shakespeare, who makes several references to mandrake (11,12). The play which most closely suggests the use of the mandrake in *Romeo and Juliet* with its concept of sleeping for two and forty hours and awakening 'as from a pleasant sleep' (13) but the plant which Friar Laurence used is not specified; however the mandrake is mentioned elsewhere in the text (14). In contemporary herbals the mandrake is portrayed in its human form and frequently the dog is shown attached to the root. The man is also frequently shown blowing a trumpet.

Turner, who might be classed as the anti-establishment maverick, was very scathing about the various shrieks which were supposed to accompany the harvesting of the mandrake. He was a herbalist who had travelled widely, particularly in Italy, and had spent some time in the Physic Garden at Bologna (15) and he boasted of having uprooted many mandrakes without suffering any ill effect (15). It has been suggested that part of the continuation of the myth was the reasonable economic desire to protect a valuable plant (16). Though drawn in the various plates of the old herbals it is difficult to ascertain how common the plant was. In the stone carvings of the Chapter House of Southall Cathedral, which was decorated at the end of the 13th century there are some marvellous botanical carvings one of which resembles the mandrake. When L'Obel visited Bristol he was given a plant of a ripe mandrake, as L'Obel had been a Physician to a Dutch King and was Botanist to an English King he was an important man and so the present would have been special (17).

Assuming that there have been no great climatic changes the absence of the mandrake from fairly standard books on Botany suggests that the plant was rare, although there is a plant in the Chelsea Physic Gardens.

The fact that the mandrake root has a characteristic smell was mentioned in the Old Testament (6). Recently the effective principle which has been found in the roots are tropane based alkaloids and consist mainly of l-hyoscyamine, l-scopolamine and a small amount of another alkaloid—mandragorine. Originally all these tropane alkaloids were lumped together and known as mandragorine (18). Consequently the active principle from the anaesthetic point of view is that of hyoscine on memory (19).

A further use for the mandrake might be in the treatment of witlessness though the dosage would have to be suitable as Lucrezia Borgia was alleged to have used the plant as a poison (20). I am thinking of the use as described in the Herbarium of Apuleius, which is one of the Anglo Saxon Herbals, where

'For witlessness, that is devil sickness or demonical possession, take from the body of this same wort mandrake by the weight of three pennies, administer to drink in warm water as he may find convenient—soon he will be healed.' (15)

Acknowledgments

I would like to thank Dr Christopher Woollam who has supplied me with slides of some of the pictures of the mandrake in the old herbals, and to Miss Rebecca Flowers for secretarial assistance.

References

(1) Bowes JB. New ties. *Anaesthesia Points West* 1977; **10**: 55–6.
(2) Claus EP, Tyler VE. *Pharmacogonosy.* London: Henry Kimpton, 1965: 237.
(3) Polunin O, Huxley A. *Flowers of the Mediterranean.* London: Chatto & Windus, 1972.
(4) Allegro J. *The sacred mushroom.* Abacus Edition. London: Sphere Books Ltd, 1973: 66.
(5) Bible, Genesis, 30:14.
(6) Bible, Song of Solomon, 7: 13.
(7) Frazer JG. *The golden bough* (Abridged Edition). London: Macmillan, 1950: 11–12.
(8) Mez-Mangold L, *A history of drugs.* Basle: Hoffman LaRoche, 1975: 45.
(9) Bible, Proverbs, 31:6.
(10) Rhode ES. *The old English herbals.* London: Minerva Press, 1972.
(11) Shakespeare W. *Othello,* III, 3, 334.
(12) Shakespeare W. *Antony and Cleopatra,* I, 5, 4.
(13) Shakespeare W. *Romeo and Juliet,* IV, 1, 106.
(14) Shakespeare W. *Romeo and Juliet,* IV, 3, 48.
(15) Rhode ES. *The old English herbals.* London: Minerva Press, 1972.
(16) Emboden W. *Narcotic plants.* London: Vista, 1972: 132.
(17) White JW. *The flora of Bristol.* Bristol: Chatfield House Press, 1972, 49.
(18) Holmes HC. In: Manske RHF, Holmes HC, eds. *The alkaloids.* New York: Academic Press, 1950, Vol. 1: 313.
(19) Pandit SK, Dundee JW. Preoperative amnesia, the incidence following the intramuscular injection of commonly used premedicants. *Anaesthesia* 1970; **25**: 493–9.
(20) Emboden W. *Narcotic plants.* London: Vista, 1972, 133.

3.3 Hog beans, poppies and mandrake leaves—a test of the efficacy of the medieval 'soporific sponge'

MARK INFUSINO[1], **YNEZ VIOLÉ O'NEILL**[1] and **SELMA CALMES**[2]
[1]Medical Center, University of California, Los Angeles*,
[2]Kern Medical Center, Bakersfield, California, USA*

For centuries, the medical literature of the Middle Ages described and endorsed a curious anaesthetic device, the soporific sponge. Texts on it survive from every century from the 9th through the 13th, and it was still described from the 14th through the 17th centuries, though with increasing warnings about contraindications. Eventually they mention the sponge only as a fact of history, a memory from a time when 'surgeons were more merciful' (1).

Modern comments on the soporific sponge reveal how difficult it is for scholars to take seriously a device the main ingredients of which include 'hog beans, poppies, mandrake leaves', and black nightshade. The mention of such names seems instantly to trigger a reaction like the one we find on the first page of Gaddum's introduction to pharmacology, 'The old pharmacopias consisted mainly of plant and other preparations that were harmless and that have subsequently been found to have little pharmacological activity. Their use is to be attributed mainly to their supposed magical properties' (2).

It took only a fairly cursory test of this recipe by Marguerite Baur in 1927 (1) to confirm an opinion that the effects of the soporific sponge were, in her words, 'a legend in the history of anaesthesia, or rather an ideal'. Baur assembled the recipe from the dried stock of local herb shops, placed sponge moistened with the mixture into a bell jar with a series of guinea pigs, and awaited results. Almost none came. Relying, apparently, on a slightly garbled account of Baur's study, a later historian characterized the sponge recipe as a 'medieval goulash' that 'wouldn't even make a guinea pig nod' (3).

Such discussion of the sleep sponge as has gone on in the last 60 years has proceeded on the assumption that it did not in fact work and that it was legend, rumour, or misunderstanding that generated the recipes. We want to approach the question from an opposite assumption: that it did work, that a procedure endorsed for 4 centuries, not only by anonymous 9th-century monks but by practical medical men like Theodoric of Cervia and his father, Hugh of Lucca, must have had an effectiveness of some sort.

The question would then be: *How* did it work? At least four general hypotheses are available none of them exclusive:

(1) *The 'quality control needed' hypothesis*. The recipe as given in the texts did produce narcosis or at least heavy sedation if the herbal sources were potent enough and the mixture was carefully processed.

(2) *The 'mysteries of the craft' hypothesis*. The recipe as stated in the text is a bare outline that was extensively supplemented and adjusted to local and particular circumstances by pharmaceutical and medical practitioners.

(3) *The 'too drunk to care' hypothesis*. The sponge was applied as a final touch after a strong 'wound draft' of opiated wine.

(4) *The 'trance inducement' hypothesis*. The sponge was accompanied by hypnotic techniques that induced a trance, perhaps aided by the highly developed aura of authority around the physician and the mystique of the particular drugs this recipe contained.

Analysis of recipes from various sources

The most well known version of the recipe, the one offered by Theodoric in his *Cyrurgia*, Book 4, ch. 8, a 13th-century work is given below as adapted and corrected from the Campbell-Colton translation (4) with reference to the 1498 edition (5), Daems (6), and Raper (3).

*Research for this publication was supported in part by funds from the UCLA Aesculapians.

Table 1

The order in which ingredients appear in collected recipes

Opium	1st	75%
	2nd	9%
	1st or 2nd	84%
Iusquiamus	3rd or above	60%
(Henbane—*Hyoscyamus*	4th	17%
niger)	4th or above	77%
Mandragora	2nd	25%
(Mandrake—	3rd or 4th	25%
Mandragora	5th	17%
officinarum)	9th	17%
	4th or above	50%
Coconidum	3rd	25%
(Hemlock—	4th	25%
Conium maculatum)	4th or above	50%
Solanum	1st	9%
(Nightshade—	2nd or	
Solanum nigrum)	3rd	36%
	3rd or above	45%
Hedera		
(Ivy—	5th or 6th	33%
Hedera helix)		
Lactuca	5th	9%
(Lettuce—	7th	33%
Lactuca serriola)	8th or 9th	17%
	7th to 9th	50%

Table 2

Frequency with which various ingredients are mentioned in recipes

	Number of mentions in 12 recipes	Per cent
Opium	11	94%
Mandragora	10	85%
Coconid(um?)	10	85%
Iusquiamus	9	75%
Solanum	7	60%
Lactuca	8	66%
Hedera	6	50%
Morus (Mulberry)	2	17%
Rubus (Blackberry)	1	9%
Lapathum (Patience Dock—Rumex Patientia	1	9%
Assorted succulents	1	9%
All others	—	<9%

'The composition of a savour for conducting surgery, according to Master Hugo, is as follows: take of opium, and the juice of unripe mulberry [probably a textual mistake for black nightshade] hyoscyamus [henbane], the juice of hemlock, the juice of leaves of mandragora, juice of climbing ivy, of lettuce seed, and of the seed of the lapathum [dock] which has hard, round berries, and of the water hemlock, one ounce of each. Mix all these together in a brazen vessel, and then put into it a new sponge. Boil all together out under the sun during the dog days, until all is consumed and cooked down into the sponge. As often as there is need, you may put this sponge into hot water for an hour, and apply it to the nostrils until the subject for the operation falls asleep [he who must go under the knife—literally "be cut into"]. Then the surgery may be performed and when it is completed, in order to wake him up, soak another sponge in vinegar and pass it frequently under his nostrils. For the same purpose, place the juice of fennel root in his nostrils; soon he will awaken.'

Recipes did vary over the centuries. To help us judge which materials in the recipe were most emphasized over the seven-hundred year course of the tradition, and to begin to generalize about their active ingredients and examine the potency of the recipe as given, we constructed a database (Tables 1 & 2) analysing texts of the recipes recorded between 900 and 1600 (1), (7).

From the earliest surviving recipe for the soporific sponge, in the Bamberg antidotary of the 9th century to the last echoes of it in the works of 16th-century physicians like Jean Canappe and Juan Fragoso, the most constant and most emphasized ingredient in the sponge remained opium (usually mentioned first). It was in every sense, the primary ingredient, with henbane, nightshade, mandrake and hemlock usually coming next, all of which can be classed as secondary materials. Most of the other ingredients seem to have been at least implicitly recognized as tertiary in importance, although wild lettuce (the source of old-fashioned *lactucarium* (8), (9) or 'lettuce opium', which possibly contains significant levels of scopolamine) does seem to waver between the secondary and tertiary lists. All the secondary ingredients except hemlock contain atropine and scopolamine in varying amounts. Thus looking at texts representing the whole history of the soporific sponge, we find that the primary and secondary ingredients are almost always significant sources of morphine and scopolamine, which are drugs used as pre-medication in modern anaesthetic procedure (10).

Experimental method

We decided it would be worthwhile to use these drugs to repeat Baur's experiment of 60 years ago. We speculated that the materials Baur obtained were not as strong as the medieval *materia medica*, that practitioners found some way (perhaps using alcohol) to dissolve opium into the sponge solution, and that they used fairly potent batches of henbane, belladonna, and mandrake.

We exposed five female rats (Sprague Dawley's strain) to a sponge soaked with 50 μg of sublimase, to simulate the primary ingredient, opium in its dissolved state, with standard adult (human) dosages of atropine and scopolamine, to simulate the secondary ingredients of the medieval sponge (the henbane, belladonna, mandrake, and lettuce extracts).

Results

The first subject pointedly avoided the damp sponge and became quite unresponsive after a few moments, and seemed sedated, but we observed no drop in rate of respiration over the 10 minutes of exposure; nor did it increase after 10 minutes with an unmoistened placebo sponge. Interestingly, there was no avoidance of the placebo sponge.

The second subject, though more active overall, did seem slightly sedated during the 10 minutes with the moistened sponge, but again, no significant drop in respiration rate could be established.

The third subject was a very active and aggressive specimen with a very rapid respiration rate which was difficult to count, but one that was somewhat lower during exposure to the moistened sponge.

About one hour into the experiment all three rats which had been exposed to the sponge and returned to the cage were more active and responsive than those not exposed. Was this an after-effect of exposure to the drug, or merely to handling? We are not sure.

The fourth rat was relatively sedate when removed from the cage and displayed negligible change in behaviour or respiration. The fifth rat was less active while exposed to the moist sponge, but no effect beyond this slight sedation was observed.

Finally taking cognizance of the vagueness of the recipe with respect to the route of the anaesthetic, we finally made a brief test of the nasal mucosa as a route. We repeatedly swabbed the nasal area of the first rat with a well-moistened sponge for 30 seconds. Some sedating effect was observed, but three of the 10 minutes of close observation under the bell jar were spent in fairly vigorous exploratory activity. In the 10 to 15 minutes after close observation, this rat was the most active of those in the cage, leading us again to suspect a delayed stimulating effect. We also tried similar direct application to the especially active individual (the third rat), but it showed no sedation even after 60 seconds of direct application to the nasal area.

Discussion

Aside then, from the slight sedating effect observed in three of the five rats, the results of this preliminary experiment do seem to confirm those of Baur, and tend to diminish the likelihood of the first hypothesis (that only good quality control was needed to make the recipe work). It must be admitted, however, that at least three possible factors in this hypothesis remain to be evaluated:

(1) A synergistic effect of coniine in hemlock (which we did not test) might have made the solution effective;

(2) The route of this anaesthetic may have been the mucous membranes of the nostrils or eyes, a route we were not able to test adequately;

(3) Longer exposure may have yielded more results.

Our experiment, in its use of dissolved opium, necessarily combined hypotheses (1) and (2) to some extent, in that we postulate among the 'mysteries' of the mediaeval art of medicine, a method of dissolving the opium using alcohol (thus allowing the normally-gummy opium to penetrate the body more readily). Of course the testing of hypotheses (2) and (3) ('mysteries of the craft' and 'too drunk to care') would be quite open-ended, and would need to be supported by closer reading of the mediaeval texts. Two texts in our database do closely associate the sponge recipe with a potion recipe involving dissolved opium in wine, such as the dose one can see administered to the monk in an illustration of Diebold Schilling's *Swiss Chronicle* (1513) (11).

Lest hypothesis (4) ('the trance inducement' hypothesis) seems to be merely a desperate or flippant 'fall-back' explanation, we would refer to reliably reported cases of serious surgery, even amputation, under trance, especially when aided by religious and cultural preconceptions (12).

How closely herbs could be linked to religious culture may be indicated by *The Book of Hours* of Anne of Brittany (13). This work includes in its borders lovingly precise colour *trompe l'oeil* renderings of over 330 herbs labelled in both French and Latin and is a more reliable botanical guide that many medieval and Renaissance herbals. This *Book of Hours* sometimes places herbs in contexts which suggests their cultural associations; for instance, nightshade (*Solanum dulcamara*) is placed opposite a full-page rendering of shepherds struggling to keep awake in the night. It seems to evoke that deep wearisome night of the first Christmas during which the shepherds were aroused by an angel. A systematic study of this book along such lines might reveal much about the mystique of individual herbs.

The mystique of mandrake, of course, is well known. It was thought to contain some quasi-human essence and considered so potent that it should not be pulled out of the ground by a human hand, but rather by the leap of a hungry dog tied to it, since its shriek could madden or kill.

Such associations may have aided a process of hypnosis. Some (1) have argued the possibility of a medieval practice of medical hypnosis, and point to illustrations of God the Creator inducing sleep in the second creation story of Genesis, a thesis that also deserves further investigation.

Conclusion

We differ with some of the recent investigators who wish to argue that history is a purely intellectual discipline and that physical experimentation has no place in it (6). While one cannot establish or prove the historicity of events or procedures by re-enacting them, one can certainly illuminate the possibilities. We hope that others will make suggestions for more effective ways of studying the soporific sponge, this venerable and elusive anaesthetic device.

References

(1) Baur M. Recherche sur l'histoire de l'anésthesie avant 1846. *Janus* 31; 1927: 24–39, 63–90, 124–37, 170–82, 213–25, 264–70.

(2) Gaddum Sir J. *Gaddum's Pharmacology*. 9th ed. Revised by ASV Burgen and JF Mitchell. Oxford: Oxford University Press, 1985: 'What are Drugs?', 1, 'General Anaesthetics', 95–101, 'Opiate Analgesics', 105–17.

(3) Raper HR. *Man against pain: the epic of anesthesia*. New York: Prentice Hall, 1945: 3–23.

(4) Campbell E, Colton J. *The surgery of Theodoric; ca AD 1257. Translated*. New York: Appleton-Century Crofts, 1960. II, 213.

(5) Theodoric. *Cyrurgia*, Book 4, Ch. 8, f. 146. In: Chauliac, G de. *Cyrurgia Guidonis de Chauliaco, Et Cyrurgia Bruni Theodorici* [*etc.*]. Venice: Bonetus Locatelli for Octavius Scotus, 1498.

(6) Daems WF. Spongia somnifera: Philologische und pharmakologische Probleme. *Beitr Gesch Pharm* 22, no. 4; 1970: 25–6.

(7) Moulin D de. *Heelkunde in de vroege Middeleeuwen*. Leiden: EJ Brill, 1964: 121–5.

(8) United States Pharmacopoeial Convention, Washington, 1900. *The Pharmacopieia of the United States of America: Eighth Decennial Revision*. Philadelphia: Board of Trustees, U.S. Pharmacopoieal Convention, 1905: Lactucarium, 253, Syrup of, 442–3, Tincture of 472–3.

(9) Wood GB, Bache F. *The dispensatory of the United States of America*, 19th ed. Philadelphia and London: JP Lippincott, 1907: Lactucarium, 686–9, Syrup of, 1229–30, Tincture of, 1274–5.

(10) Weiner N. Atropine, scopolamine, and related muscarinic drugs. In: Goodman L, Gilman A, Rall TW, Murad F, eds. *The pharmacological basis of therapeutics*, 7th ed. New York: Macmillan, 1985: 130–44; and earlier editions, especially Innes IR, Nickerson M. Drugs inhibiting the action of acetylcholine on structures innervated by postganglionic para-sympathetic nerves (antimuscarinic or atropinic drugs). In: 4th ed., 1970: 524–48.

(11) Keys TE. *The history of surgical anaesthesia*. New York: Dover Publications, 1963: 4–5 and Fig. 1.

(12) Agnew LRC. An 18th century amputation. *Lancet* 1983; **2**: 1074–5; and Poulin J. L'Anésthesie avant l'emploi du chloroforme et de l'ether. Doctoral thesis, Faculty of Medicine, Paris, 1931: 73–87, 101–7.

(13) Harthan J. *The book of hours*. New York: Park Lane, 1977: 126–33 on BN, Paris, *ms. lat. 9474*; and the key commentaries *Le livre d'heures de la reine Anne de Bretagne, tr. du latin et accompagné de notices inèdites par M. l'abbé Delaunay, catalogue des plantes par J. Decaisne*. Paris, L. Curmer, 1841 [i.e. 1861, a facsimile]; and *Les heures d'Anne de Bretagne; Bibliothèque nationale (manuscrit latin 9474) Texte par Emile Mâle . . . Legendes par Edmond Pognon; Verve, revue artistique et litteraire* 4, nos. 14 et 15; Paris, Editions Verve, 1946.

3.4   The mandrake legend

JOHN L. COUPER
Medical University of Southern Africa, Republic of South Africa

Mandrake is the common name of a plant and the word is derived from man, probably an allusion to the man-like form of the root of the plant, and drake or dragon alluding to the magical properties of the plant. It is a member of the genus Mandragora which is one of the potato family in the order Solanacea (1).

The genus Mandragora has very short stems, thick, fleshy, often forked roots, and large sinuately toothed leaves. The flowers are purplish to pale violet or white and the globular berries are golden or yellow. It has little horticultural merit and contains poisonous narcotic and emetic principles that cause it to be featured in many herbals. There are several species native to Europe and the Mediterranean. The particular species called the mandrake is *Mandragora officinarum* which contains atropine, scopoletin, hyoscyamine, hyoscine and other solanaceous alkaloids. The herbals distinguished a male and female form in the plant kingdom as in animals. It was Linnaeus in 1732 who clearly explained the difference in function of the stamens and pistils which obviated the need to have two sexes of plants (2).

Mandrakes and fertility

Mandrakes were highly prized as a fertility agent. This is borne out in the account in Genesis, chapter 30, of the barren Rachel who bargained for the mandrakes given to her sister Leah by Leah's son Reuben; as a result Rachel later bore her first-born Joseph. Some authorities have argued that the mandrake was not used as a love potion or stimulant to pregnancy, but for the relief of labour pains during delivery of the babe. Frazer in his *Folklore of the Old Testament* writes that a later Jewish version of the story has it that Reuben tied his father's ass to a root of mandrake while harvesting was in progress. When he returned to the ass he found it was dead. Having struggled to get loose it had uprooted the mandrake and succumbed to its fatal screams (3). Frazer suggests that Reuben was attracted to the mandrake plant by its peculiar but not unpleasant odour. He plucked the round yellow fruit which he tasted and found it to be juicy and sweet. He then gathered a lapful of the berries (about the size of a plum) and took them home to his mother Leah.

Mandrakes were highly prized as love charms particularly by childless women and by the 17th century were so sought after that effigies were made and sold for large amounts (4). Clark (4) states that mandrake roots are still imported by orthodox Jews of Chicago and New York by childless women to insure fertility. In Baghdad amulets of the root are worn by men to stimulate virility and in Attica young men and girls carry pieces of mandrake about with them as love charms.

The facilitation of pregnancy is featured in the account of the Elephant in the Bestiaries. In the Book of Beasts (5) it is stated that the Elephant has no desire to copulate while Physiologus (6) maintains that their copulating is free from wicked desire. If the elephant wishes to produce young he goes with his mate to the East towards Paradise where there is a large tree called the mandrake. She first takes of the tree and then gives some to her spouse. After he has eaten they join together and she immediately conceives in her womb. It is interesting to follow this story for when the time comes for her to give birth she walks into water up to the udders and gives birth. The calf then swims around, finds her thighs and suckles at her teats. Meanwhile the male stands guard to ward off or trample the serpent who is the enemy of the elephant and who would steal and devour the calf if it was born on land. To Ursus, the Bear, the mandrake was poisonous. Should they eat the fruit they die, unless they hurry off for fear that the poison should grow strong enough to destroy them, and eat ants to recuperate their health (7).

An investigation under the Ayurvedic (Medical) Research Council of India found that mandragora was capable of controlling the sex of the prospective child. This is administered in the second month of pregnancy, the male form being used to beget a son and the female form to produce a daughter. 'The sex of every unborn child has hitherto been believed to be determined by X and Y, two types of spermatozoa at the instant of conception'. The secretary of the Council reported that the results are ninety percent positive after testing on thousands of cases (8).

Use as an oral soporofic

The account of the use of mandrake in Genesis may not be the earliest mention of the use of the root. The Count Palatine reported that mandrake roots have been found in the royal tombs at Thebes (9). An ancient Egyptian legend tells that Ra, the Sun God, sent Mathor to earth to punish mankind who had displeased him. Mathor slew so many men that Ra took pity on the human race and forced Mathor to drink the blood of his victims mixed with mandrake root. This put Mathor into a drugged sleep and when he awoke he had forgotten why he had been sent to earth, and so the slaughter ceased (9).

Several authors state that mandrake was used by the ancient Babylonians and Egyptians as a narcotic and the root is included in ancient Persian and Mesopotanian texts. Demosthenes (382–322 BC) is reported as saying the lethargy of the Athenians resembled 'sleep induced by mandragora or some other narcotic' (10).

Pliny the Elder in *Historia Naturalis* (77 AD) advocates mandrake for diseases of the eye. Although the juice is a dangerous poison it can be used as a narcotic before incisions are made in the body, and also for snake bites, and as an emetic (10,11). Pliny also gives directions for gathering the plant and extracting the juice.

Dioscorides, whose *De Materia Medica* was the foundation of western materia medicae for sixteen centuries went further than Pliny (from whom he undoubtedly drew some of his material). He advocated that the wine of the bark of the root be given before cutting or cautery so that the patient will not apprehend the pain because he will be overborne with dead sleep (12). Thereafter mandrake, for its soporific effect, was included in pharmacopoeias and herbals until the end of the 17th century. In 1748 Pomet stated in his complete history of drugs that mandragora was formerly esteemed to have a strong narcotic quality but is now never used.

The soporific sponge

There is uncertainty as to the originator of the spongia somnifera for the production of surgical anaesthesia. This was made by steeping a decoction of many herbs including mandragora, opium, hyoscyamine, lettuce seed, hemlock and mulberry juice. A fresh sea-sponge was soaked in the mixture and allowed to dry in the sun. When required for use the sponge was dipped into warm water and then applied to the nostrils whereupon the patient would quickly go to sleep. The application to the nostrils implied that the effect of the herbs was through inhalation but none of the ingredients were volatile so its effect could not be through inhalation (10). Even more interesting is the recommendation in the *Antidotarium* of Nicolas of Salerno, that to awaken the patient apply the juice from the root of the fennel and he will soon bestir himself (13). Fennel contains two major ingredients, anethole and fenchone, which are used today as flavouring agents and carminatives (14). Theodoric instructed his patients to breathe deeply when he applied the soporific sponge under the nose. When he wanted to revive the patients he held sponges filled with vinegar under their noses (13).

It has been suggested that the contents of the sponges was absorbed through the buccal mucous membrane or that the concoction was administered as a draught. Armstrong Davison (10) believes the spongia somnifera is one instance of many in which magic and superstition were part of therapeutics in the Dark Ages. It certainly appears that the spongia somnifera could not have produced a satisfactory state of anaesthesia as we know it today. The fact that it went out of use before the end of the 17th century and that illustrations of surgical operations do not convey the impression of an anaesthetized or painless patient, gives credit to this scepticism.

Probably the earliest description of the spongia somnifera appeared in the *Antidotorium* of Bamburg about 850 AD and in the *Codex* of the Abbey of Monte Cassino (10) of about the same time. Thereafter the account of the sponge appeared in materia medicae and surgical treatises.

Avicenna (980–1037 AD) in his *Canon of Medicine* includes the recipe for the sponge as well as the method of procuring the mandrake, but thought poppy extract a better soporific. Jasser (15) maintained that the Arabs were credited with the introduction of inhalational anaesthesia by using the 'anaesthetic or sleeping sponge'. He quotes from Sigrid Hunke on the sponge: 'the science of medicine has gained a great and extremely important discovery and that is the use of general anaesthetics for surgical operations . . . the art of using the anaesthetic sponge is a pure Arab technique which was not known before'. The earliest account I can trace of the sponge by an Arab is that credited to Avicenna about 250 years after the Antidotorium of Bamburg.

The *antidotoriums* compiled by two famous physicians of the Salerno school, that of Nicolas in the 11th century and that of Michael Scot about the year 1175 advocated taking equal parts of opium, mandragora and henbane to prepare the mixture for the soporific sponge. Subsequent writers appear to have copied these descriptions, with one or two additional herbs added. Among these were Theodoric (1205–98), son of Hugh of Lucca, famous father and son surgeons of Bologna and Guy de Chaulliac in his Churiga Magna. Neither of these writers actually stated that they themselves had used the sponge. Guy disapproved of the pre-operative use of opium juice because some patients who had been given it had gone mad and subsequently died (10). John Ardene, the English counterpart of Guy de Chaulliac, used the mandragora and many other herbs to compound an ointment for producing surgical anaesthesia. Ambrose Paré disapproved of mandragora.

Keys (13) suggests that, because there was no standardization of the drugs used, the action of the sponge was uncertain and fell into disuse. Often a drugged sleep resulted in death and this discouraged many medical men from attempting to relieve the pain of surgery.

Other medical uses of the mandrake included feverish headache, eye diseases, body rashes and skin infections.

Gathering the root

The gathering of the mandrake root was quite a ritual. Shakespeare alluded to this when Juliet, pausing before she drinks the sleeping potion in contemplation of the horrors of the vault (*Romeo and Juliet*) Act IV Scene 3), says:

> *'What with loathsome smells*
> *And shrieks like mandrakes torn out of the earth*
> *That living mortals, hearing them, run mad?'*

Theophrastus, in the 3rd century BC, wrote that it was necessary to trace a circle thrice round the mandrake with a sword, then cut it facing westwards (3). Pliny repeated this advice but added that it would be advisable to keep to windward because of the very unpleasant smell.

The earliest reference to the use of a sacrifice to uproot the mandrake appears in the 5th century Herbarium of Apuleius. While the plant is being uprooted it moans, howls and shrieks so horribly that the digger dies on the spot. Although there are several versions of the traditional rites for obtaining the root, the essential procedure is to stop the ears with wax so that the gatherer may not hear the deadly yell. The gatherer had to go out on a Friday night with a black dog (some accounts say a white and black dog), make three crosses round the mandrake, then loosen the soil about the roots (some accounts say no iron tool to be used for this, others stipulate ivory should be used) and tie the root to the dog's tail. The gatherer must go out of earshot and throw bread or meat near the dog. The dog, which should be hungry, runs at the food, drags out the root and falls dead, killed by the horrible yell of the plant. The root can then be taken up by the gatherer, washed in wine, wrapped in silk and laid in a casket. It must be bathed every Friday and clothed in a little white smock every new moon.

If the mandrake is treated kindly the owner would have no enemies, could never be poor and would not be childless. If money was laid beside the mandrake it would be doubled overnight. When the owner died the mandrake was passed on to the youngest son who had to place a piece of bread and a coin in his father's coffin before burial.

Another belief was that the mandrake only grew under gallows or at crossroads where suicides had been buried. It was natural in the medieval mind to make herbs grow out of graves—beneficent and friendly herbs spring from those of holy men, while plants associated with witches and magic grew under gallows or over suicide.

Turner in his *Herball* written in the middle of the 16th century records that he had taken out the roots of mandrakes on numerous occasions without hearing any groans or shrieks (16).

Heraldry

It is surprising that the mandrake has not been used in heraldry by physicians. The (British) Anaesthetic Research Society has the mandrake as its symbol and they have a very attractive tie depicting the plant. The only English family to use the mandrake is Bodyam or Bodyham of Essex, granted arms in the middle 16th century. The arms consist of three male demi-mandrakes and the crest a she-mandrake. A French family, de Camps of Niverais and branches of this family have five mandrakes on their arms (17).

In literature

Shakespeare mentioned mandrakes on six occasions. In *Anthony and Cleopatra* when the Queen bemoans the absence of Anthony

Cleopatra: *'Ha Ha! give me to drink mandragora'*
Charman: *'Why Maddam?'*
Cleopatra: *'That I might sleep out this great gap of time.*
My Anthony is away.'

and in Othello when Iago is hatching his foul plot

Iago: *'Look where he comes. Not poppy nor mandragora*
Nor all the drowsy syrups of the world
Shall ever medicine thee to that sweet sleep
Which thou awd'st yesterday.'

Shakespeare also used it in contempt of the physical appearance of man for example when Falstaff alluding to the diminutive stature of his page says 'Thou whoreson mandrake, thou are fitter to be worn in my cap than to wait at my heels'.

Conclusion

The mandrake arrived on the scene in Genesis as a love plant that brought blessing on infertile women. It protested violently when uprooted but this may have been in self-defence. It lived on the rotting flesh of criminals, demanded milk, food and constant baths. It was the familiar of witches and killed those that spurned its evil associations or drove them to madness. It may have had healing and analgesic properties and have been capable of inducing soothing sleep but these attributes were unlikely to have been achieved in the manner described.

References

(1) *The World Book Encyclopaedia*, Vol 13. Chicago: World Book—Childcraft International, 1982: 103.
(2) Anonymous. The legend of mandragora. *Ann Med Hist* 1917; **1**: 102–5.
(3) Frazer JG. *Folk-lore in the Old Testament*. Vol 2. London: Macmillan, 1919: 372–97.
(4) Clark HF. The mandrake fiend. *Folklore* 1962; **73**: 257–69.

(5) White TH. *The book of beasts*. Gloucester: Alan Sutton, 1984: 25–6.
(6) *Physiologus*. Translated by MJ Curly. XX. On the Elephant. Austin: University of Texas Press, 1979: 29–32.
(7) White TH. *The book of beasts*. Gloucester: Alan Sutton, 1984: 47.
(8) Raj H. New light on mandrake. *Med Hist* 1962; **6**: 342.
(9) Trew CJ. *The herbal of the Count Palatine*. London: Harrap, 1985: 36.
(10) Armstrong Davison MH. *The evolution of anaesthesia*. Altrincham: John Sherratt and Son, 1965: 36–49.
(11) Nuland SB. The origins of anesthesia. Birmingham: *The classics of medicine* 1983: 6–12.
(12) Guthrie D. *A history of medicine*. London: Thomas Nelson and Sons, 1945: 116–7.
(13) Keys TE. *The history of surgical anesthesia*. New York: Robert Krieger, 1978: 5–11.
(14) Trease GE, Evans WC. *Pharmacognosy*. 11th Ed. London: Baillière Tindall, 1978: 414–7.
(15) Jasser MT. Anaesthesia in Arab medicine. *Middle East J Anaesth* 1978; **5**: 125–8.
(16) Murdoch JE. *Album of science: antiquity and the middle ages*. New York: Scribner, 1984: 193–4.
(17) Dennys R. *The heraldic imaginations*. London: Barrie and Jenkins, 1975: 129–30.

3.5   Anaesthesia with mandrake in the tradition of Dioscorides and its role in classical antiquity

ULRICH VON HINTZENSTERN
University of Erlangen, German Federal Republic

Little is known about Dioscorides. Presumably he descended from Anazarbos in Cilicien, a landscape in Minor Asia. Like many Greeks in Roman duty he accepted the name of a patrician family and then he called himself Dioscorides Pedanius. He wrote his famous work *Materia Medica* probably in the year 77 AD. About the life of Dioscorides we know only what he wrote in the preface of his *Materia Medica*. From youth he showed much interest in pharmacological and botanical studies and during his warfare career (presumably as a Roman military physician) he saw many foreign countries.

Dioscorides' *Materia Medica*

Materia Medica became a pharmacological and pharmaceutical standard work soon after its publication. Contrary to his predecessors Dioscorides chose a functional and systematic classification for his work. The author says in his preface that only a part of his knowledge is due to his own observations but a large amount of knowledge is derived from different sources starting at Diocles, including especially the works of Sextius Niger and Crateus. *Materia Medica* was—partly in Latin translation, recension, addition and Arabic versions—held in great esteem throughout the middle ages, in the Orient as well as in the Occident. In the latter, the developing natural sciences made this work gradually dispensable, from the beginning of the 16th century. By the Oriental physicians it was considered as the incarnation of the complete pharmacological knowledge till the end of the 19th century (1).

In chapter 76 of the 4th book we find something about the preparation of both the female and male species of mandrake (mandragora) for anaesthesia:

'. . . some are boiling down the roots with wine to one third, then filtering and removing
it. In case of sleeplessness or excessive painfulness they ingest a cup of it. They proceed
in the same manner with those who undergo surgical procedures. From the bark of the
root they are preparing a wine without boiling. Then 3 minae (1 mina = 436.6 g) of that
are mixed with 1 metretes (1 metretes = 39.36 litre) of sweet wine. Three cups of this
preparation are given to those who are to be cut or burnt because they do not feel any
pain in their sleep.'

Additionally Dioscorides describes a third species of mandrake which he knows only by
hearsay:

'An amount of one dram (1 dram = 3.411 g) drunken or ingested with barleys in bred
is resulting in deep sleep; man is sleeping for 3 to 4 hours without sensation—you must
know—in the same position in which he incorporated it. This preparation is also used
by physicians for cutting and burning.' (2)

The chemical composition of mandrake

For better understanding of these described actions one has to consider the chemical content
of mandrake. The plant is a member of the family of Solanacae. The narcotic properties of
the roots are based on the concentration of 0.3 to 0.4% of tropanalalkaloids. According to
Wentzel's examination it is composed of several bases which essentially consist of hyoscyamine-
like Atropa Belladonna (3). Furthermore little hyoscine (scopolamine) or atropine is found,
the latter resulting from chemical change of hyoscyamine. Tropanalalkaloids are esters of the
tropanal with various acids. Reabsorption is rapid in mucosa as well as in skin. Hyoscyamine
and atropine have similar actions. Low doses inhibit peripheral parasympathetic neuron-
synapses. Relatively high doses cause central actions which stimulate especially the cerebrum,
mid-brain and medulla oblongata. Subsequently the stimulation of narcotic-like paralysis
appears, leading in some cases to coma and lethal paralysis of breathing. With scopolamine,
central paralysis predominates from the beginning, in the course of which the respiration is
suppressed, in higher doses irreversibly paralysed. The actions of mandrake described above
are clearly explicable by natural sciences. In 1888 the English physician Richardson experimented
with mandrake to investigate its pharmacological actions, known since classical antiquity (4).
He obtained a root of mandrake from Greece and prepared a tincture by having the root
macerated for 4 weeks then pulverized and diluted in alcohol five times. He carried out
experiments mainly with small animals such as rabbits and pigeons using narcotic doses of
this wine of mandrake produced in accordance with the original recipe. He experimented with
human beings only with subnarcotic doses. His conclusions are:

'The wine of mandragora is a general anaesthetic of most potent quality. The action
no doubt depends on the presence of an alkaloid like, . . ., atropine, . . ., and which
would, I have no doubt, be one of the most active anaesthetics we have yet discovered
. . . the alkaloid might, under necessity, be once more employed, as in the olden time,
to deaden the pain of a surgical operation, and that, too, with comparatively little risk
to life.' (5).

Use of the mandrake as an anaesthetic

The somniferous action of mandrake was considered its chief quality in classical antiquity.
Otherwise the Roman lexicographer Hesychios would not have mentioned under the catchword
'mandragora', a kind of plant, being poisonous and somniferous and under the catchword
'hypnotic', mandrake. If one looks for remarks about the propagation of mandrake as a general
anaesthetic in classical antiquity, one finds actual literature with some comments and references,
but on closer examination these publications derive almost always from second hand experience.
The texts will not bear close examination in comparison with the original sources. Regarding
the precise prescriptions and quantitative details given by Dioscorides for the preparation of

the wine of mandrake, both the female and the male species (the third one was known simply by hearsay), one could assume, that Dioscorides or who ever wrote these lines originally, must have had knowledge of the practical use of mandrake as a general anaesthetic. The original text says that only a few used this preparation. The reason might be the difficult dosage of this dangerous drug. To get more detailed information concerning the actual use of mandrake in anaesthesia, Randolph studied more than 150 references in Greek and Latin, dealing with surgery (6). He could only find general hints with regard to anaesthesia, but no mention of another narcotic. He found no remark about the frequency of anaesthesia using mandrake or any reference describing the application of the wine of mandrake in a particular individual during a surgical procedure. Quotations are found such as the following one, written by the Roman encyclopaedist Celsus in the preface of book 7 of his work *De Medicina*:

> *'The surgeon should be imperturbable in his mind and have just so much sympathy with the patient that he wants him to be healed. On the contrary the crying of the patient should not urge him to hurry more than necessary or to cut less than appropriate. He should rather act as if the patient's wimpering could not touch his mind.'* (7).

In summary we could say that mandrake has a very high general anaesthetic quality, its application as a narcotic agent was known and practised in classical antiquity, that probably no other narcotic agent was used and that frequent application was not encouraged because of the risk of overdosage with possibly lethal consequences.

References

(1) Wellman M. Dioskurides. In: Ziegler K, John W, eds. *Paulys Realencyclopädie der classischen Altertumswissenschaft 5/1.* Stuttgart, 1905: col 1131–42.
(2) Wellmann M, ed. *Pedanii Dioscuridis Anazarbei de materia medica libri quinque.* Berlin, 1906–1914.
(3) Wentzel M. *Ueber die chemischen Bestandteile der Mandragorawurzel.* Berlin. Friedrich-Wilhelms-Universität zu Berlin, 1900. Dissertation.
(4) Anonymous. The anaesthetic of the ancients. *NY Med J* 1888; **47:** 684–5.
(5) Richardson BW. *Asclepiad* 1888; **5:** 174 ff.
(6) Randolph CB. The mandragora of the ancients in folk-lore and medicine. *Proc Am Acad Arts Sci* 1905; **40:** 487–537.
(7) Daremberg C, ed. *A Cornelii Celsi de medicina libri acta.* Lipsiae, 1859.

| 3.6 | The role of atropine in antiquity and in anaesthesia |

MONIKA ADT[1], PETER SCHMUKER[1] and IRIS MÜLLER[2]
[1]Deutsches Herzzentrum, Berlin and
[2]Ludwig-Maximilians-Universität, Munchen, German Federal Republic

---

This study serves to describe the historical importance of atropine during the centuries and its role in modern anaesthesia.

Atropine in antiquity

Archaic medicine, dating from 8000 to 3000 years BC, is still practised by primitive nations. According to native belief, illness and pain never occurred without a reason,

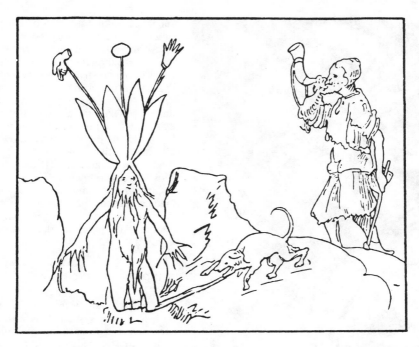

Figure 1   This drawing, dating back to the Middle Ages, shows the removal of the mandrake root. (Original, Germanic Museum, Nuremberg).

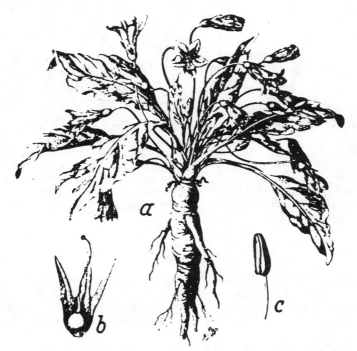

Figure 2   A schematic illustration (approx. 1910) of the mandrake plant (Mandragora autumnalis).

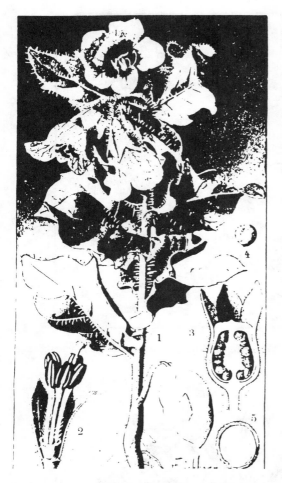

Figure 3 Hyoscyamus niger *(black henbane).*

such as breaking a taboo or blasphemy of a god. The actions of the magician or priest, to perform a cure, were of mystic and ritual character. For minor illnesses, herbs were known to the women who had the task of preparing the meals, and this knowledge was passed on from mother to daughter (1). As the art of writing did not exist, we have no indication as to which herbs were used (2). It is well known, that all the primitive tribes consumed liquids made from mandrake (Figs. 1 and 2), jimson weed or henbane (Figs. 3 and 4), or mixtures of similar plants, not for medical reasons, but to achieve a state of delirium (3). All the plants mentioned contain 'atropine' as the main active agent.

Egyptian medicine

As the Egyptians were the first nation with a writing system, it is possible to reconstruct their healing methods. Of course, mystic medicine still existed, but the Egyptians distinguished between the powers of the priests and the powers of the physicians (4). It is supposed, however, but not proved, that the Egyptians were also familiar with opium and cannabis (5,6).

According to an old Egyptian myth of the Gods, Queen Hathor had begun to exterminate the whole human race. God Re, however, served her beer, and added the juice of mandrake fruit. After drinking the beer, Hathor became 'delightedly drunk, and did not recognize her people'. Hathor's picture was decorated with blossoms, possibly from the mandrake tree (7).

An intoxicating drink was produced from mandrake fruit, but not for medical purposes. Therefore, it appears to us that the hallucinating properties of mandrake were known and applied in the Egyptian period. In the Mesopotamian period, some 250 medical herbs were known, mostly difficult to identify. Among them were henbane, mandrake, opium and cannabis (8,9).

Greece

In Greek medicine, religion lost its importance in pathogenesis, as well as prognosis and treatment of diseases, yet mandrake, opium and cannabis were still known as analgesic and hallucinogenic drugs (10). Female priests were in charge of the Oracle of Delphi, but before making their prophesies they presumably took a prepared drink of henbane and thus created a state of ecstasy (11).

Circe, the Greek sorceress, and her attendants used mandrake preparations to bewitch travellers and sailors who visited their island (12). The old Romans prepared a pain-killing liquid for surgical purposes, which is described as being a derivative of mandrake roots:

'A wine is prepared from the bark of a root, without boiling and 3 pounds are put into a cadus (about 18 gallons) of sweet wine, and 3 cyathea are administered to those requiring to be cut or cauterized: when being thrown into a deep sleep, they do not feel any pain'. A preparation of mandrake was also taken against sleeplessness (13).

John Snow's investigations

John Snow investigated the efficacy of the Roman prescriptions in 1858. He verified that mandrake, a relative of deadly-nightshade, can cause unconsciousness, especially after intoxication with this drug (14).

The Christian era

The growth of Christianity resulted in a setback for the development of medical methods and drugs. Pain and illness were interpreted to be God's punishment for crime and sin. Not medical treatment, but only prayers and humility were tolerated (15). In 391 AD, fanatical Christians burnt down the library of Alexandria, the hellenistic centre of medicine and natural science.

In the Middle Ages, the monks took care of the sick. The abbeys were centres of science, which strictly controlled all knowledge. However, ordinary people, mostly women, knew formulas for

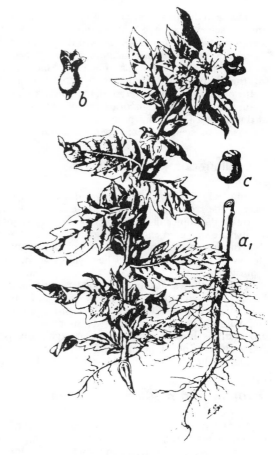

Figure 4 Hyoscyamus albus *(white henbane).*

soporifics and analgesics. In the early days of Christendom, physicians died as martyrs. Later, preparations of 'spongia somnifera', probably originating from Alexandria, were used for premedication, prior to surgical operations. Juices from poppy seed, mandrake leaves, aconite and various other plants were mixed. The sponge was then dipped into the juice and dried. Prior to use, the sponge was moistened and placed under the nose of the individual. It is suggested that it was not the vapour that was responsible, but the fluid contained in the sponge, that was consumed in order to achieve a satisfactory effect (16). As lethal complications had also occurred following the use of 'spongia somnifera', this method was abandoned (17).

It was also evident that solanaceae were used in non-medical fields: an old Bavarian law regarding the brewing and distribution of beer states: It is not forbidden to add salt, juniper berries and caraway seed to the beer, but the addition of any other herbs and seeds, especially of henbane, will be punished. The German name for 'henbane' is Bilsenkraut and names of cities, such as Pilsen, Bilsengarten and Bilsdorf indicate that henbane was formerly cultured in these regions (18,19).

Witchcraft

In the 14th to 16th centuries, the belief in witches was widespread in Europe. In the true context, the women who were said to be witches, in reality used 'black magic' methods. However, there is evidence in the literature, that a group of socially outcast women routinely used hallucinogenic drugs to achieve a state of hallucination. One of the main, orally consumed drugs was mandrake; more attention, however, was paid to the preparation and administration of ointments, made from mandrake, henbane, aconite and other herbs, mostly on a basis of animal fat or the fat of infants (20). The effect of aconite, especially on the sensitive nerve endings of the skin, together with the hallucinogenic effect of mandrake, could exert the impression that a coat of fur or feathers was enveloping the body, and, therefore, establishing the belief, by means of autosuggestion, of transformation into an animal or a bird. It is pointed out by the advocates of this theory, that such women were drug addicts of a low social standing, who did not have the means to acquire more expensive hallucinogenic drugs (21).

Miscellaneous medical usage

In John Ray's *Historia Plantanum* dated 1686, it is stated that during the treatment of an ulcer in the region of the eye, a fresh leaf of deadly-nightshade was placed over the ulcer; overnight the pupil enlarged and did not react to light (22). Later, in all parts of Europe, deadly-nightshade was used externally against cancer, especially cancer of the breast. The drug was also consumed to support diuresis and purgation and it also had a sedative effect on the stomach. However, Thomas Gatacker, the royal surgeon, questioned the benefit of deadly-nightshade against cancer (23).

In later centuries, deadly-nightshade was administered against epilepsy and abdominal spasms. It was also used in ophthalmology. In 1833, Liebig analysed atropine chemically and found the formula $C_{17}H_{23}NO_3$. In the 19th century, atropine was used as a mydriatic for therapeutic and diagnostic ophthalmology, as a suppressant of increased salivation and perspiration, for broncholysis during bronchial asthma, against constipation, against intestinal paralysis, ileus and incarceration of hernia, and as an antidote against morphine intoxication to prevent respiratory arrest (24). The side-effects of the drug prevented more frequent use.

Atropine and modern anaesthesia

In the early stages of ether and chloroform in anaesthesia, it was well known that salivation was augmented. John Snow says: 'The inhalation of ether causes an increased flow of saliva in many cases; quite as frequently, in fact, as chloroform' (25). Statistical investigations show that death occurred in one out of 3000 chloroform anaesthesias. In contrast, death due to ether anaesthesia occurs in 1:14 000 cases. The cause of sudden death during chloroform anaesthesia is very often cardiac syncope, probably due to an overdose (26). Nevertheless, atropine was not used in this period of anaesthesia to prevent such complications.

Johann N. Nussbaum seems to have been the first surgeon who combined a subcutaneous injection of morphine with a chloroform anaesthesia. His method was modified by two French surgeons, who injected morphine prior to the commencement of anaesthesia in order to reduce the anxiety of the patient. This seems to be the beginning of preanaesthetic medication (27). A Bohemian physician named Franz von Pitha used the extract of deadly-nightshade, applied per rectum to achieve prolonged anaesthesia and analgesia. He seems to have been the first person to administer atropine concomitant with anaesthesia, but this appears to be an exception to usual practice (28).

In 1930, Ernst von der Porten, recommended, in a detailed publication regarding the problems of anaesthesia, the preparation of the patient prior to induction of anaesthesia with morphine and atropine administered subcutaneously. He cited the following reasons: morphine ameliorates psychical shock during induction of anaesthesia and reduces the consumption of anaesthetic drugs, while atropine eliminates salivation and reduces post-anaesthetic vomiting. He also recommended premedication with morphine and atropine for children (29).

The purpose of atropine, as a premedication drug, was to prevent side-effects of the anaesthetic (salivation) and of premedication (respiratory depressant action of morphine). Although anaesthetic drugs have changed over the years, atropine has remained an essential component of premedication. In the nineteen sixties a discussion about the benefit of atropine in premedication took place, because it is now known that atropine has arrhythmogenic properties (30).

When cardiac surgery is performed, especially in patients suffering from coronary artery disease, atropine-induced tachycardia is not desirable (31) and consequently nowadays, a great number of operations in patients with coronary artery disease are undertaken without premedication with atropine. Premedication itself has also changed. The administration of a tranquillizer is supposed to be the most comfortable preparation for a patient prior to major surgery. It seems to us, that the use of atropine can be avoided—at least in adults.

References

(1) Sigerist HE. *A history of medicine.* Vol I, New York: 1951: 114.
(2) McKenzie D. *The infancy of medicine.* London: 1927: 182–4.
(3) Kuhlen F-J. *Zur Geschichte der Schmerz-, Schlaf- und Betäubungsmittel in Mittelalter und früher Neuzeit.* Stuttgart: 1983: 172.
(4) Sigerist HE. *A history of medicine.* Vol I, New York: 1951: 264.
(5) Leca A-P. *La médicine egyptienne.* Paris: 1971: 436.
(6) Grapow H. *Wörterbuch der ägyptischen Drogennamen.* Berlin: 1929: 490.
(7) *Dioscordes, Pedanius: Arzneimittellehre in fünf Büchern (De materia medica).* Übers. u. mit Erkl. vers. v. J. Berendes. Stuttgart 1902.
(8) Haupt. Zschr. Assyr. Vol 30: 60–66. Justin Zehnder: Le pavrot et son usage chez les assyriens. Soc. Helvet. Sc. Nat. Lausanne (1928), Sect. de Pharmacie.
(9) Albright WF. Assyr. martakal "Haschisch" and amartinnu "Sidra". *Zsch Assyr* 1926; **37**: 140.
(10) Kuhlen F-J. ibid, p. 99.
(11) Seemann O. *Mythologie der Griechen und Römer.* Leipzig. 1910: 37.
(12) Kuhlen F-J. ibid. p. 175.
(13) Snow J. *On chloroform and other anaesthetics.* London: Churchill, 1858: 2.
(14) Snow J. ibid, p. 3.
(15) Lichtenthaeler Ch. *Geschichte der Medizin.* Köln. 1982: 284–285.
(16) Snow J. ibid, p. 6.
(17) Keys TE. Die Geschichte der chirurgischen Anästhesie. In: *Anesthesia and Resuscitation* 1968; **22**: 24.
(18) Fühner H. Solanaceen als Berauschungsmittel. Eine historisch-ethnologische Studie. In: *Naunyn-Schmiedebergs Arch exp Pathol Pharmakol* 1926; **111**: 292.
(19) Hofler M. *Volksmedizin und Aberglaube in Oberbayern,* München: 1893: 135.
(20) Kuhlen F-J. ibid, p. 314.
(21) Fühner H. ibid. pp. 281–94.
(22) Buess H. *Zur Geschichte der Atropa Belladonna als Arzneimittel in Gesnerus* 1953; **10**: 37–52.
(23) Buess H. ibid. pp. 41–2.
(24) Eulenberg. *Reale Encyclopädie der gesamten Heilkunde* Wien–Leipzig 1907: 76–84.
(25) Snow J. ibid. p. 361.
(26) Snow J. ibid. p. 343.
(27) Nussbaum JN. *Über die Chloroformwirkung.* Breslau 1884: 40.
(28) Puschmann Th. *Handbuch der Geschichte der Medizin.* Jena 1905: 61–2.
(29) Porten v. d. E. Das Narkoseproblem in der Praxis. In: *Die Medizinische Welt* 1930; **52**: 1855–9.
(30) Goodman L. S., Gilman A. *The pharmacological basis of therapeutics*, 7th Edition. New York: Macmillan, 1985: 134.
(31) Tarnow J. Prämedikation. *Anästh Intensivmed* 1985; **26**: 174–81.

3.7   Anaesthesia 1000 years ago

ADNAN A. AL-MAZROOA and RABIE E. ABDEL-HALIM
University Hospital, Jeddah, Saudi Arabia

Pain is a subjective experience which requires the presence of consciousness. Over the ages there has been a demand for methods of relief. In this paper, we present a brief report about the use of narcotics for pain relief from antiquity up to the Renaissance.

Greek and Roman medicine

Though Celsus (1) in the 1st Century used opium and mandrake for pain relief, Galen in the 2nd Century (as stated by Cumston (2) and De Moulin (3)) recommended great care with the use of powerful narcotics such as opium, considering it a dangerous drug. According to Campbell (4) and Cumston (2), Galen was looked upon as one of the great physicians. He summarized the knowledge accumulated in Greek medicine up to his time and studied every aspect of medicine. In cases of colic or other very violent pains, he used only opium.

After Galen, Greek medicine produced four writers who did not contribute any advancement. Their works mainly consisted of quotations from Hippocrates and Galen (4). As a consequence the strong narcotic drug mandrake used by Celsus (1) seems to have fallen into neglect; confirmation of this is that Paulus (5) in the 7th Century, who is regarded as having summed up all medical knowledge accumulated up to his time, did not use it in the trochisci as an anodyne.

Paulus did not give the toxic dose or details of the specific actions of either mandrake or opium. It seems that there was no standardization or regulation of dosage (6,7). It was therefore impossible to standardize the results (6,8,9) and, attempts at the conquest of pain were sporadic (10).

The Middle Ages

In the Middle Ages Christian Europe was in a state of intellectual stagnation (2,4,7,11,12) and the theological doctrine that pain serves God's purpose and must not be alleviated, militated against the improvement in methods of narcosis (4,6,7). Nuland (7) points out that the Middle Ages in Europe were dark ages so far as advances in the pharmacology of anaesthesia was concerned. However in the East, with the firm establishment of the Muslim supremacy between the 9th and 16th Century, the study of medicine along with other branches of science revived and acquired a truly scientific nature (2,4,13,14).

Therefore, not only Avicenna (16) but also Al Razi (17), Al Bagdady (18) and Ibn El Kuff (19), paid great attention to the phenomenon of pain (3). They attributed it not only to the breach of continuity, as stated by Galen, but also to a sudden change of temperament (by only heat, cold or dryness) with or without abnormal humours. Hence, for pain relief, they stressed the treatment of the underlying cause and they subsequently developed a large number of analgesics with variable modes of action. The anaesthetics they described included a wide range of medical plants as well as ice or very cold iced water as an efficient and safe mode of local anaesthesia even though there might be an increase in the pain at the beginning. Refrigeration anaesthesia which is considered by some to be a modern discovery thus had its origins in the medicine of the past.

They attributed the anaesthetic action of the various medical plants used to a specific poisonous property of variable strength, and thus according to Avicenna (16), opium is the most powerful, then mandrake, papaveris, henbane or hyocyamus, hemlock, solanum and wild lettuce. These drugs, especially opium, were used as local anaesthetics in dental cases, earache, eye pain and joint pain (especially in gout).

In dentistry, they used opium, mandrake root or henbane juice in the form of pastes, patches or fillings. Gargles from decoctions of mandrake root, henbane root or seeds or the root of solanum were also used.

Opium drops in rose oil, infusion of root of solanum, decoction of papaveris, oil or juice of henbane and angelica juice were used for earache. The relief of eye pains was achieved by either using dressings from mandrake leaves or mixing the eye medicines with mandrake tears or juice of hemlock. Embrocations of the juice of henbane leaves or seeds were also used on the eye and, for joint pains, dressings from mandrake leaves or embrocations from opium, hemlock, henbane or cannabis.

In addition, because it was noticed that severe pain may lead to death, the soporific action of these drugs was employed especially pre-operatively in the cases of amputation, cautery, circumcision and lacerations. They were administered by ingestion, inhalation or rectally. Infusions of solanum, cannabis, opium and mandrake were given orally or rectally on a plug which has to be changed hourly. Opium, mandrake and henbane were also used by inhalation in the form of odorants.

The wild lettuce has a mild soporific effect. It was used either fresh or boiled as an adjuvant to any of the previous medications or alone in cases of insomnia.

These physicians not only determined the required dose in each drug precisely but also were able to fix the length of time which the anaesthesia was to last with great precision. Avicenna for example, gave a dose of one 'mithkal' of mandrake for 3–4 hours of general anaesthesia.

Unlike Paulus (5), Avicenna (16), Al Razi (17), Al Bagdady (18), Ibm El-Kuff (19) and Ibn El Bitar (20), in the light of their own experiments and observations, described the general and special botanical characters of the plants in detail as well as indicating their habitats and what was best selected from each. They also specified methods for obtaining the active ingredient whether as juice or in the various medical forms that can be prepared as infusions, decoctions or dressings.

They also described the specific actions and side effects on the various systems of the body and stated with great accuracy the required dosage from juice, bark or decoctions as well as the toxic dose. Finally, they outlined the action of antidotes, adjuvants and alternative remedies.

The Muslims must be given the credit for developing the science of botany (12,13,21). Ibn El Bitar is one of the greatest Arabian botanists (2,20,22,23). His book *Al Gami Al Kabir* is the most original among the Arabic *materia medica* texts of the mediaeval period. Arabic *materia medica* had a considerable impact on European herbal and antidotarium authors from the 12th to the 17th century (2,4,24,25). Constantine wrote nothing original; all his books are plagiarisms or skilfully disguised translations from the Arabic. The medicinal remedies reported by Dioscorides are thus of Islamic origin (2). The same may be said of the work of Celsus which was hardly noticed by the Greeks and overlooked in the Middle Ages (26). In the section on emollients (Vol. II) Celsus describes one of them as the invention of a certain Arab, and some of his recipes are based on Arabic *materia medica* with its tables of weights and measures (pound, dirham and dinarium or dinarii).

Conclusion

The only conclusion possible is that the writings of the Muslim scholars in their Latin form influenced European medical thought over a very considerable period.

References

(1) Celsus. *De Medicina*. London: Heinemann; Cambridge: Harvard University Press, 1938, Vols 1–3.

(2) Cumston CG. *An introduction to the history of medicine from the time of the Pharoahs to the end of the XVIII Century*. London: Dawsons, 1968.

(3) De Moulin D. A historical phenomenological study of bodily pain in Western man. *Bull Hist Med* 1974; **48**: 540–70.

(4) Campbell DC. *Arabian medicine and its influence on the middle ages*, 1st Ed. (reprint). Amsterdam: Philo Press, 1974.

(5) Paulus Aegineta. *The seven books of Paulus Aegineta*, translated by F. Adams. London Sydenham Society, 1844–1847, Vols 1–3.

(6) Keys T. *The history of surgical anaesthesia* New York: Schuman's, 1945.

(7) Nuland SB. *The origins of anaesthesia*. Birmingham: The Classics of Medicine Library, 1983.

(8) Tallmadge GK. Some anaesthetics of antiquity. *J Hist Med All Sci* 1946: **1**: 515–20.

(9) Horine FE. Episodes in the history of anaesthesia. *J Hist Med All Sci* 1946; **1**: 521–6.

(10) Kitz RJ, Vandam LD. A history and the scope of anaesthetic practice. In: Miller RD ed. *Anaesthesia*, Vol 1, 2nd ed., New York: Churchill Livingstone, 1986, 3–25.

(11) Bickers W. Adventures in Arabian medicine. *J Roy Coll Surg Irl* 1969; **5**: 5–14.

(12) Desnos E. The history or urology up to the latter half of the nineteenth century. In: Murphy LJT, ed. *The history of urology*. Springfield: Thomas, 1972.

(13) Dickinson EH. *The medicine of the ancients*. Liverpool: Holden, 1875.

(14) Kirkup JR. The history and evolution of surgical instruments. I. Introduction. *Ann Roy Coll Surg Engl* 1981; **63**: 279–85.

(15) Sigrid Hunke. *Allah's sonne uber dem abendland unser Arabische erbe*, Arabic Translation by F. Baidoon and K. Dosoky, 6th Ed. Beirut: Dar Al-Afak Al-Jadida, 1981.

(16) Ibn-Sina. *Kitab Al-Qanun fi T-tibb. (The Canon of Medicine)*. Beirut: Dar Sadir, reprint of Cairo Boulak edition, 1877.

(17) Al-Razi. *Kitabul Hawi Fi T-tibb (Rhazes Liber continents)*, Vol 23, 1st Ed. Hyderabad: Osmania Oriental Publications, Osmania University, 1961.

(18) Al-Bagdady. *Kitab Al-Mukhtarat Fil Tibb*, Vols 1–4, 1st Ed. Hyderabad: Osmania Oriental Publications, Osmania University, 1942–1944.

(19) Ibn El Kuff. *Al-Omda Fil Jiraha*, Vol 1–2, 1st Ed. Hyderabad: Osmania Oriental Publications, Osmania University, 1936.

(20) Ibn El Bitar. *Jami Mufradat Al-Adwia Wa Al-Aghzia (A Dictionary of simple drugs)*— manuscript No. 3979, Chester Beatty Library Dublin-Microfilm at Imam Ibn Saud University Library Riyadh—1399.

(21) Margotta R. In: Lewis, P, ed. *An illustrated history of medicine*. Feltham: Hamlyn, 1968.

(22) Hamerna SK. *Tareekh Al-Tibb Wa Assaidala Endal Arab*, Vol 1–2, Cairo: 1967.

(23) Ibn Abi-Usaybia. *Uyunal-Anba Fi tabaqat Al Atibba (The sources of the knowledge of classes of doctors)*. Beirut: Dar Maktabat al-Hayat, 1965.

(24) Garrison FH. *An introduction to the history of medicine*, 3rd Ed. Philadelphia and London: Saunders, 1924.

(25) Dunlop DM. Arabic medicine in England. *J Hist Med* 1956; **2**: 166–82.

(26) Guthrie D. *A history of medicine*. London: Thomas Nelson, 1945.

3.8   Anaesthesia in the history of Islamic Medicine

M. TAHA JASSER
University of Aleppo, Syria

Science and medicine do not belong to any one ethnic or national group. Of the innumerable scientific discoveries made by man, only a few are really the work of a single person, nation, locality and generation. Often a medical discovery is the summation of many contributions made by scholars throughout the ages.

It is unfortunate that leading historians have ignored the achievements of the orient as a whole and of Moslems in particular, in the various fields of science and medicine. It will suffice to mention the names of but a few great Arab and Moslem scientists, whose gigantic contribution to the progress of civilization is presently enjoyed by all mankind. The description of the pulmonary circulation by Ala Aldeen Ibnul Nafiess antedated the discoveries of the renaissance period, by 300 years (1). Ibn El-Heitham was the founder of optics and El-Khawaremi the originator of algebra. The purpose of this paper is to highlight the discoveries of Arab and Moslem scientists in the field of anaesthesia.

Anaesthesia in Islamic medicine

The delay in the introduction of pain allaying drugs is attributed to the old belief in the west, that pain and suffering was the price paid by humans for their sins (2). Humanity is indebted greatly for the introduction of modern anaesthesia to Morton, Wells, Simpson and others, (3) but most textbooks suggest that inhalational anaesthesia was not known previously, although there may have been some attempts at anaesthesia by Greeks and Romans who are reported to have used magic and superstition, hypothermia and oral analgesic mixtures (4).

The physicians of Islamic civilization were familiar with surgery and undertook a number of operations including amputations, tonsillectomies, and excisions of tumours (5). Such extensive surgery could not have been performed without some method of allaying pain. In addition, one of the reasons why the Moslems could make their way into the field of anaesthesia was the fact that the concept of pain as punishment from God had no place in their belief and tradition.

There is evidence that Moslems used to administer sedatives and analgesic mixtures before a surgical operation. A quotation from Avicenna reads:

> *'A patient who wants to have an amputation of one of his organs must have a drink prepared from a mixture of mandragora and other sleeping drugs.'* (6)

Other plants used for the same purpose were: Indian cannabis (Hashish), opium poppies (El-Khishkash), hemlock (Shweikran), and hyocyamus.

The Moslem scientists can also be credited with the introduction of inhalational anaesthesia by using the 'anaesthetic sponge'. A quotation from Sigrid Hunke reads:

> *'. . . the science of medicine has gained a great and extremely important discovery and that is the use of general anaesthesia for surgical operations, and how unique, efficient and mercyful, for those who tried it, the Moslem anaesthetic was. It was quite different from the drinks the Indians, Romans and Greeks were forcing their patients to take for relief of pain. There had been some attempts to credit this discovery to an Italian or to an Alexandrian, but the truth is, and history proves it, that, the art of using the anaesthetic sponge is a purely Moslem technique which was not known before. The sponge used to be dipped and left in a mixture prepared from cannabis, opium, hyoscyamus and a plant called Zoan.'* (7)

Ether

In the field of chemistry, the ether bond $(-O-)$ which is the basic radical in a group of anaesthetics in common use today (diethyl ether, methoxyflurane, enflurane and isoflurane) deserves special consideration. There seems to be some disagreement as to who synthesized ether first. Some sources credit Valerius Cordus who is said to have described the technique of its manufacture in his book *Annotation on Dioscorides* printed in 1561, and called it 'sweet vitriol'. Other sources claim that Paracelsus described the synthesis of ether in his *Opera Medico-Chemica Sive Paradoxa* (printed 1605) and reported its use in a chicken (8).

There is evidence, however, which indicates that physicians of Islamic medicine were the discoverers of alcohol and probably unknowingly of the ether radical $(-O-)$. It is well documented that alcohol was distilled by El-Kindi (9). The word alcohol is pure Arabic, coming from the original word derived from the Arabic *'Al-Goul'* which means something which knocks down the brain, and it is mentioned in the Holy Quran, describing the wine of paradise as being 'Free from Al-Goul and those who will try it will not suffer hangover' (10). Despite this there have been some attempts to credit the introduction of the word to western authors. Eric J. Holmyard (1937) came up with the following statement:

> *'It was Paracelsus who first gave the name alcohol to the spirit of wine. Originally signifying the black eye-paint used by eastern women, Al-Kuhl or Al-Kohol had gradually acquired the meaning of any very finely divided powder; thence by a natural transference it came to mean the best or the finest part of a substance. Possibly Paracelsus regarded spirit of wine the best part of wine and therefore named it alcohol of wine or simply alcohol.'* (11)

Another study by M. Y. Hashimi (1968) adopts the view of Holmyard and he even goes further stating 'Alcohol is plural of Al-Kuhl' (12). Both views are in fact far from the truth. There is no such word in Arabic as alcohol according to all Arabic dictionaries, encyclopaedias and literature. Al-Kuhl is a remedy put in the eye for treatment and there is no plural of this word. An Arab proverb says 'Fine as Al-Kuhl' for solid substances, and certainly not for the liquids and there is evidence that the word 'alcohol' is a deformed conversion of Al-Goul, a derivative of El-Ightial which means knocking down swiftly or assassination, the characteristics of wine as mentioned in the poetry of some Arab poets before Islam (13).

There is also evidence that sulphuric acid was discovered by El-Razi (14). They used to distil alcohol by treating it with sulphuric acid. Considering that diethyl ether can be produced by the extraction of water out of alcohol: $(2C_2H_5OH + H_2SO_4 = H_2O + C_2H_5-O-C_2H_5 + H_2SO_4)$; it becomes likely that the old Moslems were first to lay down the basis of the synthesis of this essential anaesthetic substance.

Resuscitation

In the field of resuscitation, the use of bellows for respiratory resuscitation is credited to the Society of Resuscitation of Drowned Persons of Amsterdam in 1767 and to the Royal Humane Society of London in 1771 and some even credit the use of bellows to ventilate the lung to Paracelsus (1493–1541) (15). However, there is evidence that Moslems of the 13th century AD were familiar with resuscitation of respiration by using the bellows. The following abridged anecdote is taken from Ibnu-Abi Usibi'a *Classes of Physicians* (16) written in the 13th century. The author was a learned physician and oculist who lived chiefly in Cairo and died in 1270 AD (18). Ibnu-Abi Usibi (17) tells us, 'El-Rashid (Emir El-Mou'mineen or Prince of Believers) would not eat unless his physician Gabriel Ibn Boukhtaishou was present. One day Gabriel arrived late for dinner and begged the forgiveness of El-Rashid saying that he was busy trying to give medical care to the cousin of the Emir (Ibrahin Bin Saleh), who was very ill and that he did not think that the cousin would survive longer than the time of sunset prayers. On hearing this, The Grand Vizir Jafar Ibn Yahya intervened and said: 'Great Emir El-Mou'mineen, I know one by the name Saleh Bin Bahla who is familiar with the Indian way of medicine and I would suggest seeking his services.' Saleh Bin Bahla was summoned and ordered to examine the Emir's cousin Ibrahim and report back to the Emir. On completing his examination, Saleh Bin Bahla reported saying: 'Be humble enough your Highness, Prince of Believers to be my witness that if your cousin expires tonight, every animal I own will be sacrificed to god, and whatever fortunes I have will be gifted to the poor.' When the time of the evening prayer came, the death of cousin Ibrahim was announced. On hearing the news, El-Rashid started to blame Saleh. Saleh kept silent for a while and then shouted: 'Allah! Allah! Your Highness, Prince of Believers, I urge you not to bury your cousin alive. Your cousin is not dead. Please allow me to see him again.' Permission was granted, Saleh brought a bellows and a snuff called El Kundus, and started to inflate through the nose of Ibrahim for around twenty minutes. Soon the body of Ibrahim began to shake, then he sneezed and sat up in front of El-Rashid. Ibrahim subsequently married El-Rashid's sister, Princess El-Abbassa and was appointed governor of Egypt and Palestine.'

Conclusion

Science has no native home of its own and every person has the right to ask for it. When the talents and circumstances exist, new horizons can be discovered. The Moslems are the first in the list of nations who had the honour of holding the torch of civilization for quite a while and made a great contribution to basic sciences, upon which modern technology and progress is raised. In the field of anaesthesia and resuscitation, the contribution of Islamic civilization is enormous and the discoveries made have laid down the foundation of modern practice.

References

(1) Haddad FS. Ala-Aldeen Ibnul Nafiess. *MEJ Anaesth* 1974; **4**: 223–4.
(2) Davison MHA. The history of anaesthesia. In: Gray TC, Nunn JF, eds. *General anaesthesia*, 3rd Ed. Vol I. London: Butterworths, 1971: 708–10.
(3) Atkinson RS, Rushman GB, Lee AJ. *A synopsis of anaesthesia: The history of anaesthesia*. 8th Ed. Bristol: Wright, 1977: 1–10.
(4) Davison MHA. The history of anaesthesia. In: Gray TC, Nunn JF, eds. *General anaesthesia*, 3rd Ed. Vol I. London: Butterworths, 1971: 716–18.
(5) Avicenna AE (980-1036 AD) El-Kanun Fil Tibb. A new print by El-Musanna Bookshop, Bagdad, Offset from Boulak print 1294 AH and 1877 AD: Vol II-371, Vol III-132, 134, 137, 229.
(6) El-Shatti, Sh. About cancer in Arab medicine. *Proc Fourteenth Science Week*, Damascus: Publication of High Council of Sciences. 1974.
(7) Hunke S. *Allah Sonne Uber Abendland, Unser Arabische Erbe*, 2nd Ed. Arabic text, Beirut: The Trading Office, 1969: 279–280.
(8) Davison MHA. The history of anaestheia. In: Gray TC, Nunn JF, eds. *General anaesthesia*, 3rd Ed. Vol I, London: Butterworths, 1971: 711.
(9) El-Kindi J Ib Is (796–873). *Chemistry of perfume and distillation*. Arabic text, Leipzig: 1948:50.
(10) The Holy Quran, El Saffat Verse. Chapter-23, Aiet-47 (7th Century).
(11) Holmyard EJ. *Makers of chemistry*. Oxford: 1937: 111–2.
(12) El-Hachimi MH. Sur L'histoire de L'Alcool. *XII Congress International D'Histoire de Sciences*. Albert Blanchard, 1968.
(13) Ibnu Manzour (630–711 AH—13th/14th Century) Lisan El-Arab. Beirut: Sader House. Vol XI: 584–7.
(14) El-Razi EB (850–932 AD) *Kitab El-Esrar*. Milli-UNESCO Dar Iran, Shamara Commission Publication, Jib Khana, Hydari, 1343 AH: **4**: 109–110.
(15) Herholdt JD, Rafn CG. *Life saving measures of drowning persons*. Copenhagen: 1796. Reprinted by Scandinavian Society of Anaesthesiologists. Aahus: 1960.
(16) Ibnu Abi-Usibi'a (1203–1269 AD). *Classes of Physicians*. Wahbiye Press, 1922.
(17) Ibnu Abi-Usibi'a. (600–668 AH) *Tabakat El-Atibba*, Arabic Text. Beirut: Dar El-Hyatt publication, 1965: 475–7.
(18) Hassan K. *Encyclopaedia of Islamic medicine*. Cairo: General Egyptian Book Organization, 1975: 711.

3.9	Background of scientific law to the discovery of surgical anaesthesia

B. RAYMOND FINK

University of Washington School of Medicine, Seattle, Washington, USA

The social, ethical and scientific developments which led up to the discovery of anaesthesia have been much discussed. As analysed by Greene (1), these included the evolution of a humanitarian ethic, the advent of rational chemical and medical science, and the ready availability of a suitable, safe substance, ether. Caton (2) inquired why Morton (1819–1868) succeeded where others failed; he suggested that Morton's predecessors presented the concept of surgical anaesthesia before its time had come—that is, before the amelioration of pain was seen as a societal goal and before pain and suffering had lost their religious connotations and become biological phenomena open to management.

This paper takes a somewhat different approach, emphasizing the accelerated growth of science and technology during the two decades between Hickman (1800–1830) and Morton. It attributes to this the contrast in the receptions accorded these two men. It cites as evidence of a changed outlook the emergence during the 1840s of the third great conservation law of nature, the principle of the conservation of energy (3)—the previously discovered laws being, of course, the conservation of momentum expressed in Newton's third law of motion in 1687 and the conservation of mass stated by Lavoisier in 1789.

On the political plane, fundamental changes in public attitude had occurred with the revolutions in America and France (4). These intensified the feeling of civilized mankind for intellectual and moral liberty and for the dignity and importance of all human labour, and aroused general hopes for betterment, summarized in Napoleon's ringing promise, 'La carriere ouverte aux talents'—opportunity for all!

Scientific and technical advance in the first half of the 19th century

In the ground so prepared, from about 1830 onwards scientific and technological progress accelerated spectacularly. Steam was one of the most powerful forces shaping civilization. By the 1840s steam ploughs and steam threshers were replacing the labour of man, but the decisive change came with steam locomotion—both by land and by sea. Steamships were now crossing the Atlantic in seventeen days instead of forty by sail. Where rails were laid, telegraph systems were constructed alongside—Morse invented the electric telegraph in 1844. News and letters could now be carried cheaply and swiftly, an intensified mobility of ideas at least as important as the newly speedy movements of people and goods.

It is true that the developments in industry, commerce and trade, which brought vast new wealth, at the same time created in Western Europe a rootless working class and vehement intellectual protest. But the arousal of social conscience against specific evils led to legislation regulating the hours and conditions in the factories and mines and the large-scale hazards to health. Water purification by filtration through sand was introduced in London in 1829, although poor engineering in the distribution system often resulted in recontamination. Fundamental documents of public health appeared in 1840 in Paris, in 1842 in Great Britain and in 1845 in New York (5).

In general, the mood at the approaching mid-century was one of optimism and unbounded confidence in progress, nurtured above all by the spectacular advances in scientific knowledge and its applications, grounded in experimental physics and chemistry and no longer pursued by gifted amateurs but rather by professional workers and researchers.

An outline of the principal gains in the years between Hickman and Morton may suitably begin by mentioning the publication in 1824 of *Réflexions sur la puissance motrice du feu* (6), the analysis by Sadi Carnot (1796–1832) of the factors involved in the production of mechanical energy from heat. This masterpiece laid the foundation for the new science of thermodynamics. The British Association for the Advancement of Science was formed and held its first annual meeting in 1831. The word 'scientist' was invented by Whewell (1794–1866) to describe those present at the meeting in 1833 (7). The year 1831 also saw the invention of those two harbingers of the coming electrical revolution, the mechanical generation of electric current by Faraday (1791–1867) in England (8) and the invention of the electric motor by Henry (1797–1878) in the United States. This was barely thirty years after Volta (1745–1827) had devised the first chemical electric battery. 1830–1833 saw the publication of the famous three volumes by Lyell (1797–1875), *The Principles of Geology*. Lyell's work firmly established the validity of the uniformitarian principle originated by Hutton (1726–1979), that the forces now operating to change the earth's surface had been operating in the same way and at the same rate throughout all earth's past. Lyell extended the age of the oldest fossil bearing rocks to the unheard-of figure of 240 000 000 years.

Astronomy

Vast expansion also took place in man's knowledge of space.

In 1838 Bessel (1784–1846) achieved the centuries-old dream of determining the distance to a star. He succeeded in measuring the parallax of 61 Cygni and calculated that the light from this star took more than six years to reach the earth. 1842 was the year in which Doppler (1803–1853) explained the change in the pitch of sound when source passes the observer, and predicted a similar effect for the colour of light. Then, in September 1846, the German astronomer Galle dramatically found the planet Neptune almost at the exact spot that had been calculated by Le Verrier (1811–1877). At a stroke this nearly doubled the known size of the planetary solar system. Incidentally, it is fortunate that Neptune, like Uranus, is too faint to have been discovered by the Babylonians, or the world might have been saddled with a nine-day week!

Chemistry

1839 saw the advent of photography, a chemical wonder achieved by Daguerre (1789–1851) with silver salts deposited on a copper plate and subsequent treatment with hyposulphite. Organic chemistry, another new science, was soon bearing highly important fruit. Chevreul (1786–1889) in 1825 patented the manufacture of candles from fatty acids. The fatty acid candles were whiter, harder, brighter, and less smelly than the old tallow ones, and represented a major improvement in the amenities of life to men of the mid-nineteenth century. In 1827 Prout (1785–1850) divided the components of foodstuffs into carbohydrates, fats, and proteins (9) and in 1828 Woehler (1800–1882) synthesized urea, thereby undermining the vitalist belief that organic compounds could be produced only in living plants and animals. The decisive blow was delivered by Kolbe (1818–1884) in 1845, with the synthesis of acetic acid from completely inorganic materials. Organic chemistry was now defined, not as the chemistry of living systems but as the chemistry of carbon compounds. This was to a large extent due to Liebig (1803–1873), who in the early 1830s perfected the technique of analysing organic compounds and was soon asked by the British Association for the Advancement of Science to draw up a Report on the State of Organic Chemistry. He responded in 1840 with his hugely popular book, *Organic Chemistry in its Application to Agriculture and Physiology*, which stimulated the growth of a commercial fertilizer industry. Liebig maintained that the chief factor in the loss of soil fertility was the consumption by plants of the mineral content of the soil. Liebig's next book, *Animal Chemistry, or Organic Chemistry in its Applications to Physiology and Pathology*, dating from 1842, was the first formal treatise on the subject. It developed the concept of metabolism, treated the nature and role of food materials at considerable length and proclaimed the principle that the working of the living body is to be sought in the chemical actions going on within it.

Biology

Biologists, meanwhile, had been investigating the nature of the cell. In 1831 Brown (1773–1858) discovered the cell nucleus. In 1836 Cagniard de Latour (1777–1859) observed microscopic globules in beer yeasts and also in wine, and proposed that the globules belonged to the vegetable kingdom and were responsible for the formation of carbon dioxide and alcohol (9). By 1839 Schwann (1810–1882) had extended to animals the cell theory enunciated by Schleiden (1804–1881) for plants in 1837, the theory that all living things are made up of cells or of materials formed by cells, and that each cell contains a nucleus and is surrounded by a membrane. It was Schwann who coined the term 'metabolism' to represent the overall chemical changes taking place within living tissue.

Neurology

Last in this catalogue, but not least, is the remarkable growth of understanding of the nervous system. It may be recalled that Gall (1785–1828) in 1810 was proposing the importance of grey matter for intellectual processes, that Levallois (1770–1840) in 1812 had located the respiratory centre in the medulla oblongata, and that Magendie (1783–1855) in 1822 proved the separate sensory and motor functions of the posterior and anterior roots of the spinal nerves. In 1824 Flourens (1794–1867) stated that animals that survive removal of the cerebral hemispheres 'lose perception, judgment, memory and will, therefore the cerebral hemispheres are the sole site of perception and of all intellectual abilities.' In 1825 Magendie discovered the cerebrospinal fluid. The 'law of specific nerve energies', that a sensory nerve always produces the same kind of sensation no matter what the stimulus, was enunciated by Mueller (1801–1858) in 1826 and gained currency in the 1830s, after Marshall Hall (1790–1857) described the spinal reflex. In 1842, Flourens distinguished three major functional regions of the brain, the cerebral hemispheres, the medulla, and the cerebellum, respectively having sensory, vital, and motor roles. Finally, in 1843 Du Bois-Reymond (1818–1896) demonstrated a negative electrical variation in nerve during activity and thus discovered the action current.

The energies of nature and the discovery of anaesthesia

It is clear even from these sketchy notes that, compared with those of the 1820s, the mental horizons of the mid-1840s had been enlarged and diversified to an unprecedented extent. The innovations were transforming thought and existence at a rate and to a degree exceeding anything on record and naturally inspired immense new confidence in the power of science to ameliorate man's lot. The leap in understanding achieved in two decades is epitomized by the somewhat diffused emergence of an entirely new concept concerning the variety, interconvertibility, and equivalence of the energies of nature. Indeed, the word energy in its present strict sense was not available, and no little confusion arose at the time from the indiscriminate use of the term 'force' to do duty for it. For a similar reason there must have existed a corresponding lack of clarity concerning the possibility, let alone the nature, of the phenomenon of anaesthesia, until it was observed and named. Davy (1778–1829) from self-observation spoke of 'the destruction of pain' (10), Hickman, of 'suspended animation', Wells (1815–1848), of the 'influence of gas', Morton (1819–1868), of 'ether sleep' (11). Long (1815–1878) had no term at all but retrospectively used 'anaesthesia', in itself a confession of why he did not pursue the lead he had opened up.

It is worth following the mental process, described by himself (12), that led the German physician Julius Robert Mayer (1814–1878) to the first formulation of the principle of the conservation of energy in 1842. It provides a fascinating insight into the state of medical science and practice in 1840, when Mayer was a ship's surgeon aboard a Hamburg freighter bound for Java. Venesection was still a principal standby of treatment in those days. In the tropics Mayer noticed that the crew's venous blood had an intense red colour. He thought that the temperature difference between the inside and outside of the organism regulated the amount of animal heat produced from the oxidation of blood and hence determined the colour difference between arterial and venous blood. In northern Germany the temperature difference was 15°C, on the Java coast only 5°C. Mayer concluded that in the tropics not as much oxidation was necessary to maintain body temperature as in northern Germany, because in the warm air less heat was lost by radiation, and for this reason tropical venous blood hardly differed in colour from arterial blood. But, reasoned Mayer, there is another way in which the body can warm the surroundings, and that is by work, for work always eventually produces heat. This too must have been produced by the oxidation of the blood. And since in both cases the heat produced is proportional to the oxygen consumed, so also must be the mechanical work which temporarily takes the place of one part of it. Heat and work must therefore be equivalent and mutually convertible in some fixed ratio. This is the essence of the conservation of energy. So Mayer suggested that mechanical forces, chemical forces, and heat are interconvertible. He conducted no experiments of his own. But, guided by what was then known about the difference in heat absorption by gas heated at constant pressure and gas heated at constant volume, he ingeniously calculated a value for the mechanical equivalent of heat. Since the quantity of heat required to raise the temperature of a given mass of gas is less at constant volume than at constant pressure (where the volume increases), Mayer assumed that the difference can be equated to the work done by the gas as it expands against the constant external pressure. It is both impressive and amusing (and apparently not previously noted) that such a profound insight was achieved starting from erroneous physiological premises. The brightness of the venous blood was of course not a consequence of decreased metabolism but of vasodilatation; however, vasomotor control had not yet been discovered, the notion of a basal metabolic rate lay far in the future, and the true site of bodily heat production had not yet been traced to the cells.

Medical science was in fact a late and very slow starter and in 1846 was still in an essentially preventive phase, curative therapeutics having barely progressed at all in the preceding decades (13). Indeed, anaesthesia was only the second major advance of the modern period, the first having been Jennerian vaccination in 1796, and both of these were preventive in character. Yet, as has been pointed out by others (1,2), in 1846 anaesthesia was an idea whose time had come. Presumably the discovery itself came in the new world and not in the old because that is where the incentives and the 'can do' spirit of the age most insistently beckoned on the horizon.

Conclusion

The progress of technology between the middle 1820s and the middle 1840s nurtured optimism and confidence in the power of the mind. The drumbeat of the first great march of science stimulated unlimited human aspirations to control nature, to increase comfort, and to prevent pain. It is no huge coincidence that this movement brought forth almost simultaneously a splendid new insight into natural law and a grand victory in the war on physical evil. In this light one may read the events in the Ether Dome on 16 October, 1846, as signalling the spread of that movement to the healing arts, amid a feeling of excitement close to that of William Wordsworth at the commencement of the French revolution (14):

> *'Bliss was it in that dawn to be alive,*
> *But to be young was very heaven!'*

References

(1) Greene NM. A consideration of factors in the discovery of anesthesia and their effects on its development. *Anesthesiology* 1975; **42**: 117–26.

(2) Caton D. The secularization of pain. *Anesthesiology* 1985; **62**: 493–501.

(3) Wightman PD. *The growth of scientific ideas*. New Haven: Yale University Press, 1953: 495 pp.

(4) Wright E. *History of the world. Vol 2, The last five hundred years*. London: Newnes Books, 1984: 768 pp.

(5) Rosen G. *A history of public health*. New York: MD Publications, 1958: 211, 237, 252.

(6) Carnot S. *Reflexions sur la puissance motrice du feu.* Edition critique par Robert Fox. Paris: Vrin, 1978: 371 pp.

(7) Knight DM. In: Bynum WF, Brown EJ, Porter R, eds. *Dictionary of the history of science.* Princeton: Princeton University Press, 1981: 381.

(8) Asimov I. *Asimov's biographical dictionary of science and technology.* 2nd Ed. New York: Doubleday, 1982: 939 pp.

(9) Ihde AJ. *The development of modern chemistry.* New York: Dover, 1984: 851 pp.

(10) Davy H. *Researches, chemical and philosophical; chiefly concerning nitrous oxide or dephlogisticated air and its respiration.* London: Johnson, 1800: 580 pp.

(11) Duncum BM. *The development of inhalation anaesthesia.* London: Oxford University Press, 1947: 77–129.

(12) Lindsay RB: *Julius Robert Mayer.* Oxford: Pergamon Press, 1973: 238 pp.

(13) Warner JH. *The therapeutic perspective.* Cambridge: Harvard University Press, 1986: 117.

(14) Wordsworth W. *Selected poems.* London: Oxford University Press, 1913: 196 (The World's Classics).

3.10   Metaphysical conclusions derived from
                                     a proposed mode of anaesthetic action

SAMUEL TIRER
University of Pennsylvania, Philadelphia, USA

Approximately two years ago, I purchased a book whose title intrigued me. It was called *L'âme. Demonstration de sa réalité déduite de l'étude des effets du chloroforme et du curare sur l'économie animale* (1). This translates as 'The Soul. The Demonstration of its Reality Deduced from the Study of the Effects of Chloroform and Curare on the Animal Economy.' It was written in 1868 by Ramon de la Sagra.

A year passed before I decided to undertake the task of translating the book and discovering how de la Sagra went about carrying out his goal. This proved to be quite challenging. Ferreting out biographical data concerning de la Sagra was an adventure with multiple phone calls to many libraries.

This article is organized into three sections. The first outlines what de la Sagra stated in his text, some biographical information follows and the paper concludes with a summary of the philosophical and scientific background in France which stimulated the appearance of this work.

De la Sagra's thesis

Purpose

De la Sagra's goal is to prove the existence of the soul. He is motivated in his book (1) to do this as a reaction against the popularity of the antireligious scientific philosophies of materialism (pp. 14 & 15) (1) and positivism (p. 3) (1) which are considered in detail later in this paper.

He sets out to accomplish his purpose by citing the results of studies and case reports of anaesthesia which bolster his arguments. Although the title of the book specifies the effect of chloroform, de la Sagra liberally uses information from studies performed with ether. He takes great pains not to impugn the reputation of the scientists whose works he is quoting.

He states that his arguments are not *ad hominem* but only counter the beliefs held by these scientists and thinkers (pp. 9–10) (1).

The conclusions that he draws from the data are usually at odds with those of the original authors. He states that he is examining anaesthetic phenomena from a 'psychological' point of view, overlooked or misinterpreted by others (p. 8) (1). He also wishes to correct the terminology used which also reflects the popular contemporary scientific theories and philosophies.

De la Sagra's view of sensation is close to that of modern physiology. He states that organs or tissues are not inherently sensitive or 'sensible' as he terms it. Outside stimuli cause impressions in the tissue which are then transmitted via the sensory nerves to the brain. The sensory nerves are not themselves sensitive but only transmit impressions. In the brain, perception of the impression occurs, an act of the intellect. Similarly, motor nerves do not move but transmit impulses which cause the muscles to contract (pp. 17–18) (1).

Anaesthetics act peripherally by blocking the impressions from arriving at the brain where they would be perceived. The brain centres are unaffected by ether. He rails against the idea that the various areas of the brain possess different functions which are affected by anaesthetics (pp. 89 & 98–99) (1).

De la Sagra criticizes the work of two important physiologists of the 19th century (pp. 39–41) (1). The first is Marie-Jean-Pierre Flourens (1794–1867). He was a physician who studied at Montpellier and devoted his career to the study of the physiology of the nervous system (2).

Flourens' theory (3) of the action of anaesthesia is based on data derived from the ablation of different areas of the brain. The function of the cerebral hemispheres followed sequentially by that of the cerebellum, spinal cord, and finally medulla is eliminated by anaesthesia. In animals who are etherized (this term is also used with agents other than ether), loss of consciousness, of feeling, of movement and finally, of life are observed. He was the first to localize the respiratory centre to the medulla.

The other major authority is François Achille Longet (1811–1871) who studied in Paris (4). His textbook of physiology which appeared in 1842 is considered a classic. Longet's idea of anaesthetic action (5) is similar to that of Flourens. The cerebral lobes, cerebellum, pons, spinal cord and medulla are the areas sequentially affected. He bases this on the observation of two distinct stages of anaesthesia in animals and on physiological studies of the nervous system. In the first stage, the animal falls over unconscious with no spontaneous movement. However, there is a withdrawal response to a stimulus such as pinching. This is the period of anaesthesia of the cerebral hemispheres, cerebellum and other areas except the pons and medulla. With prolonged inhalation, the second stage is attained and the animal ceases to respond and thus the pons is now anaesthetized. Both physiologists opine that the intellect is first affected by anaesthesia, then sensation (3) (5). De la Sagra strongly disagrees in his book (pp. 94–95 & 98–9) (1).

De la Sagra's belief in the peripheral action of anaesthetics is based on several lines of evidence. First, he outlines studies where nerves immersed in ether are, not surprisingly, shown to undergo morphological changes along with the loss of ability of transmitting impulses (pp. 100–110) (1). Secondly, the hypaesthesia reported by patients and physicians as an early sensation during induction is another proof of the local effect (pp. 81 & 111) (1). His third point is that the topical application of ether causes prolonged analgesic action at the affected site (pp. 127–128) (1). Electrical stimuli of sensory and motor nerve become ineffective when the nerves are respectively under the influence of ether and curare given systematically (p. 132) (1). De la Sagra uses the curare as a motor nerve analogue of ether and chloroform.

Finally, he devotes a large section to the effects of anaesthetics on the *mimosa pudica* or sensitive plant which exhibits the property of folding its leaves when touched. Ether and chloroform suppress this reactivity. This is not only proof of the peripheral action of anaesthetics but as plants do not possess a brain, then this organ cannot be involved in the anaesthetic process in the higher animals including man (145–147) (1).

Clinically, he bases his premise on cases reported in the literature where the patient undergoes anaesthesia and is able to speak during the procedure, cooperate with the surgeon, or manifest function of the intellect in other ways (pp. 53–55, 64, 114 & 115) (1). He also discusses reports by physicians who have administered anaesthetics to themselves and become analgesic although they were still able to think lucidly (57, 114 & 115) (1). The authors attribute this to incomplete or light anaesthesia. It is evident to de la Sagra that if patients are able comfortably to undergo surgery by means of an anaesthetic but manifest intellectual activity, then anaesthetics are not affecting the brain but act peripherally.

He divides the anaesthetic process into three stages. Initially, the being is isolated by alterations of the nerves. Sensation is subsequently modified with the gradual loss of pain. Finally, other sensations are lost (pp. 77 & 78) (1).

What one is then left with is the intellect, isolated from the external world by the elimination of sensory input. The intellect is a vital force and a property of the soul. Simply because there are no outward manifestations does not mean that intelligence is not functioning. Even if the patient struggles and moans during the surgery, this is not evidence of pain (pp. 94 & 95) (1). What one is observing is solely reflex activity (pp. 113, 167, 174 & 175) (1) or irritability (pp. 170–172) (1) and when the patient is questioned afterwards, he either remembers nothing or dispassionately recalls details of the procedure (pp. 64, 114 & 115) (1) or recounts the experience of rapturous dreams. Amnesia is not an explanation as many of the patients recount vivid dreams but deny painful sensations (p. 165) (1). Since the patient can recall dreams or the procedure just undergone, then his intellect and therefore his soul is functioning.

De la Sagra begins with the assumption that the soul exists and that the intellect is a vital force and property or faculty of the soul (p. 15) (1). Impressions are physical and material. Sensation is metaphysical and spiritual. Sensitivity is the act of perception of impressions. Perception including that of pain requires intelligence. Therefore anaesthesia cannot ablate intelligence before sensation (pp. 70–71) (1). Anaesthetics being material cannot affect intelligence (p. 213) (1). The immaterial nature of the intellectual faculties unaffected by anaesthesia bolsters the idea of the existence of the soul, itself immaterial.

De la Sagra does not go into great detail with regard to the proof of the reality of the soul. He refers the reader to a forthcoming unabridged book (p. 158) (1) which he is in the process of writing. It is unknown if this tome ever appeared in print.

What does this isolated soul do during anaesthesia? First, it acts on sensations from within. Second, it acts on ideas from the past. Third, it can act on ideas acquired by unknown means since it is detached from the senses (p. 176) (1).

What are the ramifications of this detached soul? Thought accelerates because external impressions are not present to provide a time reference. The nature of the thoughts are rapturous. This is to be expected as the soul, unfettered by its earthly ties, expresses its true joyful nature (192, 193 & 203) (1). The corollary is that the intellect functions by different means than the organism and is semi-independent of it (p. 208) (1). The senses are faulty intermediaries to study the world with. The soul is the only absolute reality (p. 209) (1).

Biography

De la Sagra was born in Corunna, Spain on 7 December, 1798 (6) (7) or 1801, (8) depending on the source. He spent his youth in Havana, Cuba. He studied in Madrid and became Director of the Botanical Garden of Havana and Professor of Botany at Havana University from 1820 (8) or 1822 (7) to 1832 (6) or 1834 (7). In 1837 (6), he was named correspondent to the Académie des Sciences of Paris.

He amassed a large collection of Cuban flora and sent specimens around the world to various institutions. He was also interested in the development of agriculture, public instruction, and public institutions such as prisons and orphanages. He felt that education and religious and moral instruction of youth would lead to social reform in the future. He opened a class in agricultural botany and founded a model farm (8).

He travelled widely and visited the United States in 1835. His visit to Baltimore, where he met Dr Robley Dunglison, is noted in an article which appeared in 1974 (9). He spent several years in Paris and then went to Madrid where he founded a magazine and devoted himself to the study of political economy. In 1848, he went to Paris and took part in the revolution. From 1854 to 1856, he was a deputy in the Cortes (7).

His scientific work was supported by the Spanish government. In 1867, de la Sagra wrote an article in an obscure French journal which advocated the emancipation of the slaves in

Cuba. He lost the support of Queen Isabella and became destitute (8). He died at Cortaillod, near Neuchâtel in Switzerland on 25 May, 1871.

De la Sagra wrote a number of books. These include *Historia económica, política, y estadística de la isla de Cuba* (1831), *Historia física, política, y naturel de la isla de Cuba (2 volumes, 1837–42)* (8), and *'Cinco meses en los Estados Unidos* (1836) (7) (10).

None of these references list the book which is the subject of this present paper. A glance at the National Union Catalogue shows that it is in only two major libraries in the United States, Harvard University and the National Library of Medicine. It was written after he had fallen out of favour and one can only surmise that it may have been a form of protest for the fate which had befallen him. As the world was careening away from the genteel and more ordered era of the early 19th century, de la Sagra may have felt compelled to provide some religious stability to an increasingly disordered and alien time.

Philosophy

Paris was the centre of the medical and scientific world in the first half of the 19th century. The French Revolution was partly responsible for this state of affairs. The health and hospital system had been reorganized and centralized to three major centres; Paris, Strasbourg, and Montpellier. Medical education had been revamped with both surgeons and physicians now attending medical schools. Medicine was transformed from a scholastic, theoretical art to a clinical and laboratory science.

Today, scientific philosophy is not a major concern to those working in the field. However, the philosophical underpinnings and implications of the discoveries made at the time were of great importance to those involved in scientific work (11).

Iatrophysics and iatrochemistry

From the third to the 16th century, the humoral concept of pathology had reigned supreme. In the 1700s, there arose two new schools of thought (12). The first, iatrophysics, was championed by René Descartes. He proposed that man was a machine except for the rational soul which resided in the pineal gland and operated spiritually. The soul separated man from animals and fostered sensation and self-awareness. Iatrophysics was popular in southern Europe where discoveries by Galileo, Borelli, and Toricelli strengthened the basis of physics. The last major iatromechanical text was *Haemostatics* written by Hales in 1733.

Iatrochemistry (12) was the other philosophy, although never as well accepted due to the more primitive state of chemistry at the time. Sylvius of Leyden classified diseases according to acidosis or alkalosis. All problems were due to chemical imbalances.

Reductionism or mechanism

This is the term used to describe a philosophical outlook which was important in 19th century science. It is the belief that the functions of the body are reducible to the laws, rules, and assumptions of physics and chemistry (11). There was a resurgence of popularity in this idea during the 1840s due to the Industrial Revolution and developments such as the Voltaic pile and advances in the thermodynamic study of animals (13). There is much overlap between mechanism and materialism.

Vitalism

In contrast to mechanism, vitalism is the doctrine that states that there is present in a living system a substantial entity that imparts to the system powers possessed by no inanimate body (14). George Ernst Stahl (1660–1734) stated that the sensitive soul or anima inhabited all parts of the organism and prevented the natural process of putrefaction. Stahl was also responsible for the phlogiston theory which existed until Lavoisier disproved it. The school of Montpellier advocated vitalism in France (12).

A more scientific view of vitalism was expressed by Xavier Bichat (1771–1802) (12), (15) who was the first to localize pathology to the level of the tissues. He regarded vitalism like gravitation, as another force to be quantitated. The vital force could not ultimately be understood but experimentation could still go on. He postulated the existence of two vital properties, sensibility and contraction. Sensibility was decentralized where each organ received and retained its own impressions. A blow against vitalism was the synthesis of urea which was performed in 1824 by Frederick Wohler. Up to that point, one of the mainstays of vitalism was the belief that living matter reduced to its most basic components possessed an irreducible vital element that could not be duplicated in the laboratory. In other words, compounds produced by living things shared the same vitality (13).

Materialism

Materialism was a German philosophy. The Germans regarded the organism as subject to forces which act according to blind necessity and inherent in matter itself. The original force was a product of the Creator but it now ran autonomously like a planetary system. This was a mechanistic form of materialism. German physiologists hoped to reduce the discipline to biophysics and biochemistry. The ultimate expression of materialism was summarized by Moleschott: "Der Mensch ist, was er isst"—man is what he eats (16). Supporters of this philosophy were often persecuted since they opposed the divine right of kings and were political revolutionaries (13).

Materialism was embraced by the French, although altered to some degree. Many of the French were vitalistic materialists. Man was an animal. Mental activities were simply due to sensation. This belief fostered vivisection as a means of studying the animal with its vital principle intact (16).

Sensualism

Sensualism was the philosophy of Condillac (1715–1780) Ideas were derived from the impressions we receive through our external sense organs. The soul felt and the organs of the body were its agents (17).

Idéology

Idéology was a philosophy of the late 18th century that lasted to the middle of the 19th. It was the successor to sensualism. The salon of Madame Helvetius (56) was the meeting place for the adherents of this philosophy. Among the visitors to this salon were Benjamin Franklin, Thomas Jefferson, and Antoine Lavoisier (17).

Two basic premises were the major tenets of Idéology. Sensations are the primary data of cognition. All faculties of understanding (e.g. perception, judgement, etc.) are compounds of sensations which can be resolved by analysis into components. Ideas are created from experience which is derived from sensation (18).

The two major proponents were Destutt de Tracy (1754–1836) and Cabanis (1757–1808). Cabanis felt that the brain was an organ that digested impressions and secreted thought. Idéology made the mind a mere function of the body and is therefore considered by some to be a subset of materialism (17). Internal impressions accounted for instinctive actions. The passions, thought, and will were due to internal and external sensations (16). Sensation was a biological phenomenon or attribute of matter. However, vitalism did play a role in their philosophy as an unknowable force. For Cabanis and Destutt de Tracy, feeling was a biological phenomenon or even a property of matter. The soul did not play a part. The physiologist, Bichat, supported Condillac's sensualist view with the soul essential to the act of feeling. François Magendie (1783–1855) who succeeded Bichat as the foremost physiologist of France, agreed with Cabanis (17).

Positivism

Positivism was a designation for what we now call the scientific method. Science is the only valid knowledge and facts are the only possible objects of knowledge (19). Magendie became an advocate but the most famous adherent was Claude Bernard (1813-78). It was a pragmatic philosophy and did not delve into the essence of life. Repeatable results derived from controlled experiments were paramount. Bernard wanted physiology to be an autonomous science. Mechanists possessed data but the nature of the organism as a whole was beyond them. Vitalists regarded this nature as inscrutable. Therefore, both philosophies were dead ends (13).

De la Sagra's philosophy

Armed with the preceding philosophical primer, we can now examine de la Sagra's thesis. He deals with two interrelated topics; the physiology of the nervous system and the mechanism of action of anesthetics. He states from the beginning that he is fighting materialism (pp. 14 & 15) (1) and positivism (p. 3) (1). His outlook is obviously vitalistic. The soul is central.

However, in focusing on the philosophical tenets of any of the figures of the time, we often see an element of the eclectic. Very few of the cited authorities have a pure philosophical viewpoint. For example, Bichat's work combined vitalism and sensualism with an element of materialism (12) (15). The Idéologues did not exclude the soul from their thinking but simply pushed it to the background (17).

De la Sagra's concept of the mechanism of sensation is also eclectic. Bichat believed that tissue had vital properties. De la Sagra's vitalism resides in the more traditional soul which transcends the body. However, he does accept Bichat's idea of the sequential transmission of impressions from the peripheral senses to the brain, then to the soul where pain or pleasure is elicited (17). However, de la Sagra does not express the notion that the brain is passing on information to the soul. Acquisition appears to be simultaneous.

Bichat believed in the 18th century concept that peripheral tissues themselves were sensitive (i.e. impression and perception occurring peripherally). Magendie, Flourens and Cuvier articulated an opposing viewpoint in the early 19th century. Sensation was not peripheral. Impressions were received peripherally and transmitted by the nervous system to the brain where they became sensations. Cuvier went further and supported the idea that the entire brain was the material instrument of the unitary soul (20). De la Sagra echoes this view. Where he differs is that it was the soul rather than the brain which possessed the faculty of sensation. This is a concept taken directly from sensualism. Ironically, he rejects the positivistic reasoning by which Magendie, Longet and Flourens reached their conclusions. They looked at overt signs of pain in animal experiments. De la Sagra rejects this as reflex movement. Overt signs of pain mean little. De la Sagra believes that it is an error to judge phenomena by appearance (p. 185) (1). Movement can occur without pain just as pain can exist without movement (pp. 188 & 8) (1).

De la Sagra's ideas regarding the mechanism of action of anaesthetics are at odds with the views of Longet and Flourens. He also disagrees with Flourens' and Longet's ideas that pain sensation is referable to certain parts of the brain since it is the soul that interprets pain. Intelligence and the different areas of the brain are not affected by anaesthetics. There is no seat of intelligence. However, by relying on the rare cases of manifestation of intelligence under anaesthesia, he seeks to bolster his concept of the central function of the soul.

How did la Sagra's views fit in with the controversy regarding the safety moral implications of the use of anaesthetics which were extant during the first 20 to 30 years after the Morton demonstration? Many of those in opposition used vitalistic arguments (21). They regarded pain itself as the vital force or the spur to the vital force. Some considered pain as separate from the vital force but anything that could overcome pain could also overcome the vital spark. Therefore, suppression of pain had mortal implications for the patient.

De la Sagra sidesteps the entire issue with the idea of the peripheral action of anaesthesia. Anaesthetic phenomena are a means of demonstrating his philosophical viewpoint. He is an enthusiast and wholeheartedly praises this medical advance (p. 11) (1). However, his ideas do not represent any prevalent thought of the period. His was very much a lone voice.

Conclusions

Ramon de la Sagra wrote an unusual work (1) in the declining years of his life after having lost the support of the Spanish monarchy. In an increasingly alien and atheistic world, he was seeking to establish an oasis of religious rational thought. His attention was caught by early accounts of the administration of anaesthetics. The phenomena described appeared to support his views that intelligence and hence the soul was central to the act of sensation and anaesthetics acted peripherally.

One wonders how his book was received. Although he was a correspondent to the Académie des Sciences, it is notable that no mention was made of his death in their journal (*Les Comptes rendus des séances de l'Academie des sciences*). He stated that he wished to avoid causing offence. Were the contrapuntal views of this botanist and political economist cause for umbrage?

De la Sagra is an enigma. On the one hand, he was a participant in the royal establishment of Spain to the extent that he received their patronage. He was also a religious conservative. In contrast, he was a social reformer and participated in the revolution of 1848.

The idea of the intellect functioning under anaesthesia is not entirely lost. Aside from articles describing cases involving muscle relaxants, there are rare articles that postulate the occurrence of this phenomenon (22).

Perusing the anaesthesia literature rarely provokes any philosophical thoughts on the part of the majority of readers. De la Sagra has given us a glimpse of a fruitful and tumultuous era in the history of medicine and science (1).

Acknowledgments

I would like to thank the following people for their assistance: Edward Mormon, McIver W. Edwards, Jr, Tom Horrocks, College of Physicians of Philadelphia, Philadelphia; Roy Goodman, American Philosophical Society, Philadelphia; Janet Evans, Pennsylvania Horticultural Society, Philadelphia; Sylvia Baker, The Academy of Natural Sciences, Philadelphia; and Anita Karg, Hunt Institute for Botanical Documentation, Pittsburgh.

References

(1) De la Sagra R. *L'ame. Demonstration de sa réalité de l'étude des effets du chloroforme et du curare sur l'économie animale.* Paris: Germer-Ballière, 1868.

(2) Kruta V, Flourens Marie-Jean-Pierre. In: Gillespie CC, ed. *Dictionary of scientific biography.* Vol 5. New York: Charles Scribner and Sons, 1972: 44–5.

(3) Flourens P. *Archives générales de médecine.* 4ième série. 1847; **13**: 391–2.

(4) Neuberger M. *The historical development of experimental brain and spinal cord physiology before Flourens.* Trans. by E. Clarke. Baltimore: The Johns Hopkins University Press, 1981: 339.

(5) Longet FA. *Bulletin de l'académie royale de médecine* 1846–7; **12**: 361–70.

(6) *Bulletin de la société botanique de France* 1871; **17**: 188–9.

(7) Ramon de la Sagra. In: Wilson J, Fiske J, eds. *Appleton's cyclopaedia of American biography.* Vol 5. New York: D. Appleton and Company, 1888; 367–8.

(8) *Annual Report of the Board of Regents of the Smithsonian Institution* 1875: 162–3.

(9) Carrol D. A Botanist's Visit to Baltimore in 1835. *Md State Med J* 1974; **23**: 49–55.

(10) Ramon de la Sagra. In: Stafleu F, Cowan R, eds. *Taxonomic Literature.* 2nd Ed. Utrecht/Antwerp: Bohn, Scheltemac, Holkema, 1983: 1056–7.

(11) Mendelsohn E. Revolution and reduction: The sociology of methodological and philosophical concerns in nineteenth century biology. In: Elkana Y, ed. *The interaction between science and philosophy.* Atlantic Highlands: Humanities Press, 1974; 407–26.

(12) Ackerknecht E. *A short history of medicine.* Revised Edition. Baltimore: The Johns Hopkins University Press, 1982.

(13) Coleman W. *Biology in the nineteenth century.* New York: John Wiley and Sons, 1971.

(14) Beckner MO. Vitalism. In: Edwards P, ed. *Encyclopedia of philosophy*. Vol 8. New York: Crowell, Collier, and Macmillan, 1967: 253–6.

(15) Lesch J. *Science and medicine in France. The emergence of experimental physiology, 1790–1855*. Cambridge: Harvard University Press, 1984; 50–79.

(16) Temkin O. Materialism in French and German physiology of the early nineteenth century. *Bull Hist Med* 1946; **20**: 322–7.

(17) Temkin O. The philosophical background of Magendie's physiology. *Bull Hist Med* 1946; **20**: 10–35.

(18) Rosen G. The philosophy of ideology and the emergence of modern medicine in France. *Bull Hist Med* 1946; **20**: 328–39.

(19) Abbagno N. Positivism. In: Edwards P, ed. *Encylopaedia of philosophy*. Vol 6; New York, Crowell, Collier and Macmillan, 1967: 414–9.

(20) Gross M. The lessened locus of feeling: A transformation in French physiology in the early nineteenth century. *J Hist Biol* 1979; **12**: 231–71.

(21) Pernick MS. *A calculus of suffering*. New York: Columbia University Press, 1985; 278.

(22) Mostert, JW. States of awareness during general anesthesia. *Perspec in Biol and Med* 1975; **19**: 68–76.

Chapter 4
THE INTRODUCTION OF MODERN ANAESTHESIA IN THE USA AND THE SPREAD OF THE GOOD NEWS TO THE UNITED KINGDOM

4.1 The start of modern anaesthesia

LEROY D. VANDAM
Harvard Medical School, Boston, Massachusetts, USA

Somewhat like an apprentice in the atelier of a renowned artist, I shall add some brush strokes to the portrait begun by Dr Nunn (Paper 3.1) of the origins of anaesthesia. My role is to depict the start of modern anaesthesia. 'Modern' conveys the idea of a contemporary event or something that has taken place in the immediate past. Nonetheless, in the historical context surely it is permissible to interpret as modern some happenings that occurred about 145 years ago when anaesthesia first became of clinical consequence; after all, is the time span that great when we know that the species, *Homo sapiens*, began to appear about two million years ago, and that the least visible galaxy in the firmament is billions of light years away?

The first and second medical revolutions

For the moment, however, permit me to convey the idea that modern anaesthesia as we know it actually arose about 45 years ago, to coincide with medicine's second revolution. According to Lewis Thomas (1) the first revolution occurred sometime in the 1800s when physicians began to question the centuries old practice of doing something forceful about an illness, according to the Galenic, humoral theory of disease. The physician proposed, then, not to meddle and by means of the physical examination and experience with signs and symptoms, to make a diagnosis, offer a prognosis and stand by the patient to await the crisis—an attitude of therapeutic nihilism. The few effective drugs available comprised digitalis leaf, quinine, morphine, and arsenic and mercury for the treatment of syphilis. This was the useful pharmcopoeia when I graduated from medical school in 1938. Having relinquished chloroform, anaesthesia possessed nitrous oxide, ether, procaine and newly synthesized thiopentone and cyclopropane. The second revolution began with the introduction of sulphanilamide, penicillin and streptomycin for the treatment of bacterial infection. With the first use of tubocurarine and the study of the pharmacokinetics of thiopentone, anaesthesia began its modern phase. Thus, as propounded by sociologist, Peter Caws (2), 'the development of science is a stepwise process: nobody starts from scratch and nobody gets far ahead of the rest.'

The background to the introduction of inhalational anaesthesia in the 1840s

Caw's comment (1) redirects me to the main theme, the start of anaesthesia, and therefore the relevant biographies of the innovators. I shall attempt to conform to the current practice of historiography where the social, philosophical and even geographical elements are brought to bear on a theme. Why was it that clinical anaesthesia was first tried over a span of several years, independently by several people? We know that Priestley, Davy and Hickman had the idea, so too did several others, in addition to Long, Wells and Morton. According to the sociologists, questions about origins are said to belong to the, 'context of discovery, and the devising of hypotheses is ascribed to genius, intuition, imagination, chance or any number of other extralogical processes.' (2) Arthur Lovejoy remarked that, 'whatever definition of man be true or false, it is generally admitted that he is distinguished among the creatures by the habit of entertaining ideas. And ideas are the most migratory things in the world' (3). But why so many people with the same idea? Owsei Temkin adds, 'sociologists of science have cited in evidence for social causation the multiple appearance of the same discovery—'multiples' in the language of Robert Merton. The independent use of anaesthesia by Long, Wells and Morton is a well known example. Though discoveries are not necessarily ideas, both are spoken of as being 'in the air' or 'ripe for their time' (4). Both regional and intravenous anaesthesia have similar histories. W. Stanley Sykes in an unpublished chronicle of the development could list some 30 events that preceded the start of modern anaesthesia (5).

Why in America and not England, France or Germany where the scientific foundations already existed? In England, to paraphrase Duncum (6), the year 1846 followed a peaceful quarter century, but this was a time of intensive industrialization, urbanization and overcrowding, with their attendant social and political problems. The country was prosperous and had begun to institute reforms relating to public health and medical care. There were in addition to the old hospital foundations based on voluntary contributions, hospitals for the poor and destitute and specialized infirmaries. Medical education was entirely clinical at the bedside at the major medical centres. As the central figures, the general practitioners were given the major hospital appointments. A tendency to specialize in medicine had begun along with a reluctance to accept change. Fellowship in the Royal Society was exclusive and there was little exchange of ideas. The conclusion might be drawn that the country was preoccupied with other matters and the medical system too highly structured to venture or accept new ideas. In France, which was undergoing the transition from monarchy to republic, hospitals were under state control but there was free exchange of ideas in the scientific community; probably that was why Wells petitioned the French Academy to acknowledge his priority for the discovery, as in Prussia and Austria, medicine was too deeply steeped in the study of chemistry and physics. Finally, we scrutinize America, still in the stages of internal development but prosperous, with its frontiers edging ever westward. General standards of medicine had deteriorated in the process even though the Eastern practice of teaching and learning was patterned after that of Edinburgh. Everything had to be done in the quickest and most expedient manner; thus it fell to the lot of a general practitioner and two dentists to make the move toward anaesthesia.

Overriding all intellectual and geographical factors, however, was a burgeoning humanitarianism, largely manifest in England and extending toward America, so that secularization and relief of pain became major considerations for society (7,8). For this reason, in the face of strong opposition from the medical establishment and elements of the church, anaesthesia achieved immediate acceptance the world over.

In this setting and without any attempt to resurrect the controversy over priority, an examination of the personal characteristics of three young men might explain how the drama unfolded and how it ended. All three had rural upbringings, ranging from Vermont through Massachusetts to Georgia, near to the East Coast, and differing in the quality and quantity of their education. John F. Fulton (9) depicted the story of the introduction of surgical anaesthesia as typifying the vision and daring of youth. In 1842, Long was approaching 27 years of age, Wells in 1844 was 29 years old and Morton 27 in 1846. James Venable, an academy student, and Edward Gilbert Abbott, a printer, the first to be anaesthetized other than for dental extraction, had hardly reached their twenties.

Crawford Williamson Long (1815–1878)

According to Beaton (10), Crawford Williamson Long was born in Danielsville, Georgia, on 1 November, 1815, of Scottish, Irish Presbyterian lineage. His parents lived a happy and rather luxurious plantation life and none of the family wanted for worldly possessions. At age 14, he enrolled at Franklin College (later to be the University of Georgia) where his roommate was Alexander H. Stephens, subsequently the Vice President of the Confederacy. Upon graduation, second in his class, Long taught for a time in the local academy and read medicine with Dr Grant of Jefferson. He studied for a year at the Medical Department of Transylvania University, in Lexington, Kentucky. The school had a distinguished faculty including the professor of surgery, Benjamin Winslow Dudley, one of the world's best known lithotomists, such was the nature of surgery at the time. Nearby in Danville, resided Ephraim McDowell, the first successfully to perform ovariotomy, even as his patient read prayers from the Bible. From 1837 to 1839, Long was a student at the University of Pennsylvania, the second school in the colonies, next to the College of Physicians and Surgeons, to grant a degree in medicine[1].

Long's instructors included George Wood and Hobart Hare, both of whom wrote and spoke of nitrous oxide and ether (11). At the time, ether enjoyed wide use at the Pennsylvania and Philadelphia General Hospitals as a therapeutic agent after the manner of its employment at the Pneumatic Institute in Bristol. Although some may challenge the inference, Long surely witnessed many an ether frolic there.

After graduation from Pennsylvania, in 1839, Long 'walked' the hospitals in New York City for 18 months where he garnered a reputation as a promising surgeon. Subsequently, yielding to his father's entreaties, Long settled into general practice in Jefferson, Georgia. I shall not delve into the details of the operation performed under ether anaesthesia on James Venable, 30 March, 1842, with several witnesses present and a special inducement for the patient in the form of a reduced fee for the procedure, two dollars, and a charge of 25 cents for the cost of the ether.

The perennial question in everybody's mind is why Long waited so long to proclaim his discovery. As in so many aspects of anaesthetic history, W. S. Sykes cogently addressed this enigma in his essay, 'The Reticence of Dr Long.' (12). Actually, Long himself supplied the reasons in his report to the *Southern Medical Journal* for 1849 (13) published three years after Morton's demonstration. Sykes was hardly convinced by Long's explanations. These were; that he was too busy with a country practice to find the time; that he still had doubts about priority; that it was mere negligence on his part; that he subsequently had too few opportunities to give ether anaesthesia (only three times at first and until October of 1846 only a total of eight cases); that, although he did not believe in mesmerism or hypnosis, he was aware of many instances where painless operations had thus been accomplished, and he had to prove to himself that etherization was genuine; that he had not had the opportunity to employ ether for a major operation; and, lastly his isolation in an environment where he could not share his experiences and thoughts with others. In disagreement with Sykes, I find these explanations to be eminently logical. Long may have been the first to give ether for obstetric delivery when his daughter, Frances, gave birth on 27, December, 1845. Sykes goes on to say, 'If only Crawford Long had the self confidence of a Morton or a Simpson he would have been a worthy contender to the end' (12).

Horace Wells (1815–1848)

Horace Wells was born in Hartford, Vermont, on 21 January, 1815. I find it to be a striking geographical coincidence that it was indeed the town of Hartford, and that Gardner Quincy Colton should come from Georgia, but in this case, the town in Vermont. From 1821 to 1834, Wells attended some of the select academies in the area, and for a while, like Long, was a teacher of reading and writing in a district school (14). At one time he contemplated entering the ministry. It is well known that from 1834 through 1844, he studied dentistry in Boston and practised both there and in Hartford, Connecticut. Over that period he wrote several articles for dental journals and became William Thomas Green Morton's mentor, as his day book repeatedly shows. Then came that fateful encounter with Gardner Quincy Colton on December 10, 1844, followed the next day by his own tooth extraction while 'under the influence'. By circumstance, all of the accounts of their thoughts and actions supplied by Long, Wells and Morton, were, to be sure, retrospective, undoubtedly embellished and biased. For example, in 1847 Wells (15) wrote:

> *Reasoning by analogy I was led to believe that surgical operations might be performed without pain, by the fact that, an individual, when much excited from ordinary causes*

[1]It is of interest that in 1794, Joseph Priestley who had migrated to America to escape religious persecution, was offered, but refused the professorship of chemistry at Pennsylvania. After Priestley's rejection, James Woodhouse accepted the post. He was perhaps the most brilliant American chemist of his generation who knew of Priestley's discovery of nitrous oxide and of Davy's experiences.

may receive severe wounds without manifesting the least pain; as for instance, the man who is engaged in combat may have a limb severed from his body, after which he testifies that it was attended with no pain at the time, and so on.'

This passage is somewhat redolent of Humphry Davy's expression, perhaps in keeping with our current concepts of the actions of endorphins.

Wells had some of the educational advantages that Long enjoyed, he was not given to duplicity and though he sought pecuniary award, that was not his main thrust. However, this well meaning, modest and religious man undoubtedly showed the stigmata of a manic-depressive temperament as revealed by his reaction to the failed nitrous oxide demonstration ('The excitement of this adventure brought on an illness from which I did not recover for many months, being thus obliged to relinquish entirely my professional business.'). Having been associated with Morton for so many years, and having been abetted by Morton in the abortive nitrous oxide demonstration of 1845, one can easily imagine what transpired in Wells's mind when the news of the ether demonstration was conveyed to him; thus, he literally went to pieces and took his life while in psychotic turmoil.

Again, our sage commentator, W. S. Sykes, portrays Wells in the essay, *De Profundis* (5), by asking why he had such an unhappy and unsuccessful life and such a tragic death ('As I see it, he was a man easily depressed and discouraged, too easily led and influenced by others: for after one partial public failure, he completely abandoned his attempts to publicise nitrous oxide anaesthesia which had already been satisfactory in his hands in a number of cases. We know that he was irresolute, wayward and volatile, for he kept abandoning his dental practice to make a living in strange and unusual way: buying pictures in Paris to sell in the US and other queer ventures.'). These enterprises included amongst others Wells's 'panorama of nature'—a series of entertainments on natural history—and the manufacture and sale of portable shower baths, stoves. Sykes continues

'He was in fact the exact opposite of the phlegmatic Morton, who fought tooth and nail for his discovery against the persistent encroachments of Jackson; the exact antithesis of the rock-like Simpson who thrived on controversy and dearly loved a fight. Only death itself silenced Simpson'.

William Thomas Green Morton (1819–1868)

As for the third figure, William Thomas Green Morton, even in the face of his stellar accomplishments, there has always been the tendency toward disparagement; for example, this quotation is typical: 'Dr Morton's talent of recklessness fitted by nature with those qualities of mind, being reckless and bold, untrammeled by education.' Much of what we know about Morton's life was in essence dictated by him as he later waged his campaign for recognition and award. Designated as materials for a biography of W. T. G. Morton, the accounts of his early existence given first to Benjamin Perley Poore (16), then to Nathan P. Rice (17), are both replete with inaccuracies and contradictions. True, his forebears had emigrated from Scotland early in the 1700s, at first settling in Salem, Massachusetts, then in various Quaker settlements in Rhode Island, with a brief sojourn in New Jersey. Morton was born in Charlton, Massachusetts on 9 August, 1819. The description of his birthplace does not fit the image of what is now believed to be the actual dwelling, a brick structure. According to Rice, it is depicted as a large, square, old fashioned, wooden manse with an immense stone chimney in the centre, a brook by the door, and each room with a fireplace. That edifice is alleged to have burned to the ground but a brook could not have meandered to the top of the hill. The description may have been a composite of another dwelling, the Waters-Morton house, to which the family moved in 1827; the brook is there. Morton presumably attended the academies in Charlton, Leicester, Oxford and Northfield (academies were in those days the equivalent of our present secondary schools) but his education progressed no further because of familial economic stringency. At age 17, he went to work for a bookseller in Boston, then betook himself to Baltimore to study at the newly established College of Dental Surgery, although no record exists of his having been there. A diploma given him was an honorary one presented to him several years after the demonstration. No doubt exists that he studied with Wells, attended lectures given by the Harvard Medical Faculty and that he was a domiciliary student with Charles T. Jackson, the eccentric and paranoid chemist, who was not a member of the faculty. Morton did not receive the MD degree although it was often affixed to his name.

Most propitious, however, were Morton's relations with some of the more renowned surgeons of the era. There was John Collins Warren who had received his degree at Edinburgh and successively, over the first several decades of the 19th century, became Dean of the Medical School and Professor of Anatomy and Surgery, and, with the physician James Jackson, and others, rejuvenated the Massachusetts Medical Society, founded the *Boston Medical and Surgical Journal* (now the *New England Journal of Medicine*), the Boston Medical library and the Massachusetts General Hospital, and helped to compile the first pharmacopoeia in the colonies. Moreover, Morton had access to Henry Jacob Bigelow, son of Jacob Bigelow, who arranged both the nitrous oxide and ether demonstrations, later to become America's foremost orthopaedic surgeon. Also noteworthy were the associations with Augustus Addison Gould believed to have been Morton's ghost writer, and with the redoubtable Oliver Wendell Holmes. Morton, his wife Elizabeth Whitman and their newborn son, William James, resided with the Goulds after the estrangement from Jackson. These were the professional associations of which neither Long nor Wells had the advantage.

Morton wrote a good deal more than either Long or Wells whose literary output was sparse. His publications were first in relation to dentistry and later, after the demonstration, largely polemical. Morton's pamphlet written late in 1847 (18), which was possibly edited by Gould, is a succinct narrative, apparently not influenced by Bigelow's earlier description (19) but revealing a knowledge of the history and an acquaintance with John Snow's, *On the Inhalation of the Vapour of Ether* (20). Although Morton does not describe the signs or stages, nor could he possibly possess the clinical observational powers of Snow, he does, however, emphasize the need for the purity of ether, stresses the advantages over the original glass globe of a bell-shaped sponge applied directly to the face, the hazards of entraining too little atmospheric air which might lead to asphyxia, the various anaesthetic depths required for various procedures, and as a dentist might, the need for preliminary examination of patients, plus organization and efficient use of surgical instruments.

W. Stanley Sykes (5) failed to analyse in detail Morton's characteristics and temperament as he did those of Long and Wells, although he does refer to Morton many times in passing. Probably, Sykes would have got around to doing so had he survived. Overall, although Morton's education was truncated, his self-teaching was more than adequate. One cannot disregard his keen native intelligence, relative emotional stability (Sykes called it 'phlegmatic') tempered by aggressiveness, and entrepreneurship, little of which the others displayed. Fulton (9) asked 'What would have happened if the first patient receiving ether at the Massachusetts General Hospital, had died under the anaesthetic. Few of the other eventual claimants would have risen to support the Boston dentist had a calamity occurred—and how long would it have been for anaesthetization to become a reality if the death had occurred?

Had there been more time allotted to me, surely I would have given John Snow all the credit for having introduced professionalism to anaesthesia, in every sense of the term, as so admirably documented by his successor and biographer, Benjamin Ward Richardson (21).

References

(1) Thomas L. Medicine as a very old profession. In: Wyngaarden JB, Smith LH Jr. eds. *Cecil text book of medicine.* Philadelphia: WB Saunders, 1982: xli–xliii.
(2) Caws, P. The structure of discovery. *Science* 1969; **166**: 1375–80.
(3) Lovejoy AO. Reflections on the history of ideas. *J Hist Ideas* 1940; **1**: 3–23.
(4) Temkin O. The historigraphy of ideas in medicine. In: Clarke E, ed. *Modern methods in the history of medicine.* London: Athlone Press, 1971.
(5) Sykes WS. De profundis. Chapter 11. In: *Essays on the first hundred years of anaesthesia.* Vol II, Edinburgh: E & S Livingstone. 1961: 144–7.
(6) Duncum BM. *The development of inhalation anaesthesia. With special reference to the years 1846–1900.* London: Oxford University Press, 1947: 1–21.

(7) Greene NM. A consideration of factors in the discovery of anesthesia and their effects on its development. *Anesthesiology* 1971; **35**: 515–22.

(8) Caton D. The secularization of pain. *Anesthesiology* 1985; **62**: 493–501.

(9) Fulton JF. The vision and daring of youth: the story of the introduction of surgical anesthesia. *Yale J Biol Med* 1946; **19**: 207–16.

(10) Beaton A. Crawford Williamson Long. *Yale J Biol Med* 1946; **19**: 189–93.

(11) Eckenhoff JE. *Anesthesia from colonial times. A history of anesthesia at the University of Pennsylvania.* Philadelphia: J. B. Lippincott, 1966.

(12) Sykes WS. *op cit.* Chapter I. The reticence of Dr Long. Vol III. 1982: 1–13.

(13) Long CW. An account of the first use of sulphuric ether by inhalation as an anaesthetic in surgical operations. *South Med Surg J* 1849; **5**: 705–13.

(14) Archer WH. Chronological history of Horace Wells, discoverer of anesthesia. *Bull Hist Med* 1939; **7**: 1140–69.

(15) Wells H. *The history of the discovery of the application of nitrous oxide gas, ether, etc. to surgical operations.* J. Gaylord Wells: Hartford, 1847.

(16) Poore BP. *Historical materials for the biography of W. T. G. Morton, M.D., discoverer of etherization with an account of anaesthesia.* Washington: G. S. Gideon, 1856.

(17) Rice NP. *Trials of a public benefactor, as illustrated in the discovery of etherization.* New York: Pudney and Russell, 1858.

(18) Morton WTG. *Remarks on the proper mode of administering sulphuric ether by inhalation.* Boston: Dutton and Wentworth, Printers, 1847: 44 pp.

(19) Bigelow HJ. Insensibility during surgical operations produced by inhalation. *Boston Med Surg J* 1846; **35**: 309–17.

(20) Snow J. *On the inhalation of the vapour of ether in surgical operations.* London: John Churchill, 1847.

(21) Richardson BW. Memoir of the author. In: Snow J. *On chloroform and other anaesthetics, their action and administration.* London: John Churchill, 1858.

4.2   Early ether anaesthesia:
the news of anaesthesia spreads to the United Kingdom

RICHARD H. ELLIS
St Bartholomew's Hospital, London, UK

Professor Vandam (Paper 4.1) has ably described how and why inhalation anaesthesia was introduced in the United States; but this—as it were—was just a beginning. If anaesthesia was to become established in medical practice after 1846 it was important that the news should be spread to other mature medical centres in Britain, in Europe, and further afield. If anaesthesia was to develop it was unlikely that this would have been achieved by merely spreading the news within the United States itself, for, in the late 1840s it was a very different country from the one we know now (1).

The background to the introduction of inhalational anaesthesia from the United States to the United Kingdom

The United States in the 1840s was much smaller, and less united than the super power of today. It did not extend from coast to coast. Much of the land in the far west was Spanish, and not even owned by the United States. Beyond the Mississippi it was still in the process of being settled. Further east it was securely settled, but given over to farming, and there were few important towns or academic centres. And so in the 1840s the main developed areas were along the Atlantic seaboard, and it was here that the centres of population, commerce, industry, trade, culture and learning were to be found; but the states of the eastern seaboard, themselves, were not particularly united. Their division was mainly because of slavery—the norm in the southernmost, cotton producing states, but abhorrent to those in the north. In 1846 the northernmost states were the more sophisticated, and were the seats of commerce, learning, culture and sophistication. The principal cities in this area were Baltimore, Boston, New York, and Philadelphia. Each was characterized by its insularity and independence, and there were enormous rivalries between them.

Happily, however, in the mid-1840s, Boston itself provided an ideal environment for the reception, nurturing and dissemination of the news of anaesthesia's discovery. For Boston was an academic city (2). Its well-to-do citizens were used to informing themselves about all manner of scientific advances mainly by forming small, learned scientific societies or discussion clubs. Most Bostonians involved in the ether story belonged to one or more of these societies, such as the American Association for the Advancement of Science, the Boston Society of Medical Improvement, the Warren Club, the Thursday Club, the Saturday Club, and the 'new' club. In the months preceding the introduction of ether these clubs had discussed such topics as the New Medical College in Boston, Daguerrotypes, the Dynamics of Moving Bodies, Schönbein's newly discovered explosive called gun-cotton, and—most excitingly of all—the recent discovery of the unseen planet we now know as Neptune (3).

So it's understandable that the discovery of ether anaesthesia—on their own doorstep—came to be appreciated so quickly by the medical and lay intelligentsia of Boston, most of whom had close links with Britain and Europe. In 1846 these links were straightforward because Samuel Cunard's steamships maintained a regular, fortnightly mail service between Boston and Liverpool (4). Clearly, if the news was to be relayed abroad it had to be sent to, or by way of the United Kingdom.

The first successful use of anaesthesia outside the United States was in the United Kingdom. It was James Robinson—a London dentist—who was the first to use it in England. This was on Saturday 19 December, 1846, at a private house in central London. The anaesthesia was given by James Robinson, who also performed the operation which was the extraction of a molar tooth (5). It seems that anaesthesia was also used on the same day in Dumfries, in Scotland at The Royal Infirmary (6), although there is no satisfactory evidence to prove that this actually happened.

In London, two days later—on 21 December, 1846—anaesthesia was first used in England for major surgery. This was at University College Hospital (5). The anaesthesia was given by William Squire and the operation was performed by the famous London surgeon Robert Liston. He amputated a leg. This was the event which established ether anaesthesia in Britain.

The classical account of the spread of the news to the United Kingdom

The previously accepted view (7,8) is that the news of ether anaesthesia first arrived in Britain on 16 December, 1846, and that the news was brought across the Atlantic by the steamer *Acadia* which left Boston on 1 December, and arrived in Liverpool 15 days later on the 16th. But it now appears that this classical view is not correct, and that the first news of ether arrived in Britain more than 4 weeks earlier than has hitherto been recorded.

The beginning of things was Morton's use of ether on the 16 October, 1846, at the Massachusetts General Hospital in Boston. Morton gave the ether, and Professor John Collins Warren operated while his surgical colleagues looked on (9). Of those surgical colleagues the most important, for our present purpose, was Henry J. Bigelow (10). He encouraged Morton to persist with his early experiments, and also defended the controversial attempts made by Morton to patent ether anaesthesia for himself. In addition he read papers on ether anaesthesia to two scientific societies in Boston. The first was to a meeting of the American Academy of Arts and Sciences—at which both Jacob Bigelow, and a man named Edward Everett was present (11). The second was a longer detailed paper read before the Boston Society of Medical

Improvement. This second paper was published in full by the *Boston Medical and Surgical Journal* (12) and—on the following day, 19 November—it was reprinted, word for word, in the *Boston Daily Advertiser* (13) which was then one of Boston's leading newspapers.

It was the *Boston Daily Advertiser* of 19 December, 1846, in which Henry Bigelow's paper was reprinted for the general public. It deserves our attention because it was a copy of this newspaper which was sent to England to provide a detailed account of the subject. It was sent by Henry Bigelow's father, Professor Jacob Bigelow. Jacob Bigelow wrote a letter to London on 28 November, giving his own enthusiastic views about ether. To his letter he added a copy of the *Boston Daily Advertiser* containing his son's article. The letter was written to one of Jacob Bigelow's close friends who was then living in London and whose name was Dr Francis Boott (14). Boott received Jacob Bigelow's letter on Thursday, 17 December, and immediately did three things. Firstly he informed the British medical press, secondly he informed Robert Liston, then London's leading surgeon, and finally he himself brought about the first use of ether in England. This took place on Saturday, 19 December, at Boott's home in Central London where he had arranged for a trial of ether for dental extraction. For this he enlisted the help of his friend and neighbour—the dentist James Robinson (5). Robert Liston was invited to see Boott and Robinson at work, and immediately made plans for the first use of ether in England for major surgery. This was for the leg amputation on Monday, 21 December, 1846 (15).

Soon after these two events, and solely as a result of Francis Boott's actions, ether anaesthesia received widespread publicity in Britain, its use spread rapidly throughout the country and it soon became firmly established. Thus there can be no doubt that Jacob Bigelow's letter to Francis Boott was the principal way in which the news of ether's discovery was sent from America to Britain. This is the accepted and orthodox view, and it must be stressed that none of the new information which is presented below should be interpreted as diminishing the facts on which it is based.

Earlier communications from the United States to the United Kingdom

There were, however, 17 or 18 other separate ways in which the news of ether's discovery arrived in Britain either before or at the same time as Jacob Bigelow's letter to Francis Boott. In addition to Jacob Bigelow those involved in Boston were Dr William Fraser, Robert H. Eddy, Edward Everett, Professor John Collins Warren and Dr John Ware. Particular attention should be paid to the contribution of Mr Eddy and Mr Everett, both of whom wrote about ether to correspondents in the United Kingdom. The existence of their letters has, to all intents and purposes, been overlooked.

The despatch and arrival dates of these letters can be ascertained accurately because, in 1846, the only means of transport between America and Britain was by sea. Only 4 vessels sailed from the United States to Britain in the interval between the first public use of ether at the Massachusetts General Hospital, and its first use in Britain just over two months later (16). Three of the vessels were Cunard's mail steamers which travelled between Boston, and Liverpool. Perhaps significantly for the Canadians they all went by way of Halifax, Nova Scotia. On 1 November, the *Caledonia* left Boston and arrived in Liverpool on the 15th. She was followed by the *Britannia* which sailed on 16 November, and arrived on 1 December. The next vessel to sail was the *Acadia* which—according to the orthodox view first conveyed news of ether to Britain by means of letters carried aboard her, and also (if the Dumfries episode is true) by her ship's surgeon Dr William Fraser. (One other vessel, the sailing boat *Joshua Bates*, also completed the journey within the time. She was not an official carrier of mail, and I doubt that anything significant was sent aboard her.)

There can be no doubt, though, that at least one letter about ether was aboard the *Caledonia* when, just two weeks after Morton's famous demonstration, she steamed out of Boston on 1 November. Having touched, on the following day, at Halifax the *Caledonia* arrived in Liverpool on 15 November, and the letter was delivered in London one day later—that is on 16 November. Thus it was delivered 31 days earlier than was Jacob Bigelow's letter to Francis Boott: indeed it was delivered in London 12 days before Jacob Bigelow, in Boston, even wrote his letter to Francis Boott.

The earliest letter, and the English Patent

On 28 October—12 days after ether's first public use—Robert H. Eddy, a Boston patent lawyer advised Morton to apply immediately for ether to be patented overseas, firstly in England and then in Europe (9). Morton agreed and Eddy wrote with details to an American lawyer named James Dorr who was then living in London. Eddy's letter was, without doubt, aboard the *Caledonia* when she left Boston on 1 November, 1846.

James Dorr, in London, received the letter on 16 November, and immediately contacted Moses Poole who was London's most experienced and efficient Patent Agent. Moses Poole obtained the Patent, in his own name but on Morton's behalf. It was granted to Poole on 21 December, 1846 (17). In 1846 the procedure for obtaining a patent was extremely complicated and usually took at least 6 weeks to complete. But there is firm evidence to show that, for an extra fee, Moses Poole would complete the process in 5 weeks, but never in a shorter time (18). Significantly, the interval which elapsed between Dorr's receiving his instructions from Mr Eddy and the issuing of the English Patent to Moses Poole was exactly 5 weeks. Thus, the earliest news to reach Britain about ether's successful use in Boston arrived on 15 November—31 days earlier than Bigelow's letter to Boott—and that it was sent specifically to obtain an English Patent for ether on Morton's behalf. Understandably, the information was not made public until the Patent had been secured.

Edward Everett's letters to Dr Henry Holland

Two weeks later, on 2 December—again well in advance of Bigelow's letter to Boott—another letter about ether arrived in London. It was written by Edward Everett to a prominent London physician named Dr Henry Holland.

Everett was a distinguished American (19), with a well established New England family background. From 1841 until 1845 he had lived in London as a most successful United States' Ambassador to Britain. On leaving this diplomatic post he returned to Massachusetts and, in 1846, was elected President of Harvard University. In the same year he also became a Vice-President of the American Academy of Arts and Sciences. It was in this last capacity that he (with Professor Jacob Bigelow) was present to hear Henry Bigelow deliver his first paper on ether anaesthesia in Boston (11).

Everett wrote about ether to at least 12 different people in Britain. His earliest ether letter was written on 14 November, and sent to Dr Henry Holland, who received the letter in London on 2 December. Between the 27 and 30 November, he wrote at least 12 more letters about ether to various people in Britain, France and Germany. On this occasion I would like to describe those letters which were sent by Everett to Dr Henry Holland (to whom he was writing for the second time), The Reverend Dr Whewell, Sir Benjamin Brodie and Dr Francis Boott. All these letters were received in Britain on 17 December.

Fortunately for us as historians of anaesthesia Everett was a methodical man and made fair copies of most of his letters before sending them off. Most of these copies still survive. As far as I know only one of these has ever been publicized, and the others are discussed below in the United Kingdom for the first time since they were written just over 140 years ago.

Everett's first ether letter was to Dr Henry Holland (20). His fair copy of this letter, of 14 November, 1846, is the oldest surviving document relating to anaesthesia's spread from Boston to Britain. That unique document is now in the Archives of the Massachusetts Historical Society in Boston where it has lain, seemingly overlooked, since it was penned some 140 years ago. The letter is three pages long, and virtually the whole of it was devoted to ether. After a brief introduction Everett wrote:

> *'My immediate object in writing to you today is to inform you that a real promising discovery has lately been made here in your professional province, viz. the application of a Narcotic gas to facilitate the performance of surgical operations . . .'*

He went on to say that he had learnt about ether from Henry Bigelow at the American Academy of Arts and Sciences, and then described ether's introduction in Boston. He gave details of various cases in which it had been used, and began to close his letter by writing of the few difficulties which had so far been encountered.

> *'These do not appear', he wrote, 'in the opinion of our Physicians, to throw any serious doubt over the prospect of its being a most valuable auxiliary of surgical operations.'*

Within a fortnight, on 27 November, Everett wrote a second, long and detailed ether letter to Dr Holland (21). It began 'Since I last wrote to you I have witnessed the operation of sulphuric ether . . .' and went on to describe, in his own lay terms, what had happened when Charlotte, his daughter, had gone to Morton to have a tooth removed under ether. The extraction was difficult and prolonged, and she had to be anaesthesized three times in quick succession before the whole tooth was removed. Everett was enthusiastic, and his letter concluded 'Is this not something very important? I shall try to get you one or two pamphlets in which it is mentioned to send you by this steamer.'

One of the pamphlets he referred to was the latest *Boston Medical and Surgical Journal* containing Henry Bigelow's article on ether (12). The other was the published version (22) of the speech which Everett had made at the recent Opening Ceremony of the new Medical College in Boston.

Dr Henry Holland, the recipient of those two early and important letters about ether from Everett, presents something of a paradox as far as anaesthesia is concerned. He was a successful London physician (23) with a very fashionable medical practice amongst the social élite of London. He had travelled widely throughout the world and, medicine apart, had a broad range of scientific interests. Indeed his scientific attainments were such that he had been elected to two of Britain's most prestigious scientific offices. He had, for a while, been President of The Royal Institution and he was also a Fellow of The Royal Society. Despite these academic attainments, however, Holland was medically unimpressive.

When Everett wrote to Holland on 14 November, and again on the 27th, he may have had every reason to suppose that the early information he was giving to Holland about ether would have been acted upon promptly to spread the news of anaesthesia to Britain. Everett would have known only too well of Dr Holland's high standing amongst the social and scientific élite of Britain. And surely Holland, because of these connections, was in an excellent position to either use of disseminate the early information he had received about ether. But he chose to do nothing except, predictably, write back to Everett to ask if the inventor was famous, and whether or not he had met him during a recent visit he had made to Everett in Boston (24). Thus, the unique opportunity which Everett had presented to Holland was wasted.

Everett's letter to The Reverend Dr Whewell

Everett also wrote, on 30 November, to the Reverend Dr Whewell, the Master of Trinity College, Cambridge, in England. Everett had come to know Whewell very well during his time as Ambassador to Britain. The original of that letter is now housed in the archives of Trinity College, Cambridge. It is fascinating to have come across both this original document in Cambridge, England (25), and also the fair copy (preserved in Boston) which Everett made at Harvard in Cambridge, Massachusetts (26). The letter itself was without effect on the introduction of ether in the United Kingdom but its existence is worth noting since, to the best of my knowledge, Edward Everett's letter to Whewell is the oldest surviving original document in Britain relating to the spread of the news about ether from Boston to Britain.

Everett's letter to Sir Benjamin Brodie

Another letter which Everett wrote about ether was to the eminent British surgeon, Sir Benjamin Brodie. This was written on 28 November, and Brodie received the letter in London on 17 December. Everett wrote 'My present object in writing to you is to convey a number of the *Boston Medical and Surgical Journal* in which you will find an authentic account of a method of producing a temporary suspension of sensibility by inhaling sulphuric ether . . .'. He then gave more details about the discovery and finished by noting 'Our best physicians and surgeons appear to anticipate the most important benefits from the discovery (27).' Brodie was not impressed, however, and wrote 'I had heard of this before. The narcotic properties of ether have been long known. . . . I have tried it on guinea-pigs whom it first set asleep and then killed. One question is whether it can be used with safety.' (28)

Surprisingly enough Brodie was right, for he had investigated ether some 25 years earlier. Not only that, he had done so in the Royal College of Surgeons of England where this Symposium was held. In 1821 Brodie had given a long series of lectures at the College. In one of these he had dealt with the subject of poisonous gases. His lecture notes still survive in the Library. During the course of his lecture he said 'Ether is said to have intoxicating properties if swallowed. What are the effects if respired? Ether being volatalized at low temperatures this is easily ascertained.' He then put guinea-pigs in bell jars full of ether vapour, whereupon they became unconscious. Some recovered fully when removed from the ether but others died. Brodie concluded 'I attribute these effects to the specific action of the ether—not to suffocation.' (29). Sir Benjamin Brodie, in 1821, had no thought of ether as anything other than a poison, but his unenthusiastic reaction to the news of ether's deliberate use for anaesthesia 25 years later is understandable.

Everett's letter to Dr Francis Boott

Edward Everett also wrote a letter about ether to Dr Francis Boott who received the letter at about the same time as he received Jacob Bigelow's letter with the *Boston Daily Advertiser* containing Henry Bigelow's article on ether insensibility. Boott had been a near-contemporary of Everett's at Harvard, and the two men met each other during the four years of Everett's ambassadorship to Britain where Boott, for a while, served as physician to the American Embassy (14).

Everett wrote his letter to Boott on 27 or 28 November, and, with it, enclosed a copy of the Address which—as President of Harvard—he had made on 4 November, at the Opening of Boston's new Medical College. Boston's new Medical College was just a few hundred yards away from the Massachusetts General Hospital and their senior medical staff moved freely between the two institutions.

Everett's speech was a great success and was published as this pamphlet soon afterwards (22). By the time it was published Everett had added an enthusiastic postscript about ether which ended:

> '*I understand great confidence is placed in this effectual method of inducing complete insensibility under the most cruel operations. It seems not easy to overrate the importance of such a discovery.*' (22)

Of all the 14 or so early ether letters which Everett sent to Britain this was the only one to be publicized—by Boott in *The Lancet* of 2 January, 1847. Francis Boott included a copy of Everett's letter and his Medical College speech with all the other material about ether which he sent to *The Lancet*. As a result of Boott's actions *The Lancet* was able to place an enormous amount of information before the medical profession and, indirectly, the lay public on 2 January, 1847 (5). This told of Boott's enthusiasm for what he had heard from Boston, and of Henry and Jacob Bigelow's confidence in the new invention; both were well known in London medical circles. By publishing the detailed copy from *The Boston Daily Advertiser*, *The Lancet* conveyed the general approval of ether in Boston, and Everett's letter confirmed its ready acceptance by the city's lay intelligentsia. The communication also reported Boott and Robinson's own successful trial of ether, as well as Robert Liston's successful use of the agent for major surgery and, for good measure, the Editor of *The Lancet* added an enthusiastic editorial (30).

The extensive coverage which Francis Boott obtained for ether in the British medical press virtually guaranteed that it would be taken seriously in the United Kingdom. It is nonetheless, at first sight surprising that of all the 17 or 18 letters sent from Boston to Britain, only the two letters which Jacob Bigelow and Edward Everett had written to their expatriate friend Dr Francis Boott were effective in publicizing ether. The reasons for this paradox make a fascinating study, but this is beyond the scope of the present paper.

Even so, it is clear that Francis Boott received from Bigelow exactly the same information which was sent by Everett to Brodie and he received from Everett far less information than Everett had earlier sent to Dr Holland. While Brodie and Holland did nothing Boott immediately grasped the significance of the discovery of ether anaesthesia and promoted its use in the United Kingdom. He responded to the news effectively, with great modesty, absolute selflessness and absolute rectitude. It was entirely because of his actions that ether was so readily adopted in Britain, and it was because it was so readily adopted in Britain that it eventually was accepted in France, then in other European countries, and then even further afield.

Paradoxically, Boott (in London) also helped to sustain ether anaesthesia in the United States as a whole, for he relayed the news of its ready adoption in Britain back to his medical friends in Boston. This news then helped to confirm the usefulness of ether anaesthesia in the United States where (outside Boston, and as a result of the rivalries which I mentioned at the beginning) it had received a mixed welcome and got off to a very hesitant start (28).

This hitherto overlooked point was clearly recorded in the writings of both John Collins Warren (30) and Henry J. Bigelow (31), each of whom, as leading Boston surgeons, was excellently placed to know the true position about ether's acceptance in the United States. But the point was, however, most clearly articulated by the perspicacious John Snow. In his preface to his famous book on chloroform he wrote:

'Considerable opposition was made to the inhalation of ether in America soon after its introduction, and it seemed likely to fall into disuse when the news of its successful employment in the operations of Mr Liston, and others in London, caused the practice of etherization to revive.' (32)

Anaesthesia was solely an American invention, but, in 1846, its validity could only be assessed, and its use guaranteed, by its acceptance in Britain, Europe and beyond. This paper has presented some entirely new information concerning the spread of the news about anaesthesia from Boston to Britain.

References

(1) Brogan H. *The Pelican history of the United States of America*. Harmondsworth: Penguin, 1986.

(2) Morse JT. *Life and letters of Oliver Wendell Holmes*. London: Sampson Low, Marston and Co., 1896.

(3) Edward Everett Papers. Diary, Volume 253, 1846 Oct 8: Massachusetts Historical Society, Boston.

(4) Grant K. *Samuel Cunard, pioneer of the Atlantic steamship*. New York: Abelard-Schuman.

(5) Boott F. Surgical operations performed during insensibility. *Lancet* 1847; **1**: 5–8.

(6) Baillie TW. *From Boston to Dumfries*. Dinwiddie: Dumfries, 1969.

(7) Duncum BM. *The development of inhalation anaesthesia*. London: Oxford University Press, 1947.

(8) Sykes WS. *Essays on the first hundred years of anaesthesia, Vol 1*. London: Livingstone, 1960.

(9) Rice NP. *Trials of a public benefactor*. New York: Pudney and Russell, 1859.

(10) Bigelow WS. *A memoir of Henry Jacob Bigelow*. Boston: Little, Brown and Co., 1900.

(11) Edward Everett Papers. Diary, Volume 253, 1846 Nov 3: Massachusetts Historical Society, Boston.

(12) Bigelow HJ. Insensibility during surgical operations produced by inhalation. *Boston Med Surg J* 1846; **35**: 309–317.

(13) Bigelow HJ. Insensibility during surgical operations produced by inhalation. *Boston Daily Advertiser* 1846 Nov 19, page 2, cols 2–4.

(14) Ellis RH. The introduction of anaesthesia to Great Britain: 2 A biographical sketch of Dr Francis Boott. *Anaesthesia* 1977; **32**: 197–208.

(15) Squire W. On the introduction of ether inhalation as an anaesthetic in London. *Lancet*, 1888; **i**: 1220–1.

(16) Lloyd's Lists, London. October 16–December 21 1846.

(17) Moses Poole. Specification for administering the Vapour of Ether to the lungs for medical or surgical purposes. 1846, No. 11, 503. The Great Seal Patent Office, London.

(18) Minutes of Evidence from the Report from the Select Committee on the Law relative to Patents for Inventions. Ordered by the House of Commons to be printed 12 June, 1829.

(19) Frothingham PR. *Edward Everett: orator and statesman.* Boston: Houghton Mifflin, 1925.

(20) Edward Everett Papers. Correspondence. Volume 159. Letter to Dr Henry Holland, 14 November, 1846. Massachusetts Historical Society, Boston.

(21) Edward Everett Papers. Correspondence. Volume 159. Letter to Dr Henry Holland, 27 November, 1846. Massachusetts Historical Society, Boston.

(22) Everett E. *Address delivered at the opening of the new Medical College in North Grove Street, Boston.* Boston: William Ticknor and Co., 1846.

(23) G.T.B. Sir Henry Holland. *Dictionary of national biography*, 1891; **27**: 144–5.

(24) Edward Everett Papers. Correspondence. Volume 159. Letter to Dr Henry Holland, 31 Dec 1846. Massachusetts Historical Society, Boston.

(25) Whewell Papers. Everett E. Add M.S. a, 203 (109). Trinity College, Cambridge, England.

(26) Edward Everett Papers. Correspondence. Volume 159. Letter to Reverend Dr Whewell. 30 November, 1846. Massachusetts Historical Society, Boston.

(27) Edward Everett Papers. Correspondence. Volume 159. Letter to Sir Benjamin Brodie. 28 November, 1846. Massachusetts Historical Society, Boston.

(28) Bigelow HJ. Etherization—A compendium of its history, surgical use, dangers, and discovery. *Boston Med Surg J* 1848; **38**: 229–37.

(29) Brodie BC. MS Lecture Notes on 'Poisonous Gases—Vol 1. London: Royal College of Surgeons of England, 1821.

(30) Warren JC. *The influence of anaesthesia on the surgery of the nineteenth century.* 2nd Ed. Boston: Privately printed, 1906.

(31) Bigelow HJ. *Surgical anaesthesia, addresses and other papers.* Boston: Little Brown and Co., 1900.

(32) Snow J. *On chloroform and other anaesthetics: their action and administration.* London: Churchill, 1858.

4.3   A quick look at the first London etherists

BARBARA M. DUNCUM
*Honorary Member History of Anaesthesia Society,
26 St Edmund's Terrace, London NW8, UK*

On a Monday afternoon four days before Christmas 1846, Professor Robert Liston, briefed with the news from Boston by Francis Boott, became the first surgeon in Europe to do a major operation on an etherized patient (1). The etherist was one of his students, William Squire, and over the weekend William's pharmacist uncle Peter Squire, briefed by Liston, had purified some ether and assembled an inhaler. He used a flat-bottomed conical flask with an outlet near the base—part of Nooth's apparatus for making soda-water. In the neck of the flask Squire put a funnel containing sponge for the ether, and he fitted one of Read's flexible valved inhaling tubes into the lower opening. The tube ended in an ivory nozzle to be held in the patient's mouth while his nostrils were pinched together by the etherist (2). Such inhalers were in everyday use for medicating the lungs.

There were a lot of spectators in the theatre at University College Hospital when Liston's patient, a 36-year-old butler named Churchill, began inhaling under young William's guidance. After two or three minutes Churchill seemed to be insensible, and during the next 25 seconds Liston cut off the man's leg through the thigh. According to the dresser looking after the case, Churchill showed no signs of distress although he was not unconscious. When the arteries were tied Churchill was questioned. Half sitting up he said drowsily that he had heard voices and felt something being done to his limb, but no pain; and he was wholly unaware that his leg was already off (3,4). To everyone present painless surgery was now a reality.

Because of Christmas the news didn't spread far until the following week. Then the journals in the New Year increasingly carried reports of etherizing and there was a flush of improvised inhalers. At the big London hospitals, operating sessions intended for students and visiting medical practitioners but open to hospital patrons and patients' friends were suddenly as popular as music-hall turns. At Guy's in mid-January, after word got round that a major operation would start at one o'clock, a crowd began collecting at half-past eleven, and when the theatre doors opened there was a stampede for seats and standing-room. Within minutes even the passage from the wards was crammed with sightseers and some found their way to a skylight and peered down. Hemmed in by so many people the patient, a boy of 14 about to undergo lithotomy, was terrified. At the Westminster Hospital pupils angrily complained they couldn't see what the surgeon was doing because of the pack of visitors round the table (5).

James Robinson (1813–1861)

More often than not at these public sessions the etherist was James Robinson, the dentist Dr Boott had at once invited to help him devise an inhaler and to give the ether on the very first occasion in England: the painless extraction of Miss Lonsdale's tooth on Saturday, 19 December, 1846. Robinson now used an improved version of the original inhaler, much like Squire's but having a mouthpiece like a baby's dummy with a padded rim which fitted snugly over the lips, and a spring-clip to close the nostrils (6). In Robinson's capable hands and with his call of 'Patient ready!', anaesthesia usually went without a hitch. Less experienced etherists were apt to run into difficulties.

John Snow (1813–1858) and other contemporaries

The failures of etherization did not surprise John Snow, a 33-year-old general practitioner interested in respiration. Soon after Christmas, Snow was at a demonstration Robinson gave for a few friends at his house in Gower Street. Despite Robinson's efficiency Snow saw that etherizing needed a proper physiological and practical basis. The etherist must know the appropriate strength for the ether-air mixture inhaled and be able to control it. He therefore began experimenting, working from the known fact that at different temperatures 100 cubic inches of air would take up different percentages of ether vapour. He also kept clearly in mind the design of an inhaler invented in 1836 by Dr Julius Jeffreys for treating bronchitis with moist air. This was a small metal drum with an air inlet and an inhaling tube in the lid. Inside the drum a spirally-coiled baffle-plate, the key factor, caused the air drawn in to circulate several times over the surface of warm water in the bottom, to be well moistened before being inhaled (7).

On 23 January, 1847, at a meeting of the Westminster Medical Society, Snow introduced his ether inhaler adapted from Jeffreys's prototype with ether under the baffle. Snow placed his vaporizer in a basin of water at around 65°F, which generated an ether–air mixture containing about 47% ether vapour—not unpleasant to breathe and reliably producing anaesthesia in from three to four minutes. The Society was impressed and the inhaler was written up in *The Lancet* (8).

Encouraged, Snow offered his services as etherist to the surgeons at St George's Hospital. His first session there was on 28 January, 1847, and at the end of the next session a week later the senior surgeon Mr Caesar Hawkins addressed the crowd. He and his colleagues wanted to thank Dr Snow publicly, he said, adding that Dr Snow's instrument was very much superior to those they had previously used (9).

During February there were two notable innovations. Dr Thomas Smith in Cheltenham, having tried various inhalers, announced he had given them up in favour of a sponge moistened with ether and held above the patient's nose and mouth allowing him to breathe naturally (10). At the Nottingham General Hospital Dr Francis Sibson was using a modified Snow's inhaler to relieve facial neuralgia with ether. He too wanted his patient to breathe freely. Discarding Snow's mouthpiece but keeping the valved inhaling tube he improvised a facepiece out of a sixpenny mask from a toyshop, cutting away the middle and using the sides to support a mackintosh cup fitting over nose and mouth and secured by a strap round the neck (11). Pleased with his facepiece Sibson sent one to Snow who tried it out during the late spring while evolving his own.

Snow's metal facepiece had a triangular opening for nose and mouth bordered by a wide surround of sheet-lead, covered outside in glove-leather and lined with oiled silk. It was pliable enough to be pressed closely over the patient's features. A ¾-inch (2 cm) calibre inhaling tube opened into the floor of the mask through a lightly-balanced valve, and a vent at the back was covered simply by a flap of rubber on a pivot, turned aside when fresh air was needed (12). Anyone still using an inhaler quickly added a facepiece; but a good many people following Smith's example had already opted for the free and easy use of an ether-soaked sponge (13).

Early in May, 1847, Snow, using a very compact version of his inhaler, began etherizing for Liston at University College Hospital and in Liston's private practice. Soon Liston was recommending him to other surgeons in private practice. This was important; a hospital was a place where one might make a name but private practice was where one made a living. By the end of the summer Snow was steadily building up the first professional anaesthetic practice, and much of the most interesting and demanding work in London was being offered to him (14).

In September, Snow published his 88-page monograph on ether. Some six weeks later James Young Simpson published his pamphlet on chloroform. But that's another story.

References

(1) Boott F. Surgical operations performed during insensibility, produced by the inhalation of sulphuric ether. *Lancet* 1847; **1**: 5–8.
(2) Squire P. On the inhalation of the vapour of ether, and the apparatus used for the purpose. *Pharm J* 1847; **6**: 350–3.
(3) Palmer E. Entry for 21 December, 1846, in Liston's Casebook No. XI. MS in University College Hospital Medical School Library.
(4) Forbes J. On a new means of rendering surgical operations painless. *Br For Med Rev* 1847; **23**: 309–12.
(5) Anonymous. Painless surgical operations: hospital reports. (a) *Med Tms* 1847; **15**: 310–11. (b) *Lancet* 1847; **i**: 500.
(6) Robinson J. *A treatise on the inhalation of the vapour of ether*. London: Webster, 1847: 5–6, 7, 16–18.
(7) Jeffreys J. On artificial climates: the atmospheric treatment of the lungs. *Lond Med Gaz* 1841–2; **1**: 814–22.
(8) Anonymous. Westminster Medical Society: report of meeting on 23 January, 1847. *Lancet* 1847; **i**: 120–1.
(9) Anonymous. Painless surgical operations: hospital reports, St George's. *Lancet* 1847; **i**: 158, 184.
(10) Smith T. Oleum ethereum, with ether, in surgical operations. *Lond Med Gaz* 1847; **4**: 395.
(11) Sibson F. On the treatment of facial neuralgia by the inhalation of ether. *Lond Med Gaz* 1847; **4**: 358–64.
(12) Snow J. A lecture on the inhalation of vapour of ether [sic] in surgical operations. *Lancet* 1847; **i**: 551–4.
(13) Anonymous. Review of Snow J. *On the inhalation of the vapour of ether in surgical operations*. London: Churchill, 1847. *Lond Med Gaz* 1847; **5**: 814.
(14) Richardson BW. Memoir. In: Snow J. *On the inhalation of chloroform and other anaesthetics*. London: Churchill, 1858: xiv–v.

4.4   The first anaesthetics in St George's Hospital, London

D. D. C. HOWAT
St George's Hospital, London, UK

In 1733, some physicians and surgeons broke away from the Westminster Hospital over a disagreement about where its new site should be. They set up a new hospital, St George's, in the seat of the Earls of Lanesborough at Hyde Park Corner, which was then a salubrious spot in the country just outside London (1,2). The present building, with its attractive Georgian façade, was built in 1833 and was occupied until just over seven years ago, when the hospital removed to its present site in South West London about seven miles away.

One of the frustrating aspects of research into the early days of anaesthesia in this country is the indifference with which it appears to have been treated by many medical men of that time, for their diaries and papers often reveal little. The medical and surgical staff of St George's Hospital were no exception.

As is well known, the first ether anaesthetic was given in London by the dentist James Robinson in Dr Boott's house in Gower Street, and two days later William Squire gave another for Robert Liston's famous operation in what is now University College Hospital. Reports of other operations under ether anaesthesia then began to appear in the *Lancet* and the *Medical Gazette* and in the lay press. Dr Boott described a modification of Nooth's ether apparatus in the *Illustrated London News* of 9 January, 1847 (3). The London *Times* of 4 January, reported the use of ether for an operation in Bristol two days previously and reports soon followed of ether anaesthetics given at University College Hospital on 4 January, at King's College Hospital on 11 January, and at Guy's Hospital and in Liverpool on 12 January (4,5).

The use of ether at St George's Hospital

The use of ether in St George's Hospital was first recorded in the *Times* of 15 January, and had taken place the previous day (6). In a lecture given to the London Hospital Medical Society in 1898, Probyn-Williams, who was an anaesthetist at that hospital, quoted from this report (7). Three operations were to be performed under ether anaesthesia in a public demonstration. The surgeons were named as Caesar Hawkins (son and grandson of famous surgeons of the same name), Edward Cutler and Henry James Johnson. It was not stated who administered the ether.

The first patient is described as a 'weakly lad of 19 to 20 years of age, labouring under disease of the great toe'. 'All attempts, however, to inhale the ether were fruitless. What with fright, and what with coughing, he always stopped before a sufficient effect could be obtained.' The surgeon (Caesar Hawkins) had to abandon the operation.

The description of the next administration will strike a chord in the memory of anyone who has induced a patient with ether:

> *'The second person who was brought in was a robust young man, a patient of Mr Cutler's with a diseased finger. He set about the inhalation* con amore, *and carried it on, with some persuasion and an occasional struggle to abandon it, for ten minutes at least. He appeared to suffer a great deal from it, turning very red, or rather purple, in the face, and resisting at times somewhat violently. The effect on the bystanders was anything but favourable, several declaring that the ether was as bad as the operation, or worse. At last, the seeming insensibility, and concurrent circumstances, warranting a resort to the knife, Mr Cutler proceeded to remove the finger. The patient was at once restored to his senses, and shouted so loudly, and snatched his hand from the operator so vigorously, as to leave no doubt that he suffered pain as acutely as if no steps had been taken to deaden it.'*

The report states 'this case then was a total failure'.

'The third and last patient was a young man of powerful frame, who laboured under disease of the ankle joint. He was a patient of Mr Henry James Johnson, who exhorted him earnestly to inspire the ether until he felt its full effect. The poor fellow followed the advice implicitly, and, in three or four minutes, insensibility having taken place, Mr Johnson at once performed amputation below the knee. The operation was executed with much dexterity, and with such rapidity that in less than a minute the limb was off. The patient regained his senses while the saw was applied to the bones, when he remarked that he felt the instrument. During the cutting of the skin and muscles he did not evince the slightest consciousness of pain, and altogether the case was very satisfactory.'

Probyn-Williams did not mention two further comments in the *Times* report. Mr Johnson, obviously pleased with his successful operation, 'addressed the spectators in a short speech, which was received with much applause. In it he reviewed the circumstances of the case, and pointed out its favourable character.'

Eminent spectators

Probyn-Williams did not mention a connection with Napoleon Bonaparte either. Amongst the spectators were Benjamin Brodie, Robert Liston and Jerome Bonaparte. The latter was the son of Napoleon's younger brother, also called Jerome, the ex-King of Westphalia, by his second wife, Catherine of Wurtemberg (8,9,10). He had escaped from prison in France the previous year and come to England to stay with his friend Louis-Napoleon, later Napoleon the Third. He was a favourite in London society and was familiarly known as 'Plon-Plon', said to be his first childish effort to say 'Napoléon'. It was quite common at that time for gentlemen who had an interest in scientific matters to attend such demonstrations and other names which are mentioned in press reports of the time are Lord Walsingham, Lord Falkland, Lord Morton, Sir Henry Mildmay and Sir George Wombwell. I have been in touch with the descendants of three of these individuals, but none has any record of his ancestor's recollections of such demonstrations. Nor do the writings of Benjamin Brodie, Robert Liston or Jerome Bonaparte reveal anything.

Hospital reports

The Annual Reports of St George's Hospital, the minutes of the meetings of the Board of Governors and the reports of post mortem examinations for the years 1846 and 1847 make no reference to anaesthetics or their administrators or to the public demonstration of 14 January. Benjamin Ward Richardson, in his biographical preface to John Snow's book on chloroform, relates how Snow came to give anaesthetics in St George's Hospital, first in the outpatient dental department and later in the operating theatre 'upstairs', but Snow's own diaries do not start until July, 1848 (11,12). In his book *On the Inhalation of Ether*, Snow states that he first gave ether for three major operations in St George's Hospital on 28 January, 1847 (13); however, the earliest record in the hospital archives is in the minutes of the weekly meeting of the Board of Governors for 2 May, 1849.

'It was moved by Mr Charles Hawkins—seconded by Mr Morley and agreed to—That the duty of administering chloroform or ether to Patients in the Hospital be entrusted to the Assistant Apothecary.
    It was moved by Mr Powell and seconded by Mr Currie and unanimously agreed that it be recommended to the next Quarterly or Special Board to elect Dr Snow as Honorary Governor of this charity for services to the Hospital.' (14).

A year later, the Assistant Apothecary, Mr Potter, was commended by the Board for 'the careful manner in which he performed that duty to the entire satisfaction of the surgeons' and his salary was raised from £60 to £80 a year (15). His duties included 'cupping' and it was not until 1860 that dressers took over this duty.

In 1866, it was laid down that the House Physician should give anaesthetics when the Apothecary was absent. The Apothecary resigned in 1871, but it was not until 1879 that a qualified doctor, William Bennett, who had been house surgeon and surgical registrar to the hospital, was appointed chloroformist (16); he later became a well-known surgeon and was knighted by Queen Victoria.

John Snow himself relates how Mr Bumpstead, a house surgeon, administered ether in four emergency cases in 1847 and it seems likely that, as Snow's services became more and more in demand at other hospitals and in private practice, many of the administrations of ether and chloroform, particularly after Snow's death in 1858, were given by whoever was available, until the Assistant Apothecary was given that duty nearly a year later. In later life, Bumpstead related how he remembered using Snow's original apparatus, which was first shown at a meeting of the Westminster Medical Society on 23 January, 1847 (17). Unfortunately, there is no record of the name and status of the administrator of the first anaesthetic at St George's. Was it perhaps that eager druggist, mentioned by Benjamin Ward Richardson, whom John Snow met coming out of one of the hospitals—it might well have been St George's—and who bustled along with a large ether apparatus under his arm, saying he was 'getting into quite an ether practice', and who gave John Snow the idea of trying it himself?

References

(1) Peachey GC. *The history of St. George's Hospital*. Vol 1. London: John Bale, Sons & Danielsson, 1910.
(2) Blomfield J. *St. George's Hospital 1733–1933*. London: Medici Society, 1933.
(3) *Illustrated London News* 1847. Jan. 9th, 28th, 30th, Feb 6th.
(4) *The Times* 1847. Jan 4th, 11th, 12th, 15th, 16th, 21st.
(5) *London Medical Gazette* 1847, **39** (N.S.4), 156–157.
(6) *The Times* 1847, Jan 15th, 3 (col 2).
(7) Probyn-Williams RJ. London Hospital Gazette 1898; **4**: 196.
(8) Melchior-Bonnet B. *Jérome Bonaparte ou l'Envers de l'Epopée*. Paris: Librairie Académique Perrin, 1979.
(9) Holt E. *Plon-Plon. The Life of Prince Napoleon (1822–1891)*. London: Michael Joseph, 1973.
(10) Flammarion G. *Le Prince Napoléon (Jérome: 1822–1891)*. Paris: Editions Jules Tallardier, 1953.
(11) Snow J. *On chloroform and other anaesthetics*. London: John Churchill, 1858; xiv.
(12) Snow J. *Diaries* 1848–1858.
(13) Snow J. *On the inhalation of the vapour of ether*. London: John Churchill, 1847: 56.
(14) Minutes of the Board of Governors of St George's Hospital, 1849, May 2nd; 629.
(15) Minutes of the Board of Governors of St George's Hospital, 1850. June 5th; 858.
(16) Crellin JK. Apothecaries, dispensers and nineteenth century pharmacy at St George's Hospital, London. *Medical History* 1962; **2**: 131–145.
(17) *Lancet* 1847; **1**: 120–1.

Other Sources
Duncum B. *The developments of inhalation anaesthesia*. London: Oxford University Press, 1947.
Edwards G. 1st John Snow Lecture. *Anaesthesia* 1958; **14**: 113–26.
Fraser I. John Snow and his surgical friends. *Anaesthesia* 1968; **23**: 501–14.

Chapter 5
THE KNOWLEDGE SPREADS THROUGH EUROPE

5.1 The news extends across the European continent

J. RUPHREHT
Erasmus University, Rotterdam, The Netherlands

After the defeat of Napoleon in 1815, Europe thrust out into the colonial world, impelled by the force of its own industrialization. America followed this lead and conquered the last expanses of its indigenous empire. The tempo of change during the 19th century was greater than that of the total previous millennia. During the nineteenth century the earlier agricultural society was transformed into an urban, industrialized, technocratic one which, currently, has almost conquered the last remnants of the past.

In the three leading industrial areas—the United Kingdom, Germany and the United States—the population had increased almost five-fold in the preceding one hundred years. This increase was fostered by improved industrial and agricultural methods, coupled with efficient communications. Advances in social conditions, and medicine, resulted in a dramatic decrease in mortality from cholera, smallpox, tuberculosis and other contagious diseases. The population not only expanded rapidly, but it became more mobile than ever before. The reasons for these movements were both political and economic. From the poor under-developed totalitarian areas people poured into more liberal, promising and developed countries.

With the extension of the railway systems, Europe was decisively propelled into the industrial age. By 1850 the railway networks of England and Belgium were virtually complete, and Germany had established most of its main lines. Trains transported not only industrial goods but also printed information and provided mobility of learned people. Together with the improved economic and social climate and the possibility for rapid exchange of information, by 1840, the setting was complete for further developments—indeed technological innovations, progress in chemistry forced the medical world to improve its age-old methods.

Improvements to old methods must, necessarily, be preceded by new ideas. New ideas, in turn, are not generated by one isolated sector of society. The great changes in thinking and developments in medicine were a reflection of the cultural and social unrest in Europe at the start of the 19th century. The French Revolution had been a great catalyst of change. Liberalism all over Europe was the initial echo of this change and was also the source of a developing nationalism. This new nationalistic trend weakened the imperial order in Europe and eventually led to national states and an expectation of satisfactory international cooperation. Although this line of thinking proved to be an illusion, it provided a stimulus to make Europe a place ripe for the acceptance of new ideas. Anaesthesia was one of them.

All developments are related to the general social, economic and intellectual life of a country and Professor Mushin has stated that anaesthesia is no exception (1). Although the discovery of anaesthesia was almost accidental, by the middle of the 19th century the quality of life had already softened to the extent that relief of pain during surgery became an important consideration. This discovery was enthusiastically put into practice within a few weeks, or even days, after the news reached any developed community. Due to excellent communications throughout most parts of Europe, news about anaesthesia spread like fire and initiated a wave of clinical applications, apparatus design and physiological and pharmacological studies. There was some opposition to its widespread acceptance but there was no major obstruction to the introduction of pain relief in surgery. The relief of pain was considered important but, strangely, being overwhelmed with the new discovery, very few people realized that the introduction of anaesthesia was essential for the further development of medicine.

Public opinion concerning anaesthesia

Newspapers were a very important medium in the dissemination of news concerning anaesthesia. Most surgeons learned about the discovery from their columns. It is therefore no surprise that, in 1847, European professional writing had a pronounced popular touch, for the benefit of the lay public. Famous and learned exponents of surgery produced popular booklets, one example being J. F. Dieffenbach's *Der Äther gegen den Schmerz* (2).

The public became interested in the discovery of anaesthesia from the very first reports. In several countries, every interested reader of newspapers could have learned everything known about anaesthesia by the end of February, 1847. There is an interesting parallel to this phenomenon in our own times—it is probable that an interested reader of the popular press, with a good memory, is certainly more up-to-date on knowledge about acquired immune deficiency syndrome (AIDS) than the average member of the medical profession.

At times, and 1847 was no exception, the public may be critical and impatient when the medical profession does not immediately embrace new ideas. Such an attitude often proves to be transitory but it does give a consensus for further development. In 1847 this was manifested by a great willingness to undergo anaesthesia and there is much data and statistics showing the dramatic increase in surgical procedures in the few months and years following 1846. It was, perhaps, in Paris that the discovery and application of anaesthesia caused the greatest sensation (3). A similar situation occurred in Vienna, where public demonstration of anaesthesia in animals was given by F. Ragsky (4) and lay persons demonstrated inhalation of ether in restaurants, on a commercial basis. The public was warned against this type of practice, but it is difficult to assess whether this had any influence.

As is characteristic of public interest in something new, the excitement surrounding anaesthesia, judged by articles in the popular press (3) was not long-lasting. A considerable number of reports on anaesthesia in German newspapers started towards the end of January, 1847, and culminated in mid-February. A month later, other subjects on wider issues almost completely replaced reports on anaesthesia. The unfortunate habit of preferential reporting on anaesthetic mishaps must have started in those days and has persisted ever since. Observed retrospectively, the practice of anaesthesia spread throughout Europe with an almost universal acclaim.

This new medical treatment changed the attitude to surgery among both lay people and professionals. The method known as etherization came into general practice as fast as the means of communications would allow.

Timing and geographical factors

It is a tedious job to compile chronological tables of places where the so-called 'first' anaesthesias were performed. The subject becomes slightly more interesting only when one discovers yet another 'first' anaesthesia in a certain place. Such endeavours are of purely academic interest because the variation in dates may involve only a few days or weeks at the most. A compilation of places and dates where anaesthesia was tried and introduced in early 1847 can be useful as an indicator of the state of organized and developed medicine, however. Generally speaking, in 1847, Paris, Vienna and Berlin were considered centres of medical developments while the 'Golden Prague' enjoyed the fame of a 'Medical Mecca' (5). These cities remained the strongholds of medical excellence and science for a further eighty years.

Secher produced a most useful table of first known anaesthesias in various places (6) which has served to provide an overall impression of the spread of anaesthesia throughout Europe. Several places and names have since been added (Table 1). But overemphasis on the importance of the 'first' anaesthesia has led to difficulties. In Yugoslavia for example, for many years the earliest known anaesthesia was attributed to the city of Zadar, performed by I. Bettini (7). A special medal was named after Bettini to commemorate this achievement. However, at a later date yet another 'first' anaesthesia was traced in the same country (7).

The news and application of anaesthesia spread from the western coast of Europe to the east and south and, as mentioned, railways and newspapers played a major role. *The Augsburger Allgemeine Zeitung* reported on anaesthesia on 10 January, 1847, deriving information from

Table 1

Table 1

Dates on which various European cities were attributed earliest known anaesthesias

1846	Dumfries, Scotland	19 December	William Scott (1820–87)
	London, England	19 December	Francis Boott (1792–1863)—
			J. Robinson (1813–1861)
	London, England	21 December	Robert Liston (1794–1847)
	Paris, France	22 December	A. J. Jobert de Lamballe
			(1799–1867)
1847	Bern, Switzerland	23 January	Hermann A. Demme (1802–67)
	Erlangen, Germany	24 January	J. F. Heyfelder (1798–1969)
	Vienna, Austria	25 January	F. Schuh (1805–65)
	Munich, Germany	25 January	F. Chr. v. Rothmund (1801–1891)
	Riga, Latvia	c. 25 January	B.F. Baerens (?)
	Timişoara, Austria	5 February	Musil & Siesa (?)
	Prague, Czechoslovakia	6 February	Joseph Halla (1814–87)
	Berlin, Germany	6 February	H. W. Berend (1807–73)
	Stockholm, Sweden	c. 6 February	E. G. Palmgren (1910–55)
	Krakow, Austria	6 February	L. Bierkowski (1801–1860)
	Moscow, Russia	7 February	Fedor Inozemcev (1802–1860)
	Gothenburg, Sweden	11 February	C. Dickson (1814–1902)
	St Petersburg (Leningrad), Russia	14 February	Nikolaj I. Pirogoff (1810–81)
	Madrid, Spain	14 February	Diego de Argumosa y Obregón (1792–1865)
	Warsaw, Russia	15 February	L. Koehler (1799–1871)
	Copenhagen, Denmark	20 February	Søren Eskildsen Larsen (1802–90)
	Ljubljana, Austria	24 February	L. Nathan (?)
	Christiania (Oslo), Norway	4 March	Christen Heiberg (1799–1872)
	The Hague, The Netherlands	5 March	A. T. C. Schoevers (?)
	Helsingfors (Helsinki), Finland	8 March	L. H. Törnroth (1796–1864)
	Zadar, Austria	13 March	I. Bettini (?)
	Lisbon, Portugal	12 April	Gomes B. A. (?)

Countries following the name of a city denote political dependence in 1847.

several London papers and a medical journal (3). *Basler Zeitung* brought the news on 18 January, and the *Zürcher Zeitung* on 20 January, 1847. In Holland, S. J. Galama produced a remarkable review on etherization and also mentioned numerous newspapers as sources of information on anaesthesia (8).

According to B. M. Duncum, news about Morton's discovery reached France directly from America (9). A young American doctor, Francis W. Fisher from Boston, received the news and tried to arouse Velpeau's enthusiasm, but without success (10). He did manage to try etherization on Jobert de Lamballe's patient, at Hôpital St Louis (Table 1).

By 12 January, 1847, Malgaigne reported on several successful operations under ether. Some controversy accompanied the introduction of ether at Paris, but this completely escaped the attention of another American doctor, Henry Bryant. He wrote back to Boston, that ether 'has taken its rank among medical agents, and it is quietly and firmly established as if it had been known for centuries' (11).

In France, the earliest anaesthesia-related systematic pharmacological and physiological studies were begun, later to be continued in Russia and Great Britain (12,13). In fact Flourens described the anaesthetic actions of chloroform, but no-one heeded his reports. This was the same Flourens who had isolated the respiratory centre in the medulla, as early as 1842. Pirogoff started studies of ether in Russia early in 1847, followed by experiments with animals (14).

Acceptance of anaesthesia in Europe

Both the public and medical profession were aware in 1847 of the desirability of finding means to alleviate surgical pain. The success of Mesmer could be attributed to his fulfilling the need for something like anaesthesia. Thus, it can be assumed that Mesmerism played an important role in paving the road for the acceptance of anaesthesia (15).

The importance of public enthusiasm has already been mentioned. Fortunately, several great men in the medical profession realized the importance of Morton's finding. In France, Velpeau read a paper to the Academy on 17 January, 1847, stating his reservations towards the use of ether, but by 1 February, he had become most enthusiastic about it (16). Velpeau correctly emphasized that ether inhalation would profoundly affect not only surgery, but also physiology, chemistry, and even psychology. The day after the meeting of the Academy, on 2 February, 1847, ether was introduced into all surgical services in France.

In Germany, von Siebold carefully paved the road to anaesthesia. It is interesting to note that, at this stage, the authorities quickly started to establish rules for the new medical treatment. As early as 6 April, 1847, the Hannoverian Ministry of the Interior passed a law forbidding the use of ether in operations performed by barber-surgeons and dentists unless a qualified physician was present (17). Similar measures were soon taken in other German territories.

Following the initial enthusiasm about anaesthesia, opposition and warnings were forthcoming, but never succeeded in halting the use of ether. The public interest in anaesthesia, that began to wane by April, 1847, was revived later the same year following reports of Simpson's use of chloroform.

It is worth recalling here, two wise thoughts of the great French savant, Flourens, which later became famous aphorisms in anaesthesia:

'L'éther qui ôte la douleur, ôte aussi la vie, et l'agent nouveau qui vient d'acquérir la chirurgie est à la fois merveilleux et terrible.'

This quotation is from the early stages of the use of etherization in France. His other observation ridiculed the uncritical praise of chloroform as an anaesthetic when compared to ether:

'If sulphuric ether is a marvellous and terrible agent, chloroform is a more marvellous and more terrible agent.'

In Holland, the use of anaesthesia was widely accepted, opposers were slow to react and unsuccessful. Galama (8) was rather too hesitant when summarizing the virtues of ether at the end of 1847 stating:

'The fate of etherization will be alike to that of most newly found agents: at first highly praised, assiduously applied and recommended—only all too soon to be rejected by others as dangerous. Then the time comes when, through experience, the truth about its virtues and merits will emerge.'

In Spain, the opposition to anaesthesia was considerable from within medical circles. Santos Guerra opposed the use of anaesthesia on the basis of reactionary vitalism, 'An operation is painful but not enough to necessitate tortures and dangers of chloroform' (18).

It can be said that by the end of 1847 anaesthesia had been introduced throughout all civilized Europe. However, a sound physiological understanding of the actions of ether and chloroform was still far away.

Early anaesthetic apparatus in Europe

Initially, there was much controversy, concerning the ability of ether to produce insensibility to surgical pain. In France, at a given moment, all doctors of medicine in Toulon declared that: 'the action of ether nearly always is satisfactory, seldom incomplete, and never completely absent' (Gazette Médical de Paris, 14: 256–9, 1847).

Different findings regarding the potency of ether were probably due to different or inadequate design of the apparatus used, or to its incorrect use. It was, in fact, not possible to construct a good vaporizer for ether and administer it correctly as there was little appreciation of the physiology of respiration, and the pharmacology of ether had yet to be elucidated.

Within a few months after the introduction of anaesthesia a wide choice from a myriad of modifications to the original Morton's glass apparatus, or from clever innovations, was available. The early reviews on ether anaesthesia usually contained long lists of apparatus. The greatest praise was usually given to apparatus designed and produced by Charrière of Paris. In fact, any apparatus was good enough as long as it provided free access of air, prevented rebreathing, provided heat for evaporation of ether and had little resistance. Other requirements of inhalation anaesthesia techniques, that we are currently familiar with, could have been only a dream in 1847. Later, apparatus for application of ether became even more primitive, though more effective than those that had been used in the beginning. It seems that the age which saw the introduction of anaesthesia was not yet ripe for sophisticated anaesthetic apparatus.

References

(1) Rupreht J. Prof. William W. Mushin about anaesthesiology. An interview. In: Rupreht J, van Lieburg ML, Lee JA, Erdmann W eds. *Anaesthesia: essays on its history*. Berlin, Heidelberg, New York, Tokyo: Springer-Verlag, 1985; 388–92.
(2) Dieffenbach JF. *Der Äther gegen den Schmerz*. Berlin, 1847.
(3) Walser HH. *Zur Einführung der Äthernarkose in deutschen Sprachgebiet in Jahre 1847*. H. R. Sauerländer & Co., Aarau, 1957; 9.
(4) Kronner VN. *Der Scwefel-Äther*. Vienna, 1847.
(5) Sonderegger L. *Selbstbiographie und Briefen*. E. Haffter, ed. Frauenfeld, 1898.
(6) Secher O. The introduction of ether anaesthesia in the Nordic countries. *Acta Anaesthesiol Scand* 1985; **29**: 2–10.
(7) Soban D. Zgodnja uporaba anestezije v deželni civilni bolnici v Ljubljani (24. februarja 1847). *Zdrav Vestn* 1986; **55**: 599–601.
(8) Galama SJ. Over de uitwerking der inademing van zwavelaether. *Nieuw Practisch Tijdschrift voor de Geneeskunde* 1847; **26**: 393–435.
(9) Duncum BM. An outline of the history of anaesthesia. *Br Med Bull* 1946; **4**: 120–8.
(10) Fisher FW. The ether inhalation in Paris. *Boston Med Surg J* 1847; **36**: 109–13.
(11) Bryant H. Inhalation of ether in Paris. *Boston Med Surg J* 1847; **36**: 389.
(12) Flourens MJP. Note touchant l'action de l'éther sur les centres nerveux. *CR Acad Sci (Paris)* 1847; **24**: 340–4.
(13) Pirogoff N. *Recherches pratiques et physiologiques sur l'éthérisation*. St Pétersburg, Imprimerie française, 1847.
(14) Strunsky M. *Die Entwicklung der Anästhesiologie in Russland und in der UDSSR*. Die Freie Universität, Berlin, 1981.
(15) Rosen G. Mesmerism and surgery. *J Hist Med* 1946; **1**: 527–50.
(16) Neveu R. The introduction of surgical anesthesia in France. *J Hist Med 1946;* **1**: 607–10.
(17) Frankel WK. The introduction of anesthesia in Germany. *J Hist Med* 1946; **1**: 612–7.
(18) Santos Guerra M. Breve reflexiones sobre la eterización y chloroformización. *Bol Med Cir Far* 1848; **3**: 99–101.

5.2   First years of anaesthesia in the Netherlands

J. RUPREHT

Erasmus University, Rotterdam, The Netherlands

For centuries, The Netherlands has been a major gateway to the mainland of Europe. It is therefore not surprising that no one has been able to precisely determine how the news of anaesthesia reached this particular region. One assumes that most doctors learned about anaesthesia primarily from newspapers, as was the case in other European countries. Dr S. J. Galama wrote an extensive review on ether anaesthesia towards the end of 1847 and mentioned several English newspapers as sources of information, as well as referring to a large number of medical journals (1).

At the height of public interest in anaesthesia throughout Europe, Dr C. B. Tilanus reported on ether anaesthesia at a medical meeting in Amsterdam on 17 February, 1847 (2). He said that 'this etherization' was attracting much interest among surgeons in nearly all European lands. Lacking personal experience on the matter he was unable to formulate an informed opinion.

The first known and successful ether anaesthetic administered in Holland was given on 5 March, 1847, in The Hague by A. T. C. Schoevers to a patient undergoing correction of contractures of the joints (3). In the same month, successful ether anaesthesias were given in the cities of Alkmaar, Amsterdam, Kampen and Aardenburg. In Utrecht, the first anaesthesia was given for amputation on 16 March, by A. C. van Woerden, a surgeon and obstetrician (4). For several decades this was to be considered the first 'real' anaesthesia as the procedure was accompanied by bleeding. However, van Woerden had accomplished anaesthesia earlier. He anaesthetized a young volunteer on 26 and 27 February, and was convinced that the young man became insensitive to needle prick stimulus. The name of the volunteer was not recorded. The apparatus used for this anaesthetic was designed by J. R. Seilberger who, according to his report, was convinced that his apparatus was better than those of others (4). This may indicate that doctors were very well informed of all developments in the field of recently discovered anaesthesia. Seilberger also mentioned that he had produced several modifications to his simple and inexpensive apparatus. The clinical description of van Woerden's procedure does not differ from that of earlier anaesthesias: it took nine minutes before the patient was anaesthetized for an amputation procedure that lasted, surprisingly, three and a half minutes.

In 1847, besides Schoevers and Seilberger, no other Dutch doctor had written extensively in the professional press about his own experiences with ether anaesthesia. Schoevers warned that an overdose of ether might lead to death, analogous with an excess of alcohol. Surprisingly, he considered that the use of ether for 'small procedures' was not justified. He also recorded that ether could be of use in non-surgical treatment, for example for hydrophobia or tetanus. He stressed that there had been no unfavourable reports from abroad but warned that only further experience would enable the formulation of an informed opinion on the use of ether. Schoevers also stressed that the patient should not re-breathe during anaesthesia. Interestingly, G. Wassink used ether in the Dutch East Indies on 24 November, 1847. His report on the use of ether was written on 13 July, 1848, in Soerabaja but was not printed in Holland until 1849 (5).

Early controversies in Holland on the use of anaesthesia

In the Netherlands, the first serious scientific controversy concerning the action of ether was published in 1847. A physiologist from Groningen, I. van Deen, described his own experiments with ether and criticized the views of a Belgian veterinarian T. A. Thiernesse, regarding the action of ether on respiration (6,7). Van Deen emphasized that the action of ether reflects depression of brain activity and that the medulla oblongata is the last part to become inactive.

Judging from the relative scarcity of original works on ether in the Dutch medical press of 1847 one might get an erroneous impression that the Dutch medical profession was rather slow to embrace the wonder of anaesthesia. C. B. Tilanus from Amsterdam, however, remarked that one should not rely on 'somebody else's experience and achievements'. This may imply that much more work on ether was performed than may seem apparent when compared with the number of written reports (8).

Within one year following the introduction of anaesthesia in Holland two review studies attempted to evaluate the application of the new method. J. Sarlius from The Hague translated J. Schlesinger's booklet on ether from the German language, and wrote a foreword in which he stated that the lack of professional publicity on ether was a reflection of traditional Dutch cautiousness in evaluating something new (9).

Chloroform and the use of anaesthesia in obstetrics

L. Ali Cohen made an incomplete report on anaesthetics in a lecture on 26 January, 1848, in Groningen. He mentioned the early use of chloroform, on 17 December, 1847, by van Woerden of Utrecht (10). There are various reports on the use of ether or chloroform, in obstetrics to be found in the Dutch medical journals of that time. Besides the thirteen medical journals, scientific publications were found in various yearbooks. Reviewing the application of anaesthesia in Holland in 1847, one has the impression that there were few reservations as far as surgical patients were concerned. In obstetrics, however, the introduction of anaesthesia met with considerable resistance, primarily on religious grounds. In addition, considering the backgrounds of doctors who applied anaesthesia in Holland in the period 1847–1848, one can assume that no specific promoting role was played by the established University centres.

H. Schorrenberg reported on rectal administration of ether on 15 April, 1848 (11). In January of the same year, F. H. van Dommelen anaesthetized a horse whereupon he felt so sick that he decided to reserve the administration of ether to horses only in extreme need (12). In the same year, L. Ali Cohen warned against free availability of chloroform 'as this agent was so suitable for accomplishment of a murder'.

Conclusion

From our current knowledge about the very first years of anaesthesia in The Netherlands we can conclude that it readily found application in medicine, but with somewhat less visionary acclaim than in some other countries. Based on reports in the medical press of that time (13), there is evidence that development of apparatus took place and there was an investigatory echo in the fields of chemistry, physiology and pharmacology following the introduction of anaesthesia. It must be stressed, however, that many more exciting facts may emerge from a detailed study of the lay press of that time. Such a study is certainly needed in order to obtain a complete picture of the spread of anaesthesia in the western part of Europe.

References

(1) Galama SJ. Over de uitwerking van zwavelaether. *Nieuw Practisch Tijdschrift voor de Geneeskunde* 1847; **26**: 393–435.
(2) Anonymous. Verhandelingen van het Genootschap ter Bevoordering der Genees- en Heelkunde te Amsterdam. 1848; **1**: 112.
(3) Schoevers ATC. De aether inademing. *Boerhaave T Geneesk. Heel-, Verlos- en Artsenymengkunde* 1847; **6**: 444–56.
(4) Seilberger JR. Mededeling omtrent een zeer eenvoudigen een doelmatigen toestel ter inademing van den zwavelaether. *Boerhaave T Geneesk. Heel-, Verlos- en Artsenymengkunde* 1847; **6**: 456–9.
(5) Wassink G. Waarnemingen van onder aanwending der aetherisatie verrigte heelkundige kunstbewerkingen. *Nw Pr T v Geneeskunde* 1849; **28**: 139–49.
(6) Deen I van. Iets over aetherisatie. *Nw Archief* 1847; **2**: 207–18.
(7) Deen I van. Eenige aanmerkingen op de door den heer Thiernese uit zijne aetherisatiproeven gemaakte gevolgtrekkingen. *Nw Archief* 1847; **2**: 324–32.
(8) Anonymous. Verhandelingen van het Genootschap ter Bevoordering der Genees- en Heelkunde te Amsterdam 1848; **1**: 122.
(9) Schlesinger J. Over den invloed der inademing van zwavelaether op menschen en dieren. Translated by J. Sarlius. Den Haag, 1847.
(10) Ali Cohen L. De anawending van den aether en de chloroform in ons vaderland (uit eene voorlezing van de Redact. bij het Genootschap ter Bevoordering der Natuurwetenschappen te Groningen gehouden den 26 januari 1848). *Nw St G Jaarboek* 1848–49; **2**: 616–20.
(11) Schorrenberg H. Beschrijving ener kunstbewerking, ter grondige genezing der inbrengbare liesbreuk, met aanwending van de zwavelaether per anum. *Lancet* 1848–1849; **4**: 177–84.

(12) Dommelen FH van. Eenige aanmerkingen over het aëtheriseren onzer grote huisdieren. *Repertorium* 1849–1850; **3**: 125.

(13) Vandewalle EM. Literatuuronderzoek aangaande de introductie van de anesthesie in Nederland. Stage verslag. Instituut voor Medische Encyclopedie. Vrije Universiteit, Amsterdam, 1986.

5.3   Theodoor Hammes (1874–1951):
the first professional anaesthetist

J. J. DE **LANGE**
Free University Hospital, Amsterdam, The Netherlands

Theodoor Hammes was born on 3 October, 1874, in Andijk, a small village in the northern part of Holland. He was the son of the local general practitioner (1). In 1892 he started his medical education at the University of Amsterdam (2). During his study he met several artists, who stimulated his feeling for arts; several articles in the famous student's journal *Propria Cures* witness that he was an able writer (3). Hammes graduated M.D. on 4 May, 1901. He decided to become a surgeon and became a resident in the surgical clinic of the famous Professor J. A. Korteweg (4). During his residency he was one of the founders of the 'Nederlandse Vereniging voor Heelkunde' (Dutch Surgical Society) in February, 1902 (5).

The start of a career in anaesthesia

Later in 1902 it became evident to Hammes that the study of anaesthesia was more attractive than surgery. He therefore decided not to become a surgeon and travelled to London to learn the newest anaesthetic techniques including the application of nitrous oxide.

He returned to Amsterdam in 1903 and started in practice as a specialist in anaesthesia. The famous gynaecologist H. Treub gave him the nickname 'the municipal stupifier', (6) a nickname he retained, even in the newspapers, until his death (7).

Hammes's original contributions 1903–1908

From many lectures and articles it is clear that Hammes was very innovative even in the first years of his practice. As early as 1903 he gave a lecture for the 'Nederlandsche Tandmeestersvereniging' (Dutch Dental Society) about the benefit of nitrous oxide anaesthesia (8).

Nitrous oxide was not used in The Netherlands before 1903 because in 1870 the pharmacologist Stokvis had declared that the anaesthetic effect of nitrous oxide was due to asphyxia (9). Hammes asserted suffocation should always be avoided, although he believed that all inhalation anaesthetics had a toxic effect leading to general anaesthesia. He stated that nitrous oxide does not cause asphyxia if used in combination with oxygen, that the gas was indicated for short surgical procedures and that foreign statistics showed that the mortality rate was zero (10).

Ethyl chloride

Hammes regarded ethyl chloride as a good drug for the general practitioner in the countryside, especially for surgical procedures less than 20 minutes (11). Hammes himself used ethylchloride as an induction agent for ether anaesthesia and reported that the mortality rate of this technique was 1 to 17 000 from English reports. Later he advocated ethyl chloride for longer lasting procedures because it seemed to be less damaging to renal function than chloroform and ether (12). He had himself used it for 600 cases.

Chloroform

At the start of his career Hammes preferred chloroform to ether for long surgical procedures but the gynaecologist Van de Velden preferred ether in obstetrics, because there was more bleeding after childbirth, a higher mortality rate and more renal damage due to chloroform (13). Hammes contested these beliefs and argued that the higher mortality rate after chloroform was the consequence of what he called 'primary syncope', which did not occur in the obstetric patient. Although he recognized the higher mortality rate in general surgery due to chloroform, he saw the relationship between ether and chloroform anaesthesia as 'less dangerous against more beautiful anaesthesia'.

There were many theories about the cause of death during or after chloroform anaesthesia but Hammes believed in only one cause 'primary syncope'. Chloroform was primarily toxic to the myocardium and he described nine cases of chloroform syncope from his own experience (14). All these patients survived due to a very slow and careful induction and subcutaneous injections of camphorated ether. Interestingly in this connection he wrote in a later article that chloroform was always very easily blamed for this primary syncope (15) and argued with the aid of a case report that the cause of primary syncope can also be a surgical stimulus; this theory was very revolutionary at a time in which every acute death during operation was thought to be due to the anaesthetic.

Deaths under anaesthesia

Hammes discussed the causes of death during anaesthesia in another article, which concerned two cases from the literature, one during chloroform and one during ethyl chloride anaesthesia. In both cases it was reported that the cause of death was due to the anaesthetic. Hammes thought that the cause could be apoplexy due to the excitation of muscle activity causing hypertension. He proved that there were blood pressure increases during labour and exercise at a time that blood pressure measurement was not the general practice (16).

The textbook 'De Narcose'

The textbook *De Narcose* was published in 1906 as a manual of anaesthesia practice (17,18). It describes historical and chemical aspects of anaesthesia and also theories about the mechanism of general anaesthesia. Different anaesthesia techniques are detailed and Hammes demonstrates his ability as a clinician. The shortest chapter is the last entitled: 'Who is allowed to give anaesthesia?' The contents read: 'He is allowed to give anaesthesia, who, if it would be possible, would give anaesthesia to himself; he is allowed to give anaesthesia to other people—and what you do not want to happen to you, do not do to other people.'

The second edition of the textbook was published in 1911 (17). The major difference from the first edition was so drastic that Va Capellen in Hammes's funeral oration in 1952 wrote: 'To him is the honour that he substituted the dangerous chloroform anaesthesia for the better and safer ether anaesthesia' (3).

Hammes also introduced scopolamine–morphine–ether anaesthesia in this edition, but Arrias, another prominent anaesthetist in the Netherlands at the time criticized this opinion (18).

The third edition was published in 1919 (19). In this Hammes warned against the use of morphine and scopolamine by the less experienced and recommended half the dose of morphine–scopolamine. This edition keeps up to date with the development of German anaesthesia equipment but it appears that Hammes stood still in the development of his speciality. New American developments, like the new theories in the prevention of shock and the combination of local anaesthesia with general anaesthesia, are not mentioned (20). He stated that 'Injection of cocaine in the lumbar canal and subcutaneous injections of scopolamine and morphine are not able to replace inhalation anaesthesia.'

This was Hammes's last original publication about anaesthesia. In later years he refused to accept all new developments and, for example, he detested the use of curare after the Second World War (21).

Hammes's later conservation

All Theodoor Hammes's articles and lectures were published in *Het Nederlansch Tidschrift voor Geneeskunde* (The Dutch Journal of General Medicine between 1903 and 1908 and the last edition of the textbook in 1919. The question arises why Hammes terminated his innovating work at such an early time although even the University recognized him as an authority (4). Perhaps there are several reasons. Hammes was a soloist in his speciality. There is no indication that he had ever had contact with anaesthetist colleagues from his own country nor from outside the Netherlands after his visit to London. He adopted a superior attitude in discussions with other medical practitioners in his speciality and, even when there were several practising anaesthetists in Holland, there was no professional group or society. It is significant that Hammes did not participate in the foundation of 'De Nederlandse Anaesthesisten Vereniging' (Dutch Society of Anaesthetists) in 1948 (22).

Is it amazing that a man in such an isolated position inclined towards conservatism? In addition, after the publication of the last edition of his book his interests in medical politics and in the arts were to the detriment of his interest in writing about anaesthesia (23). In 1924 he became vice-chairman of the Amsterdam section of the 'Maatschappij der Geneeskunst' (society of Medicine) and on three occasions (1928, 1929, 1935) he was chairman of the board of the 'Maatschappij'. He was also one of the authors of a book about medical ethics and from 1934–1941 he was a member of the editorial board of 'Het Nederlands Tijdschrift voor Geneeskunde' (24).

Hammes's individualism, his unwillingness to train others and his lack of professional contact with his colleagues are probably the reason that his scholarly activities about anaesthesia ended about 1920. One should also realize that there was no interest at all in anaesthesia in the Netherlands in that time. The Dutch medical historian Schoute wrote in 1947, 'As a mark of our national character the public applauded our lack of interest in anaesthesia' (25).

The foundation of the 'Nederlandse Anaesthesisten Vereniging' in 1948 was 36 years after he stopped publishing. Maybe this is the reason that Hammes was not the founder of modern anaesthesiology in the Netherlands, but always remained 'the municipal stupifier'.

References

(1) Hammes Th. Private archive Hammes's family.
(2) Persoonlijkheden in het Koninkrijk der Nederlanden in woord en beeld. Nederlanders en hun werk. Amsterdam-Holkema: Warendorf 1938; 599–600.
(3) Van Cappellen D. In memoriam Th. Hammes. *Ned Tijdschr Geneeskd* 1952; **96**: 37–9.
(4) Lindeboom GA. *Dutch Medical Biography*. Rodopi 1984: 778–79.
(5) Nederlandse Vereniging voor Heelkunde 1902–1977. Utrecht, Bohn, Scheltema: Holkema, 1977: 70.
(6) Faber LA, Th. Hammes, 75 jaar. *Medisch Contact* 1949; **4**: 621–3.
(7) Het Parool, newspaper of the city of Amsterdam. 3 oktober 1949.
(8) Hammes Th. Iets over anesthesie en asphyxie. *Ned Tijdschr Tandheelkd* 1903; **10**: 253–64.
(9) Tilanus JWR, Stokvis BJ. Discussie over het protoxydum ozoti. *Ned Tijdschr Geneeskd* 1870; **24**: 240.
(10) Hammes Th. Iets over lachgasnarcose. *Ned Tijdschr Geneeskd* 1903; **47**: 652–9.
(11) Hammes Th. Aethylchloride als anaestheticum inhalatorium. *Ned Tijdschr Geneeskd* 1903; **47**: 1439–51.
(12) Hammes Th. Verlengde chlooraethylnarcose. *Ned Tijdschr Geneeskd* 1905; **49**: 1372–5.

(13) Van de Velde H. Chloroform of aether in de operatieve Verloskunde? *Ned Tijdschr Verloskd Gyn* 1904; **15**: 69–72, 84–92.

(14) Hammes Th. Over chloroformsyncope. *Ned Tijdschr Geneeskd* 1904; **48**: 1444–59.

(15) Hammes Th. Syncope door shock of door chloroform. *Ned Tijdschr Geneeskd* 1908; **52**: 838–70.

(16) Hammes Th. Spierarbeid, resp. excitatie-bloeddrukverhoging resp. apoplexie. *Ned Tijdschr Geneeskd* 1906; **50**: 403–6.

(17) Hammes Th. *Leerboek der Narcose.* Scheltema Holkema's Boekhandel Amsterdam 1906, 1911, 1919.

(18) Arrias E. Boekaankondigingen: De Narcose, Leerboek door Th. Hammes. Tweede verbeterde druk. *Ned Tijdschr Geneeskd* 1911; **55**: 749–50.

(19) Hammes Th. In: Lamertin H. *La narcose, theorie et pratique.* Bruxelles 1913.

(20) Arrias E. Boekaankondigingen: Leerboek der Narcose door Th. Hammes. Derde verbeterde druk. *Ned Tijdschr Geneeskd* 1921; **65**: 2197–98.

(21) Roelofsz-Hammes Y. Personal communication. Amsterdam 1985.

(22) Mauve M. Personal Communication. Utrecht 1986.

(23) Hammes Th. *Dr. Samuel Coster en zijn betekenis voor de cultuurgeschiedenis van Amsterdam.* Amsterdam: J H de Bussy, 1950.

(24) Van Loghem JJ. Th. Hammes. *Ned Tijdschr Geneeskd* 1949; **93**: 3328–83.

(25) Schoute D. Over de invoering der narcose in ons land honderd jaar geleden. *Ned Tijdschr Geneeskd* 1947; **91**: 941–46.

5.4   The development of regional anaesthesia in the Netherlands

J. M. VAN KLEEF
University Hospital, Leiden, The Netherlands

The meeting of the European Society of Regional Anaesthesia and the American Society of Regional Anaesthesia which was held in Vienna in 1984 commemorated the introduction of cocaine into clinical practice as a local anaesthetic. Carl Koller was the first physician to use the drug for topical anaesthesia of the eye twenty-four years after the isolation of cocaine by Niemann.

The interest in this form of anaesthesia was so great that even in the first year following Koller's discovery, more than one hundred publications on the use of cocaine as a local anaesthetic appeared in print. The practice of regional anaesthesia flourished at the turn of the century, but subsequently enthusiasm waned with the improvement of general anaesthesia. The early history of regional anaesthesia in the Netherlands followed a similar pattern.

1884–1910

Nijkamp (1) published an original Dutch article on cocaine (*Solutio Cocaini Muriatici als Anaestheticum*) in the 'Nederlands Tijdschrift voor Geneeskunde' (*Dutch Journal of General Medicine*) only three months after Brettauer's demonstration of Koller's discovery at the international conference in Heidelberg. The author discussed a few of his cases in which he had painted an aqueous cocaine-solution (5%) on the pharynx, larynx and the tongue. This resulted in excellent anaesthesia.

On 30 April, 1885, Römer (2) defended his thesis on cocaine (*Over Hydrochloras Cocaini*) at the University of Leyden. Like Koller Römer used the drug as a local anaesthetic for the eye.

Infiltration anaesthesia was first discussed in 1896 by Römer (3). The author went into the subject of the technique as described by Schleich in 1894. Local anaesthesia was produced by means of 'oedematizing' the tissues with a solution consisting of: 0.1% cocaine in 0.2% saline (solution 1) or, 0.2% cocaine in 0.2% saline (solution 2).

Solution 1 was sufficient for most cases, however in areas of inflammation solution 2 was preferable. The fact that the low pH in inflamed tissues causes a greater proportion of the drug to be ionized and therefore was unable to diffuse through nerve membranes, was not known in 1896, but the mere fact that the solution had to be more concentrated in areas of infection strongly suggests that the clinical implications were already known.

Perineural injection was studied by van Lier in 1903 (4). He injected the local anaesthetic solution (eucaine) into or close to the sciatic nerve. He concluded that the injection should be administered near to, but never into the nerve.

Regional anaesthesia was described by van Eden in 1904 (5). He, like Aulhorn (6), made the distinction between infiltration anaesthesia and regional anaesthesia. 'Infiltration anaesthesia' affecting the peripheral endings of the sensory nerves could be either 'direct' (into the tissue of the incision) or 'indirect' (into the area surrounding the incision).

Regional anaesthesia, was the blockage of conduction in a peripheral nerve. The local anaesthetics that were advocated at the time were cocaine and eucaine.

Use of adrenaline. Sikemeyer (7) published an article on the use of adrenaline (epinephrine) during infiltration anaesthesia. According to him the vascular spasm caused by adrenaline would stop the circulation at the site of injection and would thereby localize the local anaesthetic by slowing absorption and it was already well-known that slowing absorption resulted in diminished central nervous action of the drug especially when cocaine was used.

Novocaine Sikemeyer (8) referred to the work of Heineke and Laẅen on the use of novocaine (monochlorohydrate of para-amino benzoyl ethylaminoaethanol) in 1905. According to Sikemeyer novocaine (procaine) was five times less toxic than cocaine, two to three times less toxic than stovaine, clearly less effective than cocaine and approximately as effective as stovaine. A 1% solution of novocaine was recommended for regional anaesthesia and a 10% solution for spinal anaesthesia.

Spinal anaesthesia was first reported in the Dutch literature by Sikemeyer in 1905. He discussed the use of solutions of tropococaine, eucaine and stovaine. Further articles on spinal anaesthesia were published by van Lier in 1906 and 1907 (9,10). Because the side-effects of cocaine, eucaine alypine and novocaine were so prominent that the advantages of spinal anaesthesia were minimal. According to van Lier a dose of stovaine sufficient to provide reliable anaesthesia often resulted in side-effects like vomiting, headache and/or paralysis. Tropococaine was then the drug of choice because side-effects were less frequently observed as well as being less serious. Van Lier published a list of the properties of an ideal local anaesthetic drug in 1908, the application of which would result in excellent anaesthesia without causing unpleasant side effects. Some other important pronouncements made by van Lier were:

1. *'It is strongly advisable to take the same precautions in the preoperative period for spinal anaesthesia as for general anaesthesia. In case of a failed spinal one can then easily switch over to general anaesthesia.'*
2. *'The patients should be informed that shortly after the drug is injected the sensation to pressure may still be present even though sensation of painful stimuli is absent.'*
3. *If anaesthesia spreads above the umbilicus, circulatory collapse and respiratory depression may occur.'*

Finally the author gave a survey of the literature related to complications up until that time (1907).

c. 1910 to *c.* 1930

The period *c.* 1910 to 1930 saw the consolidation of some old techniques and the discovery of several new ones. These included splanchnic block (11), sacral block (12) and lumbar epidural block (13).

Regional anaesthesia flourished in the Netherlands in this period but warnings of the need for moderation and caution were heard. Despite this some investigators recklessly continued to practise new techniques in inappropriate situations, and, not surprisingly, complications occurred. For example in 1930 Hulst (14) published a case where the injection of a novocaine and adrenaline solution resulted in a fatal outcome. His conclusions may be considered as important for the time in which ester-type local anaesthetics were the only ones that were available. He stated that the severity of any allergic reaction would be minimized by first injecting the patient with only 0.5 ml of a 0.5% novocaine solution, then waiting five minutes and subsequently injecting the remainder of the dose if no allergic reaction occurred.

In 1929 Koch (15) advised the use of a combination of general and regional anaesthesia. If there were no contra-indications to either of the techniques, both could benefit from each other.

1930 to 1948

This period represented a decline in the use of regional anaesthesia not only in the Netherlands but also in Germany, England and France. This was not only a reflection of the increasing safety and efficacy of general anaesthesia, but also a consequence of reports of serious complications caused by regional anaesthesia.

The development of more efficient sterilization techniques and disposable equipment has had much to do with the revival of the use of local anaesthesia in the period after 1948.

References

(1) Nijkamp. Solutio Cocaïni Muriatici als anaestheticum. *Ned Tijdschr Geneeskd* 1884; 1139.

(2) Römer JA *Over Hydrochloras Cocaïni.* Academisch Proefschrift. Leiden, 1885. (Ph.D. Thesis, University of Leyden).

(3) Römer R. Infiltration-anaesthesie. *Ned Tijdschr Geneeskd* 1896; **II**: 858.

(4) Lier EH van. Regionaire anaesthesie. *Ned Tijdschr Geneeskd* 1903; **I**: 507.

(5) Eden V. Locale anaesthesie. *Ned Tijdschr Geneeskd* 1904; **II**: 1148.

(6) Aulhorn E. Erfahrungen mit der lokalen Anästhesie in der poliklinischen Praxis. *Münch Med Wochenschrift* 1904; **35**: 1544.

(7) Sikemeyer EW. Ervaringen omtrent het opereeren onder cocaïne-adrenaline-anaesthesie. *Ned Tijdschr Geneeskd* 1904; **II**: 1430.

(8) Sikemeyer EW. Ned Tijdschr Geneeskd 1905; **II**: 7163.

(9) Lier EH van. Over ruggemergsanaesthesie. *Ned Tijdschr Geneeskd* 1906; **II**: 1434.

(10) Lier EH van. Medullaire anaesthesie. *Ned Tijdschr Geneeskd* 1907; **I**: 1216.

(11) Haas WG de. Plaatselijke gevoelloosheid bij buikoperaties. *Ned Tijdschr Geneeskd* 1920; **I**: 2334.

(12) Schellekens WMJ. Over pijnverdooving bij de baring. *Ned Tijdschr Geneeskd* 1921; **II**: 2060.

(13) Bouwdijk Bastiaanse MA van. Lumbale en epidurale anaesthesie vooral bij verloskundige kunstverrichtingen. *Ned Tijdschr Geneeskd* 1930; **IV**: 6013.

(14) Hulst IPL. Een geval van novocaïne-adrenaline inspuitingen met doodelijken afloop. *Ned Tijdschr Geneeskd* 1930; **I**: 2884.

(15) Koch CFA. Plaatselijke anaesthesie. In: *Uitgaven van het Rijksinstituut voor Pharmacotherapeutisch Onderzoek.* Meededelingen no. 17. NV A.W. Sijthoff's Uitgeversmij., Leiden, 1929.

5.5   Anaesthesia in the Netherlands from the thirties to 1948

M. MAUVE
Laren, The Netherlands

This paper is an account of my personal experiences in the nineteen thirties and forties. I was born in 1912 and studied medicine from 1930 until 1938. I then set up as a general practitioner but, after the war, I specialized as an anaesthetist and I practised in that specialty until my seventieth year.

The influence of other European countries on Dutch medical practice

My country is a small country situated between France, Germany and the United Kingdom. There have always been important international contacts, political and commercial as well as artistic and scientific. Medicine has been no exception. In the course of the nineteenth century we were influenced by the French, after that by the Germans and representatives of the Viennese school. Between about 1870 and 1910 many Germans and Austrians (surgeons in particular) were appointed to professorial chairs in The Netherlands. When I was a medical student textbooks were more often in German than in our own language. After the war this changed and until now Anglo-American influences have prevailed. As a result our medical jargon is now interspersed with English words and phrases but, nevertheless, some expressions are still reminiscent of the French and German influences.

Anaesthesia in The Netherlands in the nineteen thirties

In the thirties the German system deeply affected daily routine in surgical departments and particularly in operating theatres; as a kind of after-effect this was noticeable after the war too—in fact it took a generation before cooperation between surgeons and anaesthetists on a footing of equality became a real possibility. Before that the surgeon was the undisputed central figure, the only one to know everything, to be able to do everything and to decide everything. Anaesthesia was part of his competence too. Local and regional anaesthesia were administered by him, for general anaesthesia he needed assistants. These used to be nurses, some of whom became highly experienced and carried out their tasks excellently. In teaching hospitals the youngest trainee was charged with anaesthesia. There were general practitioners that anaesthetized too, sometimes for extra earnings, sometimes because they liked it. All of them acted upon the surgeon's orders. Usually ether anaesthesia was given but in some cases, for example when there were pulmonary affections, chloroform was administered still. Although generally the ether versus chloroform battle was decided in favour of ether, I know of a paediatric hospital where until 1950 a nurse administered chloroform anaesthesia exclusively. Finally there were some professional anaesthetists, four in all, who have been discussed in Dr de Lange's paper (5.3). I myself never saw them in action.

Personal experience in the period 1935 to 1946

My personal experience of anaesthesia began in 1935 when I was still a medical student. I was appointed to a job in the laboratory of the department of gynaecology and obstetrics of the University Hospital at Leyden and, although far from being a qualified physician, I was charged with the administration of anaesthesia. The only reason for this was that I had joined the staff most recently; as far as I can remember this consideration did not surprise me as it was the usual practice and, besides, I was keen to be involved in the treatment of patients. It should be explained that the first five years of the study of medicine were entirely theoretical at the time and, consequently, I had come into contact with patients for the first time only three months before in the medical department. All I know about anaesthesia was remembered from an early surgical lecture. It was not considered to be necessary for me to study a book about anaesthesia, an older trainee would instruct me.

I vividly remember that instruction. The patient lay waiting on a stretcher in a room off the theatre; on a side-table there were a big Juliard ether-mask, some bottles and a towel. The older trainee, dressed in the red rubber apron for scrubbing up, told me what to do. First I had to measure 5 ml of ethyl chloride from a small syphon into a measuring-glass, then to pour this into the mask and put it on the patient's face and immediately begin to drip on the ether. In the meantime my instructor was crying 'breathe Madam, breathe deeply!' and he firmly held the resisting woman with a nurse until she stopped moving. After that it was all left to me. At the professor's request, 'Come in!' I wheeled the patient into the theatre. There he stood with four students, ready for the vaginal examination, first by the professor, then by the others. They threw me many angry looks for the patient had not relaxed. The woman was then laid on the operating table, catheterized, disinfected and draped at high speed. Without forewarning the table was turned to a steep head-down position and the operation began. When the abdominal cavity was opened the bowels protruded. Once again their looks told me I was to blame—'The muscles have not relaxed, quickly more ether!' I was told. In what manner this proceeded I do not remember exactly now. The surgeon succeeded in closing the abdomen. The operation was soon over and before the last stitch the next patient lay waiting.

This was my training and after that I had to anaesthetize with the help of whatever nurse happened to be available. I cannot deny that in the long run I did acquire some dexterity at anaesthetizing, but the results were often meagre. Over and over again the professor would call out, 'Come in!', the muscles would fail to relax sufficiently, the bowels would protrude and every time I was the one to be blamed. After a few weeks, when the professor said to an assistant during an operation: 'He will never learn!', I thought that that was just reproach and I felt very stupid.

There used to be two sessions a week, each with nine or ten operations, among which at least four laparotomies. At about noon it was all over and done with and we had coffee in the professor's room. There the atmosphere was always kind and nobody seemed to be worried by my failures any longer. Later, when I visited the room to see the patients who had been operated upon, I entered an inferno watched over by a domineering nurse. She thought I had no business there and would hardly admit me at all. It was dark, there was a smell of ether and sour vomit and a complex sound of vomiting, groaning, snoring and soft cries of 'Nurse, nurse!'. I soon left this place of horror and did not often return.

I still have some other horrible memories. I recall a young woman whom I had to anaesthetize in the delivery room who suffocated in her vomit. In the fifties this was still a relatively frequent occurrence, as can be seen in Wylie's report in 1956 concerning 'Deaths associated with anaesthesia'. Then again I have known the professor forbid me to anaesthetize a patient because she had been weakened too much by loss of blood in consequence of a placenta praevia. Without any anaesthetic a caesarian section was performed at once and, when the woman screamed too loudly, he prodded her firmly in the ribs crying: 'Be quiet, it is a matter of life and death now!'. How she survived I do not know, perhaps the haemorrhagic shock protected her.

I have not dealt with this at such length in order to commiserate or to indicate how hard it is, if not impossible, to relax the muscles with ether within a short space of time. I wanted however, to give some idea of the system of those days and of the way people set to work, and, of the low status of anaesthesia—not to mention the virtual absence of monitoring. I also remember with distress the brutal manner in which patients were handled as objects having to undergo treatment without any say in the matter and many of them behaved accordingly. I have to admit that conditions were somewhat archaic in our department but, nevertheless, that is what happened and it was probably the same elsewhere a few decades before.

I handed the administration of anaesthesia over to a new junior a year later. I was convinced at the time that I would never have to administer anaesthesia again. I was mistaken, however.

I became a general practitioner and met a surgeon who invited me to assist at his operations and later even to administer anaesthesia. He was a patient man, allowing me ample time for my work and I came to enjoy it. I used an old anaesthetic machine dating from 1928 and I mastered gas–oxygen anaesthesia with positive pressure. The surgeon, was one of the first to practise pulmonary surgery in The Netherlands but, in this expert company I shall not enter into the problems presented by anaesthetizing a patient with bronchiectasis for a thoracotomy, using spontaneous respiration and without an endotracheal tube. Every one of you can imagine them for himself.

Practice after 1946

I worked in this way until 1946. In October of that year I learned that a professional training in anaesthesia was available in the surgical department of the University Hospital at Amsterdam, supervised by a British anaesthetist who had lately been engaged. I gave up practice as a general practitioner and started as her first trainee in January 1947. In 1948 the Netherlands' Society of Anaesthetists were founded and shortly after that anaesthesia was officially recognized as a medical specialty. In the course of years some ten training centres were set up and many anaesthetists have been trained.

Conclusion

If I have succeeded in giving you an impression of the former anaesthesia problems and if you have succeeded in visualizing them, then you may imagine my amazement on entering the world of modern anaesthesia. It was my teacher, Doreen Vermeulen-Cranch, the mother of anaesthesia in The Netherlands, who opened this new world for me.

5.6   History of pain control in dentistry in The Netherlands

D. M. E. VERMEULEN-CRANCH, CBE
University of Amsterdam, The Netherlands

The pattern of the history of pain control in dentistry in the Netherlands differs from that in Britain or America. This fact became clear to me when comparing my first years in anaesthesia in Britain with those spent after the war in the Netherlands, training Dutch doctors in anaesthesia and lecturing to dental students. What factors influenced the differences and how does the situation compare nowadays with elsewhere?

By the law of 1818 (1) chirurgijns (surgeons) and tandmeesters (dentists) were both licensed to draw teeth. They advertised pain-free extractions widely. Their success was based on suggestibility and speed. Undoubtedly the stoic, phlegmatic character and Calvinistic background of the Dutch made them less sensitive to pain or more ready to submit to it.

The Act of 1823 offered hospital training to the chirurgijn and his status began to improve, but not so the tandmeester. His status sank back with his lack of education and lowly task. The discovery of anaesthesia made no great or lasting impact on the relief of pain in dentistry. No Morton, Simpson or Snow came forward.

By 1865 it was decided that dentistry required a medical training in order to administer an anaesthetic and to arrest haemorrhage. It was believed that there would be medics enough to perform all the dentistry required and that any addition to their education would be superfluous. Only the established tandmeesters could continue to practise.

In 1875 the situation was described as critical. The remaining sixty tandmeesters were doomed to extinction, yet only four medics had taken up dentistry, two of whom had been able to learn from their tandmeester fathers. The medics were obviously uninterested in the lowly tasks of dentistry and their minimal training was outdated.

A year later by the Act of 1876 the Act of 1865 was repealed, out of sheer necessity, but not without protest from the medics. Tandmeesters would now attend theoretical and practical training in dentistry, together with the medical students, to be followed by a State, non-academic examination, judged by professors of medicine. The latter were however minimally aquainted with the requirements of dentistry. Practice was limited to purely local treatment of teeth, sockets, gums, orthodontics and the fitting of artificial teeth.

Prescribing or administering any drugs which could have a generalized effect was forbidden. It is not surprising that students who were dissatisfied with their teaching and exams, chose to train abroad and take their exams on returning if in a position to do so.

An interesting historical situation ensued (2) because a foreigner had been and was practising unlawfully in the Hague as tandmeester. It was generally known that he treated the aristocracy and royal family, that he was a modest, unpretentious man and skilled in relieving pain. He was 'protected' by recognition of a training abroad, yet his diplomas were never produced. According to Dr Dentz, he was none other than the 'great Picnot' (1820–1910), of English origin, who with Dentz, founded the Dutch Society of Dentistry in 1879 and who did much to raise the status of tandmeesters and the standard of dentistry. The law of 1876 explains why Picnot worked with a medical narcotiseur and his exclusive clients explain why his fees were high. Extractions, 5 Dutch guilders; with nitrous oxide and a doctor in attendance, 15 Dutch guilders.

In 1877 Dr Th. Dentz, being medically trained and trained by his father as tandmeester was appointed Lector at the University of Utrecht. He allowed trainee tandmeesters to attend his classes provided they had passed the required theoretical exam and had followed a preliminary general education of five years.

However, the accommodation and equipment available were totally inadequate. With the help of money raised by tandmeesters and students a new Institute was opened in 1895. The waiting room was planned as far away as possible from the treatment room, so that the screams of patients would not penetrate.

In his opening address Dr Dentz drew attention to the progress made in dentistry in the last 30 years. He said, however, that general anaesthesia with nitrous oxide was rarely used, first because its use by tandmeesters was illegal and secondly because the doctors, who would be allowed to use it, were completely unknowledgeable concerning its use (3).

In the museum in Utrecht there are a number of masks for giving chloroform, ether and ethyl chloride but whether these were ever used by the tandmeesters is not clear. Ethyl chloride spray was used officially as a local 'cold' analgesia in the mouth but probably had some general effect as well.

It is not surprising that suggestion and hypnotism were advocated as a means of relieving pain (4).

Historically important examples of syringes dating from 1876, used for implanting morphine into tissues for pain relief and of syringes for administering cocaine around 1890 can be seen in the Utrecht Museum. Tandmeester Otté working closely with the professor of surgery in Groningen made successful intra-osseous injections of cocaine under pressure in 1896 (5).

Dentz, the father of Dutch dentistry, retired in 1908, having striven to improve the training and status of tandmeesters. It is interesting that his students had, in 1897, founded the first and most well-known dental students' Society in Utrecht (6), named after John Tomes, the English dentist and dental anaesthetist, who had achieved so much for dentistry in Britain.

There were few medics interested in anaesthesia and fewer in dental anaesthesia. The most famous was Dr Hammes, who was appointed Tutor in Narcology in 1906 to the University of Amsterdam. He became a member of the Dutch Dental Society, contributing translations of the history of anaesthesia to the *Dutch Journal of Dentistry* in 1907 and 1908. Hammes visited the National Dental Hospital in London in 1902 and carried out 700 successful dental anaesthetics there (7). He used Hewitt's apparatus and endeavoured to introduce the use of nitrous oxide and oxygen for short surgical operations and for dentistry.

It had practically never been used in the Netherlands, in the mistaken belief that its only action was that of asphyxia. He devoted a chapter in his book, published in 1906, to its safe use. His colleague Arrias in the Hague, who had also visited Britain for experience with nitrous oxide, supported him (8). Occasionally tandmeesters did administer nitrous oxide themselves. In the legal proceedings which followed Hammes disapproved strongly. A few country doctors used nitrous oxide for extractions, but its use was minimal.

The records of the Amsterdam Sickness Insurance company since 1848 (9) reveal that the medic was paid 70 cents to extract teeth without anaesthesia. In 1908, novocaine having been discovered, it was suggested that an extra charge of 50 cents—1 guilder be made for local analgesia and 3–5 guilders for anaesthesia given by a medic. However, from 1908–1919 the extra money received for pain relief amounted to only 4.7% of the total.

Strictly speaking using local anaesthesia was illegal according to the law of 1876, but its use was condoned. Sepsis was not considered, a contraindication to injection, although there was evidence of infection spreading. It was, however, advised to inform the patient beforehand not to expect entirely pain-free treatment under such circumstances, since the patient might otherwise lose faith in the injection technique of his tandmeester! A patient's fear of the injection was also ignored.

About 1937 in the *Dutch Journal of Dentistry* some tandartsen (by then the name had changed) were reprimanded for using nitrous oxide, analgesics, sedatives and hypnotics (10,11). Court proceedings, with support from Hammes (12), suppressed this violation of the 1876 Act. Articles in the *Journal* by tandartsen (13,14) on nitrous oxide anaesthesia followed, either condemning its use altogether in view of possible dangerous complications, or advocating its use, with a medical practitioner, for pain relief under certain indications. The editors of the *Journal* scathingly reminded the tandartsen of the law and that the need for anaesthesia for dentistry was exceptional and that local analgesia should be used only with a good indication.

In 1946 tandarts Van de Kamer wrote (15) that he considered nitrous oxide, used as an anaesthetic, unsatisfactory but that as an analgesic for conservative dentistry it offered important advantages to anxious patients and to the tandarts. It enabled the anxious patient to undergo treatment and continue regular treatments. It gave adequate pain relief if local anaesthesia was ineffective and it also saved the tandarts' time and both his and his patient's nerves. He had for several years personally treated patients using a McKesson's nitrous oxide oxygen graduated in percentages, analgesia-on-demand apparatus, whereby the patient could squeeze a rubber ball for more effect. This was an early Dutch report of dental analgesia, recognizing that patients were not always pain or fear free during conservative treatment and that the dentist was capable of administering analgesia with nitrous oxide–oxygen as occurred in America and Britain, to alleviate it.

It was becoming clear that there had been gross underestimation over the years by the government, by the medics, by some tandartsen and by the public of the value of a high standard of dentistry to the general health and well being of the community, as reflected in the low educational standards set, the severe limitations of practice, the inadequate financing and facilities, and the sluggish, indecisive reactions of the authorities to the protests of the tandartsen to the 1876 Act.

Change eventually came in 1947 with the new dental Act. Dentistry became a full academic study of 6 years, with license to practise dentistry to its full extent. As is the case with medical training, it would provide the dentist with such knowledge, experience and sense of responsibility as to enable him to assess his own limitations. Five dental sub-faculties were set up within 20 years. It changed very little regarding the practice of the relief of pain. Tandartsen had never been taught to give general anaesthetics themselves and now they had no good reason to wish to do so, especially after the introduction and more general use of lidocaine.

But in the 1950s dubiously qualified persons set up premises in large cities, advertising total extractions under 'Evipan narcosis' and immediate fitting, in one session, of dentures. It was pure commercial exploitation without clear dental indications or after care. However, people with a fear of dental treatment flocked there, because unfortunately this fear had mostly been disregarded by the tandartsen who considered it cowardice.

In Amsterdam, by teaching dental undergraduates the negative effect of anxiety on pain control, and by starting a post-graduate course on the use of nitrous oxide as a sedative (16), seven years later the Ministry of Health approved its use as a sedative by the tandartsen who had successfully followed the course. It is good to see that the dubious commercial institutes have, since last year, come under closer control.

Considering the training and responsibilities of the dentist in the Netherlands, control of pain has achieved a point in development which now compares well with that in other countries, namely:

General anaesthetics are given by an anaesthesiologist in a hospital.

Intravenous sedation is given by an anaesthesiologist.

Inhalation sedation is given, as an adjuvant to behaviour management and adequate local analgesia, by the dentist qualified to use it, when indicated.

References

(1) de Ranitz CJA. De ontwikkeling van de opleiding en de bevoegdheid van tandartsen in de Nederlandse wetgeving. *100 Jaar Tandheelkundig Onderwijs in Nederland 1877–1977*. Amsterdam: 't Koggerschip, 1977; 37–44.

(2) Buisman PH. De ontwikkelingsgang der Tandheelkunst in ons land. *Ned Tijdschrift v. Tandheelk* 1969; **3**: 166–99.

(3) Buisman PH. Ontstaan en ontwikkeling v.h. Tandheelkundige Onderwijs (1877–1940). *100 Jaar Tandheelkundig Onderwijs in Nederland 1877–1977*. Amsterdam: 't Koggerschip, 1977; 45–154.

(4) Renterghem AW. Chirurgische anaesthesie langs psychische weg verkregen. *Tijdschr v. Tandheelk* 1912; **19**: 182–205.

(5) Otté J. Intra-ossale Cocaine Injectie. *Tijdschr v. Tandheelk* 1896; **3**: 251–5.

(6) Fuhring MJBH, Wabeke KB. De tandheelkundige Studentenvereeniging 'John Tomes'. *100 Jaar Tandheelkundig Onderwijs in Nederland 1877–1977*. Amsterdam: 't Koggerschip, 1977; 237–52.

(7) Hammes, Th. Iets over lachgas narcose. *Ned Tijdschr v. Geneesk* 1903; **11**: 652–9.

(8) Arrias E. Het toedienen van lachgas-zuurstof door middel van Paterson's neusmasker. *Ned Tijdschr v. Geneesk* 1906; **2**: 1020–31.

(9) Leclerq WL. Tandheelkundige Hulp. Geschiedenis v.h. Algemeen Ziekenfonds v. Amsterdam 1847–1947. 1947; 99–109.

(10) Inspecteur v.d. Volksgezondheid Putto. Toepassing van lachgasnarcose door Tandartsen. *Tijdschr v. Tandheelk* 1937; **44**: 1116.

(11) De Hooge Raad. Het afleveren van Geneesmiddelen. *Tijdschr v. Tandheelk* 1937; **44**: 1025.

(12) Hammes Th. Voor het gebruik van lachgas Veroordeeld. *Tijdschr v. Tandheelk* 1939; **46**: 297.

(13) Hamer R. Waarom zouden wij ook in Nederland in de tandheelkunde lachgas gaan gebruiken? *Tijdschr v. Tandheelk* 1937; **44**: 996–1000.

(14) Van der Klei JH. Waarom zouden wij in Nederland in de tandheelkunde geen lachgas gebruiken? *Tijdschr v. Tandheelk* 1938; **45**: 67–73.

(15) Van de Kamer HJ. Honderd jaar lachgas als anaestheticum. *Tijdschr v. Tandheelk* 1946; **53**: 103–11.

(16) Makkes PC, Vermeulen-Cranch DME *et al, Inhalatie Sedatie in de Tandheelkunde I* 1980; **87**: 415–8 and *II* 1980; **87**: 448–52.

5.7   The development of anaesthesia in Malta

N. AZZOPARDI
Consultant Anaesthetist, Malta

Malta is an island in the middle of the Mediterranean sea forming part of a 120 square mile archipelago made up of three other islands and at present inhabited by a third of a million people.

This archipelago is steeped in documented history left by Phoenician, Greek, Roman, Carthagenian, Byzantine, Arab, Norman, Spanish overlords until Charles V of Spain ceded it to the Knights Hospitallers of St John of Jerusalem. True to their name the Knights Hospitallers built a huge hospital in the capital city Valletta that served as a Military, Civil and Medical School Hospital.

In 1798 the Knights were shown the way out by Napoleon Bonaparte on his Egyptian expedition and after two years the Maltese revolted against the occupying French force, shutting them up in the capital city, Valletta. Admiral Nelson of the British Navy, a good opportunist, offered help to the besieging Maltese by blockading the archipelago and gradually following the Navy, a British Army occupied Malta. After the surrender of the French force the islands were taken over by Britain as the Treaty of Vienna was signed in 1814.

The Island's hospitals

During the French occupation of Malta the Knight's Hospital in Valletta was used exclusively for the occupying force and their families. The Maltese patients in this hospital were transferred to the small church of St Mary Magdalen also in Valletta. There were three other civilian small hospitals in the island, one in Rabat just outside the old capital city of Mdina, a small hospital run by a religious order in Zebbug and a small hospital in the island of Gozo. When the British forces entered Valletta they took over the Knight's Hospital and used it as a combined Army and Navy one for a few decades. A separate Naval hospital was planned and built on a promontory facing the Knight's Hospital but on the other side of the Grand Harbour. This new Naval building opened its doors in 1832 and was called the Bighi Hospital. The Army and Navy hospitals were staffed by young British doctors seeking a career with the armed forces and always keen to try out new medical discoveries and make a name for themselves. Both the Knight's Hospital (now the Army one) and the Bighi Hospital (now the Navy one) exist to this day as the Mediterranean Conference centre and the other unfortunately is in a derelict state.

The civilian population and the medical school had to wait till 1852 to get a new hospital in Floriana—the Civil Hospital built outside the walls of Valletta. This Civil Hospital is today the Police Headquarters.

Ether inhalation

The new Bighi hospital was the site where ether anaesthesia was first tried in Malta. Etherization had been heard about by the local medical people since 26 December, 1846, when *The Malta Times*, an English paper published daily, reported that in Boston, USA a dentist, Morton, tried using inhalation of sulphuric ether for 200 dental sessions and had had uniform success. He used inhalation of ether through a soaked sponge for two minutes and produced unconsciousness for another two minutes, just enough for a quick dental operation. In the same issue it is reported that in the UK Dr Heyward of the London Hospital had cut off the leg of a patient for white swelling using ether inhalations and the amputation was painless. The article above reported ends in a note of caution probably appended by a local medical reporter '. . . it has in a few cases failed owing probably to the peculiarity of the patient's constitution or temperament or want of skill in the administrator . . .'

During January and February, 1847, *The Malta Times* reported what the British press had to say about the new discovery and I could find quotations from *The Cambridge Adventurer*, *The Observer* and *The British Journal*. From France I found a quotation from the *Journal des Debats* where caution is called for when a lighted candle is used to illuminate the operating field during etherization, with the grave possibility of an explosion occurring inside the patient's chest. On the 9 March there is a report that Mr Hughes of Godstone UK used ether for shodding a horse—the first mention of anaesthesia used for veterinary purposes.

But the important confirmation of use of ether locally comes in a report of *The Malta Times* dated 23 March, 1847. Under the heading 'Etherization' it reported that a Mr Wells, RN had on 16 March successfully performed eye surgery for squint on two patients at the Bighi Hospital. The local Societa Medica d'Incoraggiamento at its monthly meeting tried out etherization when the same Mr Wells administered the drug to two local doctors using Hooper's Inhaler. This inhaler brought from the UK consisted of two communicating glass globes each containing a sponge. One globe opened to air and the other to a mouthpiece. Ether had been poured to saturate the sponge of the first globe and the patient inhaled air and ether through the second globe.

It is reported that the local doctors differed in their reaction to ether. One of them, a tall frail chap, Dr L. Callejja, 'turned red in his face, lacrimated profusely, felt his sense of touch diminish, felt his head spinning round and passed out. He was unconscious for a few minutes and complained of severe headaches when he recovered consciousness'. The other one, a Dr F. L. Gravagna, 'became red in the face, had a fixed stare and while his face assumed a stupid expression burst out laughing. He said that he did not lose consciousness but could feel no pain to pinprick'. His failure to pass out and the fact that he had a terrible headache after the ether administration is attributed to his temperament as he was known to be a heavy wine drinker.

An interesting advert in *The Malta Times* of 6 April, 1847, advises that at 40 Strada San Zacharia in Valletta teeth can be extracted without pain through the inhalation of ether vapour administered by an experienced British surgeon.

A few words about the ether administrator Dr Wells. This is none other than the famous surgeon Sir Thomas Spencer Wells who started his medical career as a Naval surgeon and spent six years in Malta at the Bighi Navy hospital. He was already a Fellow of the Royal College of Surgeons and was also enrolled as a member of the local Societa Medica d'Incoraggiamento. His expertise with ether was called for on the 15 June, 1847, when a Maltese woman from Senglea had hydrophobia following a cat bite some four months before. It was hoped that etherization would also cure the rabies convulsions but unfortunately the woman died after three days. It is not reported whether the convulsion improved under ether influence.

The Maltese readers of *The Malta Times* were alarmed by reports from London, Vienna, Paris and Rome about the dangers of unprofessional tampering with the drug. At Colchester Hospital it was reported in *The Essex Standard* of 23 March, 1847, that a surgeon, Mr R. S. Nunn, operated on a Mr T. Herbert for lithotomy and after recovering from the etherization unfavourable symptoms appeared that killed the patient in 24 hours from exhaustion. A Dr James Pickford reporting in *The Morning Chronicle* of the 6 July, 1847, noted that 'ether can produce tuberculous consumption of the lungs and that in thirty cases of death after use of ether at the Dublin Hospital the cause of death could be traced to recent tubercules believed to be a product of ether'.

This same doctor reported that 'the insensibility ether produces is due to a chemical alternation of the vital constituents of the blood which is deprived of oxygen, and the power of coagulation, and the corpuscles where fibrin is formed are acutely dissolved. After etherization blood takes a long time to regain its life supporting flesh forming character, wounds refuse to heal and the patient sinks in death'.

All these warnings influenced the local medical fraternity and militated against the rapid acceptance of ether as an anaesthetic and many doctors still preferred their patients to suffer excruciating pain than take advantage of the most wonderful discovery of the day.

Chloroform inhalation

A Dr J. Y. Simpson of Edinburgh specializing in obstetrics reported in 1847 that ether could be safely used during labour and that the contractions of the uterus were not inhibited while the pain was abolished. Despite opposition from the Clergy he continued experimenting and on 10 November, 1847, introduced chloroform 'chloric ether' as a new anaesthetic agent, a substitute for sulphuric ether in surgery and midwifery. *The Malta Times* of 4 January, 1848, reported about chloroform as 'a new therapeutic agent in place of inhalation of ether. It can be used with greater rapidity and success than ether . . . no particular instrument or inhaler is necessary . . . all that is required is to diffuse a little of the liquid into a hollow shaped sponge or even a pocket handkerchief and apply the same on the mouth and nostrils as to be fully inhaled'. This method of administering 'chloroform a la reine' impressed the local medical colleagues after Queen Victoria accepted it from John Snow at the birth of Prince Leopold in May, 1853.

This year marked the opening of the Crimean War and the full utilization of the Bighi Naval hospital facilities as well as the Army one. These hospitals were full of wounded soldiers and sailors which were shipped over from the Crimean War zone on the insistence of Miss Florence Nightingale. This valiant lady was impressed by the discipline, cleanliness and the administrative capabilities of the Sisters of Charity who cared for the sick in Germany where she trained. She took some of the German sisters with her to work in Scutari and copied most of their rules so reforming the role of nurses and patient care in military and later in Civil hospitals.

Anaesthesia using ether or chloroform as practised in Malta Hospitals, mainly for amputation of limbs, and it is documented that two surgeons were in charge of the anaesthetized patient, one to administer chloroform or ether and the other to monitor the pulse.

On the 20 April, 1855, it is reported in *The Malta Times* that a 35-year-old labourer, having an amputation of a finger at the private home of a British practitioner Dr F. Sankey had 'trembling of the pulse, blood ceased to flow and the patient expired without a groan and despite all efforts, to restore suspended animation the patient was declared dead'. This setback was instrumental in diminishing the popularity of chloroform use as the sole agent for anaesthesia in Malta.

Nitrous oxide gas

In 1868 nitrous oxide gas was used in London at the Royal Dental Hospital in Soho Square by a Dr Evans. This gas was imported from France in iron bottles and released into a bag held over the anaesthetist's shoulder and delivered to the patient through a nasal or oronasal mask.

In the USA a chemist, Colton, had since 1846 struggled to make the gas popular as a safe and efficient anaesthetic for short operations. In 1876 this gas was used by Dr Clover in the UK as a precursor of ether inhalation so bypassing the disagreeable smell and violent struggles of ether inhalations.

Chloroform controversy

Starting in 1879 chloroform use was suspect even in the UK. The British Medical Association Committee meeting in Glasgow came to the conclusion that the drug lowered the blood pressure and depressed heart action. This view was contested by the Nyzam of Hyderabad Commission that in both sessions cleared chloroform inhalation of its reported side effects. As this view was not at all accepted by the British Medical Association Committee chloroform use in Europe remained controversial. However in Malta it was made popular again for gynaecological and obstetric use as the professor in the speciality, Joseph Schembri, found it useful for his patients. Laparatomies and lower segment caesarean sections were performed under anaesthesia at the Civil Hospital between 1890 and 1891 with good results; the chloroform administration entrusted to one of four medical officers employed as chloroformists.

The First World War

In 1914 Malta's hospitals were overflowing with invalid British, Anzac and Indian soldiers shipped over from the Dardanelles war zone. Not only were the Army and Navy hospitals fully utilized but six other temporary hospitals were established to care for the wounded. Many Maltese doctors, surgeons and anaesthetists were welcomed into the RAMC and there they perfected their learning and practised alongside the hard pressed British medical staff. At the time Malta was dubbed 'The Nurse of the Mediterranean'.

The first recorded appointment of a full time anaesthetist in Malta's Civil Hospital occurred on the 20 June, 1919. Dr Emmanuel Vella had gained experience at the Army Hospital working with Sir Charles Balance, a British Army Colonel surgeon. Although Dr Vella was only aged thirty four at the time he had seen foreign service in the First World War in France attached to the Royal Army Medical Corps of the British Army.

Dr Vella described how hard it was to anaesthetize the hardier country type of patient using only rag and bottle chloroformization. He was also required by the Royal University of Malta to organize a voluntary course on the theoretical and practical instruction in the administration of anaesthesia to graduates.

Dr Vella retired due to ill health after three years and was succeeded by Dr George Busuttil another RAMC man.

From then onwards anaesthesia progressed in Malta alongside its development in the UK, especially at St Bartholomew Hospital London whose anaesthetic staff led by Dr F. T. Evans— the Dean of the Faculty of Anaesthetists of the Royal College of Surgeons—served as 'foster parents' to the young Maltese trainees. Also they learnt about the Boyle's machine from Dr Boyle himself, intubated under chloroform with Sir Francis Shipway and learnt the use of Stovaine 5% for spinal analgesia from Mr Arthur Barker, FRCS.

In 1920 a young Maltese surgeon Dr P. P. Debono studying for the FRCS in London also learnt the art of spinal analgesia and on his return used to practise single handedly in the Civil Hospital, relying on his own anaesthetic and surgical expertise for the successful outcome of both analgesia and the operation. Another surgeon practising in London in the 1930s was both an Ophthalmologist and a Count. Luigi Preziosi learnt the technique of local analgesia for ophthalmic surgery working at the Moorfield Eye Hospital.

The Second World War

The occurrence of war always stimulates medical research and as the UK was the foremost world power any new anaesthetic agent or technique was surely to be found both in the UK and in its war ravished frontiers.

In 1945 a severe polio epidemic beleagured the island. This polio epidemic started in Canadian airmen who had been flown to Malta to prepare for the Sicilian campaign, the invasion of mainland Europe. From the Mtarfa air force hospital this disease spread to the local population and the few iron lungs available could not cope with the number of patients suffering from respiratory paresis. The Royal Navy brought additional iron lungs on loan from the London Hospital. Intermittent positive pressure ventilation using a simple endotracheal tube and relays of students, ventilating patients through a modified Water's cannister was carried out and many lives were saved.

At that time too curare was used locally only three years after its discovery in Canada by Harold R. Griffiths and Enid Johnson. It was used at the newly opened St Luke's Hospital to produce muscle relaxation for surgical operations by the Belfast trained civilian anaesthetist and lecturer Dr Charles Podesta, FFARCS, my teacher.

The future

The further development of anaesthesia in Malta reflects the influence and trends that the speciality registers world wide.

Bibliography

The Malta Times 1846, 1847, 1848.

Bellamy Gardner H. *A manual of surgical anaesthesia* 2nd Ed. London: Ballière Tindall and Cox, 1916.

Cassar P. *Acta Anaesthesiol Melitensia*; **1** (2): 13–8.

5.8　The development of anaesthesia and intensive therapy in Poland

MARIAN KUŚ[1], MAREK SYCH[1] WITOLD JURCZYK[2], and ZDZISLAW RONDIO[3]
[1]Medical Academy, Krakow, [2]Medical Academy, Poznán and
[3]Institute of Mother and Child, Warsaw, Poland

In the 19th century Poland was occupied by Russia, Prussia and Austria. Vienna was one of the leading medical centres in Europe. The news of the first ether anaesthesia on 25 January, 1847, in Vienna spread most quickly through the Austrian part of Poland (1). On the 6 February, 1847, in the surgical clinic of the Jagiellonian University in Kraków under the supervision of Ludwik Bierkowski, professor of surgery, ether was used as an anaesthetic in two operations, of funicocoele and for incision of a large abscess, following successful trials with ether on three volunteers.

The information on this event reached all the three parts of the country at an amazing speed. A few days later in district hospitals of the Austrian part of Poland surgical operations were performed under ether anaesthesia (on 8 February, in Rzeszów and before 15 February, in Lvov). On the 15 February, Ludwik Koehler used ether in the Evangelical Hospital in Warsaw (the Russian part of the country). During 1847 ether anaesthesia became popular in the whole country even in small hospitals. The first trials of ether anaesthesia were also made in dentistry and obstetrics.

In Warsaw on the 11 December, 1847, Alexander Le Brun, head of the biggest department of surgery in Warsaw, used chloroform anaesthesia for the first time in Poland and a year later he had recorded over two hundred cases. Soon chloroform almost entirely replaced ether in operating rooms. In 1856 Hipolit Korzeniowski published the first monograph on anaesthetics in Polish.

In 1858 the first death under chloroform anaesthesia was reported.

The scientific activity of the Polish physician Stanisław Klikowicz deserves particular attention. He introduced a method of pain relief during labour by administration of a mixture of nitrous oxide and oxygen (2). He used it with success in Petersburg in 25 women in labour. Following this Heliodor Swiecicki in Poznań constructed an inhaler for obstetric analgesia with nitrous oxide and oxygen. He presented it during an international congress of obstetricians in 1890 where it had a favourable reception.

On the 15 March, 1877, in Warsaw endotracheal anaesthesia was used for the first time in Poland for laryngectomy, using the Trendelenburg device. It was the tenth operation of this type in the world.

One should also keep in mind the original experimental studies carried out by Jan Prus, professor of Lvov University in the years 1899–1900. He performed direct cardiac massage and artificial ventilation of the lungs in dogs suffering from asphyxia, electric shock or chloroform overdose (3). He demonstrated the efficacy of those procedures in restoring all functions of the central nervous system.

At the beginning of the 20th century general anaesthesia was gradually replaced by various forms of local analgesia. In this respect the surgical clinic in Lvov particularly should be mentioned. In 1921 R. Rodziński published the results of post-mortem studies on the determination of extradural space volume. He punctured the extradural at different levels including the cervical one. In the same clinic in 1925 an original approach to brachial plexus block was developed by Hilarowicz.

During the congress of Polish surgeons in 1926 benefits from the work of doctors 'specialists in anaesthetizing' were recognized for the first time in Poland. This concept became more popular in the thirties when numerous Polish physicians visited Great Britain and the USA and for the first time were brought into contact with professional anaesthesiology.

After World War II, anaesthesiology in Poland developed in a similar way to other countries in central Europe. There were two main factors that particularly contributed to the recognition of Anaesthesiology as an independent specialty: 1) The urgent need for the development of thoracic surgery. 2) The direct contact of many Polish doctors with anaesthesiology in the Allied Forces during World War II.

In addition, after the War, equipment for anaesthesia such as Heidbrink and McKesson machines became available in Poland. Curare was introduced in Poland by Stanisław Pokrzywnicki as early as 1947.

In 1949 regular postgraduate training for doctors specializing as anaesthetists was organized in Warsaw (Mieczysław Justyna) and in Łódź (Stanisław Pokrzywnicki). The system of postgraduate training courses designed to meet the needs of the hospitals developed successfully: in 1986 46 courses for basic training in anaesthesia and for advanced training in special topics were organized in Poland.

Two levels of examinations in anaesthesiology, to a large extent similar to the British system, were introduced in 1958. In 1952 anaesthesiology was recognized as an independent specialty and a national consultant in the Ministry of Health in anaesthesiology was nominated (4).

On the 18 November, 1959, the Polish Society of Anaesthesiologists was organized, which soon joined the World Federation of Societies of Anaesthesiologists (5). In Poland ten national anaesthesiology congresses have taken place including two international ones for Eastern Europe (1967 in Poznań and 1979 in Wrocław). At present the Polish Society of Anaesthesiology and Intensive Therapy (a new name) is organized in 11 regional branches that cover the whole country. Six specialist sections have also been organized for emergency care, paediatric anaesthesia, pain research and treatment, anaesthesia nursing, neuro-anaesthesia and neuro-orientated intensive care. In 1986 in Kraków a symposium on the history of Polish anaesthesia took place and a section of history of anaesthesiology was established.

In the fifties and early sixties anaesthesiology developed mainly in medical schools. In 1961 the first Chair of Anaesthesiology in the Military Medical Academy in Łódź was established (Chairman, Professor Stanisław Pokrzywnicki). In 1962 the Poznań Medical Academy followed: the first independent Department of Anaesthesiology was established (Chairman, Professor Witold Jurczyk). At present all twelve medical schools have independent departments and clinics in anaesthesiology and intensive therapy. In 1965 the first full professor of anaesthesiology was nominated (Professor Stanisław Pokrzywnicki) and now there are 14 professors and 29 associate professors (docents).

The first dissertation for a Doctor's Degree on the use of curare in surgical anaesthesia was submitted in 1949. An important factor that contributed much to the development of research was the establishment of the Committee of Pathophysiology of Anaesthesia and Resuscitation affiliated with the Polish Academy of Sciences. In 1969 a quarterly entitled *Anaesthesia and Reanimation* the official organ of the Society of Anaesthesiology and Intensive Therapy was published. This journal was also edited in English from 1973 to 1975.

In the sixties and seventies anaesthesiology developed in regional and county hospitals, where according to the instruction of the Ministry of Health independent departments of anaesthesiology and intensive therapy were established. At the moment there are about 2500 anaesthetists in Poland but the needs are twice as high.

References

(1) Kuś M. The history of anaesthesiology in Poland. *Bull Polish Med Sci Hist* 1970; **13**: 182–7.
(2) Richards W, Parbrook GD, Wilson J. Stanislav Klikowich (1853–1910). Pioneer of nitrous oxide and oxygen analgesia. *Anaesthesia* 1976; **31**: 933–40.
(3) Bożek K. Jan Prus (1859–1926). *Biogram Anest Inten Ter* 1983; **15**: 199–207 (in Polish).
(4) Jurczyk W, Pokrzywnicki S. The development of anaesthesiology in 30 years of the Polish Peoples' Republic. *Anest Inten Ter* 1974; **6**: 301–7 (in Polish).
(5) Rondio Z. 25th Anniversary of the Polish Anaesthesiologists (general reflexion). *Anest Inten Ter* 1984; **16**: 5–10 (in Polish).

5.9   The history of anaesthesia in Jordan*

M. S. M. TAKROURI
Jordan University, Amman, Jordan

There is an established idea that modern anaesthesia practised in the Middle East is due to western civilization contact with the sleeping East brought to 'Bilad Asham' (natural Syria) as a result of Ibrahim Pasha's conquest in the 19th century. As a consequence the Western knowledge acquired during Napoleon's conquest of Egypt in 1798 was transmitted.

This is only one face of the truth. The other face is that the Middle East area was not at all a complete vacuum; there was an inherited wealth of medical tradition and knowledge.

Jordan, for example, was on the way of warrior nations; many battle fields and many castles are scattered on its land. So there must have been some surgical practice, certain forms of traditional therapy and methods.

The earliest surgical thoughts recorded from this land are to be found in Ibn Al Koff's book: '*Al Omdeh, Fi Sinaat Al Jiraha*'. Abul Faradj Ibn Mouafek Eddin Yakoub Ibn Issaac Ibn Al Koff was born in 1232 A.D. in Karak. His father was in the service of King Al Nasser Yousef Ibn Mohamed and that explains his migration from Karak to Sarkhad, Damascus, Ajloun then Damascus.

In his book, he has shown a great knowledge in surgical, medical, physiological fields and even in accurate measurement. He wrote a complete chapter on pain relief. In his chapter on pain, he described the use of opium (Afune), hyoscine alkaloids and others (Al Banj).

While in Al Zahrawi's book (Abulcasis) the description of the patient under surgical interference never mentioned the use of anaesthesia since the patient was held awake by two or four servants, we see that Ibn Al Koff, on the contrary, has made reference in his book to pain relief: '. . . You should know that pain relief is of two types: true and untrue. The first is what opposes the cause of the pain . . . while the untrue pain relief is "*the Anaesthetics*" which the surgeon needs in this situation . . . the first type of pain relief is the true one and the one with good sequence while the second is untrue because, although the pain is relieved or the ability to treat is obtained and as it reduces pain, it decreases the force and fixes the painful matter to the organ. So the surgeon should use it only for great tasks and Allah is the most knowledgeable'.

This quotation indicates without doubt that pain relief only without treatment of the cause is not a cure, but the surgeon may refer to it in serious conditions during therapy.

When we study the drugs described as 'anaesthetics', we find opium and hyoscine which he described as producing sleep when given by all routes.

His meticulous classification of measures and pharmacological properties leave no doubt that this is the first true mention of anaesthesia in Jordan, since Ibn Al Koff was born in Karak (1232 AD–630 Hegire) and he was the surgeon of Ajloun Castle. His book is a serious document of medical knowledge in his era.

Ottoman Empire era

Jordan followed the Ottomanic state politically, scientifically, military and economically which meant that the scientific movement lost its originality and was restricted on following the heritage of previous Islamic product.

Medicine in particular followed 'Salajic' period for Medical Education during the 5th, 6th and 7th Hijrah century. Medical lectures were theoretical; then what was learnt was applied in the (Madrasah). Medical pupils were trained and practised in Hospital. The theoretical knowledge was acquired from Avicina's 'Al Canon' and Ali Ibn Al Abbas's 'Al Kamel'.

*Reproduced from the *Middle East Journal of Anaesthesia*, 1987; **9**: 141.

During the reign of the Turkish Sultans, Mohamad the conqueror Bayazid (1481–1512), and Soliman the great (1512–1520) the Medical Education in the Ottomanic schools was comparable to those of other famous European medical centres. Physicians and scientists from Arab countries, Persia, and Turkistan taught in the Ottomanic medical schools.

This represented the prosperous period but when the state started to weaken, medical schools deteriorated as well and fell behind European medical education specially during the reign of Soliman Al Kanouni (1520–1566).

This state of things continued as professors inherited their teaching posts from their fathers and the title of scientist was given to those who were not fit for it. The number of physicians was small but there were also surgeons and pharmacists.

During the reign of Sultan Mahmoud the second (1808–1839) a school of Medicine was founded (Toubanah) and another for surgeons (Jirahanah). The latter was transformed into a Faculty of Medicine in 1911.

We conclude from this history that whatever happened to the Ottomanic empire, happened to the people under their reign, including the Arabs. As for Jordan, there were no universities nor Faculty of Medicine. This situation prevailed until the beginning of this century.

Napoleon and Mohamad Ali in Egypt were considered as the first important line of communication with western civilization; and, although Ibrahim Pasha occupied the Jordanian city of Karak in 1848, there were no traces or known influence on medicine or anaesthesia as a result of it.

Historical landmarks

Napoleon conquest of Egypt	1798
Ibrahim Pasha in Karak	1840
Ether in America and Britain	1846
Ether in France	1847
Chloroform in Scotland	1847
Chloroform in Lebanon	1863
N_2O in Lebanon	1906

We have accepted that the early contact with Western medical science occurred in the area surrounding Jordan, but even so we may cast a great doubt on its real influence. Clout Bey was Ibrahim's Pasha physician; he has accompanied him in all his advances against Syria and if we look to what he has written in his medical book in 1835, we will find that medical instruction did not exceed what the early Arab islamic teaching left. He instructed the surgeon to give hyoscine, opium and mandrak during surgery and advised the pressure on limbs or nerves to relieve pain. He also advised that surgery should only be performed if the surgeon's skill and the patient's endurance permit it; it should be postponed until the child is old enough; it might stop if the patient cannot tolerate it and, if he loses consciousness, cold water and sniffing ammonia or vinegar were used to wake him up.

Modern times

The Jordanian region is unique in regard to civilization's influences. The Jordanian Kingdom was politically founded in 1922. Parts of Palestine which influenced Jordan were occupied in 1948. The rest was occupied in 1967. This has affected the development of its indogenous medical traditions.

On the other hand there are only few documents which give historical data concerning the period we study, so we had to rely upon personal interviews with people who lived at that period and upon personal history of medical practitioners.

The first modern Arab doctor was Dr Tawfik Kanan in Jerusalem who graduated in 1911. By 1920, four doctors existed in East bank of Jordan: Dr Souran the Armenian, Singhial the Indian, Khaled Al Khatib the Syrian and Dr Khoulousi the Turk. By 1921, Dr Mouzhar Arslan was appointed as health Consultant; Dr Rida Tawfik was the first health Director; Dr Halim Abu Rahmah was the first Director of the Department of Health appointed by British mandate governor in Palestine. He held that post until 1939 then he was followed by Dr Jamil Toutonji.

A contemporary person, Hamad Shihab, mentioned that Dr Singhial the Indian came to Jordan in 1923 and practised in Irbid and then in Amman at the site of the Italian Hospital. This surgeon used chloroform and worked in his barrack in the presence of the patient's relatives. He died in 1934. His Majesty King Abdullah sponsored him during his illness and his last days. After his death, the Italian Hospital took over his barrack and annexed it to its land.

In 1926, the first hospital clinic was founded at the Central Prison of Amman. In 1926–1927, the Italian Hospital was founded in Amman and in 1929 an Italian Hospital was founded in Karak.

According to the records of the Department of Health there were 4 doctors in 1920, 15 doctors in 1926, 47 doctors in 1927, 48 doctors in 1928, 55 doctors in 1929 and 64 doctors in 1931. Those figures do not include Palestine. According to Health Department's records only in 1949 surgery was performed in its premises.

The Italian Hospital was inaugurated by the National Italian Society Mission founded by Professor Schiaparelli. It started in 1927 with fifty beds only; by 1950 the number of beds rose to one hundred. This hospital was under the directorship of Dr Fawsto Taizio who operated and used spinal anaesthesia. Nuns used to give anaesthesia for his patients. We mention Sister Tonina, Sister Geralda, Sister Koncheta and Sister Kozima. They used the open drop method of ether using the Schimmelbusch mask. In 1948, Sister Geralda used trichloroethylene.

Dr Risucci was the first doctor anaesthetist to practice in this hospital in 1956. That was followed by Sister Maria Alba (1954) who had formal training in anaesthesia.

The Royal Medical Services had a great role in the foundation of modern anaesthesia in Jordan. The first Jordanian anaesthetist was Dr Fayez Al Nimri who graduated in 1950. He worked with the CMS Agency with Dr Anton Sahyoun. He joined the Arabic Army in 1951 and he was sent to the British Military Hospital in Egypt; then he went to London for his training in Anaesthesia. He founded the first anaesthesia section at the Army Base in Marka, Amman.

Dr Al Nimri was the first President of the Society of Anaesthesiology. He used ether and the Schimmelbusch mask, Bellamy Gradner dropper and regional blocks. He utilized the laryngoscope and endotracheal tubes, thiopentone and muscle relaxants—tubocurare and gallamine.

The first anaesthesia technician was Mohamad Ahmad Hamdan (1922–1982).

Dr Mouafak Al Fawaz founded the first section of anaesthesia in the Ministry of Health. He trained many anaesthetic technicians and he is the present President of the Anaesthesiologist Society in Jordan.

Dr Hilmi Hijazi is considered the first anaesthetist who has obtained a higher qualification, the Fellowship of Faculty of Anaesthesia. He was the anaesthesiologist in charge of the first heart transplant in Jordan, with the assistance of Dr Sami Sghier and Dr Hamdi Badr.

5.10   The early use of ether anaesthesia in Ljubljana, Yugoslavia

DARINKA SOBAN
University Hospital, Ljubljana, Yugoslavia

The earliest history of anaesthesia in Yugoslavia is still to be investigated. For many years it has been known that I. Bettini was using ether for surgical anaesthesia in March, 1847, at Zadar, Dalmatia (1). Later studies gave evidence that L. Nathan, professor of surgery at the Medico-surgical School in Ljubljana, Slovenia, started applying ether anaesthesia even earlier, in February, 1847 (2).

The spread of the use of ether inhalation through Europe and the World after Morton's successful demonstration 140 years ago seems like an explosion especially considering the rudimentary nature of the means of communication then available (3-7).

Some geographical and historical circumstances enabled the Ljubljana hospital to keep pace with the leading European surgical centres. Among the present Yugoslav university cities Ljubljana is the most northern and the nearest to Vienna; up to 1918 it was within the Austro-Hungarian empire. Ljubljana has a long tradition in medical training. At the end of the 17th and during the 18th century a society of learned professionals existed in the town (the Academica Operosorum), which had a medical section and, in 1782 a medicosurgical school (a 'lyceum') was founded. Botany, chemistry, anatomy, medicine, surgery, obstetrics, forensic medicine and veterinary medicine were taught. The first professors included the world famous Balthasar Hacquet (1739-1815).

Slovenia became part of the province Illyria after the French occupation of the country. In 1810 Ecole Centrale (a French model university) was established in Ljubljana, with faculties for medicine and surgery among others; a period of study of five years was required. After only three years of existence of this university, Austria re-occupied the country and immediately degraded the university to the former lyceum (8). From 1816 to 1818 the lecturer at this medico-surgical institution was J. Wattmann (1789-1866), who was later, from 1824 to 1848, professor of surgery at the medical faculty in Vienna. He and his former pupil F. Schuh (1804-1864) introduced ether anaesthesia in Vienna.

Leopold Nathan and the introduction of anaesthesia to Ljubljana

A graduate of the Viennese school, Leopold Nathan (1790-1860), came to Ljubljana in 1823, as professor of surgery. He held the post until the revolutionary year of 1848—when the angry Austrian government abolished all Ljubljana lyceums (9).

Nathan's first use of ether at the Ljubljana hospital on 24 February, 1847, was given publicity as an event of upmost importance on the first page of the provincial newspaper *Illyrisches Blatt*. The course of anaesthesia, surgery and patient's condition was described in detail by the director of the hospital. It is interesting to note that the chronicler credited this 'blessing for the suffering mankind' to Jackson without mentioning Morton's name. Wattmann's modification of the ether inhaler is mentioned (10) in the newspaper article. It has not proved possible to find a description or picture of this device but, thanks to some old publications, which were kindly made available by Professor H. Wyklicky, Head of the Institute for the History of Medicine at the Vienna University, some information about the inhaler used at the same time in Vienna by Schuh is available. Schuh says, 'I used an ox bladder (containing two drachms to one ounce of ether) to which I connected a short, wide metal tube with a boat-like ending, which fits around the mouth and is kept in position by an assistant. The cock inserted in the tubing for cutting off the vapours can be replaced by the cork' (11).

Conclusion

Good professional contacts between the surgeons of Vienna and Ljubljana enabled Leopold Nathan of the Ljubljana hospital* to use ether anaesthesia as early as four months after the Boston demonstration. Nathan introduced to Ljubljana the use of chloroform in the following year. The first anaesthetic with nitrous oxide was delayed until 1877 however.

---

*Another place close to Ljubljana is worth mentioning in connection with the early history of anaesthesia. This is Idrija with its mercury mine, the place where the famous naturalist Johannes Antonius Scopoli (1723-1788) was worked as a physician from 1754 to 1769. Scopoli discovered an unknown plant in the woods around Idrija which was later given the name Scopolia carniolica Jacq. It was from this Solanacea that scopolamine was first isolated (12). Scopolia roots containing the same alkaloid as Mandragora officinalis were collected for sale as 'pseudomandragora' by people in Yugoslavia in former days.

References

(1) Drešćik A. Prve eter narkoze u dalmatinskim bolnicama (The first ether anaesthesias in Dalmatian hospitals). In: Grmek M. *Iz hrvatske medicinske prošlosti* (From the Croatian medical past). Zagreb: Zbor liječnika Hrvatske, 1954: 257–61.

(2) Borisov P. *Od ranocelništva do začetkov znanstvene kirurgije na Slovenskem* (From promitive to professional surgery in Slovenia). Ljubljana: Slovene Academy of Sciences and Arts, 1977; 235–8.

(3) Neveu R. The introduction of surgical anaesthesia in France. *J Hist Med* 1946; **1**: 607–10.

(4) Ampler H. *Joseph Wattmann. Sein Leben und Werk*. Wien: Institut für die Geschichte der Medizin der Universität Wien, 1943. Dissertation.

(5) Weiger J. *Uber Aether und Chloroform zur Erzielung schmerzloser Operationen*. Wien: Carl Gerold u. Sohn, 1850: 26. Facsimile reprint, published by Abbott for the Anaesth. Congress at Innsbruck, 1979.

(6) Frankel V. The introduction of general anaesthesia in Germany. *J Hist Med* 1946; **1**: 612–7.

(7) Secher O. The introduction of anaesthesia into Denmark. In: Boulton TB, Bryce-Smith R, Sykes MK, Gillet GB, Revell AL, eds. Progress in anaesthesiology. *Proceedings of the fourth world congress of anaesthesiologists*. Amsterdam: Excerpta Medica Foundation, 1970: 165–6.

(8) Schmidt V. *Zgodovina šolstva in pedagogike na Slovenskem II* (The history of schools and paedagogisc in Slovenia II). Ljubljana: Državna založba Slovenije, 1964: 93–9.

(9) Pintar I. *Medikokirurški učni zavod v Ljubljani, njegov nastanek, razmah in knoec* (Medicosurgical teaching institution in Ljubljana, its start, development and end). Ljubljana: University of Ljubljana, 1939. 94 pp. Dissertation.

(10) Melzer R. Chirurgische Operationen unter Anwendung des Schwefelaethers. *Illyrisches Blatt* 1847; **17**: 65.

(11) Schuh F. Erfahrungen über die Wirkung der eingeathmeten Schwefelaether—Dämpfe bei chirurgischen Operationen. *Zeitschr. d.K.K. Gesellschaft d. Aerzte zu Wien* 1847; **3**: 347.

(12) Soban D. The origin of scopolamine. In: Boulton TB, Bryce-Smith R, Sykes MK, Gillet GB, Revell AL, eds. Progress in anaesthesiology. *Proceedings of the fourth world congress of anaesthesiologists*. Amsterdam: Excerpta Medica Foundation, 1970: 193–4.

Chapter 6
EARLY ANAESTHESIA IN NORTH AMERICA

6.1	The origins of anaesthesia in Canada

J. R. MALTBY
University of Calgary, Alberta, Canada

Canada in 1846 consisted of a number of British colonies and territories collectively known as British North America. The four Atlantic colonies of New Brunswick, Nova Scotia, Prince Edward Island, and Newfoundland were independent of each other and from the Province of Canada.

The Province of Canada was formed in 1841 by the union of Upper Canada (part of Ontario) and Lower Canada (part of Quebec) (Fig. 1). The vast wilderness west to the Pacific Ocean and north to the Arctic Ocean was largely undeveloped and sparsely populated. The total population of British North America in 1850 was approaching two million (1).

The country of Canada was formed by Confederation in 1867, and the terms British North America, Upper Canada, and Lower Canada became obsolete. For the remainder of this paper the more familiar post-Confederation names of Canada, Ontario, and Quebec are used.

Communications

News travelled regularly between Canada, the United States, and Great Britain. In 1840 the Cunard Steamship Line began a fortnightly mail service, which also carried newspapers, from Liverpool, England via Halifax, Nova Scotia to Boston, Massachusetts (2). All three harbours were usually ice-free in winter. The Atlantic crossing to Halifax took approximately fourteen days, and Halifax to Boston three days.

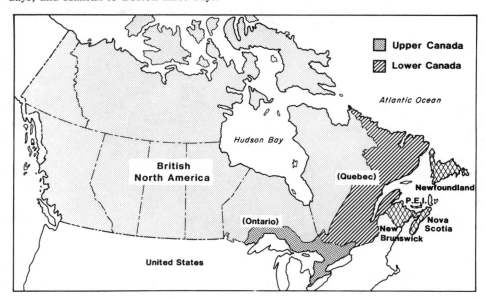

Figure 1   British North America (Canada) in 1846.

112

In 1846 mail within Canada was carried by ship or stagecoach. Although rail transport had developed in the United States, it was virtually non-existent in Canada until after 1850 (3). From Halifax, mail took up to one week to be distributed to the other Atlantic colonies and Quebec City. From the northeastern United States, mail also took up to one week to reach towns in Ontario and Quebec. Use of the electric telegraph was growing in North America during 1847–48, although it was not very reliable. Some non-medical news was transmitted by this means to a few centres in Canada.

Most Canadian newspapers were published weekly, although a few appeared three times per week or even daily. Extensive abstracting of news occurred among newspapers, which was how the public and the medical profession learned of the discovery of anaesthesia. News of painfree operations under ether in the United States reached Canada during November and December, 1846. Reports subsequently appeared from as far away as Barbados, Gibraltar, and Russia.

The only Canadian medical journal during 1846–48 was the *British American Journal of Medical and Physical Science* (BAJMPS), which was published monthly in Montreal. Its early reports of ether and chloroform anaesthesia, all of which were from Quebec, were more detailed than those in most newspapers.

Ether — earliest reports

On 3 November, 1846, the *Toronto Patriot* (4) reported W. T. G. Morton's use of ether anaesthesia in his rooms in Boston. This was two weeks before Dr H. J. Bigelow's article, 'Insensibility During Surgical Operations Produced by Inhalation', appeared on 18 November, in the *Boston Medical and Surgical Journal* (BMSJ) (5). Bigelow's paper was reprinted in the *Brockville Recorder* in Ontario on 3 December (6), and in *The Nova Scotian* in Halifax on 7 December (7).

On 12 December, *The New Brunswick Courier* in St John reported an operation under ether in Salem, Massachusetts (8). In the last week of December, three Ontario newspapers (9,10,11), reprinted Dr J. C. Warren's complete report of cases at Massachusetts General Hospital from the BMSJ of 3 December (12). The earliest reports for each province are summarized in Table 1.

Ether — first uses in Canada

Several claims for the first ether anaesthetic in Canada have been made. Most of these administrations were the first for a region and were erroneously thought to be the first in Canada.

On Saturday, 23 January, 1847, *The New Brunswick Courier* reported that on the preceding Monday (18 January) ether was administered under the direction of Adams, a dentist from Boston, when Dr Peters excised a tumour from a man's arm (16). Four days later, on Friday, 22 January, Adams administered ether again when Dr D. Millar amputated a hand (17).

Samuel Adams visited New Brunswick communities for several weeks at a time during 1846–48 to provide dental services, announcing his arrival in the local newspapers. In April, 1847, he

Table 1

Earliest reports of ether

Province	Date	City	Source
Ontario (4)	3 Nov. 1846	Toronto	*Boston Transcript*
Nova Scotia (7)	7 Dec. 1846	Halifax	*Bostn Med Surg J*
New Brunswick (8)	12 Dec. 1846	St John	*Salem Register*
Newfoundland (13)	12 Feb. 1847	St John's	*Med Times* (London)
Quebec (14)	26 Feb. 1847	Montreal	local
Prince Edward Island (15)	12 Mar. 1847	Charlottetown	local

returned to Boston to learn of further advances in anaesthesia as well as dentistry (18). He was also one of the first to use chloroform in New Brunswick (19). Dr Peters practised in New Brunswick, mostly in St John, from 1844 until at least 1882 (20).

George Van Buskirk advertised his dental practice in the *St John Evening News*, New Brunswick for six months from October, 1846 to March, 1847. In the issue on Monday, 25 January, 1847, a new entry announced that he was administering ether for dental operations. On the intervening Saturday, 23 January, the *New Brunswick Courier* published an identical notice (21).

An eminent Halifax surgeon, Dr D. McN. Parker, in his retirement speech in 1895 related how Lawrence Van Buskirk, George's brother, administered ether to him so that he, Parker, would know its effects before it was given to his patients. He performed a thigh amputation with Van Buskirk as anaesthetist and believed this was 'the first case operated on in Nova Scotia under an anaesthetic' (22). In the Faculty of Dentistry at Dalhousie University in Halifax a plaque beneath the portrait of Van Buskirk extends the claim and identifies him as the first man in Canada to administer an anaesthetic for a surgical operation (23). Parker did not give a date and, because no contemporary newspaper reference could be found, the claim to priority in Canada is neither confirmed nor refuted. It is questionable because an article in a Halifax newspaper on 29 March, 1847, reviewed the use of ether in England and made a plea for the local surgeons to start using it (24). Two more months passed before the first operations under ether in Halifax were reported, but no names were mentioned (25).

The Van Buskirk brothers were the third generation of a family of Empire Loyalists who settled in New Brunswick in 1783 (26). They both graduated in medicine from the United States and later became dentists. When Lawrence learned that ether was being used in dentistry in Boston, he went there and familiarized himself with its use (22). He was considered the leading dentist in Nova Scotia, and was the first dentist in Canada to subscribe to a dental journal (23).

Webster, a dentist in Montreal, purchased ether and an apparatus from an entrepreneur named Jones, in January, 1847. Jones was invited by Dr Horace Nelson, a surgeon, to anaesthetize two dogs to determine the animals' response to various surgical stimuli under ether. Both dogs survived extensive traumatic surgery and were allowed to recover from the ether before being sacrificed. Nelson himself inhaled ether over one hundred times and noted the symptoms it produced before allowing it to be given to a patient. On 24 February Webster, the dentist, administered ether to a debilitated woman for removal of a large thigh tumour by Wolfred Nelson, the father, assisted by Horace (27).

Horace Nelson became the editor of *Nelson's American Lancet* (28). In 1853–54 he was Professor of Surgery at the University of Vermont but returned to practise in Montreal. Although Wolfred Nelson was well known as a physician and surgeon, he was better known as a politician. He was one of the leaders of the 1837 rebellion under Papineau against what they considered British misrule (29).

Samuel Blodgett was 24 years old in 1846 when he became Ambler's dental partner (30). They practised dentistry in Ogdensburg, New York and in Brockville, Ontario, and advertised the use of letheon gas for dental surgery (31). It was Blodgett who administered ether, for which he had designed his own apparatus, when Dr Reynolds of Brockville removed a thigh

Table 2
First uses of ether during 1847

Province	Date	City	Anaesthetist	Surgeon	Operation
New Brunswick (16,21)	18 Jan. — Jan.	St John St John	Adams G. Van Buskirk	Peters G Van Buskirk	Arm tumour Dental
Quebec (27)	20 Feb.	Montreal	Webster	W. Nelson	Thigh tumour
Prince Edward Island (15)	8 Mar.	Charlottetown	Poole	Poole	Dental
Ontario (32)	8 May	Brockville	Blodgett	Reynolds	Thigh tumour
Nova Scotia (22,25)	— May	Halifax	L. Van Buskirk (?)	Parker (?)	Thigh amputation
Newfoundland (33)	— Jul.	St John's	?	Keilley	Bilat. leg amputation

tumour in May, 1847 (32). By July, 1847, a newspaper in each province had recorded one or more operations under ether anaesthesia (Table 2).

In many of the reports, the method of administration was not made clear, although an apparatus or contrivance was sometimes mentioned. The most detailed description was in the BAJMPS by Dr E. D. Worthington, a surgeon in Sherbrooke, Quebec who first used ether on 14 March, 1847:

> '*A large ox-bladder, with a stop-cock attached, a mouth-piece made of thick leather, covered with black silk and well padded round the edges, with a connecting long brass tube that had done service as an umbrella handle in many a shower, formed an apparatus that, though rude-looking, presented a very business-like and tolerably professional appearance. A couple of ounces of ether were poured into the bladder, which was then filled with air from a bellows. Not having time or ingenuity sufficient to construct a double valve, the objection to inhaling carbonic gas again into the lungs was done away with, by simply allowing the patient, after a full inspiration from the bag, to expire three or four times, when the nostrils were kept closed, and the breathing confined to the bladder.*' (34)

Worthington came from Ireland to Quebec City when he was two years old. He graduated from medical school in Edinburgh and settled in Sherbrooke (35). He gave his first ether anaesthetic at the age of 26. A year later he administered the first chloroform anaesthetic in Canada.

Chloroform—earliest reports

News of Professor J. Y. Simpson's successful use of chloroform in Edinburgh, Scotland in November, 1847, reached Canada very quickly. On 10 December, 1847, *The Guardian* in Halifax published an extract of a letter, dated Edinburgh 16 November, and signed 'C.C.', which described Simpson's chloroform experiments, his demonstration to doctors, and three minor operations under chloroform (36).

On 5 January, 1848, *The Morning Chronicle* in Quebec City reprinted an article from the Edinburgh Journal entitled The New Anaesthetic which described the advantages of chloroform over ether (37).

By the end of February, 1848, newspapers in all provinces except Prince Edward Island mentioned the discovery of the new anaesthetic (Table 3).

Chloroform—first uses in Canada

On 24 January, 1848, Dr Worthington of Sherbrooke gave chloroform to a 70-year-old lady to reduce her fractured hip (41). The following day he used it for removing a tumour on a child's hand, and then in a case of premature labour. He found chloroform preferable to ether because it was cheaper, easier to use, more agreeable, less exciting, and it was followed by less unpleasantness to the patient.

Table 3

Earliest reports of chloroform.

Province	Date	City	Source
Nova Scotia (36)	10 Dec. 1847	Halifax	*Edinburgh letter*
Quebec (37)	5 Jan. 1848	Quebec	*Edinburgh Journal*
Newfoundland (38)	18 Jan. 1848	St John's	*Caledonian Mercury*
Ontario (39)	27 Jan. 1848	St Catharines	London paper
New Brunswick (40)	— Mar. 1848	St John	*St John Courier*
Prince Edward Island	—	—	—

Less than twenty-four hours later, in the early morning of 25 January, Dr A. F. Holmes of Montreal administered chloroform to a woman in labour (42). Holmes was professor of theory and practice of medicine at McGill College in Montreal, the first Dean of the Medical Faculty of McGill University, the founder of its medical library and museum, and became president of The College of Physicians and Surgeons of Lower Canada (43).

The following week, on 1 February, in Halifax, Nova Scotia, chloroform was administered when Dr W. J. Almon amputated a woman's thumb, with Dr Parker as an observer. Almon was the third generation of a medical family which settled in Halifax after the American Revolution. He became a member of the Senate of Canada. Parker had been apprenticed to Almon's father before he went to medical school in Edinburgh. The next case was an above-knee amputation on 3 March, for which the chloroform was prepared by J. B. S. Fraser, a chemist in Pictou, 80 miles from Halifax. Fraser found the formula in a London medical journal and produced and purified the compound himself; he administered chloroform to his own wife on 22 March, for the birth of their seventh child (44).

On 17 February, in Clarendon, Ontario, Dr J. A. Sturgeon administered chloroform to ease the insomnia of a patient dying from pulmonary tuberculosis. He reported two more uses before the end of March (45). In March in St John, New Brunswick, Dr Smith performed a bilateral below-knee amputation for frostbite (40). The wording of the report infers that this was the second case in St John. In April in St John's, Newfoundland, Dr W. Carson used chloroform in a difficult obstetric case (46). No mention of chloroform was found in Prince Edward Island newspapers up to the end of July, 1848. A summary of the first administration in each province is shown in Table 4.

In contrast to the ether reports, the technique of chloroform administration was often described. An open drop method was always used. Some administrators poured it onto a handkerchief or cloth over the mouth and nose. Others placed a small sponge or some cotton in the apex of an open-ended cone or funnel which fitted over the patient's face.

Nitrous oxide

During 1846–48 no mention was found of the use of nitrous oxide in surgery or dentistry, although there were references to the gas. Horace Nelson described light ether anaesthesia for his own dental extraction as being similar to inhalation of nitrous oxide (27).

Worthington described a difficult induction with ether: 'The effect was precisely similar to that of nitrous oxide; forgetting his sore leg, the man wanted to fight . . . punched me in the side with his elbow, for a long five minutes' (41). The fact that both men compared ether with nitrous oxide suggests that the effects of inhaling nitrous oxide were widely known, at least to the medical profession.

A demonstration of the administration of 'the Nitrous Oxyde, Laughing Gas to a number of individuals showing the effect of the Exhilarating Fluid upon different constitutions' was advertised in St John's, Newfoundland on 16 November, 1847 (47).

Table 4
First uses of chloroform in 1848.

Province	Date	City	Anaesthetist	Surgeon	Operation
Quebec (41)	24 Jan.	Sherbrooke	Worthington	Worthington	Femur
Nova Scotia (44)	1 Feb.	Halifax	?	Almon	Thumb amputation
Ontario (45)	17 Feb.	Clarendon	Sturgeon	—	Insomnia
New Brunswick (40)	— Mar.	St John	?	Smith	BK amps
Newfoundland (46)	— Apr.	St John's	Carson	Carson	Obstetrics
Prince Edward	—	—	—	—	—

Discussion

News of the successful use of ether in Boston was published in newspapers in Ontario, Nova Scotia, and New Brunswick before the end of 1846. By the summer of 1847 there had been at least 80 references to ether in Canadian newspapers. The early reports of ether were enthusiastic, and some congratulated the local physicians. In Halifax, where local use of ether did not occur until six months after *The Nova Scotia* reprinted Bigelow's article, an editorial suggested that this delay was denying valuable medical treatment to the community.

Some failures were reported in which anaesthesia could not be induced with ether. In many other cases only the analgesic stage was reached. Whether this was considered desirable or was due to inexperience of the administrator is not clear. Some of those patients were awake and conversing, often in jocular vein, others described details of the operation after it was over, while attesting that they had felt no pain. Horace Nelson described his experience during a tooth extraction as '. . . perfect loss of sensation, but voluntary motion and consciousness unimpaired . . . I watched every motion of the dentist' (27).

The only administrators who took any training in Boston appear to have been the dentists Adams of St. John and Lawrence Van Buskirk of Halifax. Adams, the Boston dentist, probably learnt to give ether before he arrived in New Brunswick in January, 1847. His return visit to Boston in April included what was probably the first refresher course in anaesthesia. Whether George Van Buskirk went to Boston, or was trained locally by Adams, is not recorded; all that is known is that they both used ether in the same town in the same week in January, 1847. Lawrence Van Buskirk travelled to Boston to learn how to use ether before he became Parker's first anaethetist (22). Parker and Nelson subjected themselves to ether inhalation before allowing its use on patients. Others may have done so but did not record it. There was no report of a physician-anaesthetist visiting Boston for training.

The dental notices of Adams and G. Van Buskirk, and Nelson's inclusion of dental extractions from 'old and young persons, always with the same happy success' in his report (27) suggest that use of ether in dentistry spread quickly. Apart from dental extractions, the majority of surgical procedures were amputations for frostbite or trauma; the remainder were obstetric cases and tumour excisions.

A small number of deaths were attributed to ether and chloroform in reports from other countries. No anaesthetic deaths were reported in Canada. In a few cases ether or chloroform was given to ease the distressing symptoms of terminal illnesses, but did not contribute to the outcomes. A boy with tetanus was given ether inhalations in an attempt to control convulsions (48), and a man with advanced pulmonary tuberculosis and insomnia was given chloroform to induce sleep (45).

Having established the use of ether during 1847, each province except Prince Edward Island reported the use of chloroform in 1848 soon after its advantages over ether were described.

Acknowledgments

Copies of Canadian newspapers published in 1846–48 were either available on microfilm in the University of Calgary library, or were obtained from other sources through the interlibrary loan service.

References

(1) Kerr DGG, ed. *A historical atlas of Canada*. Toronto: Nelson, 1960: 53.
(2) Tyler DB. *Steam Conquers the Atlantic*. New York: Appleton-Century, 1939: 87.
(3) Heaton H. From confederation to the awakening of the west. In: Morrison NF, Heaton H, Bonar JC. *The Dominion of Canada*. Toronto: Nelson, 1937: 216–20.
(4) New and valuable discovery. *Toronto Patriot* 1846 Nov 3: 1(col 6).
(5) Bigelow HC. Insensibility during surgical operations produced by inhalation. *Bost Med Surg J* 1846; **35**: 309–17.
(6) For the Commercial Advertiser. *Brockville Recorder* 1846 Dec 3: 1(col 7), 2(cols 1–2).

(7) Insensibility during surgical operations. *The Nova Scotian* 1846 Dec 7: 3(cols 1–2).
(8) Accident and amputation. *The New Brunswick Courier* 1846 Dec 12: 4(col 1).
(9) Warren JC. Inhalation of ethereal vapour for the prevention of pain in surgical operations (from the *Boston Medical and Surgical Journal*). *The Globe* 1846 Dec 23: 1(cols 3–4).
(10) Warren JC. Inhalation of ethereal vapour for the prevention of pain in surgical operations (from the *Boston Medical and Surgical Journal*). *Western Globe* 1846 Dec 25.
(11) Warren JC. Inhalation of ethereal vapour for the prevention of pain in surgical operations (from the *Boston Medical and Surgical Journal*). *Toronto Patriot* 1846 Dec 29: 3(cols 3–4).
(12) Warren JC. Inhalation of ethereal vapor for the prevention of pain in surgical operations. *Bost Med Surg J* 1846; **35**: 375–9.
(13) Surgical operations without pain. *The Public Ledger* 1847 Feb 12: 4(col 3).
(14) [News item]. *The Pilot and Journal of Commerce* 1847 Feb 26: 2(col 4).
(15) Inhalation of ether. *The Islander* 1847 Mar 12 (suppl): 1(col 3).
(16) Surgical operation. *The New Brunswick Courier* 1847 Jan 23: 2(col 5).
(17) Surgery. *The New Brunswick Courier* 1847 Jan 23: 2(col 5).
(18) Dentistry. [Advertisement]. *The Gleaner* 1847 Apr 6: 207(col 3).
(19) Dental Card [Advertisement]. *The Gleaner* 1848 Jul 11: 307(col 3).
(20) Stewart WB. *Medicine in New Brunswick*. New Brunswick: The New Brunswick Medical Society, 1974: 246.
(21) Dentistical operations under the influence of the ethereal vapour. [Advertisement]. *The New Brunswick Courier* 1847 Jan 23: 3(col 1).
(22) Parker WF. *Daniel McNeill Parker, MD His Ancestry and a Memoir of His Life*. Toronto: Briggs, 1910: 394.
(23) Gullett DW. *A history of dentistry in Canada*. Toronto: University of Toronto Press 1971: 27–9.
(24) Etherism and the vapours. *The Nova Scotian* 1847 Mar 29: 2(cols 3–4).
(25) Etherism. *The Nova Scotian* 1847 May 24: 6(col 4).
(26) Eaton AWH. The History of Kings County, *Nova Scotia Heart of the Acadian Land*. Salem: The Salem Press Company, 1910: 852–3.
(27) Nelson H. Experiments with the sulphuric ether vapour. *Br Am J Med Phys Sc* 1847; **3**: 34–6.
(28) Wallace WS, ed. *The Macmillan Dictionary of Canadian Biography*. 4th rev. Toronto: Macmillan of Canada, 1978: 614.
(29) Dent JC. *The Canadian Portrait Gallery* Vol III. Toronto: Magurn 1881: 174–81.
(30) Steward DJ. The early history of anaesthesia in Canada: the introduction of ether to Upper Canada, 1847. *Can Anaesth Soc J* 1977; **24**: 153–61.
(31) "Wonders Will Never Cease" Surgical operations can be performed without pain. [Advertisement]. *St Lawrence Republican* 1847 May 3.
(32) [News item]. *Brockville Recorder* 1847 May 13: 2(col 7).
(33) Ether vapour. [Editorial]. *The Public Ledger* 1847 Jul 30: 3(col 1).
(34) Worthington ED. Case of amputation of leg—the patient under the influence of sulphuric ether vapour. *Br Am J Med Phys Sc* 1847; **3**: 10.
(35) The late Doctor Worthington. [Editorial]. *The Medical Age* 1895; **13**: 177–9.
(36) C. C. Aether superceded in surgical operations—a new discovery. [Letter]. *The Guardian* 1847 Dec 10: 186(col 4), 187(col 1).
(37) The new anaesthetic (from the Edinburgh Journal). *The Morning Chronicle* 1848 Jan 5: 3(cols 1–2).
(38) [News item]. *The Royal Gazette and Newfoundland Advertiser* 1848 Jan 18: 1(col 4).
(39) Application of chloroform to a kicking horse. *St Catharines Journal* 1848 Jan 27: 3(col 4).
(40) Amputation of both legs. *The New Brunswick Reporter* 1848 Mar 31: 79(col 1).
(41) Worthington ED. Cases of chloroform. *Br Am J Med Phys Sc* 1848; **3**: 326–7.
(42) Holmes AF. Employment of chloroform. *Br Am J Med Phys Sc* 1848; **3**: 263–4.
(43) Abbott ME. Andrew F. Holmes M.D., LL.D. *The McGill University Magazine* 1905; **IV**: 176–81.

(44) MacKenzie KA. Early adventures with chloroform in Nova Scotia. *Can Med Assoc J* 1924; **14**: 254–5.
(45) Sturgeon JA. [Letter]. *Bathurst Courier* 1848 Apr 7: 2(col 6).
(46) Chloroform. *Newfoundlander* 1848 May 4: 2(col 3).
(47) Laugh and Grow Fat! [Advertisement]. *The Public Ledger* 1847 Nov 16: 3(col 1).
(48) Crawford J. Traumatic tetanus—employment of ether inhalation. *Br Am J Med Phy Sc* 1847; **3**: 199–201.

6.2   The earliest ether anaesthetic in British North America:
a first for Saint John,[a] New Brunswick?[b]

JOSEPH A. MacDOUGALL
Saint John Regional Hospital, New Brunswick, Canada

The first use of ether anaesthesia for surgery was probably by Crawford Long in 1842 (1) in Jefferson Georgia but, two months before, in January, 1842 (2), W. E. Clarke had also administered ether for a dental extraction in Rochester, New York; however, its use did not become widespread until four years later following the first public demonstration by William Morton at the Massachusetts General Hospital when, on 16 October, 1846, he administered ether ('Letheon') to Gilbert Abbott for the excision of a neck tumour by John C. Warren (3). The news of surgical operations performed during insensibility spread rapidly. There is substantial agreement that ether was first used in Britain on 19 December, 1846, in London for a dental extraction and in Dumfries for surgery (4). There is no agreement on its first use in Canada. Matsuki, in his detailed history of ether anaesthesia in Canada gives a verified chronology (5) but on some points precise information is not given. Evidence is presented in this paper which suggests ether was first used in Saint John, New Brunswick.

The arrival of the news of the use of ether in Canada

On 1 December, 1846, the *British American Journal of Medicine and Physical Science* announced reception of the November issue of the *Boston Medical and Surgical Journal* which included H. J. Bigelow's paper on ether anaesthesia (6). This is the first information on ether published in a medical journal in Canada. In its following issue, the first of 1847, the same Journal (7), published a countervailing article, entitled 'Insensibility During Surgical Operations Produced by Inhalation'. This was extracted from the December, 1846, issue of the *Philadelphia Medical Examiner*. The medical profession, it suggested, would not be taken in by this apparent hoax. Also in January, 1847, a Montreal dentist called Webster purchased an ether inhaler and, with a Dr Horace Nelson, he experimented with ether anaesthesia in dogs. They also administered ether to each other and in March, 1847, Dr Wolfred Nelson, Horace Nelson's father removed a large tumour from a woman anaesthetized with ether by Mr Webster. The precise date is not known, but if it was before 8 March, 1847 (8), it precedes the case of Dr Worthington of Sherbrooke, who on 11 or 14 March, 1847, amputated the foot of a 30-year-old man under ether anaesthesia (9). Jacques, believed that this was the

---

[a]In the Charter of the City of Saint John the word 'Saint' is spelt in full. For many years, however, it was abbreviated by local custom to St John. In 25 April, 1925, City Common Council decided to revert to the original Saint, to distinguish their City from St John's, Newfoundland and St John, Quebec.
[b]The material published in this paper will also be included in the *Canadian Anaesthetists' Journal*.

first ether anaesthetic in Canada (10). In March, 1847, Dr James Douglass of Quebec amputated the toes of a man under ether anaesthesia (11). This precedes Dr Nelson's case and was previously thought to have been the first in Canada, the conclusion being largely on inferential from the unscientific differentiation of the terms 'lately' and 'more lately' (11).

Not surprisingly, there were also failures: A Dr Campbell at the Montreal General Hospital failed to anaesthetize a patient with ether (11). His report, together with editorial comment, appeared simultaneously (12). By 6 September, 1847, Dr J. Crawford of McGill College had attempted unsuccessfully to use ether for sedating a patient with tetanus before successfully anaesthetizing a 14-year-old boy for the amputation of a leg (13).

News of ether anaesthesia spread quickly. Dr Bigelow's paper stimulated many. Wright (14) states, 'News of ether anaesthesia had first reached Britain through the *Boston Medical and Surgical Journal* and Dr Bigelow's letter to his friend Dr Boott, which was carried in the *Acadia* from Boston to Liverpool, arriving on 16 December, 1846. Sykes (15) and Ellis (16) explored possible travel arrangements in detail.

Through Sykes we are indebted to the Cunard Shipping Line for the following information: 'We have established from our sailing records that the *Acadia*, one of the four wooden paddle steamers with which Samuel Cunard and his partners inaugurated their steamship services between Britain and North America in 1840, arrived at Liverpool on 16 December, 1846. Her voyage took just under 14 days, the average approximate time taken by Atlantic Steamers during the 1840's.' Further, the Deputy Keeper of the South Kensington Science Museum stated: 'We have a note that in 1847 The Cunard P.S. (paddle steamer) Hibernia (1843) crossed from Halifax to Liverpool in 9 days 1 hour 30 minutes at a mean speed of 11.67 knots. This was, however, a record at the time for the normal service speed of the vessel is stated to have been about 9.25 knots.'

At her usual speed, the *Acadia* would have taken about eleven and a half days from Halifax. The reference to Halifax confirms that in 1846–1847 the four ships of the British and North American Steam Packet Company sailed regularly between Liverpool and Boston, calling at Halifax, on the outward and return voyages. This is suggested in *Warden of the North* by Raddall (17). In 1846 Joseph Howe, promoting an extension of the telegraph from Saint John to Halifax, suggested that Halifax could become a clearing house for world news, 'as the first port of west bound Cunarders and the last port of the east bound.' (17).

The following documentary evidence indicates the movements of the *P.S. Acadia* in December, 1846.

> *'Cleared-Boston-Tuesday, December 1st, 1846.'*
> *'Arrived-Halifax, same day, Thursday, December 3rd, 43 hours after leaving Boston'.*
> *'Cleared-Halifax, same day, Thursday, December 3rd, 1846.'* (18).
> *'Arrived-Liverpool, December 16, 1846.'* (15)

Mail from Halifax to Saint John, which would have been cleared on Thursday, 3 December, arrived there at 10 pm, on the following Monday night five days later. Usually mail came express which took two days, but in December, 1846, the budget for this service had run out for the year and the ordinary mail was used. This took two to three days longer (19).

The first anaesthetics in New Brunswick

On Friday, 18 December, 1846, one of the seventeen Saint John newspapers (20), the *Weekly Chronicle* printed the report of the article by Henry Jacob Bigelow copied from the *Boston Medical and Surgical Journal* (3) and *The New Brunswick Courier* printed the following advertisement on 23 January, 1846:

Dentistical operations
under the influence of the
ETHEREAL VAPOUR.
Which produces insensibility to pain.

> *Mr VAN BUSKIRK has operated on several*
> *persons under the influence of the above,*
> *with complete success, and will continue*
> *it when requested.*
>
> *For further particulars please call at his*
> *rooms, Vernon's Building, Corner of King and*
> *German Streets.'*

This notice was repeated weekly until 20 March, 1847. It was also carried in the *Saint John Morning News* from 25 January, three times weekly for several months.

On Friday, 8 September, 1905, the *Saint John Globe* (21) reported a paper on the early history of Dentistry in St John, read by Dr A. F. McAvenney before the Dental Association of Halifax and subsequently published in the *Dominion Dental Journal* (22). In the fifty-seven years reviewed, between 1823 and 1880, Dr McAvenney mentions approximately thirty dentists. No details are given about eight who practised for short periods. All but two of the remainder were either from the United States or local men trained in the United States. Most were both dentists and physicians. Three were trained in New York and all the remainder were trained in Boston or Philadelphia. Dr McAvenney specifically mentions the name 'Vanbuskirk':

> *'Two brothers named Vanbuskirk practiced dentistry here in 1840. The first time ether was administered in St John for extracting teeth was in the office of the Vanbuskirks by Dr Wm. Baynard. Dr Baynard tells a very amusing story of all the precautions he took with his lady patient, and also the preperations made by the dentists in case the patient gave signs of being unruly. If she had been a raving maniac she could not have been more closely secured. . . The Vanbuskirks left St John in the early fifties, one going to Halifax, the other to Montreal.'*

The first record of the use of an anaesthetic in Saint John for general surgery, appear in *The Weekly Chronicle*, (St John), Friday, 22 January, 1847 (23).

> *'Surgical Operation.—We are informed that a tumour was yesterday removed from the arm of Mr Beatteay, of Carleton, by Dr Hunter Peters, of that place, while the man was rendered entirely insensible to pain by the inhalation of the vapor of a compound of which ether appears to form the chief ingredient—Complete sleep and insensibility were produced in three minutes by this process, under the directions of Dr Adams, of Boston, and the instant the operation was completed, an open window and a little cold water to the forehead, immediately restored the patient, who at once expressed himself as "having been very happy and quite unconscious of having felt anything" . . .*
> *The operation was performed in the presence of three Medical gentlemen, who expressed themselves perfectly satisfied with the complete and entire insensibility to pain of the patient.—Dr Adams remains a day or two in the city, when he will visit Fredericton.'*

The operation was also mentioned by a Dr Fiske in a notice in another Saint John paper the *Phoenix Advertiser* on 23 January, 1847, as an addendum to an advertisement (24):

> *'Notice.—Dr Fiske, Dental Surgeon of this City, has procured the "Letheon", a vapor administered to produce insensibility during Dental and Surgical Operations, and he will make use of it in all operations upon the mouth where it will apply. He will also direct in its use for other Surgeons, (for surgical operations) when desired.*
> *An operation was recently performed for removing a tumor from the arm at his office, by Dr Peters, of Carleton, in the presence of Drs Peters and Fitch, of this City, and other gentlemen; the result was satisfactory to all parties, and the suspension of sensibility perfect.'*

This indicates that ether anaesthesia was used in an operation which took place in Saint John, New Brunswick on Monday, 18 January, 1847, 20 days before Dr Nelson's operation in Montreal and at least 16 days before Dr Douglass's amputation, also in Montreal. It also preceded by a greater margin, Dr Worthington's amputation in Sherbrooke.

Dr Martin Hunter Peters the surgeon, was the 12th child of Charles Jeffery Peters who landed in St John on 18 May, 1783, two years after the end of the American Revolution. Charles Peters, who was born in New York, was 10 years old at the time. Dr Martin Peter's home, where the anaesthetic took place, was built for him by his father, a very successful lawyer. The house, Gothic Cottage in design, is still an attractive and interesting building (Fig. 1).

Dr George P. Peters, one of the witnesses, was a brother of Dr Martin H. Peters. Both were Edinburgh graduates. Dr George served on the Licensing Board appointed by the Lieutenant Governor to check doctors for character and competence prior to licensure. He became the Superintendent of the First Mental Hospital in British North America (25).

Dr Cyrus Fiske, a native of Salem, Massachusetts was a Harvard graduate in medicine and dentistry, one of many itinerant physicians who practised dentistry. On 19 June, 1845, he was married in St Andrews, New Brunswick, although practising medicine in Salem (26). In the *New Brunswick Courier* (NBC) of 6 December, 1845, appeared a notice informing the public that 'Dr Fiske will visit the City in a few days and will be prepared to offer all types of dental services' (27). In the NBC, 12 December, 1846, there is a description of an ether anaesthetic given by Dr Fiske in Salem (28), on Thursday, 19 November, 1846; this was copied from the Salem Register (29). In the NBC of 12 December, 1846, there is a front page notice—'Dr Fiske, Surgeon, Dentist and manufacturer of Mineral teeth—one door North of Mann's Hotel, Germain Street' (30). Dr Fiske became a successful dentist, occulist and aurist.

The NBC of 2 April, 1842, describes Dr Simon Fitch in the following notice: 'Dr Simon Fitch a graduate of Edinburgh University; member of the Medical Society of Paris and late sole house surgeon to the General Lying-in wards of Edinburgh, begs leave to offer his services in every department of his profession, to the inhabitants of Saint John and its vicinity. Residence and office in the building formerly occupied as the Post Office—corner of Germain and Princess. Advice to Poor—gratis' (31).

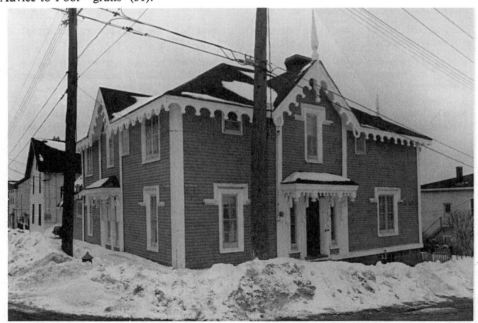

Figure 1   The home of Dr Martin Peters, corner of Watson and Gilford Streets, Saint John, New Brunswick. By kind permission of Mr and Mrs W. Foster Hammond.

The fourth physician mentioned is Dr S. Adams, a visiting consultant in anaesthesia from Boston. In a Boston directory of 1866 is listed a Dr S. Adams, Dentist; 532 Washington Street, house 3. (Boston) (32).

On Friday, 22 January, 1847 Dr Adams gave an ether anaesthetic for a partial removal of the hand by Dr David Millar of Saint John (33). On the same day, Friday, 22 January, 1847, his advertisement appeared in the *New Brunswick Reporter* and Fredericton Advertiser offering dental services and 'Etherial vapour' (34).

Wright (14), in his article, 'Early history of anaesthesia in Newfoundland,' mentions an advertisement in *The Public Ledger* (St John's Newfoundland) of 16 November, 1847, by a Dr S. Adams, a Surgeon Dentist visiting for two weeks, presumably from the mainland. On 26 November, 1847, a William L. McKay, a Chemist and Druggist, placed a similar notice in *The Public Ledger* (St John's Newfoundland), 28 November, 1847. Was this Dr S. Adams of Boston visiting again?

Ellis (16) is convinced that the news of ether was discussed during *Acadia*'s Voyage by Dr William Fraser, the ship's surgeon and some of the passengers. The news must have been spread by someone aboard for, following the vessel's arrival in Liverpool a preliminary account appeared in the *Liverpool Mercury* (16) of Friday, 18 December, 1846. It is worthy of note that in the Halifax newspaper, *The Nova Scotian* of 7 December, 1846, under 'passengers', 4 of the 43 those going from Boston to Liverpool on the *Acadia* are listed—one name was *Adams* (35).

Discussion

Information presented in the second part of this historical review became known to the author while compiling a history of anaesthesia at the Saint John Regional Hospital.

The precedence of Crawford Long and William Morton is well established, as is the sequence of events leading to the simultaneous introduction of ether anaesthesia in Scotland and England. However, bearing in mind the relative importance of Saint John in 1846, (pre-confederation) as compared to its present status, it seems reasonable to postulate that, if London and Dumfries received the news from Boston on 16 December, 1846 (4,16) carried by the *Acadia*, which called at Halifax 13 days earlier, Saint John could have and indeed did, receive the news by 10 o'clock on the night of Monday, 7 December, 1846 (19).

Early anaesthesia in Saint John was not an accident. Thousands of Loyalists left the United States for Canada following the American Revolution, (1775–1781). Saint John soon became known as the 'Loyalist City'. The immigrants were mainly from New York, New Jersey and New England. The early history of anaesthesia in the United States, Canada and England was directly associated with dentistry, and almost half of the dentists practising in Saint John between 1823 and 1880 trained in Boston. It therefore would be logical to expect early dental general anaesthesia in Saint John. While the medical profession was mainly trained in the United Kingdom and Scotland, the dental profession was almost exclusively American trained. Indeed, most were Americans. Considering the commercial, medical, dental and cultural relationships between Saint John and Boston, the presence in Saint John of some outstanding dental and Medical practitioners and the printing of Dr Bigelow's lecture from the Boston Medical and Surgical Journal in the Saint John papers following the arrival of the news in Saint John nine days before it reached Liverpool, the sequence of events seems logical. Furthermore, there is documentary evidence that ether anaesthesia was used for dentistry in Saint John in 1844 by Dr Van Buskirk and Dr William Bayard (22). Dr Daniel McNeill Parker in his memoirs, mentions that Dr Lawrence Van Buskirk gave the first ether anaesthetic in Nova Scotia (36). No date was given. Dr McAveney relates that prior to 1850 the Van Buskirks were still in Saint John (21). Support is given by Gullett who reports that George Van Buskirk of Saint John moved to Montreal in 1856 to take over the practice of W. H. Elliott (37).

The evidence presented here indicates that the first use of ether anaesthesia for general surgery in Canada was for the removal of a tumour of the arm. The patient was a Mr Beatteay of Carleton, now West Saint John. The surgeon was Dr Hunter Peters and the anaesthetist Dr Cyrus Fiske, a Saint John dental surgeon who was supervised by Dr Samuel Adams of Boston. Three medical men, one of whom was probably Dr Peters's brother and other witnesses observed.

Table 1

Names of the papers

Saint John, N.B.

The Saint John Globe
The Weekly Chronicle
The Phoenix Advertiser
The New Brunswick Courier
The Saint John Morning News

Halifax, N.S.

The Nova Scotian

The St John's Newfoundland Paper

The Public Ledger

Liverpool (England)

The Liverpool Mercury

Salem, Mass

The Salem Register

Fredericton, N.B.

New Brunswick Reporter and Fredericton Advertiser

They and the patient were perfectly satisfied with the complete and entire insensibility to pain. The operation took place on Monday, 18 January, 1847.

Acknowledgments

To the staffs of the following Libraries I am deeply grateful for their real help to a retired novice: Saint John Free Public Library, Dr Carl R. Trask Health Sciences Library, New Brunswick Museum Library, W. K. Kellogg Health Sciences Library, Halifax City Regional Library, New Brunswick Archives Department of Historical and Cultural Resources, Ward Chipman Library, University of New Brunswick, Saint John, University of New Brunswick Library, Salem Public Library, Salem, Massachusetts and The Francis A. Countway Library of Medicine, Boston, Massachusetts.

I am also grateful to Dr Ian Keith, Department of Anaesthesia, Saint John Regional Hospital, Dr Peter Toner, Professor, Department of History, University of New Brunswick, Saint John, Dr Oskar Sykora, Faculty of Dentistry, Dalhousie University, Halifax, Nova Scotia, Dr A. D. Gibbon, Frank O'Brien and Harold Wright three local historians, Mrs Barbara McCrossin, Secretary, Department of Anaesthesia, Saint John Regional Hospital, Mr Brian Daley and staff of the Media Productions Department, Saint John Regional Hospital and Mr and Mrs W. Foster Hammond (present owners of the Peters House).

Dedication

I would like to dedicate this article to my many former chiefs—Dr Wesley Bourne of St Mary's Hospital, Montreal, Dr Digby Leigh and Dr Kathleen Belton of Children's Hospital, Montreal, Dr Harold Griffith of Homeopathic Hospital, Montreal and RCAF, Dr Ned Lunney, Dr Fred

Jennings, Dr Ralph Connell, Dr Eli Davis of Saint John General Hospital and Dr Preston Leavitt, Present Chief Saint John Regional Hospital. I am blessed to have worked with such a distinguished group of physicians. May we all meet again in Heaven.

References

(1) Long CW. An account of the first use of sulphuric ether by inhalation as an anaesthetic in surgical operations. *South Med Surg J* 1849; **5**: 705–13.
(2) Keys TE. *The history of surgical anaesthesia.* New York: Schuman's, 1945: 21–2.
(3) Anonymous. Insensibility During Surgical Operations Produced by Inhalation. *The Weekly Chronicle* 1846; Dec 18: 1(col 4,5,6) 2(col 1,2).
(4) Sykes WS. *Essays on the first hundred years of anaesthesia,* Vol 1. Edinburgh, London, Melbourne and New York: Churchill Livingstone, 1982: 51.
(5) Matsuki A. A chronology of the very early history of inhalation anaesthesia in Canada. *Can Anaesth Soc J* 1974; **21**: 92–5.
(6) *Br Am J* 1846; **2**: 226.
(7) *Br Am J* 1847; **2**: 247.
(8) *Br Am J* 1947; **3**: 34.
(9) *Br Am J* 1947; **3**: 10.
(10) Jacques A. Anaesthesia in Canada, 1847–1967: 1. The beginnings of anaesthesia in Canada. *Can Anaesth Soc J* 1967; **14**: 500–9.
(11) *Br Am J* 1847; **2**: 338.
(12) *Br Am J* 1847; **2**: 304.
(13) *Br Am J* 1847; **3**: 199.
(14) Wright DJ. The early history of anaesthesia in Newfoundland. *Can Anaesth Soc J* 1979; **26**: 231–8.
(15) Sykes WS. *Essays on the first hundred years of anaesthesia,* Vol 1, Edinburgh, London, Melbourne and New York: Churchill Livingstone, 1982: 52.
(16) Ellis RH. The introduction of ether anaesthesia to Great Britain. *Anaesthesia* 1976; **31**: 766.
(17) Raddall TH. *Warden of the North.* McClelland and Stewart. 1971: 194.
(18) Shipping Intelligence. *The Nova Scotian (Halifax)*; 1846 December 7, Pg 3. col. 4.
(19) *The Morning News (Saint John)* Wednesday, December 9, 1846 p. 2. col. 1.
(20) O'Brien F. Old papers and early journalists. *The Citizen* 1985; **18**: 4(col 1,2).
(21) McAvenney AF. Early history of dentistry in Saint John. *Dominion Dental Journal* 1905; **17**: 431–8.
(23) *The Weekly Chronicle (St John)* Friday, January 22, 1847, p. 2 col. 4.
(24) *The Phoenix Advertiser,* Saturday, January 23, 1847, p. 2 col. 3.
(25) Stewart WB. Medicine in New Brunswick. *The New Brunswick Medical Society.* 1974: 286.
(26) Ward Scrapbook (Small), shelf 19, p. 91, New Brunswick Museum.
(27) *The New Brunswick Courier,* December 6, 1845, p. 2 col. 5.
(28) *The New Brunswick Courier,* Saturday, December 12, 1846. p. 4 col. 1.
(29) *Salem Register,* November 23, 1846, p. 2.
(30) *The New Brunswick Courier,* Saturday, December 12, 1846 p. 1 col. 5.
(31) *The New Brunswick Courier,* Saturday, April 2, 1842 p. 1 col. 3.
(32) *Boston Directory, City Record, General Directory of the Citizens and a Business Directory,* Boston: Sampson, Davenport & Co., 1866.
(33) Surgery. *The New Brunswick Courier,* 1847, Jan 23: 2(col 5).
(34) *New Brunswick Reporter and Fredericton Advertiser*—Friday, January 22, 1847.
(35) The Nova Scotian, December 7, 1846 p. 7 col. 3.
(36) Parker WE. Daniel McNeill Parker M.D. His ancestry and a memoir of his life. Toronto: William Briggs, 1910: 394.
(37) Gullett DW. A history of dentistry in Canada. University of Toronto Press, 1971: 29.

6.3   Anaesthesia in Quebec: the first twelve months

A. J. C. HOLLAND
McGill University, Montreal, Quebec, Canada

Morton is regarded as the 'Father of Anaesthesia' because of his successful demonstration on 16 October, 1846, of ether anaesthesia, even though Crawford Long and Horace Wells had given successful anaesthetics before him. Morton's performance (not too strong a word) was however published in *The Boston Medical and Surgical Journal* by Henry Bigelow, one of the surgeons of the Massachusetts General Hospital. The inhalation was 'a preparation' and afterwards the patient said that he was aware of the operation, although the pain was mitigated. On the following day totally successful anaesthesia for a deltoid tumour was obtained. Bigelow's article then goes on to describe four anaesthetics given by Dr Morton on that one day—all successful. In his early descriptions, Morton (or Bigelow) obviously watched the patient's pulse, respiratory frequency, and colour (1).

At the end of the article there was a real attempt to prevent the nature of his new drug from being released, and the article itself provoked a storm of controversy, both on medical and religious grounds. The story of the first year of anaesthesia in Quebec takes one from the initial introduction of ether anaesthesia, to the earliest descriptions of the use of chloroform.

Comments from the *Philadelphia Medical Examiner* following Morton's demonstration are worth quoting in full (2):

> '*From a paper by Dr H. J. Bigelow, "one of the Surgeons of the Massachusetts General Hospital," contained in the Boston Journal of the 18th of November, 1846, we derive the astounding information that Dr Warren and Dr Hayward—men at the very top of our profession—have allowed Morton to administer his "preparation"—"a secret remedy" for which he has taken out a patent—to patients on whom they were about to operate! Dr Bigelow says, in extenuation of the course pursued by Morton in taking out a patent, that "it is capable of abuse, and can readily be applied to nefarious ends;" that "its action is not yet thoroughly understood, and its use should be restricted to responsible persons" and that, one of its greatest fields is the mechanical art of dentistry, many of whose processes are, by convention, secret, or protected by patent rights. It is especially with reference to this art, that the patent has been secured.*' (2)

The Philadelphia Medical Examiner then goes on to condemn the medical profession of Boston in the following high-flown language:

> '*We are persuaded that the surgeons of Philadelphia will not be seduced from the high professional path of duty, into the quagmire of quackery by this will-o'-the-wisp; and if any of our respectable dentists should be tempted to try this new "patent medicine", we advise them to consider how great must be the influence of an agent over the nervous system, to render a person unconscious of pain—the danger there must necessarily be from such overpowering medication, and that if a fatal result should happen to one of their patients, what would be the effect upon their conscience, their reputation and business, and how the practice would be likely to be viewed by a Philadelphia court and jury? We cannot close these remarks, without again expressing our deep mortification and regret, that the eminent men, who have so long adorned the profession in Boston, should have consented for a moment to set so bad an example to their younger brethren, as we conceive them to have done in this instance. If such things are to be sanctioned by the profession, there is little need of reform conventions, or any other efforts to elevate the professional character—physicians and quacks will soon constitute one fraternity.*' (2)

In Montreal the *British American Journal* took a somewhat less sanctimonious view of the ether controversy and wrote (3):

> '*While we cannot but reprobate the method adopted by Mr Morton, a dentist of Boston, (who claims the discovery) in patenting the process, and endeavouring to render it tributary*

to his own pecuniary advantage, nor less, the encomiums passed upon it by Drs Bigelow, Warren, and Haward . . . we yet conceive that there exists ample grounds for announcing this important act, that the pain attendant, upon surgical operations may, in a great majority of cases, be very considerably alleviated, if not entirely allayed, by a recourse to the means of which we are now writing.' (3)

Communications and priorities

It is not surprising that anaesthetics were given in Quebec so soon after their initial description— after all anaesthesia, in the mid-19th century was an idea whose time had come—but what was surprising was the speed at which the news of anaesthesia spread around the world.

Only a handful of articles have been written during the last thirty years which deal with the history of anaesthesia in Canada, and to the casual reader these tend to give a somewhat confusing picture of who did what and when.

Historical priorities can be difficult if not impossible to establish and regional sensibilities may further increase the difficulty, but careful reading of the appropriate journals can often clarify points of controversy, and this is true of the early history of anaesthesia in Quebec.

It is well established that in Quebec province (then known as Lower Canada) the first anaesthetics were given in Montreal, Sherbrooke, and Quebec City by April, 1847. It seems most probable that the news of ether anaesthesia and the description of the techniques used had come from Boston by way of a number of possible combined stage-coach, railway, and packet boat routes to Montreal via Albany, Portland and Quebec City (4). An alternative route by packet boat from Boston to Halifax and then from Halifax to Quebec province by boat, rail, or stage-coach, appears not to have been used at that time possibly because of distances involved. Indeed, such was the number of ways of getting from Boston to Quebec province that it comes as no real surprise that anaesthesia was apparently given simultaneously and independently in the three largest cities of the province.

It is difficult to say with precision who gave the first anaesthetic in Quebec. By April, 1847, Dr James Douglass in Quebec City, Dr Horace Nelson of Montreal, and Dr E. D. Worthington of Sherbrooke had all reported successful anaesthetics (5,6,7).

Which of these three actually gave the first anaesthetic will probably never be known for certain because of lack of dated records and also because there was initially no clear differentiation between anaesthesia for surgical operations and anaesthesia as an experimental procedure.

Dr Campbell, at the Montreal General Hospital, had described an unsuccessful attempt at ether anaesthesia, for amputation of the leg of an alcoholic, which 'was afterwards removed in the ordinary way'. (5)

The articles on anaesthesia, in general were similar to those coming from other countries, but those from Dr Worthington and Dr Nelson, containing as they did, descriptions of the apparatus used and physiological changes in their patients, represented the beginning of the scientific study of anaesthesia in Canada (6,7).

Interestingly enough Dr J. Crawford used ether in an effort to relieve the rigidity and spasm from traumatic tetanus. This was done at the suggestion of Dr Mahony, Inspector General of Hospitals, and although unsuccessful, seems to be the first recorded instance where ether was so used (8).

Chloroform

Within twelve months, religious and medical objections to anaesthesia had largely ceased, and many of the problems with ether anaesthesia such as variability in patient requirements and difficulties in inducing anaesthesia in alcoholics had been noticed. It is interesting on reading Quebec medical journals published in 1847 and in newspapers of the time, in which anaesthetic successes or failures were recorded rather like football scores, how many Quebecers suffered from 'intemperate habits'.

The time was ripe therefore for the introduction of a drug which was apparently slightly more predictable than ether in its effect. Chloroform, which was almost certainly introduced to Quebec and the rest of Canada from the British Isles, seemed to meet this requirement.

The first chloroform anaesthetic administered in Quebec was almost certainly given by Dr E. D. Worthington (9) who had previously used and described ether anaesthesia in his surgical practice. His initial description of the use of chloroform was very enthusiastic, and he continued to use it as his drug of first choice for the rest of his life.

There were other doctors in Quebec province who gave chloroform anaesthetics independently of Dr Worthington and within a few days of his first use of this drug. Notable among these was the anaesthetic given by Dr A. F. Holmes on 25 January, 1848 (a day after Dr Worthington), in which he successfully employed chloroform for midwifery (10).

In the same journal in which Dr Holmes had described his use of chloroform, an editorial comment gave to the interested reader the name of the principal manufacturer—S. J. Lyman and Company, who also advertised widely in the Montreal newspapers of the time—together with a formula for its manufacture.

Of all the early descriptions of chloroform anaesthesia those by Dr Worthington were the most scientific in their appreciation of the drug and methods of administration (12). Not unexpectedly most of the descriptions of the use of chloroform tended to be anecdotal and there was little difference between one author and another in this respect.

At the end of the first twelve months of anaesthesia in Quebec chloroform had almost entirely replaced ether as an anaesthetic agent. It remained for a later date for the dangers of chloroform to be appreciated and for articles on religion and anaesthesia (13), and criminal assault on an anaesthetized patient, to be written (14).

The pattern of anaesthesia that was created in the twelve months after its introduction into Quebec tended to follow the British tradition. There was an important difference however, in that the vast majority of anaesthetics given in Quebec were domiciliary, and therefore chloroform, because of its portability and potency was preferable to ether for a doctor making his rounds over a great distance on horseback. Indeed chloroform anaesthesia as practised in this fashion was common in rural Canadian medical practice until World War II (15).

References

(1) Bigelow HJ. Insensibility during surgical operations produced by inhalation. *Boston Med Surg J* 1846; **35**: 309–17.
(2) Editorial comment. Insensibility during surgical operations produced by inhalation. *The Philadelphia Medical Examiner*. December 1846 (later reprinted in the *Br Am J* 1847; **2**: 247–8).
(3) Editorial. Inhalation of sulphuric ether vapour. *Br Am J* 1847; **2**: 304–5.
(4) Holley OC. *The picturesque tourist*. New York: Disturwell, 1844.
(5) Editorial comment. Employment of sulphuric ether vapour in Montreal, Quebec, and Sherbrooke. *Br Am J* 1847; **2**: 338.
(6) Nelson H. Experiments with the sulphuric ether vapour. *Br Am J* 1847; **3**: 34–6.
(7) Worthington ED. Case of amputation of leg—the patient under the influence of sulphuric ether vapour. *Br Am J* 1847; **3**: 10.
(8) Crawford J. Traumatic tetanus—employment of ether inhalation. *Br Am J* 1847; **3**: 199–201.
(9) Worthington ED. Cases of chloroform. *Br Am J* 1848; **3**: 326–7.
(10) Holmes AF. Employment of chloroform. *Br Am J* 1848; **3**: 263–4.
(11) Editorial comment. *Br Am J* 1848; **3**: 278.
(12) Worthington ED. *Reminiscences of student life and practices*. Sherbrooke: Walton and Co, 1897: 81–5.
(13) DeSola A. Critical examination of genesis III.16. Having Reference to the employment of anaesthetics in cases of labour. *Br Am J* 1850; **5**: 227–9; 259–62; 290–3.
(14) Editorial comment. Licet omnibus, licet nobis, dignitatem artis medicae tueri—The late trial of Dr Webster for a criminal assault. *The Medical Chronicle* 1858–59; **6**: 231–9; 275–81; 427–8.
(15) Gordon RA. A capsule history of anaesthesia in Canada. *Can Anaesth Soc J* 1978; **25**: 75–83.

6.4

Anaesthesia in early California

SELMA HARRISON CALMES
Kern Medical Center, Bakersfield, USA

In 1846, when surgical anaesthesia was first successfully demonstrated in Boston, California was, indeed, a very isolated country geographically and politically. Because of this isolation, California probably did not learn about anaesthesia until after many other parts of the world. At the very earliest, anaesthesia probably reached California during the Gold Rush of 1849, and it was not always used for operations, even 10 years after its demonstration in Boston.

This paper documents what I have been able to find about the introduction of anaesthesia into California. It is useful to define four separate periods. First, surgery and the relief of surgical pain in early California, before 1846, second, the period 1846 to the Gold Rush of 1849, when anaesthesia should have become known, then the period 1849–1856, when the state's first medical journal began publication and we get the first definitive evidence about anaesthesia and, finally, the years 1856–1897. This last period covers the time between proper documentation that anaesthesia was in use and the year in which the first California physician decided to specialize in anaesthesia. This was Dr Mary Botsford of San Francisco. She was not able to earn a living giving anaesthesia at that time, but she did decide to specialize.

Before 1846

The California Indians undertook surgery, such as the trephining of skulls and the repair of eviscerations resulting from battle wounds. Pain relief was with herbal preparations. The native Californian poppy was known to relieve pain. Belladonna alkaloid preparations, derived from Jimson weed, were also used for pain relief as well as to induce hallucinations for religious purposes (1,2,3).

Explorers from several countries came to California, beginning in the 16th century. But there was not much to recommend the state at the time. Spain, established in nearby Mexico, thought there were threats to California from Russia and England, both of whom were involved in fur trading along the Pacific Coast. Spain began to colonize California in 1769. It used its previously successful method, religious colonization, and formed a chain of 21 missions along the coast (4).

The first physician in the state, Pedro Prat, came that year. He was the first of the Spanish Surgeon Generals to be stationed at the Presidio (fort) in Monterey, the governmental capital for California. These Surgeon Generals were the only doctors in the state except for an occasional physician from a visiting naval or trading vessel that happened to stop (2). Only a few ships visited California, because the Spanish government forbade trade with other countries at this time. There are no records of operations by these physicians. They were probably too busy treating scurvy, which was a serious problem at the time, to operate.

Most medical care was by the mission padres, who had simple medical kits and who had been instructed in basic medicine and surgery. They even knew how to perform Caesarean sections on women who died during childbirth. Two Caesarean sections are recorded, in 1805 and 1825. They were both fatal to mothers and babies (2,5). The padres' methods of pain relief are not known, but were probably based on alcohol.

Mexico became independent from Spain in 1821, and California came under Mexican control. The missions were secularized 3 years later. Trade with other countries began to increase. This was primarily with the United States, which needed hides and tallow for the shoe and candle factories that were developing in New England. Overland travel began after 1841.

America became interested in California when it discovered that England had sent a counsel there in 1842 to work for the annexation of California to England and, also, that Mexico had offered California to England as security for a loan. America began the Mexican–American War in May, 1846, partly to acquire California. American troops landed in the state in July, 1846, and declared that California belonged to the United States. However, the Mexicans in the state put up quite a fight, and California did not surrender to the United States until January, 1847 (6).

1846–1849

So, California was thus not a part of the United States at the time of the ether demonstration, either politically or geographically. The western border of the United States was just half way across the continent. For the next 3 years (1846–1849), the period when nearly all the world learned of anaesthesia, there was not much reason for the news to reach California. First, there were hardly any physicians. There were only five trained physicians we know of, and two Army surgeons. There was no hospital, no pharmacy, no medical school, no medical society, and no medical journal (7). Travel was very difficult. It took a minimum of six months, at the best, to get there either by the Overland route or by the usual sea journey around the Horn. There was no regular mail service, either with the United States or within the state (6) and so there was little chance of the news coming quickly in a letter or by way of medical journals exchanged between physician-friends. Because of these travel difficulties, the earliest the news of anaesthesia could have reached California would have been April, 1847.

We do have a very complete record of the activity of one of the Army physicians in California during the period 1846 to 1849, and these records confirm this isolation. The diary and correspondence of Dr John Griffin cover the period from December, 1846, to 1853. He ran out of medical supplies and had to send for more, because there were none in the state, they came from Hawaii. He did not receive any medical journals until 1848, when a friend sent him some. He requested a *Dispensory* in 1847, the then equivalent of a pharmacology text, but he was told there was just one copy in the state for all the Army surgeons, and it had already been distributed.

During this period, there is no mention of anaesthesia, and there were no requisitions for it. Morphine and opium were his only methods of pain relief (7,8,9). He wrote frequently and sympathetically of his soldier patients' suffering and, if anything had been available to help them, he certainly would have mentioned it. The Griffin material documents the intense isolation of the state at that time.

1849–1856

California's isolation changed in 1849. In January, 1848, gold was discovered at Coloma, near Sacramento. Because of the isolation and travel difficulties, the news did not reach the East Coast of the United States until September and did not become widely known until December, 1848 (6). Then, in early 1849, the world rushed in! The 'forty niners' included an estimated 1300–1500 physicians (10), few of whom came to practise medicine. They came to 'strike it rich', and only practised medicine when they failed at that, as did most forty niners.

It became easier to get to California. The sea route was shortened from six months to six weeks by crossing Central America at the Isthmus of Panama or Nicaragua. Overland travel still took six months, however. Either way, travel was still quite difficult and often fatal, due to cholera, the ever-present scurvy, malaria and accidents (6). Medical communication improved, and there is evidence of the arrival of United States medical journals (11).

During the period 1849–1856, there must have been some use of anaesthetics, but this has been impossible to document precisely. The evidence is presumptive or, mostly, negative, i.e. that anaesthetics were not used. The presumptive evidence consists of information on Dr Edward Willis, an English surgeon, who was a graduate of Edinburgh and London. He somehow found his way to the tiny Gold Rush town of Placerville, where he was one of two physicians in town. In his canvas tent 'office', he displayed his microscope, a stethoscope, splints of various kinds, a huge jar of leeches and surgical instruments. A blue sign with gold letters declared 'Dr Edward Willis, MRCS. Surgery and Physic in all branches. Sets bones, draws teeth painlessly, bleeds, advice gratis' (12). Unfortunately, there is only one mention of Dr Willis. It is probably safe to presume that he was familiar with anaesthetics as an Edinburgh graduate, that he brought some anaesthetic agents with him (after all he brought his microscope and stethoscope) and that, as he promised that he could 'draw teeth painlessly', and used anaesthesia at least for that.

The rest of the evidence about the use of anaesthetics during the period 1849–1856 is negative. The first hospital built in the state had no room for surgery (13). The 1850 Fee Bill, or 'Aviso', for Los Angeles physicians, the first in the state, did not include a charge for anaesthesia (14). Most importantly, Gold Rush California was primarily a male world; there were few women and children until the mid-1850s. When anaesthesia was first introduced to America, it was used selectively, usually for women and children, the rich and educated. These were the groups that physicians of the time thought were 'sensitive' and needed pain relief. In contrast, men were thought to be strong and not need pain relief as much. Indeed, the experience of undergoing surgery without anaesthesia was thought to be helpful in achieving manhood (15). I expect the structure of California society at that time resulted in infrequent use of anaesthesia, if it was even available. There is evidence this 'macho' mentality may have lasted as long as 1858. A patient with a torn urethra after pelvic trauma underwent his operation apparently without anaesthesia: 'The operation was easily and quickly performed, and whatever pain it might have occasioned was either not felt, or not regarded, on account of his intense suffering from the accumulated urine.'

The medical literature also documented patient demand that same year, during an operation for retained placenta: 'The patient *insisting* on being rendered insensible, chloroform was administered . . .' (16).

By 1856, 10 years after the ether demonstration, California had changed markedly. The Gold Rush was over, there were families, agriculture was established and there was mail service with the United States and within the state (6). That year, California's physicians got a way to communicate, when the state's first medical journal began publication. It only lasted one year (because of lack of interest!), but, that first medical journal tells us a lot about anaesthesia which was then well established. Anaesthesia is mentioned on the very first page of the very first issue, in a report of a discussion at a Sacramento County Medical Society meeting. The case report was about the possible additive effects between morphine and chloroform. In this case, the effects may have been fatal, because the patient died (17). That same first page also described another death from chloroform.

Thirteen operations were reported in that volume. There was no mention of anaesthesia for four of these. Chloroform was used in six and ether in three. Two labouring patients received chloroform, one because the patient demanded it. So, chloroform was by far the most commonly used agent 10 years after the ether demonstration.

This volume also reported, in abstracts from other medical journals, an estimated 85–87 deaths from chloroform in Edinburgh and Boston, and the use of anaesthesia in an astounding number of other problems, including asthma, bronchitis, pneumonia, to induce sleep at night, as a local anaesthetic, in strychnine poisoning and in 'intermittent fever'.

Anaesthesia also made the popular press that year. A notorious stabbing victim in San Francisco died soon after surgery, and the following poem appeared, showing popular awareness of the hazards of anaesthesia.

> *"Who killed cock robin?*
> *I, says Dr 'Scammon'*
> *With my chloroform and gammon*
> *I killed cock robin.*
>
> *Why was it given*
> *In a smothering dose, by heaven?*
> *I refuse to say*
> *Replied Dr Gray."*

The rest of the poem included reference to the possibility of a sponge being left in the wound as well (18).

The final time period, 1856–1897, was a time of slow growth in anaesthesia. The second medical journal in the state began publication in 1858 and had pharmacy advertisements for anaesthetics, including preparations made here. In 1874, there was an article on 'stealing' children to sleep (19), which was the first English-language article on that technique. That year also brought the first mention of charges for anaesthesia services. The Alameda County Medical Society 'Fee Bill' (comparable to the present Relative Value guides) stated: 'Administration of anaesthesia in any case $5–25.' Operations, in contrast, were $100–500 for majors, $25–100 for secondary operations and minor procedures were $5–25 (20). Mortality was estimated in 1883, with deaths thought to occur once in every 2800 anaesthetics. The article ended with a plea for professional anaesthetists: 'When the administration of anesthetics becomes an isolated profession, and shall become the business of men who shall do nothing else (an example of which is the celebrated Dr Clover in London), then it is probable that the mortality will fall much under that above given' (22).

An interesting article in 1895, one year before our first specialist began work, demonstrated how far anaesthesia had come in California. This article emphasized much of what we consider today to be basic for safe anaesthetic practice. Dr Frank Bullard of Los Angeles wrote, that: 'The patient should *always* be in the recumbent position, anaesthetization should never be attempted in any other posture,' that 'eternal vigilance should be the watchword of the anaesthetizer' and 'the falling back of the tongue and closure of the epiglottis are usually prevented by keeping the jaw well forward during the anaesthesia.' He also provided statistical data on his own practice, including the incidence of complications and deaths (23).

Conclusion

This paper has briefly discussed how anaesthesia might have reached California and the early years of its use. Although the documentation is not yet perfect, the evidence so far suggests that anaesthesia did not reach the state until the Gold Rush of 1849, well after the rest of the world knew about it. This delay was because of California's geographic and political isolation. Once anaesthesia was available, it was not used for every operation until at least 1858. This probably was due to the cultural factors determining who received anaesthesia, to the male character of California's population, and to the fact that anaesthesia may not have been easily available.

References

(1) Welton J, Gratiot J, Michael P. *The medical history of Monterey County*. Monterey: Monterey Literary Association, 1969, 8–10.
(2) Bard CL. A contribution to the history of medicine in Southern California. *South Calif Pract* 1894; **9**: 287–313.
(3) Snodgrass W. *Medicine in Santa Monica: A history of medical practice in the greater Santa Monica Bay area*: Santa Monica, 1968: 9–10.
(4) Pomeroy E. *The Pacific Slope: A history of California, Oregon, Washington, Idaho, Utah and Nevada*. Seattle: University of Washington Press, 1965: 9–12.
(5) Shuman JS. *California medicine (A review)* Los Angeles: A. R. Elliott Publishing Co, 1930: 20–31.
(6) Bean WE. *California: An interpretive history*. New York: McGraw-Hill, 1973.
(7) Warren VL. Dr John S. Griffin's mail, 1846–53. *Calif Hist Soc Quart* 1954; **33**: 97–124.
(8) Ames GW. A doctor comes to California: The diary of John S. Griffin, Assistant Surgeon with Kearny's Dragoons. 1846–47. *Califor Hist Quart* 1942; **21**: 193–224 and 333–57.
(9) John S. Griffin, M.D. *Manuscript material*, Berkeley: The Bancroft Library, University of California.
(10) Jones JR. *Memories, men and medicine: A history of medicine in Sacramento, California*. Sacramento: Sacramento Society for Medical Improvement, 1950: 24.
(11) Leonard JP. Letter from California. *Boston Med Surg J* 1849–50; **41**: 394–9.
(12) Harwood J. A general practitioner in California in Once a Week, Feb 9, 1861, quoted in Lyman GD. *The scalpel under three flags in California* San Francisco: California Historical Society, 1925: 40–41.

(13) Harris H. *California's medical story* San Francisco: JW Stacey Inc, 1932: 82.
(14) Kress GH. *The medical profession in Southern California* 2nd Ed. Los Angeles: Times Mirror Printing, 1910: 8.
(15) Pernick M. *A calculus of suffering: Pain, professionalism and anaesthesia in nineteenth century America* New York: Columbia University Press, 1985: 171–96.
(16) Meigs CD. Letter from Sacramento. *Pacific Med Surg J* 1858; **3**: 187–93.
(17) NA. Abstract from proceedings of Sacramento Medical Society session of April 30, 1856. *Calif State Med J* 1856; **1**: 35.
(18) Lyman GD. *The scalpel under three flags in California*. San Francisco: California Historical Society, 1925: 54.
(19) Cluness WR. Two cases of anaesthetization during sleep. *Pacific Med Surg J* 1874; **16**: 21–2.
(20) *Alameda County Fee Bill 10/5/74*. In medical pamphlet file, The Bancroft Library, University of California, Berkeley.
(21) Lane LC. Anaesthetics. *Pacific Med Surg J* 1883; **26**: 49–68.
(22) Bullard FD. A study of anesthesia. *South Calif Pract* 1896; **11**: 281–96 and 321–8.

6.5   To keep Ether Dome a show place*

M. TVËRSKOY
Safed Government Hospital, Israel

In 1965, Ether Dome Massachusetts General Hospital was designated a Registered National Historic landmark. Evidence of this is the memorial plaque on one of the walls of the famous auditorium. Doctors of Massachusetts General Hospital contributed greatly to the development of medicine but as the eminent pioneer Schleich has said, 'All great medical discoveries are made outside the stronghold of the official guardian of science.' (1)

The world glory of the Massachusetts General Hospital was given by the unknown 27-year-old dentist, William Thomas Green Morton, whose bronze bust decorated the Hall of Fame for Great Americans in New York, since 1920. Morton's other bust, which in the past was in Ether Dome, is no longer in existence. The auditorium is now used as a regular lecture hall. The small museum which is connected to Ether Dome from the back, is a common passageway to the active doctor's office and has nothing in common with the triumph over pain. At the same time in Georgia, on the foundation of Doctor Long's original office, on 15 September, 1957, was dedicated and opened to the public the Crawford W. Long Memorial Museum in Jefferson, through which many visitors pass.

The contemporaries of those days were unable to decide who was the discoverer of anaesthesia, but it would seem that in Boston the decision has not been made in favour of Morton. But that is not the issue. It is certain that in the history of anaesthesia there was no event equivalent in importance to that which happened in Ether Dome on famous Friday morning, 16 October, 1846. The place where this occurred—Ether Dome of the old building of the Massachusetts General Hospital, is worthy of being a museum for commemorating and illustrating not only the history of the United States, but that of the entire civilized world.

Reference

(1) Schleich KL. *Those were the good days! Reminiscences*. London: Unwin, 1935: 192.

*This communication was presented as a poster.

Chapter 7
HOW THE NEWS OF ANAESTHESIA CAME TO THE ANTIPODES

7.1   The news spreads along the trade routes of the British Empire

GWEN WILSON

Australian Society of Anaesthetists, Edgecliff, New South Wales, Australia

---

This is a story of sea, of ships, and of sea-lanes. It is the story of the spread of the news of painless surgery to the far places beyond Europe.

The story began immediately after Morton's anaesthetic in Boston, when Jacob Bigelow commented 'This is something which will go round the world.'

No matter whether by sea, land or air; no matter whether it is 1847 or 1987, the routes from England to Australia and New Zealand are the longest in the world, and in 1847 a voyage to Australia of 100 days was regarded as 'splendid'. The average voyage was 120–130 days, whether it was from England or North America. Think about that; think about the isolation of those far-off colonists, still governed from England. If they wrote letters on business affairs or family matters, it was nine months before they got an answer; if the Governors of the colonies wrote to the Colonial Secretary on matters of State, it was nine months before *they* got an answer. Of wars and revolutions, economic depressions, decisions of the British government which directly concerned them, these colonists did not hear for four months. It is small wonder that the arrival of a ship carrying news caused commotion and excitement. All the ports had a series of signal stations on successive headlands and as soon as a ship hove in sight her name, port and date of departure and cargo fluttered in the flags and flashed to the towns. Rival reporters rushed to hire sailing dinghies to race down the harbour or river in an effort to be the first aboard to seize the newspapers she carried, and their editors rushed to prepare special editions.

Not until the 1890s would the number of people who had been born in Australia outnumber those born overseas, and thus, in 1847, news from England and Europe was the lifeblood of the small communities in Australia. The news might be four months old, but they had no other way of obtaining it save the ships.

The ships

What were they like, these ships which were so vital and had such identity that the news they brought was published under their names? The year 1847, the first year of painless surgery, fell precisely between two eras in shipping. When the ships which carried news of the discovery of anaesthesia to South Africa, Australia, New Zealand and the East left their ports in 1846 and early 1847, they sailed or steamed in the old era. By the end of 1847 when chloroform was introduced there were radical changes. In the steamers the screw propeller began to replace the paddle wheel, and the publication of Towson's work on great circle sailing inaugurated a new era in navigation and ship-building. In early 1847 the sailing ships were small, with limited carrying capacity, necessitating ports of call for provisioning and refitting, whilst the steamers needed auxiliary sail both to increase horse-power and reduce coal consumption. They too were small, in accordance with the power of the paddle wheels and the engines of the day, and coaling ports were another necessity.

The ships were personalities to the exiled colonists. The editors of newspapers spoke of them with familiarity and, upon arrival, the events of their voyages were noted in the newspapers in a marine shorthand perfectly comprehensible and interesting to the readers. Phrases like, 'She was held at the Downs for 6 days', or 'she spoke to the *Faerie Queen*' are mysterious to us, but were not to Australians of 1847.

Prior to 1837, when the English Post Office granted the first contract for a steamer mail service to the Iberian Peninsula to the newly formed Peninsular Steam Navigation Company, mail sailing packets left from Falmouth to avoid delays in the English Channel. Sailing vessels leaving from London could be held up for days or weeks by adverse winds or storms in the Channel, and it was the custom in such a case for them to make for more sheltered waters off Deal (or 'the Downs' as the seamen's language had it) where they anchored and waited for favourable conditions. Steamers, though then slower than sail, had the great advantage of not being dependent on winds and tides and so were in demand as mail ships since their day of departure could be advertised and relied upon.

Even today it is an event to sight another ship or plane in the vast spaces of oceans or air, and in 1847, if wind and weather permitted, the little vessels 'spoke' to each other. They hove to, boats were lowered or a line fixed between them and mail, newspapers or provisions were exchanged as necessary.

Mrs Fanny Perry, wife of the first Bishop of Melbourne, making the outward voyage in the *Stag* in 1847, kept one of the many diaries of such journeys which exist in Australian archives. The diary of the Bishop's lady gives perhaps the best description of 'speaking'. There was great excitement. If the ship was homeward bound the passengers scurried below to the cuddy to write letters to family and friends. If the ships were both outward bound, mail and newspapers were transferred to the faster ship. The fixing of the line over the heaving seas between the ships was not an experience Mrs Perry enjoyed, for they approached each other so closely she was sure they must collide. She was much amused on another occasion to see the conversation the captains carried on by the medium of signals. She writes:

'Marriott's signal-book is a most useful thing to seafaring persons; it contains an almost infinite number of questions and answers, couched in the most concise language, to each of which there is a number attached; by means of particular flags, a ship shows certain numbers and then by applying to your signal-book you see what she means and answer in like manner.'

The routes

Sailing to the East and Australia in 1847 ships used one of only three routes. The first route, and the one most commonly used, was the Cape or India Route. Ships sailed the Atlantic, provisioning and refitting at South American ports or the Canary Islands, then sailed south to latitudes 35–45°, where they encountered prevailing westerly trade winds. Turning east and sailing with these winds they made for the Cape of Good Hope. From the Cape they sailed north for Mauritius, India, Ceylon and the Far East, or eastwards to Australia. Their latter landfall was the west coast of Tasmania, whence they sailed north and through Bass Strait, or south right round Tasmania, then turning north for the east coast Australian ports and New Zealand.

The second route, across the Atlantic and south to round Cape Horn was the least commonly used on the outward journey, for, having coped with the troubles of that notorious Cape, they then faced head winds right across the Pacific. The reverse of this route was used for the homeward voyage, since the westerly winds again played their part.

The third route, which in 1847, had only recently come to prominence, was the Overland Route. This was by steamer through the Mediterranean to Alexandria, across by land to Suez, and again by steamer from Suez to Ceylon and India, Penang, Singapore (Fig. 1) and Hong Kong; from Ceylon, Penang or Singapore a sailing vessel made the passage through the Indian Ocean to Australia.

The Overland route was the fastest, and most expensive, and the one with the most interesting history. Prior to 1851 Australia was of little importance, even to its rulers in England, though a few with vision were beginning thoughtfully to note that its export earnings now totalled two million pounds. The discovery of gold, however, brought Australia before the eyes of the world. Half a million prospectors to be transported across the seas, and rich return cargoes made the maritime world sit up and take notice. When in 1845 the Peninsular & Oriental Steam Navigation Company extended its Eastern service to Penang, Singapore and Hong Kong, lobbying by the Australian colonies for further extension to Australia began at once, and items appeared in the newspapers of 1847.

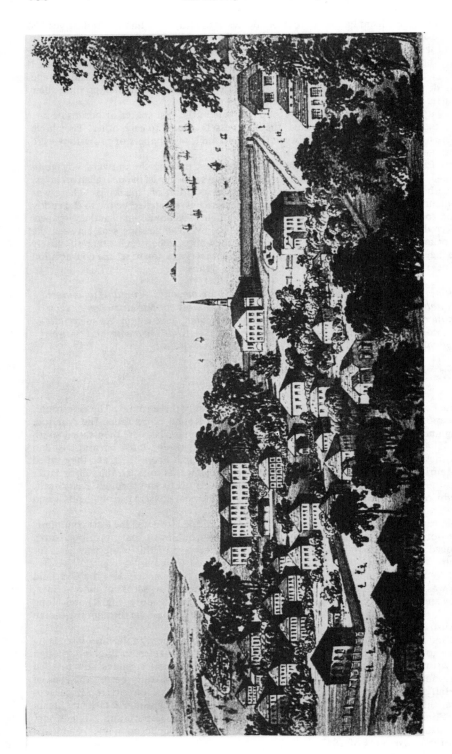

Figure 1   Singapore, circa 1847, where the news of anaesthesia arrived by the P&O steamer Braganza from the Overland Route on 14 March, 1847. Newspapers were transferred to the Lightning which reached Adelaide 3 May, 1847. Photograph from the archives, National Library of Singapore.

Prior to 1843 ships navigated according to the Mercator projections of 1569. Mercator (first to call his book of maps an 'atlas') planned his projection on the premise that the shortest distance between two points was a straight line, and ships navigated accordingly. John Towson, in his publication of 1847, postulated that the world was a globe and therefore the shortest distance around it was a great circle, and the higher the latitude, the smaller the circle. Lieutenant Maury's pilot charts, introduced in 1843 and showing the fastest routes according to winds, currents and seasons, and Towson's great circle sailing, revolutionized navigation; by 1852 the length of an Australian voyage via the Cape was 70 days or less.

The trials and tribulations of the journey

It is easy to state boldly that the ships carried the news, but it must be appreciated their voyages were long, arduous and hazardous.

The Cape route

The diaries of voyages by the Cape Route left by so many travellers have differences of emphasis, but many experiences were common to all, and most vivid impressions are left with the reader.

It needs little imagination to picture the distressing scenes of embarkation, when family and friends were being left, in most cases for ever; nor the sense of despair as the voyagers were conveyed by row boat, sail or steam tender to the ship; nor the lightening of despair to amusement as they climbed the precarious ladders to board (or were hoisted in a sling, as was Mrs Fanny Perry, the Bishop's lady, when she reached the *Stag* at Portsmouth, to sail for Melbourne on 6 October, 1847). Two days later Mrs Perry was sure she would never arrive, for the *Stag* was still tossing and tacking in wild weather in sight of Start Point on the Isle of Wight. Her passengers were seasick, weary, worn and bruised from being flung about as the ship pitched and rolled. Their nights were sleepless on many occasions from what the lady calls the 'indescribable noise', due to the creaking and clattering of the rudder, the constant reefing, taking in or setting of sails accompanied by the jigs and reels played by the ship's fiddler and then 'before dawn the pumping of water and subsequent scrubbing of the decks over our heads.' Although mentioning their presence in describing the first sight of the ship, Mrs Perry does not add to this cacophony the noises of the livestock on board these crowded ships. It was necessary to carry one or two cows for milk, several pigs and sheep, and an array of poultry in coops tied all along the ships rails. Hens and chickens on the port side, ducks and geese on the starboard side (don't ask why). The poop deck was crowded with bales of hay and stalls for the cows and sheep, whilst the pigs existed in a pen beneath one of the ship's boats, which was itself filled with marine spare parts. Mrs Perry was too much of a lady to describe the smell caused by the livestock, which came to permeate the whole ship. Other diarists were not so restrained. One and all they wanted to see the end of the poultry, and eating it was the only way, even if it was tough and stringy.

The diarists all speak of the great storms encountered when all passengers were shut below decks. The intermediate and steerage passengers waded in the water shipped into their quarters. The first class passengers had to cope with water running down their cabin walls, soaking bed linen, and mildewed clothes. The trials of the cook were many; fires were frequently extinguished and food spoilt by salt water before it could be served, if it could be served at all. They speak, too, of their envy of the sailors, who, even if they struggled on decks washed by huge waves, at least had fresh air.

Fanny Perry tells us of Sundays with prayers and sermons, of Greek testament classes and classes for the children and ship's boys in fine weather, of the wonders of waterspouts, albatrosses and flying fish as the *Stag* approached the tropics and of the calm moonlit nights when it was possible to read on deck, the light was so clear. She writes, too, of the beauties of the Southern aurora and of the heat and stillness of being, as she says 'becalmed, becalmed, becalmed', when the sailors made entertainment for themselves by swimming or catching albatrosses and dolphins. She tells us as well, as do others, of the wonderful change as the ship came to her southern latitude, turned eastwards for the Cape, propelled by the westerly winds and the great rolling seas of the 'roaring forties', and at last made for her destination under stars new to those from the north, and at much greater speed.

The Bishop's lively lady had quite a turn of phrase, and in mentioning the increased speed of the eastward run she also conveys the sense of the vast distances. The diary entry of 16 December, 1847, reads 'In October we went 2783 miles and November 3300, December up to this day 2862—making a total of 8945 miles and leaving a remainder to be done of 5600 miles.'

The *Stag* reached Melbourne on 14 January, 1848, thus most of her voyage was in the southern summer. Other diarists were not so lucky, and many speak of the intense cold of the grey stormy days in the higher latitudes, of the crew and captain's anxious watch for icebergs floating north, for even damage to the ship meant long delays on the voyage, and limping to the nearest port was always fraught with the additional danger of running out of food and water.

The overland route

Much has been written about the overland route and one could spend an hour telling of its fascinating history, for this history involves that of England, France, Egypt, the Sultanates bordering the Red Sea, and of the East India Company and the P&O line.

The P&O's remarkable accomplishment was not achieved without prodigious organization and strong resistance from the East India Company ('John Company') which, at the urging of one of its employees, Thomas Waghorn, had pioneered the Overland route some twenty years before. John Company insisted on maintaining its Suez-Bombay service in opposition to the P&O until 1852.

Before the P&O could even send its steamers round the Cape to inaugurate the Indian and Far East routes, coal had to be sent by sail to all the ports of call, and coaling facilities had to be established at Suez, Aden, Point de Galle in Ceylon, Calcutta, Penang, Singapore and Hong Kong. The Red Sea being well nigh impossible for a regular supply of coal by sail in monsoon weather, the coal for Suez had to be supplied from the Mediterranean end, and taken across the isthmus from Alexandria by huge camel trains. Suez and Aden were without water, and this regular supply had also to be initiated and maintained. The overland transport of mail, newspapers, passengers and cargo also presented enormous difficulties which had to be overcome.

Passengers disembarked at Alexandria and re-embarked on barges for transit on the Mahmoudieh canal to Atfeh on the Nile, a passage of some nine and a half hours. At Atfeh they again disembarked and transferred to Nile steamer for passage to Baulac, the Nile port for Cairo. This passage lasted 18 hours. Land transit from Cairo to Suez, across the stony desert took three days, allowing for rest periods totalling 12 hours.

Until 1843 when the P&O decided to look after its own from debarkation at Alexandria to embarkation at Suez, the land transit was managed by two Cairo agents, Thomas Waghorn and J. R. Hill. The transit was slow, costly and primitive. By 1847 the P&O had succeeded in having the Mahmoudieh Canal deepened and widened and a series of locks across the embankment between the canal and the Nile saved transhipment from canal barges to P&O's newer, faster Nile steamers to Cairo. For passengers the uncomfortable camel ride from Cairo to Suez across stony desert had been replaced by springless horse drawn carriages and a sandy road of sorts, and the rest houses in the desert had been rebuilt and were clean and relatively comfortable.

Despite the discomforts many passengers spoke with enthusiasm of the desert crossing. The horses which drew the carriages were swift and mettlesome arab steeds and their occasional escape from control constituted excitement and adventure. Then there was the desert at night; so silent, so vast, so empty, with the stars looking huge and brighter than ever before. The moonlit nights were dreamlike, with the harsh landscape softened and the occasional nomad fires giving warm red and yellow points of contrast to the silver glow of the moon. There was now no waiting for the ship at Suez, for the semaphore signal service allowed leaving Cairo at the appropriate time. Naturally, when all was running smoothly in 1847, the Egyptian government cancelled the P&O's transit permits and took over the entire Egyptian section of the route.

At Suez travellers re-embarked on P&O's large steamers *Hindostan* or *Bentinck* for the Red Sea voyage to Aden, where the ship coaled, and then Point de Galle in Ceylon. Passengers, luggage, cargoes, mail and newspapers for Penang, Singapore and Hong Kong (and after 1847, China) and Australia were transferred at Galle to *Braganza* or *Lady Mary Wood* whilst the large steamers proceeded to Madras and Calcutta. At Singapore those for Australia were again transferred to sailing vessels, such as the *Lightning*, for passage to Adelaide. It does indeed seem remarkable that, for the journey to Australia, all this could be accomplished in 100 days from England.

Passengers journeying by the Overland Route were of necessity hardy, adaptable and patient and their vicissitudes, and those of the vital English newspapers, were many.

The news travels eastward

In 1847 news from England reached Capetown in 58–62 days of sail or steam. By the Overland steamer route it reached India in 41 days, Penang in 47 days, Singapore in 49 days and Hong Kong in 56 days. Australia was about 40 days from the Cape by sail and 45 days from Singapore, for the sailing vessel usually called at Atka in the Aleutian Islands on the way. New Zealand was a further 14–18 days from Sydney.

News of the discovery of anaesthesia in Boston began to be published in England about the 21 December, 1846, and, by the last week in December, the news of the successful trial at University College Hospital (UCH) on that same date reached the newspapers. From then on, during January and February of 1847, there was an avalanche of reports in both city and provincial press, as practitioners all over England and Scotland tried their hands. The *Lancet* had its articles and editorial diatribes, *Punch* had cartoons and the *Illustrated London News* of 9 January, carried both a description of the anaesthetics at UCH and a sketch of the apparatus used.

The news of the Boston anaesthetics was the first to reach the far colonies, arriving by ships which left England before the English successes had been reported, and there seems to have been both editorial and reader hesitation to accept the 'Yankee dodge', for paragraphs in colonial newspapers were few, and no attempts at anaesthesia followed. When, however, the ships which left England in January and February brought news of English successes, a trail of admiring articles and anaesthetics in the colonies followed in their wake.

The first anaesthetics in South Africa

The Peninsular and Oriental Steam Navigation Company (so familiar to us still as the 'P&O') was inaugurated in 1837 as the Peninsular Steam Navigation Company for the fast transport of mail by steamer to the Iberian Peninsula. So successful was this service that in 1840 it was extended to Malta and Alexandria, and in 1842 (as we have noted above) it was further extended by land and steamer service from Suez to Ceylon and India thereby acquiring its new and famous name. In 1845 the *Braganza* and the *Lady Mary Wood* were detached from the Iberian and Mediterranean fleets and sailed round the Cape to Galle in Ceylon to institute the new steamer service from Suez to Penang, Singapore and Hong Kong.

It was therefore a surprise to learn that the news of the successful use of anaesthesia in North America and Europe reached South Africa in the P&O paddle steamer *Pekin* (Fig. 2) on 1 April, 1847. What was the *Pekin* doing at Cape Town (Fig. 3), way off P&O routes? Perhaps she was on her way to join the far eastern service? That this was the case was confirmed by the P&O's archivist, Mr Rabson. *Pekin*, a large paddle wheel steamer of 1500 tons, was built specially for the Hong Kong–China leg of the Overland Route, and she left England on 15 February, 1847, on her maiden voyage to inaugurate this service.

Publication of the news

Mrs Drake, the Librarian of the National Library of South Africa discovered that the news of anaesthesia was first printed in South Africa in the Cape Town *Commercial Advertiser* of

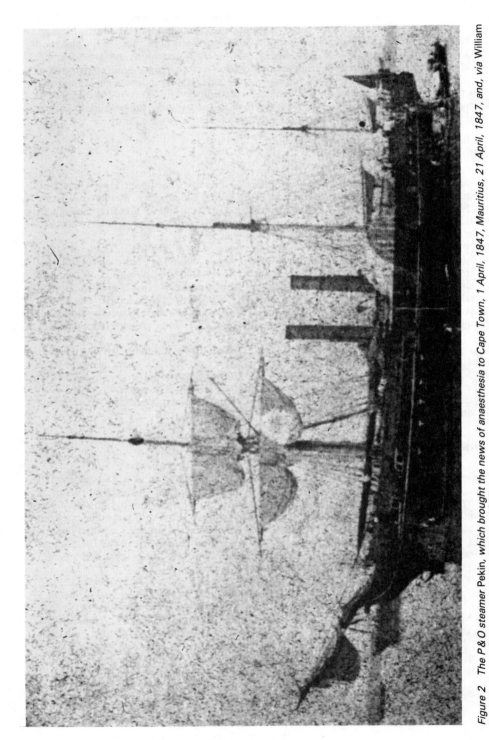

Figure 2   The P & O steamer Pekin, which brought the news of anaesthesia to Cape Town, 1 April, 1847, Mauritius, 21 April, 1847, and, via William Wise to Perth, Western Australia, 5 June, 1847.
The photograph, which dates back to 1847, was obtained from P & O archives.

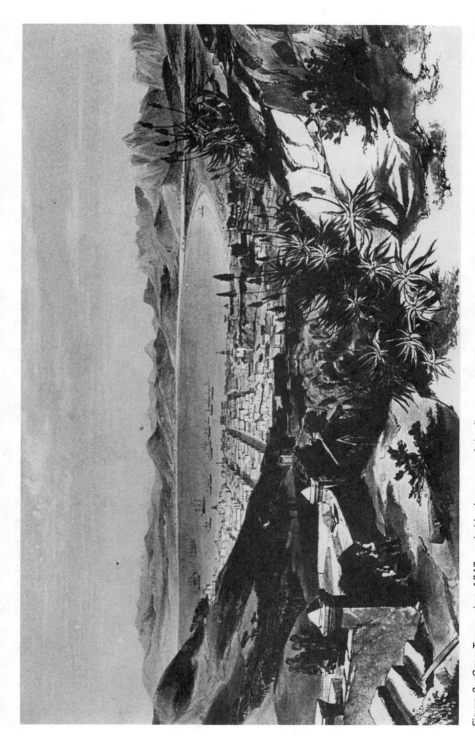

Figure 3   Cape Town, circa 1847, probably the scene of the first anaesthetic east of Europe, 17 April, 1847. Photograph from the archives, National Library of South Africa.

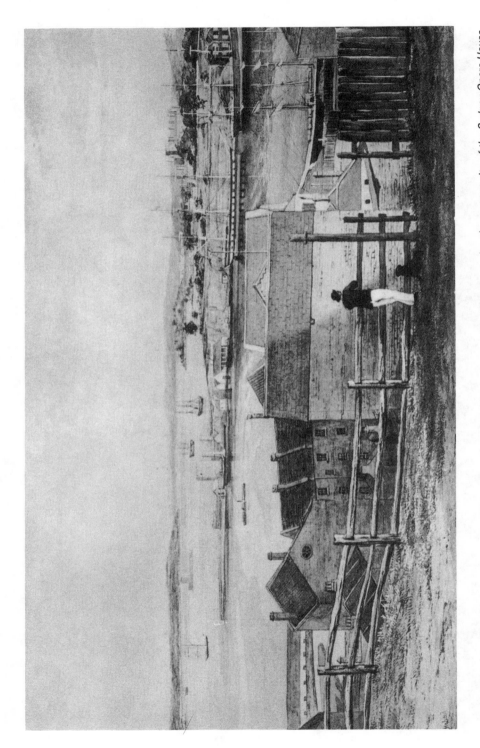

Figure 4 Sydney, N.S.W., Australia, circa 1853, showing the paddle steamer such as Thistle passing the present site of the Sydney Opera House. Photograph from the archives, State Library of N.S.W.

7 April. It was noted by the editor that the English news in this issue had been received by the P&O steamer *Pekin*, which had arrived on 1 April, 1847.

Further information supplied by the South African library indicated that there is an unsubstantiated report that news of anaesthesia had arrived earlier at the Cape, carried by a sailing vessel which had come directly from America. This surely must have been *Robert Pulsford*, outward bound to Sydney, Australia (3)—of which more later in the paper.

The first anaesthetics in Cape Town were administered a little over two weeks after *Pekin* came to the port. These were dental anaesthetics, given by the Cape Town dentist Mr Raymond on 17 April, and were reported in the *Gleaner* and the *Zuid Afrikaan* of 20 April (4,5,6). These are the first anaesthetics known to have been recorded outside North America and Europe.

The first anaesthetics in the Straits Settlements

The P&O kindly supplied a list of outward sailings for its Far East fleet for 1847, and it can be seen that the *Hindostan* left Suez for Galle (Ceylon) on 15 February, 1847, carrying the English newspapers of January, received via the overland section of the route. These were transferred to *Braganza* which left Galle on 4 March and arrived in Penang on 12 March. In the *Penang Gazette and Straits Chronicle* of the 20 March, there is the first paragraph on the introduction of anaesthesia in England.

The first anaesthetic in the Straits Settlements was given shortly thereafter on 28 April at Malacca by Dr Ratton, and was reported in the *Singapore Free Press* of 30 April (2).

The arrival of the news in Eastern Australia

Editorial reluctance to accept the Boston news is typified, we think, by lack of publication after the arrival of the *Robert Pulsford* in Sydney (Fig. 4) on 5 February, 1847. She left America on, of all dates, the 21 October, 1846, and from all ports, Boston, and she carried Boston newspapers to the date of her departure. Search of all newspapers in New South Wales, both city and country, has revealed no sign of the bombshell she must have carried, which is disappointing, for Bigelow's prediction could well have come true in the least possible time after Morton's demonstration. Sydney, right around the world from Boston, was reached by the *Robert Pulsford* in 106 days, an achievement probably made possible by the use of Maury's new pilot charts.

In the usual chatty fashion of the day it is recorded that the *Robert Pulsford* 'spoke' to the *Union* 'off St Pauls'. By this we know that she came by the Cape Route, for St Paul's island in the southern Indian Ocean was a landmark on the voyages. Her arrival in Sydney was said to be 'unexpected', as was the arrival of any ship of another nation at that time. Transport from and around Australia in 1847 was still governed by the British Navigation Laws of 1651, instituted to prevent Dutch monopoly of sea trade to the colonies. These laws meant that foreign ships were few and far between in Australian ports, for they prevented any ships other than British from carrying cargoes from and between the colonies, and so *Robert Pulsford* would have had to leave Sydney with holds empty of anything legitimate. It was a pity about *Robert Pulsford*, and you would have thought that at least one sailor might have had toothache in the week before sailing, and perhaps conveyed the news of anaesthesia by word of mouth to Sydney, for Boston must have been agog in that first week of painless surgery.

The *Mountstuart Elphinstone* left England on 23 December, 1846, and arrived in Sydney on 28 April, 1847, by the Cape Route. She certainly carried the news, for extracts from *Bell's Messenger* of 21 December, describing the Boston anaesthetics and Morton's apparatus were published; not in Sydney, be it noted, but in the *Maitland Mercury* of 8 May (1). Maitland was a small town north of Sydney and near the Hunter River port of Morpeth. To and from Morpeth to Sydney plied two small paddle steamers *Thistle* and *Rose*, making their journeys daily and carrying mail, newspapers, periodicals and passengers. *Thistle, Rose* and their sister ship *Shamrock* are of great interest, for not only did they carry news of the introduction of anaesthesia and later of anaesthetics in the colonies, but they were the first iron ships to reach Australia (in 1841) and are therefore important in Australia's maritime history.

Lightning left Singapore on 19 March, 1842, called at Atka (Aleutian Islands), and arrived at Port Adelaide on 3 May, thus sailing the last leg of the Overland Route (the particular purpose for which she was built).

The editor of the *South Australian* noted with satisfaction that the *Lightning* had brought English and European news by the Overland Route in the 'splendid' time of 100 days and he published news of anaesthesia in his issue of 4 May, 1847.

The *Prince of Wales* arrived off Sydney Heads in gathering darkness on the 10 May, 1847. Her news was printed in an extra special edition of the *Sydney Morning Herald* on the 11 May, but there was no word of anaesthesia. This did not appear until after the arrival of the *Niagara* on 15 May, although the editor of the *Herald* said *Niagara* brought no news different from that of *Prince of Wales*. *Prince of Wales* had sailed from Plymouth on 30 January, 1847, and had a fast voyage of 100 days. *Niagara* sailed from London on 11 January but was held at the Downs for 6 days by bad weather. She later 'spoke' to the *Faerie Queen* ex-Liverpool, 47 days out on her voyage, and picked up mail and newspapers to the 1 February, 1847.

The first anaesthetics in Sydney were administered in the last week of May and the first week in June, 1847, by a dentist, Dr John Belisario, and so Bigelow's prediction was at last fulfilled.

The first anaesthetics in Tasmania

The *Lady Howden* left London on 30 January and arrived in Hobart, Tasmania on 27 May. After a coach trip lasting two days newspapers reached Launceston on Tasmania's north coast, and news of anaesthesia was first published in Tasmania in the *Launceston Examiner* of 2 June.

William Russ Pugh administered what appear to be the first anaesthetics for surgical operations in Australia, at St John's Hospital on 7 June, 1847 (6).

Prince of Wales, *Niagara* and *Lady Howden* all left England at appropriate times to have on board the *Illustrated London News* of 9 January, and both Belisario and Pugh record that their apparatus was copied from its sketch.

The *Pekin*, Mauritius and Western Australia

The exploits of the *Pekin* became known in quite another fashion, but were again confirmed by the P&O company's information. In 1847 the settlements of Perth in Western Australia and its port of Fremantle, so recently seen on world-wide television during the America's Cup races, were perhaps the most isolated British colonies in the world. In June, 1847, the 1100 people in Perth and the 426 in Fremantle had received no news or cargoes for seven months, and the 'long awaited' arrival of the *William Wise* was a great event, necessitating an Extraordinary Supplement to the *Perth Inquirer* on 9 June. The third paragraph describes the introduction of anaesthesia. *William Wise's* news, so said the Editor, had been obtained from the P&O steamer *Pekin* at Cape Town.

Perth and Fremantle had a bonanza in 1847, for in late July the *Arpenteur* and the *Champion* arrived almost simultaneously. In fact *Arpenteur* stranded herself in Gage Roads and was rescued by *Champion*. *Arpenteur* brought significant news. She had come from Mauritius, via India, and it seems that, in early May, an anaesthetic was administered at Port St Louis in Mauritius, and on 23 May, at the Grand River Hospital on the opposite side of the island, another anaesthetic was given—this time for an amputation of an arm—the patient being a sailor from the *Pekin*. The *Pekin*, sailing the Indian Ocean about her business in 1847 with news of such interest 140 years later, is a ship which has entered Australian and anaesthetic history.

New Zealand

In 1847 New Zealand was in its inaugural era and it was rare indeed for ships to arrive directly from the United Kingdom and Europe. Tiny ships of 80 tons or so brought British news to Wellington across the tossing Tasman Sea from Sydney or Hobart. After the arrival of the

Sir John Byng from Sydney, news noted as having come by *Prince of Wales* and *Niagara* was published in the *New Zealand Spectator* of 2 June but there was no mention of anaesthesia. As was so often the case, minor items of news (or so the editors thought) had to wait whilst those of local importance took precedence; in this case discussion of the Queen's Charter for the new nation of New Zealand, and Maori riots in Wanganui, far outweighed what must have seemed a chancy new medical procedure. By 7 July, however, news of successful anaesthesia in Sydney had reached Wellington by the *Waterwitch*, and the new venture was briefly mentioned in the *Wellington Independent*. Interest must have been heightened by the arrival of the *Lady Leigh* from Hobart, bearing *Lady Howden*'s news, published in the *Spectator* of 10 July. Hobart newspapers carried word of Pugh's exploits in Launceston and anaesthetics given by Agnew in Hobart in June, and, on 24 July, the *New Zealand Spectator and Cook's Strait Guardian* published long articles on painless surgery. Thus the news reached the end of the long, long line from Boston.

The first anaesthetic in New Zealand was given in Wellington on 26 September, 1847 (7).

The progression of the news was of course logical given the known sea-lanes, but it is of great interest to fit the patchwork pieces of information together, and find both news and anaesthetics dotted along those lanes; in Cape Town, Mauritius, Australia and New Zealand along the Cape Route, and in Penang, Singapore and again Australia along the Overland Route.

The story of the spread of the news of anaesthesia beyond Europe is a kaleidoscope of history and colour. Certain it is that the journeys of the newspaper and mail by which it was transported were suitably exotic considering its momentous nature.

Acknowledgments

The author would like to make acknowledgment of the unfailing help provided for me in the preparation of this paper. The librarians of the National Libraries of Malaysia, Singapore, South Africa and Australia and of the State Library of NSW have been most patient and co-operative with my many requests and would no doubt sympathize with the librarian in Port Louis, Mauritius, who wrote to say 'many books have been examined, but without hope'.

Dr Richard Bailey, whose particular interest is the voyage of the *Robert Pulsford* was kind enough to do much reading and to have long discussions on its frustrating aspects, which have been a great stimulus.

Grateful thanks are also due to the author's secretary Mrs Rita Appleyard, who not only typed what seemed endless versions of this paper, but spent time in the New Zealand libraries during her holidays, procuring information about *Sir John Byng* and *Waterwitch*.

Dr Jane Baker of Dunedin, Dr Owen James of Newcastle and the photographic departments of the Royal North Shore Hospital and the Royal Newcastle Hospital were of great assistance in the preparation of the illustrations, whilst the material supplied by Mr Rabson, Archivist of the P&O Line was quite vital to the presentation.

The beautiful colour slides of the Overland Route which accompanied the verbal presentation were made possible by the loan of an advance copy of the P&O's 150 year history, issued to senior members of the staff of the P&O Line in Sydney, amongst whom was a friend, Mr Ken Huxtable.

References

(1) James OF, Vidler P. An ether anaesthesia at Stroud in 1847—A report in search of a date. *Anaesth Intens Care* 1979; **7**: 273–7.

(2) Lee YK. *The first anaesthetic in the Straits Settlements*, 1847.

(3) Laidler PW, Gelfand M. *South Africa: its medical history*, 1652–1898: pp 126–9.

(4) Laidler PW, Gelfand M. *South Africa: its medical history*, 1652–1898: p 281.

(5) Burrows E. *Quart Bull. Sth African Library* March 1954, Vol 9, 72–74.

(6) Kok OVS. History of anaesthesia in the Republic of South Africa, *Proc. 4th World Congr Anaesth* 1968; 29. *Br J Anaesth* 1972; **44**: 408.

(7) Wilson G. The pioneer anaesthetists of Australia, *Proc 1st Symp Hist Modern Anaesth* 1982; 59–64.

(8) Hutchinson B. History and development of anaesthesia in New Zealand, *Proc 3rd Asian-Australian Congr Anaesthesiol*: 494–496.

Additional bibliography

National Library of Australia, Canberra

Bradfield RA. *Serving a sea-girt land N+ 387.20994/B799.*
Ewart EA. *Hundred year history of the P&O Line.* 1837–1937, 387.09.
Fitchett TK. *The long haul,* 1980, No. 387.52/F 546.
Lubbock B. *The colonial clippers,* 3rd Ed. 1924, 656.6.
Rhodes F. *Maritime history of Australasia 1933,* M.S. Copy 994.

Mitchell Library, State Library of New South Wales

Alexander W. *Great Circle sailing with its advantages,* 527.55/1.
Anstey V. *Trade of the Indian Ocean,* S 339.05/4.
Australian Maritime History (Newspaper Cuttings) Vol 10, 32–33 F991.1/N.
Brown Cecil B. *Suez to Singapore,* DS 940.9549/55.
Carse R. *The twilight of sailing ships,* NQ 387.22/2.
Ceylon Almanac 1839, 1842, 1849, DS 351.2/4.
Chichester F. *Along the clipper way,* 910.45/36B1.
Coates W. *The good old days of shipping,* 656.509/C.
Eadie F. List of Passenger Ships arriving Wellington, N.A. 1839–1900, Bateson Q8.
Edwards HD. *Sail in the South,* Q 387.22/7, 8.
Evans EH. *Routes to Australia,* 912/E.
Farnie DA. *East & West of Suez,* N 386.43/5.
Gibbs CRV. *British passenger liners of the 5 Oceans* 1838–1963. 387.243E/2.
Hoskins HL. *British routes to India,* S 339.042/118.
Hunter Sir WW. *Imperial Gazeteer of India,* 1881, DS 954/A/10–18/19–32.
Lubbock B. *The China clippers* 339.7/2A1.
Lubbock B. *The Blackwall frigates* 656.509/21B1.
Maber JM. *North Star in Southern Cross,* N387.50994/1.
McLarty FM. *History of the Straits Settlements,* DS 959.5/18.
Maps. *Great Britain and India,* 1870–1872 Q954A/22.
Marlowe J. *The making of the Suez Canal,* 962.15E/1.
New Zealand Journal 1841–1849, Q997/N.
Robinson M. *A pageant of the sea* (Macpherson Coll. of Prints), Q 656.509/R.
The Route of the Overland Mail to India, NF 769.43/1.
Routledge, London 1853. *Voyage and venture, or perils by sea and land.* 910.4/483.
Sargent AJ. *Seaways of the Empire,* S 339.042/44.
Shipping Archives, 1846–1847, NSW, TAS., S.AUS., W.AUS., N.Z.
Towson J. *Principles of Great Circle sailing,* 1855, 527.5/T.

NEWSPAPERS

Sydney Morning Herald	Dec 1846–Aug 1847	(17 May 1847, anaesthesia)
Australian	Dec 1846–Aug 1847	(8 May, 1847, anaesthesia)
Maitland Mercury	Dec 1846–Aug 1847	
Launceston Examiner	May–Aug 1847	(2, 9 June, anaesthesia)
South Australian	May–Oct 1847	(4 May, 3 October anaesthesia)
Inquirer (W. Australia)	Jan–Dec 1847	(9 June, Aug. anaesthesia)
Penang Gazette & Straits Chronicle	20 March 1847	
Gleaner (South Africa)	20 April 1847	
Zuid Afrikaans	20 April 1847	
Commercial Advertiser	7 April 1847	

7.2   How the news of anaesthesia reached South Africa

JOHN L. COUPER

Medical University of Southern Africa, Medunsa, Republic of South Africa

In 1897 William Guybon Atherstone claimed that he had been the first person to use ether anaesthesia outside America and Europe (1). This claim is in dispute (2,3). On the same occasion he stated that the news reached him 'direct from the US by sailing vessel en route for England. I had no details whatever supplied me, and knew nothing of Simpson's work in Edinburgh' (1). Atherstone first used ether on a patient on 16 June, 1847 (4). Atherstone had been elected Honorary President of the first Medical Congress held in Grahamstown, Cape Province, South Africa, and the above statements were made before the Congress. He admitted in his address that 'in spite of my total blindness and many infirmities of age, these notes have been written in the quiet hours of the night, without my being, at all times able to follow the sequences of ideas' (1).

No account of how the news of ether anaesthesia reached South Africa could be found so a study was undertaken.

Sea communications

In the 1840s sailing vessels called in at Table Bay on their way to the East and Australia. These came from Europe mainly with only sporadic sailings from the Eastern seaboard of the United States. Vessels from the US to England would not travel en route via Cape Town. Shipping intelligence in the newspapers of the time list ports from whence ships have arrived as well as their destinations. I could find no listings of ships arriving in Table Bay from any Eastern port of the whole of the American continent bound for the Western side of the Atlantic. Atherstone's reference to the sailing vessel en route to England was the result of his infirmities of age.

In Atherstone's letters to various newspapers detailing the amputation of Frederick Carlisle's leg (on 16 June, 1847) he clearly stated he had no access to the English apparatus and so devised his own (5). This statement written at the time infers that he knew of English apparatus and had read accounts of their use and probably had even seen sketches of the equipment. The *Illustrated London News* of 9 January, 1847, reached Tasmania by 27 May, and it carried a sketch of Hooper's apparatus for the administration of ether (6). The ship carrying the mail left London on 30 January and sailed via Cape Town (7). I believe Atherstone, being a man of many interests, had seen this issue of the *Illustrated London News* as well as the many illustrations that appeared in various medical journals and that he devised his apparatus on these sketches. He wrote that he had experimented with different kinds of apparatus with and without valves (5). In his letter to the *Cape of Good Hope Examiner* he wrote 'Hot water, as recommended in the English papers to produce vaporization of the ether is not necessary' (8). This again implies that he had read various accounts of the use of ether. Cape Town newspapers, which would have been available in Grahamstown, carried several reports, copied from English newspapers, on the use of ether in each issue from early April, 1847. I believe that, as in Australia, the news of ether reached South Africa via England. *The South African Commercial Advertiser* of 31 March, 1847, states the latest intelligence from America was 8 October, 1846, and from England 28 December, 1846.

The voyage of the *Pekin*

The letter of Dr Montgomery of Mauritius published in a Cape Town newspaper (9) directed my search to the arrival of the *P.S. Pekin* in Table Bay. Dr Montgomery reported the use of ether by Dr T. Bell, of the Oriental steamer *Pekin*, using apparatus made by Mr Hooper of Pall Mall (London, England), for the amputation of the arm of a Lascar seaman.

The *Pekin* left Southampton on her maiden voyage on 15 February, 1847, bound for Point de Galle and served between India and Hong Kong. She was an iron paddle steamer built in Glasgow of 1182 tons. Her speed was 9 knots and she carried 70 first and 22 second class passengers. The *Pekin* made the fastest passage from England to the Cape, taking 45 days which included a two day call at Gibraltar and seven days at St Helena (10). She arrived in Table Bay on 1 April, and sailed on 8 April, 1847. Several Cape Town newspapers reported that the *Pekin* carried the largest mail ever to arrive at the Cape and it was after the arrival of the *Pekin* that the reports on the use of ether appeared. *De Zuid Afrikaan* of 8 April, 1847, reported, 'we now have an opportunity which rarely presents itself. The steamer *Pekin* which arrived here on Tuesday last brought us English papers to the 13 February, from which we have copied such abstracts as time permitted.'

Dr Thomas Bell: ship's surgeon

The ship's surgeon on the *Pekin* was Dr T. Bell, who administered the first anaesthetic in Mauritius. Dr Thomas Bell qualified in 1840 from Guy's Hospital with MRCS England and LSA and is listed in the London and Provincial Medical Directory of 1847 as General Practitioner, Felsted, Essex. He was 35 years of age when he joined the *Pekin*. He served the P&O steamship company on the China route being transferred to the *Ganges* in 1852 and the *Singapore* in 1853. The latest entry in the *British Medical Directory* for Dr Bell is 1865 where he is listed as abroad. I have not been able to trace any further information about Dr Bell's life.

Dr Bell was experienced in anaesthesia when he joined the *Pekin*. He had written an account of administering ether for the amputation of the leg of a pregnant woman on 25 January, 1847, in *The London Medical Gazette* (11). The patient, Mary Ann Loyd age 27, was between six and seven months pregnant, and he reported the case because he had not heard of ether inhalation ever before applied upon a patient in a similar condition. Bell used Hooper's inhaler and gave justice to Mr Hooper that 'his inhaler answers admirably the purpose for which it is intended'. He also stated in the article that he had used the inhaler with success in several cases of extraction of teeth.

Although Cape Town newspapers of the time carried reports of many meetings addressed by doctors, I can find no report of Dr Bell having addressed a meeting during the stay of the *Pekin* in Table Bay. The fact that Alfred Raymond, who administered the first anaesthetic in South Africa on 17 April, 1847, used an inhaler (12) for administering ether leads one to believe that Dr Bell met doctors during his stay in the Cape and demonstrated his inhaler or at least showed it to the local practitioners. Raymond could have had a copy made, or Bell might even have had an extra inhaler which he gave to Raymond. Raymond, through his father-in-law had a connection with shipping and so could readily have met Dr Bell (3). I also believe it likely that a medical man spending a week in Table Bay in those times would have made contact with local medical practitioners who, at that stage, were unaware of the use of ether until the mail from the *Pekin* had been distributed.

References

(1) Atherstone WG. Reminiscences of medical practice in South Africa fifty years ago. *S Afr Med J* 1897; **4**: 243–7.

(2) Kok OVS. History of anaesthesia in the Republic of South Africa. *Proc 4th World Congr Anaesthesiologists* 1970: 167–173.

(3) Couper JL. Putting the record straight—the first ether administration in South Africa. This publication, Ch. 7.3, p. 149.

(4) Atherstone WG. Sulphuric ether—painless operation. *The Grahamstown Journal*, (June 19) 1847.

(5) Atherstone WG. Sulphuric ether. *The Grahamstown Journal*, (June 26) 1847.

(6) Wilson GCM. The tyrant overcome: a review of the history of anaesthesia in Australia. *Anaesth Intens Care* 1972; **1**: 9–26.

(7) Wilson GCM. The Lady Howden. *Anaesth Intens Care* 1987; **15**: 4.
(8) Atherstone WG. Sulphuric ether—painless operation. *Cape of Good Hope Examiner* (July 2) 1847.
(9) Montgomery A. Application of ether. *De Zuid Afrikaan* (May 27) 1847.
(10) Shipping intelligence. *South African Commercial Advertiser* (April 7) 1847.
(11) Bell T. Amputation performed on a pregnant female under the influence of ether. *The London Medical Gazette* 1847; **4** (new series): 319–20.
(12) Anonymous. Inhalation of ether. *De Zuid Afrikaan* (May 3) 1847.

7.3   Putting the record straight —
                          the first ether administration in South Africa

JOHN L. COUPER
Medical University of Southern Africa, Medunsa, Republic of South Africa

---

In a paper read at the Fourth S.A. Medical Congress in Grahamstown in April, 1897, Dr William Guybon Atherstone stated that his administration of ether on 16 June, 1847, was its first use out of America and Europe (1). Atherstone administered ether to Frederick Carlisle, Deputy Sheriff for Albany for a mid-thigh amputation of his leg, assisted by his father and two other doctors. Accounts of the administration of ether for this operation were sent to and published in two Grahamstown and two Cape Town newspapers (2–6).

Early accounts of ether administration in South Africa

The account of the operation and disbelief of Carlisle that his leg had actually been amputated until he saw the dressed stump is recorded as the first use of ether anaesthesia by all authors of the history of medicine in South Africa (7–11). Some of these authors (7–9) suggest that ether may have been administered as early as April, 1847, by Dr Henry Anderson Ebden. This belief is based on an 1847 editorial in the third issue of the short-lived *Cape Town Medical Gazette* edited by Ebden (12). The editorial refers to early experiments with ether some of which were successful and some not. No actual case reports were mentioned nor whether surgery was undertaken on patients. In the fourth (October) issue of the *Gazette* (13) the editor wrote:

> *'Since we last alluded to this subject [etherization] there have been two amputations of the leg below the knee in Cape Town. In the first the patient was partly insensibile to pain while the second failed because of defect in the apparatus.'*

Schmidt (14) in his essay on the history of anaesthesia in South Africa writes that among the enthusiastic but sometimes also sceptical reports on the administration of ether before Atherstone's case, was a notice in *De Verzamelaar* of 20 April, 1847. This read

> *'Saturday last, an experiment was made by the Aether vapour by Mr Raymond Surgeon Dentist, having drawn from a Gentleman two teeth, and from an other one tooth, without causing any pain—we may therefore congratulate Mr R with the good result of his experiment.'* (15)

The only other person to credit Raymond as the first person to administer ether in South Africa was Kok who read a paper on the history of anaesthesia in South Africa to the Fourth World Congress of Anaesthesiologists in London in 1968 (16).

Table 1
Use of ether outside America and Europe 1847

	17 April	Raymond	Cape Town (15)
	24 April	Bell (Montgomery)	Mauritius (17)
	28 April	Ratton	Straits Settlement (18)
	1 May	Raymond	Cape Town (19)
±	16 May	Raymond	Cape Town (20)
	May	Belisario	Sydney (21)
	7 June	Pugh	Launceston (21)
	16 June	Atherstone	Grahamstown

There are at least seven reports of ether having been administered out of the United States and Europe before 16 June, 1847 (Table 1). These places were more distant from Europe and the US than the Cape of Good Hope and it seemed irrational that ether was not used in South Africa before this date. A search was undertaken of all newspapers published in Cape Town during 1847.

By 31 March, 1847, the latest intelligence to reach the Cape from England was 28 December, 1846, and from the United States 8 October, 1846 (22). The first report on ether appeared in the *South African Commercial Advertiser* of 7 April, 1847 (23) and, from that date onwards, most of the Cape papers reprinted reports of the use of ether from English newspapers, sometimes as many as three or four reports from different sources appearing in each issue. *De Zuid Afrikaan* of Monday, 3 May, 1847, reported that (on Saturday, 1 May)

'Mons. Raymond, Surgeon Dentist of Burg-street attended a young lady, suffering dreadfully from toothache, with his ether inhaler, and succeeded in the course of about one minute to throw the patient into a state of perfect stupor or rather unconsciousness.'
(19)

This report also stated that Raymond had a few days previously drawn teeth from two gentlemen, one belonging to the medical profession, without causing any pain to the patients. The same newspaper (20) in its edition of 20 May, carried the following communication dated St George's street 19 May, 1847:

'Last week, Mr Raymond, the highly skilful Surgeon Dentist of this Town, operated most successfully with his Ether inhaler apparatus on a mate of one of the ships then in the Bay, from whose mouth he extracted a tooth in an advanced state of decay, without his being sensible of the slightest pain whatever. Remaining still unconscious, Mr R. ventured to remove from one of his fingers a large wart which he did with a single stroke of the cutting forceps. On the patient awakening, Mr R. expressed a hope that he had not taken too great a liberty by so doing. "Far from it, Sir," he replied "you have rendered me very great service, I should long since have had it taken off, could I have been sure, as now, of its being wholly unattended with pain"!'

It is difficult to see how these reports can be regarded with scepticism as suggested by Schmidt (14). Schmidt also gives little credit to the report that one of the original patients was a member of the medical profession (24). *The Cape Town Mail* of 26 June, 1847, carried an article entitled 'New Medical Discovery', which described the discovery of ether by Morton and Jackson and its use by Liston, Robinson and Simpson. The concluding paragraph reads:

'as the writer of this notice has undergone the etherial inebriation, and during that condition had two mural teeth removed, he can add his own personal experience to the entire credibility of the facts stated here . . . the operation was performed—the first tooth being extracted without a trace of pain though it appeared to disturb the lethargic state, so that a dull pain of a trifling nature accompanied the removal of the second. Shortly afterwards the writer awoke, discovering to his complete amazement two grim-looking teeth on the table at his side. No ill effects followed.' (24)

There seems to be little doubt, this was written by the medical gentlemen whose teeth were extracted on 17 April.

The only other mention of Raymond in the Cape Town papers was a report of the Rev Mr Brown's lecture 'Sensation, action and volition' (25). At this talk Mr Raymond exhibited an improved apparatus for facilitating the process of vaporization by the application of warm water and offered to administer the vapour to anyone present. The writer of the report availed himself of the opportunity and described the sensation.

Alfred Raymond. Surgeon Dentist

Who was this Mr Raymond? All efforts to trace his existence prior to 1842 have failed. He described himself as Surgeon Dentist of the University of Paris (26) and on another occasion as a member of the Imperial College of Surgeons of Paris (27). Neither institution has any record of Alfred Raymond and the University Archivist suggests that it might be an assumed name. A Pierre Joseph Victor Raymond who was born on 13 September, 1807, in Mauritius attended the University of Paris from 1826 to 1831 when he completed his examination after attending twelve semesters. The certificate I have traced, however, does not state in which faculty he was registered nor the subjects pursued.

Alfred Raymond with wife and child arrived in Cape Town from Mauritius on the ship *Deborah* on 2 February, 1842. His wife Catherine Sophie Cauvin was the daughter of Louis Joseph Paul Cauvin (who was born in Marseilles) and Anna Johanna Bosman whose marriage was registered in the NGK Stellenbosch on 4 December, 1808. Cauvin was a jeweller, town councillor and man of property. He owned a fleet of coastal ships, and a Cauvin was the master of an 80 ton coaster plying between Mauritius and the coastal ports to Cape Town. There are very few Cauvin's listed in South African directories and letters to those listed have drawn no replies.

The Raymonds lived at various addresses during their 18 years in Cape Town. A daughter, Delphine Victoire Alfra was born on 13 December, 1842, and she was baptized in St George's Anglican Church in Cape Town on 14 August, 1843. The baptism entry is the only record that I have found of Raymond's full name—Jean Victor Paul Alfred—all other reports only give the name Alfred. It is interesting that all foreigners had to register for citizenship in the Cape, but British subjects were exempt after 1831 and they could move freely in and out of commonwealth countries. As Mauritius was a British colony in 1842, Alfred Raymond was presumably a British subject because there is no registration of citizenship.

Three more children were born to the Raymonds during their stay in Cape Town and these three were baptized in the Catholic Church. Armand Gallois was born on 15 February, 1845; Josephine Estelle on 8 January, 1847, and Amadeus Ludovicus on 11 May, 1853.

Probably in 1859 Alfred Raymond had an itinerant practice in Port Elizabeth because an advertisement appeared in the *Eastern Province Herald* in 1859: 'Mon A Raymond, Surgeon/Dentist has received by mail steamer a new composition to stop teeth. Consulting room at Mr Drinkwater's, Main Street, Port Elizabeth.' (28). The *Herald* also carried the following notice in 1860 'Mr Alfred Raymond may be expected at Port Elizabeth by the end of the month on a professional visit to the inhabitants of that community' (29). Again in December, 1862 he inserted a notice as follows:

> *'A Card. Mr Alfred Raymond member of the Imperial College of Surgeons, Paris, begs to inform his friends that he will in future devote his attention SOLELY to the operations of the Mouth and Teeth, and to the diseases of the eyes. St Mary's Terrace' (27).*

Raymond's wife, Catherine Sophie died in Port Elizabeth on 13 March, 1863, and lies buried in St Mary's Cemetery. The last entry I can find referring to Alfred Raymond is in the Port Elizabeth directory of 1881 where he is listed as A. Raymond Surgeon. In an effort to trace further details I wrote to everyone listed in telephone directories in South Africa with the surname Raymond and from the replies drew up the family tree. Only two descendents of Alfred could be traced. All the other replies from Raymonds stated they had no connection, or were first generation from England. Armand Gallois married Selena Gouch of Grahamstown and died about 1925 at the age of 80. He was a magistrate in Pretoria but the Department of Justice wrote that they destroy records after thirty years and I am still following this lead. Armand's oldest son Alfred was an alcoholic and although his wife is still alive she has lost her memory.

Trevor Gary Raymond, Armand's grandson who lives on the Witwatersrand can give no information going back before about 1910, and neither could John Armand who I have also traced. More recently I discovered that the two older Raymond girls married in the Union Chapel—Congregational Church—in Port Elizabeth. Delphine married William Robson Chalmers a clerk, son of James Chalmers a Port Elizabeth surgeon, on 16 December, 1862, and Louise married William Oswald Pullen, a farmer of King Williamstown on 3 June, 1863. So far my efforts to trace any of their descendants have been fruitless.

The only other report I have found in my newspaper searches appeared in a Bloemfontein newspaper in 1863. In the column from their Port Elizabeth correspondent appears the following paragraph:

'I am sorry to say that the Rector (of the Grey Institute in P.E., the Rev. Henry Isaac Johnson) is the victim of a very untoward event which happened last week. He had occasion to have a tooth extracted, and the operator Mr Raymond managed to extract two, together with a portion of the gum and a portion of the jaw. The Rector's suffering must have been intense.' (30)

To return to Cape Town where Alfred Raymond lived in April, 1847, when he first used ether. This was at 12 Burg street where the Saambou headquarters exist today. The site was the first office of Volkskas and it seems very likely that the building where Volkskas commenced operations could have been the same building in which Mr Raymond lived. Opposite number 12 is Keay's building and this still stands. It was at number 19 that *De Verzamelaar* was printed and published, the proprietor and editor being a Mr J Suasso de Lima. It seems more than a coincidence that the first newspaper report of ether in Cape Town was in *De Verzamelaar* yet this newspaper carried no other reports of the use of ether for many months thereafter.

The first issue of the *Cape Town Medical Gazette* included an article 'Dental Physiology' by Alfred Raymond (26). Dr Henry Ebden the editor and founder must have solicited this article from Mr Raymond. This raises the question of whether Dr Ebden, who in his editorial mentioned the experiments with ether, participated in experiments with Alfred Raymond, or he may have been referring to Raymond's successes with the vapour. To have accepted an article for the first issue of the first medical journal in South Africa Dr Ebden must have considered Raymond a reputable practitioner.

This is as much as it has been possible to discover to date, but the pursuit goes on. The quest has taken the author to the State Library and Archives in Cape Town where many days have been spent in perusing newspapers and documents; to Port Elizabeth, London and Paris. Over 500 letters have been written to glean the little information I have. I still hope to trace more information about Alfred Raymond—was he really a qualified dentist and where did he qualify (registration of dentists in the Cape was only introduced between 1882 and 1892), where was he born, where did he die and so on. The ultimate would be to find a portrait or photograph of the mystery anaesthetist, who administered the first ether in South Africa, who does not at present seem to have either a beginning or an end.

References

(1) Atherstone WG. Reminiscences of medical practice in South Africa fifty years ago. *S Afr Med J* 1847; **4**: 243–7.
(2) Sulphuric ether—painless operation. *Grahamstown Journal* (June 19) 1847.
(3) Sulphuric ether. *Frontier Times* (June 21) 1847.
(4) Sulphuric ether. *Grahamstown Journal* (June 26) 1847.
(5) Sulphuric ether—painless operation. *De Zuid Afrikaan* (July 1) 1847.
(6) Sulphuric ether—painless operation. *Cape of Good Hope Examiner* (July 2) 1847.
(7) Burrows EH. *A history of medicine in South Africa.* Cape Town: AA Balkema, 1958: 169–72.
(8) Laidler PW, Gelfard M. *South Africa: its medical history.* Cape Town: Struik, 1971: 280–3.
(9) Louw JH. *In the shadow of Table Mountain.* Cape Town: Struik, 1969: 39–40.
(10) Keys TE. Reflections after a 40 year interest in the history of modern anaesthesia. In Ruphreht J, van Lieburg MJ, Lee JA, Erdman W, eds. *Anaesthesia: essays on its history.* Berlin: Springer-Verlag, 1985: 345–51.

(11) Grobler V. *The history of dentistry in South Africa.* Pretoria: HAUM, 1977: 31-2.
(12) Anonymous. The vapour of ether. (Editorial). *Cape Town Medical Gazette* 1847; **3**: 56-8.
(13) Anonymous. The vapour of sulphuric ether. (Editorial). *Cape Town Medical Gazette* 1847; **4**: 79.
(14) Schmidt HJ. A history of anaesthesia in South Africa. *S Afr Med J* 1958; **32**: 244-51.
(15) Anonymous. *De Verzamelaar* (April 20) 1847.
(16) Kok OVS. History of anaesthesia in the Republic of South Africa. *Fourth World Congress of Anesthesiologists*, 1970: 167-73.
(17) Lee YK. The first anaesthetic in the Straits Settlements (Singapore, Penang and Malacca)—1847. *Br J Anesth* 1972; **44**: 408-11.
(18) Montgomery A. Application of ether. *De Zuid Afrikaan* (May 27) 1847.
(19) Anonymous. Inhalation of ether. *De Zuid Afrikaan* (May 3) 1847.
(20) Anonymous. Communication. *De Zuid Afrikaan* (May 20) 1847.
(21) Wilson GCM. The tyrant overcome: a review of the history of anaesthesia in Australia. *Anesth Intens Care* 1972; **1**: 9-26.
(22) Latest intelligence. *South African Commercial Advertiser* (March 31) 1847.
(23) Anonymous. Painless operation under ether. Reports from Middlesex, Westminster Hospitals. *South African Commercial Advertiser* (April 7) 1847.
(24) Anonymous. New medical discovery. *Cape Town Mail* (June 26) 1847.
(25) Anonymous. Sensation, action and volition. *Cape Town Mail* (June 19) 1847.
(26) Raymond A. Dental physiology. *Cape Town Medical Gazette* 1847; **1**: 19-20.
(27) A Card. *Eastern Province Herald* (Dec 2) 1862.
(28) Notice. *Eastern Province Herald* (Nov 29) 1859.
(29) A notice. *Eastern Province Herald* (June 15) 1860.
(30) Anonymous. This, that and the other. *The Friend of the Free State and Bloemfontein Gazette* (Sept 25) 1863.

7.4   The history of anaesthesia in Hong Kong

Z. LETT
University of Hong Kong

Many of Hong Kong's early medical records have regrettably been lost owing to the ravages of the 2nd World War and the Japanese occupation. It is consequently not known by whom—or when—the first anaesthetic in Hong Kong was administered (1). Anaesthesia in China is reported to have been introduced in 1847 by a Dr Peter Parker who, having graduated in 1843, from the Medical School in New Haven (Connecticut, USA), also became a Presbyterian minister (2).

The evolution of medical and health facilities in Hong Kong and surroundings, as well as the beginnings of medical education have recently been reviewed by Choa (3), Fang (4), and Li (5). However, information about early anaesthesia was scarce. The author is therefore indebted to Mr John Rydings, former librarian of the University of Hong Kong, for unearthing a number of references. Probably the earliest record—discovered by chance in the course of another investigation—was found in a book, *The Medical Missionary in China* by William Lockhart published in London in 1861 (6):

> '*At this period (1847), the use of sulphuric ether was first adopted in the hospital, to relieve pain in operations, according to the method of Doctor C. Jackson of Boston.*'

The hospital referred to was that of the Medical Missionary Society which moved from Macau to Hong Kong in 1843.

The development of Academic medicine in Hong Kong

To appreciate the evolution of anaesthesia in Hong Kong a look at some early (and later) events of general interest may be in order:

1841   Occupation of Hong Kong by the British.

1842   Treaty of Nanking.

1843   The Treaty was ratified and Hong Kong became a Colony. The first administrator was a captain Charles Elliot who was replaced by the second administrator, Sir Henry Pottinger. One of his early reports states:

> *'Colony was visited by a great deal of most severe and fatal sickness*
> *. . . in that year . . . 24% of the garrison force died of fever . . .*
> *also 10% of European residents (Endacott, A History of Hong Kong,*
> *Oxford University Press, 1958).'*

1843   saw the start of the Government Medical Services and the appointment of a Dr Alex Anderson as the first Colonial Surgeon. In the following five years no fewer than four Colonial Surgeons succeeded each other. This wearing out of good men was not surprising, considering their duties, which were later described by a Dr Ayres in 1873:

> *'besides general supervision of the Department, Medical Officer to*
> *the Lock Hospital, the jail which is also used as a Lunatic Asylum*
> *. . . also meteorological reporter to the government . . . also in charge*
> *of sanitary supervision of the Colony . . . also expected to attend on*
> *all those families of subordinates in the civil service drawing under*
> *£400.00 p.a. . . . also in private practice.'*

1887   Medical education began with the establishment in 1887 of the College of Medicine for the Chinese. Dr Patrick Manson who later became known as the 'Father of Tropical Medicine' was the first Dean.

1892   Graduation from this College of Dr Sun Yat-sen who later was to become the Founder of Modern China. Dr Sun was a close friend of James Cantlie, Professor of Surgery and Anatomy in the College.

1905   The words 'for the Chinese' were dropped from the name of the College.

1911   The University of Hong Kong opened and the College of Medicine was absorbed into it. The first Dean of this was a Dr Francis Clarke who simultaneously occupied the post of the Medical Officer of Health in the Government Service.

1913   Appointment of the first full-time professor (Dr H. G. Earle, physiology). Until then teaching was done by part-time doctors.

1914   Dr Kenelm Digby appointed to the Chair of Anatomy.

1915   Government Civil Hospital became the Teaching Hospital and Digby became Professor of Surgery also.

1937   Queen Mary Hospital took over as the Teaching Hospital of the University of Hong Kong.

1981   The Chinese University of Hong Kong (in Shatin, New Territories) opened its Medical Faculty and Dr Gerald H. Choa became the first Dean.

Early references to anaesthesia

1889   Dr J. M. Atkinson, Superintendent of the Government Civil Hospital wrote in Appendix B of his report about three cases of gunshot wounds. Case 2 is described:

> *'. . . the patient was anaesthesized and the wound examined . . .' The*
> *third case '. . . the patient was immediately anaesthetized, the eyeball*
> *was found to be quite disorganized and was excised . . .'*

These reports do not give any details of anaesthesia.

1892   Appendix A of the Report of the Superintendent of the Government Civil Hospital states:

> '. . . a Chinese girl aged 9 years was admitted from Wong Ma Kok on 29 October in a state of collapse suffering from . . . wounds said to have been inflicted by some wild animals . . . On admission she was in a very critical state . . . effects of shock and haemorrhage. Under the influence of chloroform the wounds were dressed . . . and the child ultimately made a very good recovery . . . discharged in February 1893'.

1898   The manuscript minutes of a meeting of the British Medical Association, Hong Kong and China Branch record that in February:

> 'Staff surgeon Wm E. Home, MD, RN read a paper on "Chloroform anaesthesia". This was followed by a discussion on the subject of "anaesthesia"'.

1900   Appendix 10 of the Report of the Acting Principal Civil Medical Officer records two mentions of the use of chloroform: one for removal of 9th rib in a case of hepatic abscess, and the other for removal of ruptured spleen from a Chinese male adult.

1903   'Adrenaline' was a topic of the talk by a Dr Stedman to members of the Hong Kong Branch of the BMA. During discussion a Dr Wm Koch stated that 'he found adrenaline useful in treating patients who collapsed during chloroform anaesthesia by placing a few drops (of adrenaline) on the patient's tongue.' In the light of present-day knowledge this practice would appear highly dangerous. From a few further mentions it seems that chloroform was the most commonly used anaesthetic between 1901 and 1904. The author is also grateful to Dr E. H. Patterson, Chief Surgeon and Medical Superintendent of the Nethersole and United Christian Hospitals in Hong Kong for unearthing relevant information amongst their records.

1896   Annual Report for 1896.

> 'Eighty-four operations under the influence of an anaesthetic were performed in the Alice Memorial and Nethersole Hospitals during 1896 with results as under: Cured 64, Improved 16, Died 4'.

1898   Annual Report for 1901.

> 'One hundred & thirty-six operations under the influence of an anaesthetic were performed in 1898—Cured 95, Improved 35, Died 6'.

1901   Annual Report for 1901.

> 'Two hundred & fourteen operations under chloroform or cocaine were performed in the two hospitals during 1901. Results: Cured 167, Improved 41, Unimproved 3, Died 3'. Of these 214 operations 119 were on the eye, which probably accounts for the use of cocaine.

Early pioneers

One of the early practitioners was the late Doctor George Thomas and the author is indebted to him for a great deal of information about that period. When he started out as an advanced medical student in 1910 and resident in the Alice Ho Miu Ling Nethersole Hospital (London Missionary Society), chloroform and ether, either singly or mixed, dropped from a bottle on an open mask, were the routine anaesthetics. Methods would depend on, the availability of drugs and personnel, and relative skill and experience of the latter. In fact, Dr Thomas thought that this was the only method known at the time. Morphine and atropine were also administered hypodermically, beforehand. A refinement was warmed ether vapour either inhaled or sometimes delivered with the aid of a pump. So lightly was the giving of anaesthesia regarded in those days that any doctor—or even a medical student—was not only allowed, but even encouraged to anaesthetize patients. Dr Thomas was admitted as a Fellow of the Royal College of Surgeons of England by Sir Arthur Porritt when he was President of the College at a unique ceremony outside England.

Another early practitioner was Dr Li Shu-fan, a surgeon who popularized spinal anaesthesia in Hong Kong. He was reputed to have been among the first Chinese doctors (with one or two others such as Dr C. H. Wan) to obtain the Fellowship of the Royal College of Surgeons of Edinburgh. He became Minister of Health in the Chinese Government of General Chiang

Kai-shek during the 1939–45 World War. He was a pioneer and an energetic advocate of the use of subarachnoid block. His brother, Dr Li Shu-pui, kindly provided the author with a copy of an article 'Spinal anaesthesia under Novocaine-caffeine Compound', which was presented at a joint meeting of the China Medical Association and the Hong Kong Branch of the BMA in 1925. Dr S. F. Li is also fondly remembered for his generous medical philanthropy, having been the founder of the Hong Kong Sanatorium, main contributor to the establishing of the pre-clinical medical science building (which bears his name) of the University of Hong Kong, the Federation of the Medical Societies of Hong Kong and many other worthwhile causes.

Dr H. P. L. Ozorio (popularly and affectionately known as 'Ozo') was the first medical practitioner in Hong Kong to undergo specialized training in anaesthesia (Oxford and London) where amongst his teachers were Sir Robert Macintosh and Bill (later Professor W. W.) Mushin. Ozo was a gentleman of many and varied talents, who also obtained postgraduate obstetrical qualifications and became an authority on tropical fish. In addition he was a gifted musician who (under his pseudonym of Hal Lorenzo) had an entertaining radio programme. Nevertheless it was his achievement in—and devotion to—anaesthesia that he will be mostly remembered by. He was fond of gadgets and invented some, such as the 'Ozorio connector' useful for operations in the mouth, or throat, where anaesthesia cannot be given through a naso-tracheal tube and an orotracheal one has to be used instead.

During Ozo's absence from Hong Kong (1948–51) and prior to the author's arrival in Hong Kong (1954), the standard and methods of anaesthesia were generally unsatisfactory and in need of improvement (7). Due to changing conditions in the private sector, Ozo decided to return to the United Kingdom in the 1960s. He continued there as consultant anaesthetist in Warrington, but his health was failing. Nevertheless he died while still in harness and glowing tributes were paid to him in obituaries in the *British Medical Journal* by Sir Robert Macintosh and also the present author (8).

Early obstetrical anaesthesia

The practice of obstetrical anaesthesia has been associated with the Tsan Yuk Maternity Hospital since its opening in 1922. The author is indebted to Professor Gordon King, OBE, FRCS, FRCOG, for supplying the information about those early days, when the range of sedative and anaesthetic drugs used during labour was rather restricted.

The tendency was to limit their use as far as possible, partly because Chinese patients seem to tolerate labour pain better than their Caucasian counterparts and partly to avoid side effects on the baby. Amongst the early drugs were potassium bromide, chloral hydrate and tincture of opium (often given in a composite mixture). During severe pain morphine 10 mg was given but not within one or two hours prior to expected delivery.

Chloroform was used on an open mask by drop method with 'plenty of fresh air', particularly during the second stage of labour. A modified Junker bottle was also available (the patient could herself squeeze a bulb which blew air through a small amount of chloroform in the bottom of a tall glass bottle which hung by the beside.) Air was delivered by a rubber tube to a mask which the patient held near her face. When she started losing consciousness, she could not squeeze the bulb until some lucidity returned. The bottle could not be overfilled, could not be spilt, and could not deliver anything but the vapour to the mask. Nitrous oxide and oxygen were later used more commonly.

Low 'spinal' analgesia was found useful, particularly for forceps delivery and stovaine was an early drug, later somewhat replaced by heavy Nupercaine—always in small doses. Such analgesia was also the choice for lower Caesarean section, internal version or other types of vaginal delivery.

Amongst alternate methods of pain relief in labour in the early days of the Tsan Yuk Maternity Hospital were 'twilight sleep' (popularized in Germany earlier this century) consisting of an intra-muscular or subcutaneous injection of morphine (10–15 mg) with hyoscine (scopolamine) 0.4 mg, early in labour. Later, pethidine was introduced. However, careful monitoring of the progress of labour and the fetal heart was essential and early forceps delivery was often embarked on. In the early stages of labour pentobarbitone sodium was found useful for sedation of the mother.

Trichloroethylene was introduced in 1948, became popular and was found equal if not superior to nitrous oxide with air. Today the Tsan Yuk Hospital provides an epidural service for parturient mothers, although the great majority of deliveries in Hong Kong take place under no—or only partial—analgesia and sedation. It has been suggested that Chinese ladies have a higher threshold for pain perception—at least while in labour (9).

Anaesthesia for cardiac surgery

Anaesthesia for cardiac surgery was first practised for operations including 'closed cardiac' surgical procedures in 1954 at the Kowloon and Queen Mary Hospitals. In 1957 the Grantham cardiothoracic centre was opened by the then Governor Sir Alexander Grantham. Dr Nancy Butt became the first full-time anaesthetist there and, gradually, full 'open heart' surgery came into its own. While the Grantham is a public hospital, recently open heart surgical facilities became available also in the private sector at the Hong Kong Adventist Hospital.

Intensive care units

Intensive care units came into being gradually and at the time of writing a great number of hospitals have good facilities. A Hong Kong Society of Critical Care Medicine has also been established. In a number of these ICUs the anaesthetists are in administrative charge, while in others the admitting unit (medical, surgical, paediatric, etc.) retain full responsibility for their patients, with consultation with others as necessary. The situation in Hong Kong remains flexible as indeed reports from other sources would also indicate (10,11).

The Society of Anaesthetists of Hong Kong

The Society of Anaesthetists of Hong Kong was founded in 1954. The co-founders were the author and the late Dr Ozorio. They were strongly supported by the few full-time anaesthetists then practising in Hong Kong, aided by a considerable number of surgeons (and others) amongst them Professor Francis Stock, Dr (later Professor) G. B. Ong, Dr Philip Mao, Dr George Choa, Dr John Chen, the late Drs John Gray and George Thomas. The then Dean of the Medical Faculty Professor Gordon King also lent his full support, and so, after a great deal of preparatory work, the inaugural meeting took place on 17 June, 1954 (after the author's arrival in April 1954), with the following doctors elected to the first Council: Drs Ozorio—Chairman, Lett, Vice-Chairman, Y. K. Poon, Hon. Secretary, Capt Donald Turner RAMC (Army) Surg. Commdr. O'Connor (Navy) Y. O. Chan, A. J. F. Eberle and Loretta Lo.

The aims of the Society, as imbedded in the constitution at the time are still valid today although they may be slightly modified when the new constitution comes into effect in 1987 or 1988. They are:

(i) to promote continued interest in the art and science of anaesthesia.

(ii) To create and maintain favourable conditions for training anaesthetists in this area.

(iii) To hold clinical meetings, lectures, scientific film shows, discussions, and conferences with special emphasis on anaesthetic and allied questions and problems.

(iv) To indirectly educate the public of Hong Kong, in a strictly ethical and professional manner, on the importance of this branch of medicine. To dispel present superstitions and wrong impressions that may prove detrimental to the advance of the science of anaesthesia and, therefore, also detrimental to the safety and well-being of the patients.

These aims remain the cornerstone of the activities of the Society. Over the years it has been host to many distinguished visitors who have passed through Hong Kong. The World Federation of Societies of Anaesthesiologists was established in 1954 and is affiliated to the World Health Organization (WHO). Hong Kong's Society was accepted for full membership in 1957. Practically every past President of the WFSA has visited Hong Kong in either official or private capacity or both.

The Faculties of Anaesthetists of the Royal Colleges of Surgeons of England, of Australasia and in Ireland maintain friendly contacts with the Hong Kong Society of Anaesthetists. The Faculty of Anaesthetists of the Royal Australasian College of Surgeons conducts the written parts of both the Primary and the Final FFARACS examination as well as the *viva voce* part of the Primary FFARACS examination in Hong Kong and also helps with a Faculty tutor for local candidates. The latter is facilitated by a grant from the Hong Kong Oxygen Company.

The 7th Asian–Australasian Congress of Anaesthesiologists was held in Hong Kong in 1986 and was regarded by many participants as one of the most successful. The Organizing Committee was under the guidance of the Congress President Dr Jean Allison having put in a great deal of hard work.

Chairs of anaesthesia in Hong Kong

The Medical Faculty of the Chinese University of Hong Kong in Shatin, New Territories, which is the younger (by far) of the two Medical Faculties, was officially opened in 1981. It has had the good fortune of attracting as its first Professor of Anaesthesia for its independent department—Professor John Andrew Thornton. Dr Jean Horton (from Cambridge, UK) and Dr Cindy Aun are the Senior Lecturers.

The Medical Faculty of the much older University of Hong Kong on Hong Kong Island did not have a Chair of Anaesthesia authorized until recently. The reason may have been partly financial but, presumably also because the Consultants (anaesthesia) from the Government Medical Services were able (and still are) to provide both service cover and teaching of students. Recently, however, interviews of suitable applicants have taken place and at the time of writing an offer of appointment has been made. A detailed account of the evolution of anaesthesia in Hong Kong has been published elsewhere (12).

References

(1) Lett Z. Anaesthesia in Hong Kong. *Anaesthesia* 1980; **35**: 993–8.
(2) Spence J. *The China Helpers (Western Advisers in China 1620–1960)*. London: The Bodley Head, 1968: 54.
(3) Choa GH. *A history of medicine in Hong Kong*. Medical Directory of Hong Kong, 3rd Ed 1985: 13–29.
(4) Fang HSY. *Hong Kong from a medical viewpoint*. Medical Directory of Hong Kong, 2nd Ed 1981.
(5) Li SF. *Hong Kong from a medical viewpoint*. Medical Directory of Hong Kong, 3rd Ed 1985: 4–12 (All 3 above published by Federation of Medical Societies of Hong Kong, 15 Hennessy Road, 4th floor, Hong Kong).
(6) Lockhart W. *The medical missionary in China*. London 1861: 166.
(7) Ong GB. Valedictory. *University of Hong Kong Gazette* 1983; **31**: 26–27.
(8) Obituary. *Br Med J* 1973; **3**: 642.
(9) Lett Z. History of anaesthesia in the Tsan Yuk Hospital. In: Daphne Chun, ed. *The first fifty years of the Tsan Yuk Hospital (1922–1972)*. Hong Kong: Cosmos Printing Press, 1972.
(10) Dudley HAF. Intensive Care: a specialty or a branch of anaesthetics? (Editorial) *Br Med J* 1987; **294**: 459.
(11) Stoddart JC. A career post—with intensive therapy. (Editorial) *Anaesthesia* 1986; **41**: 1181.
(12) Lett Z. *Anaesthesia in Hong Kong. Evolution and present position*. Hong Kong: Centre of Asian Studies. University of Hong Kong, 1982.

Chapter 8
THE ORGANIZATION OF THE SPECIALTY OF ANAESTHESIA

8.1 The Association of the Anaesthetists of Great Britain and Ireland

T. B. BOULTON

Past President, Association of Anaesthetists of Great Britain and Ireland, London, UK

The speed with which the practice of general anaesthesia spread through the World, following Morton's successful demonstration of ether at Boston in October, 1846, was truly amazing considering the means of communication available at that time (1).

The United Kingdom was one of the first countries to benefit from the new discovery and, fortunately, the tradition was quickly established that anaesthesia should only be administered by medically and dentally qualified practitioners. It may be that the introduction of chloroform by James Young Simpson of Edinburgh in November, 1847, had something to do with this. Chloroform quickly supplanted ether in the United Kingdom because of its potency, ease of administration, and more ready acceptance by patients. Chloroform is, however, a much more dangerous drug than ether and throws a greater burden of responsibility on the skill of the administrator. It was soon tacitly accepted in the United Kingdom that such a burden should only be borne by a qualified practitioner. The position was different in the United States where irritant and less potent ether reigned supreme for many years and proved relatively safe in the hands of nurses and ancillary workers, thus starting a different tradition.

Specialization also came early to the United Kingdom, even though it was limited. Men like John Snow, Clover, and Hewitt, who devoted almost all their clinical practice to anaesthesia, were to be found only in London and a few major cities. Elsewhere in the country any practitioner was expected to be capable of administering anaesthesia after an undergraduate training.

The Society of Anaesthetists

The few specialists in teaching hospitals had thus a vital part to play in developing and teaching anaesthesia. It was a natural consequence that they should feel the need to establish a corporate body for the study and development of the specialty and the exchange of information between members. The Society of Anaesthetists—the first such body in the World—was therefore formed in London in 1893 on the initiative of Dr John F. Silk of Kings College Hospital its first Secretary. The first President was Dr Woodhouse Braine who had been one of the first to introduce nitrous oxide into England.

Two-thirds of the members of the Society naturally always came from London, but the membership was, in fact, world wide and included representatives from all over the United Kingdom, Australia, Canada, South Africa, Switzerland and the United States. It also admitted lady members unlike many contemporary medical societies. The reputation of the Society prospered. It published its own Transactions and its activities were frequently reported in the contemporary press. It also exerted an influence on the academic requirements for medical degrees (2).

The Royal Society of Medicine

The Royal Medical and Chirurgical Society, had been founded in 1805 and had received its Royal Charter in 1834 from King William IVth. In 1907 it amalgamated with a number of specialist societies and became the Royal Society of Medicine. The Society of Anaesthetists joined the new Society a year later in 1908, after certain constitutional problems had been resolved. These related chiefly to the preservation of the rights of its lady members (3).

The first quarter of the 20th century

Considerable scientific progress was, of course, made over the next quarter century, but the pattern of practice of anaesthesia in the United Kingdom remained much the same well into the nineteen forties. There were specialist teachers and innovators in the university hospitals in the major cities, but only part-time general practitioner anaesthetists elsewhere. Practice in the charitable voluntary hospitals was honorary, however, and private anaesthetics were very poorly remunerated compared with surgery. Concurrent General Practice was therefore a necessity for anaesthetists—even, in many cases for those appointed to prestigious teaching hospitals.

The Association of Anaesthetists of Great Britain and Ireland

Henry Walter Featherstone (1894–1967) a Birmingham teaching hospital physician anaesthetist was President of the Section of Anaesthetics in the academic year 1930–1931 (4). He, together with a number of contemporaries, realized the need to enhance the status and training of anaesthetists, both to improve the standards of practice and to secure better pecuniary recognition for their services. A medicopolitical crusade of this kind could not be prosecuted by the Section of Anaesthetics however, because the Charter of the Royal Society of Medicine limited its activities to scientific debate; consequently, after a preliminary meeting with attendance by invitation on 27 April, 1932, the Association of Anaesthetists of Great Britain and Ireland was born on Friday, 1 July, 1932, with Dr Featherstone as its first President (5,6). Its purpose was not to replace the Section of Anaesthetics but to complement it.

Two-thirds of the first Council were London based and this was reflected in the membership. This can be contrasted to the 1987 Council, which is freely but not regionally elected, and in which less than one sixth of its members are from London.

The original membership was predominantly confined to those who devoted the bulk of their practice to anaesthesia as teaching hospital anaesthetists but, as the number of practitioners engaging in the specialty has increased, so has the scope of membership widened. There was an overseas corresponding membership from the beginning, and the unique Junior Anaesthetists' Group was inaugurated in 1967 during the Presidency of H. H. Pinkerton (1901–1982) (7).

An early factor in the process of expansion was the gradual improvement in the nature and facilities of the Poor Law Infirmaries and the creation of municipal hospital services with salaried medical staff including surgeons and anaesthetists.

The Diploma in Anaesthetics

The introduction of a qualification in anaesthesia was one of the expressed primary objectives of the Association at its formation, but the institution of a diploma could only be achieved by a chartered examining body. The Conjoint Board of the Royal Colleges of Physicians of London and Surgeons of England responded to the request of the Association to establish the Diploma in Anaesthetics (DA) in 1935—the first of its kind in the World. The Association retained an advisory role in the management of the Diploma even though it did not have the overall control of the examination.

The expansion of the specialty in World War II

There was an urgent need for a considerable number of trained physician anaesthetists for the British Armed Services on the outbreak of World War II. The Association, as the only existing official body representing anaesthetists, took the leading role in advising, training and assessing these specialists. A large number of trained and experienced physician anaesthetists were consequently available and ready to take their place in the National Health Service (NHS) when it came into being in 1948.

The National Health Service

A period of uncertainty preceded the introduction of the NHS but, ultimately after negotiations in which the Association played a prominent part, anaesthetists were accepted as consultants with equal status and remuneration to all other specialties. This crucial achievement was catalysed by the promotion by the Association of the establishment of the Faculty of Anaesthetists of the Royal College of Surgeons of England—a body dedicated to the maintenance of the training standards and the conduct of its examinations (8). The DA was upgraded to the standard of the existing British Specialist diplomas such as the Fellowship in Surgery, and, in 1953, it became the Diploma of Fellowship of the Faculty of Anaesthetists of the Royal College of Surgeons of England—a qualification the excellence of which is recognized throughout the World (9).

It is interesting and significant that, as when the Association was formed in 1932, the retiring President of the Section became the first President of the Association so the retiring President of the Association in 1948, Dr Archibald Marston (1893–1962), became the first Dean of the Faculty at its foundation (8).

The organization of anaesthesia in the United Kingdom today

There are thus now three complementary national bodies, generally working in harmony, serving anaesthesia in the United Kingdom. All three hold scientific meetings and promote learned discussion—the Section of the Royal Society of Medicine exclusively so. The Association combines with this a greatly expanded medicopolitical, general, and individual advisory roles, and the Faculty, as a component of a Chartered Royal College, is specifically responsible for the maintenance of training standards and the conduct of the examinations of the specialty.

The Association is, however, the only one of the three with a fully independent existence (a fact endorsed by the right to bear heraldic arms by Royal warrant), and now occupies its own prestigious premises at 9 Bedford Square, London W1.

Conclusion

The Association of Anaesthetists of Great Britain and Ireland has a proud record. No major development has taken place in the organizations of British or Irish anaesthesia since its foundation in 1932, which has not been either initiated or promoted unders its auspices. Whatever direction the future development of the organization of anaesthesia in the United Kingdom takes in the future, we can be sure that the advice and guidance of the Association will play an important part.

References

(1) Ellis RH. The introduction of ether anaesthesia to Great Britain, 1. *Anaesthesia* 1976; **31**: 766.

(2) Dinnick OP. The first Anaesthetic Society. In: Boulton TB, Bryce-Smith R *et al.* eds. *Progress in Anaesthesiology. Proc 4th World Congr Anaesthesiologists.* Amsterdam: Excerpta Medica Foundation 1970: 181.

(3) Davidson M. *The Royal Society of Medicine. The realization of an ideal 1805–1955.* London: Royal Society of Medicine, 1955.

(4) *Obituary*. H. W. Featherstone. *Anaesthesia* 1967; **22**: 532.

(5) Featherstone HW. The Association of Anaesthetists of Great Britain and Ireland. Its inception and purpose. *Anaesthesia* 1946; **1**: 5.

(6) Helliwell PJ. Editorial. *Anaesthesia* 1982; **37**: 394.

(7) Wishart HV, Holloway KB, Spence AA. Henry Harvey Pinkerton. President of the Association of Anaesthetists of Great Britain and Ireland 1965–1967. *Anaesthesia* 1982; **37**: 1143.

(8) Association News. *Anaesthesia* 1948; **3**: 129.
(9) Faculty News. *Anaesthesia* 1953; **8**: 210.

8.2   Faculty of Anaesthetists, Royal College of Surgeons of England

R. S. ATKINSON
Past Vice-Dean, Faculty of Anaesthetists of the
Royal College of Surgeons of England, London, UK

In 1745 the Company of Surgeons broke away from the Barber Surgeons and the first meeting of the newly created Royal College of Surgeons of London (later changed to Royal College of Surgeons of England) was held on 10 April, 1800, at No. 41, Lincoln's Inn Fields.

The present building, in which this Symposium is being held, is the result of many changes. Purchase of adjacent properties took place as the years passed, so that the address now incorporates numbers 35 to 43. It is interesting to observe in passing that No. 37 was the site of the old Duke's Theatre (approximately where the western end of the Lumley Hall and the Council Room now stand). Purcell's Dido and Aeneas received its first professional performance here in 1700, and Gay's 'Beggars Opera' was performed in Duke's Theatre many times in 1729.

In more recent times bomb damage during the 1939 to 1945 war was considerable and many of the exhibits of the Hunterian Museum were lost. Considerable reconstruction of the building was necessary after the war and in 1953 the College was honoured when Her Majesty Queen Elizabeth II laid a memorial stone.

The College itself has received a number of new Charters since its formation. The President and Council of the College constitute the ruling body.

The foundation of the Faculty

The preceding paper has explained how the Association of Anaesthetists of Great Britain and Ireland came to be formed. The need for a diploma examination became necessary as the specialty of anaesthesia grew and the Association approached the Royal College of Surgeons for help. An examination for the Diploma in Anaesthetics or DA was set up in conjunction with the Royal College of Physicians and the first examination was held in November, 1935.

Anaesthesia continued to develop and in 1948, with the inception of the National Health Service, became a full specialty in its own right. An academic body became necessary. The Council of the Royal College of Surgeons had already agreed to the formation of a Faculty of Dental Surgery in 1947 and in 1948 the Faculty of Anaesthetists was to follow. It came about because on 13 November, 1947, Council received a letter from the Association of Anaesthetists asking for a conference to discuss the matter. The report of the meeting which followed, dated 25 February, 1948, came before Council on 11 March, who wisely agreed with its recommendations.

All holders of the Diploma of Anaesthetics would be eligible to become members of the Faculty and other duly qualified practitioners could join on the recommendation of the Board of Faculty. The Board was to consist of 21 diplomates in anaesthetics with the President and the two Vice-Presidents of the College serving ex-officio. The Faculty was given powers to grant a special Fellowship in the Faculty of Anaesthetists of the Royal College of Surgeons of England. Dr A. D. Marston became the first Dean and Dr Bernard Johnson the first Vice-Dean. Within six months there were over 700 fellows.

The role and function of the Faculty

The first task of the Faculty was to raise the standards of its examinations and to introduce a Fellowship Diploma, with a Primary, (an examination in the Basic Sciences pertaining to anaesthesia), and a Final which was an examination in anaesthesia, medicine and surgery. This structure lasted, with various amendments, for many years, but in 1985 the examination was restructured. There are now three parts. Part 1 is a test of the candidates grasp of clinical medicine and knowledge appropriate to the first year of practice of anaesthesia, Part 2 a test of basic sciences, and the 'Final' Part 3 incorporates the whole spectrum of anaesthetic principle and practice.

The Faculty also concerns itself with the maintenance of standards of training and practice. Candidates are not permitted to enter the Final or Part III FFARCS examination unless they have completed posts which have been inspected by Faculty Visitors and approved by the Board. Faculty assessors sit on all appointment committees for consultant posts in the National Health Service and are able to ensure that all appointees have received adequate training not only before, but subsequent to acquisition of the FFARCS diploma. The Faculty plays an important part in the deliberations of the Joint Committee for Higher Training in Anaesthesia which regulates post-FFA or senior registrar training and recommends accreditation.

The Faculty is concerned with postgraduate education in anaesthesia. It has an educational programme and encourages local courses. It sponsors visiting lecturers from overseas and has representation on other educational bodies such as the Council of Postgraduate Medical Education.

The Faculty appoints Regional Educational Advisers in each Region and Faculty Tutors in all major hospitals and provides a counselling service through its Bernard Johnson Adviser.

The Faculty has a National Role and its remit extends throughout the United Kingdom. It has full representation on all national bodies. One of its strengths, like that of the Royal Colleges of other disciplines lies in its complete independence of government. It can therefore offer impartial advice and has considerable authority in its relationships with the Department of Health and with Health Authorities.

The Faculty has excellent relationships with its sister Faculties in Australia and in Ireland as well as with like bodies in Canada, the United States, South Africa and other countries. Many doctors from overseas seek training in centres in the United Kingdom.

The Constitution of the Faculty

The Faculty has evolved over the years within the Royal College of Surgeons of England. The Board is elected by postal vote of all its Fellows and itself elects the Dean and Vice-Dean. The Faculty now has complete autonomy within the College in the control of its affairs and has financial independence. It is subject only to the provisions of the Charter of the College and its amendments, which include its charitable status. In 1977 the Charter was revised granting Faculties the right to elect three members to serve on the College Council as full voting members, with eligibility to the offices of President and Vice-President. The office of Vice-President has subsequently twice been filled by an anaesthetist.

The future of the Faculty

In 1986 the Council of the College agreed that an approach be made to the Privy Council to consider a further amendment to the Charter to allow conferment of Collegiate Status on Faculties, without altering the relationship between these bodies within the College.

The Faculty of Anaesthetists has now been in existence for almost 40 years. Throughout this time there has been steady growth and continuous evolution of its role and function. There are now over 5000 Fellows of whom about 1200 reside overseas. The Faculty remains healthy and vigorous. Whether it remains a Faculty or evolves to Collegiate status its course is set to continue its many activities well into the 21st century.

8.3   A short history of the Canadian Anaesthetists' Society

GORDON M. WYANT[1] and RODERICK A. GORDON
[1]*University of Saskatchewan, Saskatoon and [2]University of Ontario, Toronto, Canada*

The Canadian Society of Anaesthetists 1920–1928

Few artefacts from the Canadian Society of Anaesthetists founded in 1920 survive other than the Gavel and the Seal of the Society and the programme of its first meeting held in Niagara Falls in June 1921. This was held in conjunction with the Interstate Society of Anaesthetists, the forerunner of the International Anaesthesia Research Society.

The first President was Dr Samuel Johnston of Toronto (Fig. 1), Dr William Webster of Winnipeg was elected Vice-President and Dr Wesley Bourne of Montreal Secretary-Treasurer.

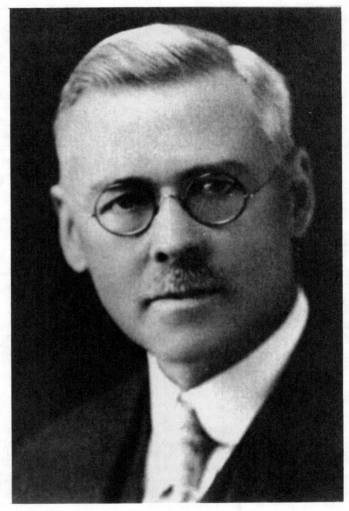

Figure 1   Samuel Johnston.

Nine other anaesthetists prominent in those days are listed as Officers of the new Society. The Society did not succeed and surrendered its charter in 1928 to become the Section on Anaesthesia of the Canadian Medical Association.

The origin of specialist certification in Canada

Widespread concern was expressed by some provincial medical associations after 1925 about the lack of adequate training of people who professed to be specialists and, while there appears to have been considerable agreement that something should be done about the situation, no agreement was reached as to which body should carry out the certification process until 1934. In that year both the Canadian Medical Association and the Royal College of Physicians and Surgeons of Canada appointed a committee and three years later (in 1937) an agreement was reached that the Royal College should undertake the certification of specialists, but anaesthesia was not a discipline deemed worthy of certification. This attitude persisted until 1942 and the Canadian Medical Association showed little interest in the problem of anaesthesia over the years and senior anaesthetists in the country therefore became convinced of the necessity to form a separate national society in order to define training and qualifications in the specialty.

The foundation of the Canadian Anaesthetists' Society

The Montreal anaesthetists undertook the incorporation of the present Canadian Anaesthetists' Society (CAS) and letters Patent for the Society as a non-profit organization were issued on 21 June, 1943. It is ironic as has been noted above, that the Royal College had finally added anaesthesia to its list of specialties in the preceding year.

The objects of the Society were defined as follows in the original charter:

'To advance the art and science of anaesthesia and to promote its interest in relation to medicine with particular reference to the clinical, educational, ethical and economic aspects thereof, to associate together in one corporate body members in good standing of the medical profession who have specialized in this particular science, to promote the interest of its members, to maintain a Society library and bureau of information, to edit and publish a journal of anaesthesia, to acquire and own such property and real estate as may be necessary to carry out effectively the purposes of this Society and to do all such lawful acts and things as may be incidental or conducive to the attainment of the above objects.'

Eligibility for membership was reserved for medical practitioners duly qualified and registered in the Country in which they practise their profession. If practising in Canada they were required also to be members in good standing of the Canadian Medical Association, L'Association des Medicins de la Langue Française de L'Amerique de Nord, or of a local or provincial medical society approved by the Council of the Society. Four categories of membership were defined, namely active members, members elect (physicians in training), associate members and honorary members.

Four divisions of the Society were recognized:

Division 1 comprised of members residing in the Provinces of Nova Scotia, New Brunswick and Prince Edward Island.

Division 2 comprised of members resident in the Province of Quebec.

Division 3 members resident in Ontario.

Division 4 members resident in the Provinces of Manitoba, Saskatchewan, Alberta and British Columbia.

Membership dues were set at $5 (Canadian) per year.

Fees

One of the first actions of the newly elected Council was to publish a schedule of fees (Fig. 2). This was an improvement over a previous national Fee Schedule suggested by the Canadian

CANADIAN ANAESTHETISTS' SOCIETY
Schedule of Fees — 1943

Any Type—(exclusive of cost of materials used).
Very Minor Anaesthetic:—
   (an anaesthetic for an operation for
which the surgical or obstetrical fee is
$15.00 or less) .... $ 5.00 & up

Minor Anaesthetic:—
   (an anaesthetic for an operation for
which the surgical or obstetrical fee
is $50.00 or less)
for first hour or fraction thereof ....$10.00 & up

Major Anaesthetic:—
   (an anaesthetic for an operation for
which the surgical fee is in excess of
$50.00)
for first hour or fraction thereof ....$15.00 & up

Prolonged Anaesthesia
   After first hour for each successive
¼ hour or fraction thereof .... $ 2.50 & up

Figure 2.

ADDITIONS 1947
Consultation and Report:
                    .... $ 5.00 & up

Diagnostic and Therapeutic Nerve Blocks
   For Stellate Ganglion block ....$15.00 & up
   For Gasserian Ganglion block ....$25.00 & up
   For Block of Cardiac Nerves ....$25.00 & up
   For Block of Single Somatic Nerve
      Root or Infiltration of Tissues .....$ 5.00 & up
   For all Other Procedures ....$10.00 & up

Specialists Schedule
   For all types of Anaesthesia, general, regional,
spinal, an increase of 25% on each item of the
minimum tariff approved by the Canadian Anaesthetists' Society. The fee is for professional services, including pre-anaesthesia and post-anaesthesia
consultation, venoclysis, plasma and blood transfusions, oxygen therapy, and all other immediate
supportive measures, and does not include the cost
of materials used.

Figure 3.

Medical Association which had recognized only minor and major anaesthetics at a fee of $5 and $10, respectively.

The new schedule recognized three levels of fees, namely 'very minor', 'minor', and major 'anaesthetics', introduced the concept of tying the anaesthetic fee to the surgical one, defined it as a minimum rather than an absolute fee, and made additional allowance for prolonged procedures. A revision in 1947 (Fig. 3) added a minimum fee for consultations and for diagnostic and therapeutic nerve blocks, as well as a surcharge for services provided by specialists. Further revisions followed in later years and indeed provincial Fee Schedules were developed which vary considerably in concept and remuneration.

Historically anaesthetists in Canada were remunerated in three ways; by fee-for-service paid by the patient, by salary as hospital employees, or by payment by the surgeon who quoted an inclusive fee to the patient. The second and third alternatives were considered improper and probably unethical and in June, 1950 the Society promulgated a statement to this effect which resulted in anaesthetists being remunerated on a fee-for-service basis throughout the country; this method still is generally applied despite provincial health insurance plans in all 10 Provinces.

Amendments to the original Constitution

These were approved in 1945 providing representation from all provinces, as well as from anaesthetists serving in the armed forces overseas. Thereafter the Bylaws of the Society remained unchanged until 1949 when the Newfoundland division was created following entry of that Province into Confederation. In 1951 the two immediate past-presidents were added to the Council to provide continuity of experience and, in 1964, the Editor of the *Canadian Anaesthetists' Society Journal* was included as well. An entire new constitution was prepared and revised in 1972 which, amongst other provisions, created an Executive Committee of the Council.

Training standards

The maintenance of standards of training and conduct of examinations has been assumed by the Royal College of Physicians and Surgeons of Canada but the Society nevertheless has continued to use its influence, and has succeeded in maintaining the principle that the length of time required for training in anaesthesia should be equal to that in all other specialties of medicine. Originally the Fellowship of the Royal College was open to anaesthetists only by examination in general medicine and a request that a Fellowship modified for anaesthesia be instituted was rejected in 1947, but eventually came into being in 1951 in the Division of Medicine.

Education

Throughout its history, the Canadian Anaesthetists' Society has promoted continuing educational opportunities through annual, regional and divisional meetings of the Society. Self-evaluation programs were devised and in 1972 a one-day review course in conjunction with the annual meeting of the Society was introduced.

The Society has remained throughout active in public relations and has designed pamphlets to be distributed to surgical patients in hospital to explain the role of anaesthetists in their treatment.

The Journal of the Society

The Canadian Anaesthetists' Society Journal has been published since 1954. In January, 1987, the name was changed to *Canadian Journal of Anaesthesia*.

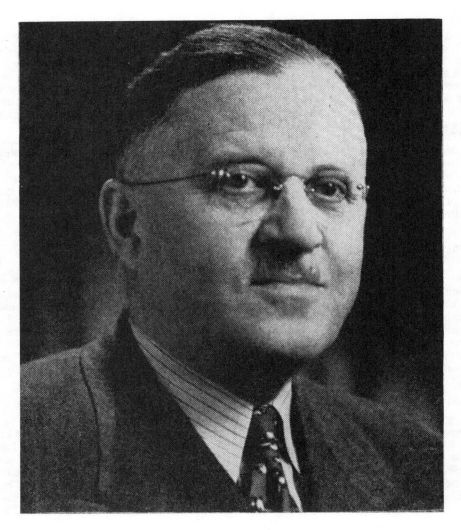

Figure 4   Dr Harold Randall Griffth.

Pensions

In 1957 Council observed that there was no organized mechanism available to self-employed physicians to provide the equivalent of pension on retirement and the Canadian Anaesthetists' Mutual Accumulating Fund Limited was incorporated as an investment vehicle in that year.

International affairs

Internationally the CAS was represented on an international committee convened in Brussels in June, 1953, to consider the formation of a world organization of anaesthetists. The WFSA came into being at a World Congress of Anaesthesiologists at Scheveningen, Holland in 1955 with the CAS as one of the founding member Societies Dr Harold Griffith of Canada was elected as first President (Fig. 4). The Society has been continuously represented on the Executive of the Federation since 1955 and hosted the Second World Congress in Toronto in 1960. In 1966 Council established a Canadian Anaesthetists' Society Training and Relief Fund to assist the teaching of anaesthesia in developing countries.

The Canadian Anaesthetist's Society Medal

The Society established the Canadian Anaesthetists' Society Medal in 1962 to be awarded to individuals for meritorius service in anaesthesia. Twenty such awards have been made to date.

Prizes and awards

Since 1967 the Society has offered prizes for the three best papers reporting original research presented by Residents in training at the annual meeting, and, starting in the same year, for the best original work by a Canadian anaesthetist published during the year in the *Canadian Anaesthetists' Society Journal* has been recognized by the award of the Canadian Anaesthetists' Society prize. In 1979 the Society established a Canadian Anaesthetist Research Foundation which made its first grant-in-aid of research in 1986.

Conclusion*

Just as the 1920 Society collapsed because, in the words of Dr Harry Shields the eminent Toronto pioneer in anaesthesia, they elected a Secretary who never wrote a letter, so did the new Canadian Anaesthetists' Society flourish because it was fortunate to have had a Secretary–Treasurer who from 1946 to 1961 devoted all his energies to the building and prosperity of the Society and its members. Dr Roderick Angus Gordon (Fig. 5), my co-author, was responsible for not only the organization of the Society, but also was the driving force behind many of the

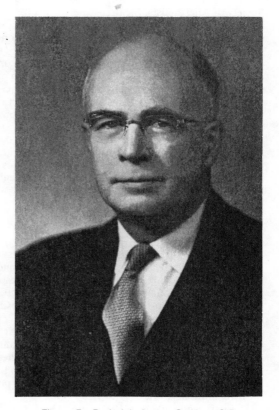

Figure 5   Roderick Angus Gordon, C.D.

activities which have been recounted, such as the journal of which he was the Editor from its inception until 1982, the Mutual Accumulating Fund, the Training and Relief Fund and many others. The CAS without Rod, as he is generally known, is unthinkable to those of us who have lived through the early and developing years of the Society.

*By Gordon M. Wyant alone.

| 8.4 | Attempts to establish anaesthesiology as a specialty in German medicine* |

W. SCHWARZ

University of Erlangen-Nürnberg, Erlangen, German Federal Republic

The German Society of Anaesthesia was founded in 1953 exactly 60 years after the inauguration of the Society of Anaesthetists of London and 48 years after the formation of the Long Island Society of Anesthetists, the first society organized for physicians interested in anaesthesiology in the USA, and the forerunner of the American Society of Anesthesiologists (1). This comparative delay seems surprising; especially if one considers that German investigators had provided a vital stimulus to the development of anaesthesia at the end of the 19th and the early years of the 20th century by pioneering contributions to local, spinal, and regional anaesthesia, intubation, open drop administration of ether, and intravenous anaesthesia (2–5). On the other hand, even before the turn of the century, voices had been heard in German medicine stressing anaesthesia as an essential part of the medical profession, and pointing to its significance in medical training (6,7). These voices were ahead of their time, however, and went unheard.

It was not before the end of World War I that the anaesthesia movement in German began to gather momentum through renewed contacts with advances made in the meantime in Britain and America. Study groups were formed by surgeons and pharmacologists interested in problems related to anaesthesia. Demands for an independent professional identity became increasingly vociferous.

E. v. d. Porten: pioneer physician anaesthetist

In 1922, E. v. d. Porten of Hamburg, the first physician in Germany claiming to be a professional anaesthetist, formulated a basic precondition for the reorganization of anaesthesia as a medical field. He emphasized that a person responsible for conducting anaesthesia should be completely familiar with the theory and practice of the subject. He therefore called for 'careful and exact instruction in the art of anaesthesia' during medical training (8).

An informative trip to Britain in 1923, and his participation in a Nottingham meeting in 1926, when v.d. Porten was mentioned in the list of participants as the only representative from continental Europe, familiarized him with anaesthesia in Britain. On these occasions he also formed personal links with leading anaesthesiologists in Britain and the USA. These experiences were to lead him to lend his support to the foundation of anaesthesia as a specialty, to the setting up a professional body, and to the publication of an anaesthesia journal based on foreign models (9).

The next steps taken in 1928 were, The foundation of the first anaesthesia journals, the journey of H. Killian and H. Schmidt to the USA, and the 'First German Anaesthesia Congress' in Hamburg.

The foundation of two anaesthesia journals

De Schmerz appeared in 1928 after three years of preparatory work. It was edited by the gynaecologist C. J. Gauss (University of Würzburg), the pharmacologist H. Wieland (University of Heidelberg), E. v. d. Porten, and the pharmacologist B. Behrens (Heidelberg). The stated goals were:

1. to maintain and promote scientific interest in narcosis as a first step towards the establishment of the anaesthetists' profession in German medicine.

*The author dedicated this paper to Professor Dr. med. H. W. Opderbecke of Nürnberg on his 65th birthday.

2. to set up an interdisciplinary platform for pain research in anatomy, physiology, pathology, prophylaxis and therapy.
3. to renew international cooperation interrupted by World War I by coopting foreign experts and scientists to the editorial board (10).

Narkose und Anaesthesie also appeared in 1928. It had similar subjectives, and was edited by the gynaecologist H. Franken and the surgeon H. Killian (University of Freiburg), the surgeon H. Schmidt (University of Hamburg), and the pharmacologist H. Schlossmann (Medical Academy, Düsseldorf).

The foundation of these separate journals reflected the situation of anaesthesiology in Germany at that time with groups still continuing to work independently of each other. But in view of the economic situation (the Great Depression of 1929), the editors of the two journals agreed to merge their publications into one journal entitled 'Schmerz, Narkose, Anaesthesie' (Pain, Narcosis, Anaesthesia) (9) during the second year of publication.

The foundation of an independent scientific journal of anaesthesiology has to be seen as an important step in the development of anaesthesiology as a separate discipline in Germany. What had previously been sporadic and isolated scientific and professional activities could now be brought together and coordinated. Hence the warm welcome extended to these two journals by international anaesthesiology (11,12). The International Anaesthesia Research Society at its annual meeting in 1928 awarded the editors of both journals the 'Scroll of Recognition' (9,13). In 1943, the journal ceased publication, 16 volumes having appeared. It had not met with the success its founders had expected (14).

The journey of H. Killian and H. Schmidt to the USA in 1928

In May, 1928, H. Killian and H. Schmidt travelled to a meeting in America at the invitation of the International Anesthesia Research Society. Schmidt had just been appointed to what was presumably the first university lectureship in Germany for 'Surgery and Narcosis' (13). The two delegates reported to the meeting on their research work and the state of anaesthesia in Germany.

In his paper, Schmidt, besides reporting on the criteria for the indication of inhalation versus intravenous anaesthetics, announced that, during a special session at the 90th Meeting of the Society of German Scientists and Physicians in Hamburg, 'we intend to form a German society of Anaesthetists' (15). The International Research Society spontaneously decided 'to send the Secretary-General to this Congress to represent Organized Anaesthesia and to be helpful in every possible way'. F. H. McMechan, the secretary-general, expressed the expectation that through this congress 'anesthesia would come into its own in Germany' (16).

Following the congress in Minneapolis, where Killian and Schmidt had been able to link up with numerous American anesthesiologists, they visited several large clinics to get acquainted with anaesthesia in the USA. Later Schmidt also travelled to Canada and Britain, visiting 53 different hospitals (18).

On their return, the two scientists reported on their experiences, Killian in a comprehensive contribution to his journal (17), and Schmidt in his paper given at the meeting of German scientists and physicians in Hamburg (18). Both were impressed by the professionalism with which anaesthesia was administered in clinics in America and Britain, serving the interest of surgeons and patients alike. Some fine distinctions, however, are made in their final assessments.

Killian stated that 'the unique character of the educational background and medical studies, and the specific economic conditions in the USA would not allow us here in Germany to copy the American organization. We will have to take account of economic and cultural conditions in Germany, and have to reorganize anaesthesiology in accordance with our own principles' (17). Killian did not describe the form this should take but he was to do so eleven years later (13).

Schmidt was so impressed by what he had seen and heard during his three months study trip that he 'decided there and then to become an anaesthetist in Germany' (18), and 'to devote himself in his clinic, at least for a time, to the improvement of anaesthetic techniques, the organization of anaesthesia services, and the training of students' (19). This he actually did for two years. Then, due to the economic crisis of the time, he came to realize that being a pioneer of anaesthesiology was too risky an enterprise and decided to continue his career as a surgeon (18).

The 'First German Anaesthesia Congress' in Hamburg, September, 1928

It was on 20 September, 1928, at the 90th Meeting of the Society of German Scientists and Physicians in Hamburg that a joint session on 'Inhalation anaesthesia and its significance for narcosis' was organized by the surgery, gynaecology, and pharmacology sections. It was hoped that this session would provide a valuable stimulus for the further development of the specialism of narcosis in Germany. McMechan, in his welcoming address, gave expression to this hope (20), and Schmidt, in his paper on 'Inhalation anaesthesia as seen by the American anaesthetist', attempted a programmatic breakthrough in the field.

He reported in detail on the structure of anaesthesia as a specialty in America and Britain, on problems of practical narcosis including patient management, on the organization of anaesthesia services, on university training, on money-making opportunities, and on the controversies with nurse anesthetists in the USA. Against this background he criticized the opinion, widespread in German medicine, that the specialty of anaesthesia was not necessary. It was his belief that 'the seriousness of narcosis was frequently under-valued which often meant a greater risk or injury to the patient than surgery'. Specialized anaesthetists would administer anaesthesia more safely and with less risk thus making the stay in hospital shorter. In consequence, the introduction of anaesthesia would pay for itself. Schmidt therefore pleaded for some degree of specialization at universities and large hospitals in Germany (18).

This plea for the consolidation of anaesthesiology both as a profession and a specialty fell on deaf ears. It had been the irrationalist fears of the older generation of surgeons, Schmidt said in retrospect, that had led them to reject unanimously 'a second, jointly responsible person placed at their side' (19).

The session, too, ended without any compelling recommendation for practical narcosis. Based on his ideas on the theory of narcosis, the pharmacologist P. Trendelenburg emphasized the general superiority of inhalation anaesthesia compared with other methods (21). The surgeon E. Rehn favoured nitrous-oxide for prolonged administration, and ether for shorter operations. Schmidt recommended combined inhalation anaesthesia using nitrous oxide and ethylene. Killian rejected narcylene due to its explosive potential. On the other hand Gauss, having introduced narcylene, preferred this substance in spite of this danger, believing nitrous oxide insufficient (9).

This confused situation at the end of a meeting supposed to point towards the future was reflected in Killian's entry in Schmidt's visitor's book: A sketch shows a group of perplexed surgeons surrounding a patient and asking themselves: 'With what shall we anaesthetize after this congress?' (19,22).

Killian's memorandum on the state of anaesthesia in Germany (1939)

Eleven years after this year of high expectations and disillusionment, Killian presented his demand for a reorganization of anaesthesia taking account of German economic and cultural conditions. At the annual meeting of the German Society of Surgery in 1939 he delivered a memorandum on the state of anaesthesia in Germany to the President of the Society. At the same time he sent the following proposals to the public health administration (23):

1. Foundation of a German Society of Narcosis and Anaesthesia.
2. Transformation of the existing journal into a national journal for narcosis and anaesthesia.
3. Training for anaesthesia teachers and anaesthesia assistants.
4. Student training in anaesthesia.
5. No anaesthesia without exact instruction and without special supervision.
6. Establishment of a central research centre with an anaesthesia museum and special library (14).

Twenty-five years later, Killian wrote in his book (23) that he had never heard what had become of these proposals. The outbreak of war, he said, had halted the reorganization of modern anaesthesia in Germany. There seems to be no obvious reason why Killian did not mention that he had in fact received an official reply to his memorandum from the 'Reichsärztekammer' (National Board of Physicians). The Ministry of Health had forwarded the record to the 'Reichsärztekammer' which was responsible for matters related to medical professionalism and specialization. This reply of 14 September, 1939, was based on an endorsement of the National-socialist Association of University Lecturers and on 'a comprehensive statement by Professor Dr Goetze from Erlangen University' [unpublished letter]. This fact indicates that the Presiding Council of the German Society of Surgery must have discussed Killian's proposals.

The 'Reichsärztekammer', in its statement, admitted deficiencies in the training of young doctors in narcosis, but: 'Your plans for the separation and over-specialization of anaesthesiology seems completely impracticable'. He was advised to present his proposals for discussion by the German Society of Surgery without organizational commitment. He published his memorandum two years later (14). It may be noted that, despite this opposition by the national health administration to a further division of the medical profession, in 1940 pathological anatomy had been adopted as a specialty for the medical profession (24).

The failure of Killian's efforts was probably largely due to opposition by the German Society of Surgery. In a letter dated 14 April, 1953, only a few days after the foundation of the German Society of Anaesthesia, Killian wrote to R. Frey, then secretary of the society, that ever since 1926 he had been pursuing the aim of founding a society, his last attempt in 1939 having been 'sabotaged' by Goetze's recommendation.

Regrettably, the records to which the letter from the 'Reichsärztekammer' refers have not yet been discovered. But Goetze's arguments may be reconstructed. In connection with a discussion with roentgenologists in 1939 on the affiliation of radiodiagnosis Goetze presented a fundamental statement on 'General surgery and specialization' (25). He argued that nearly all advances in science had been made through specialization, and to this extent general surgery and surgical specialization belong together. A surgical specialty is defined by its own comprehensive diagnostics and therapy. A specialty not meeting these criteria, e.g. radiodiagnosis, has, according to Goetze, to be classified as an ancillary science (25). We may conclude that, in accordance with these criteria, Goetze classified anaesthesia as an ancillary science, and advised against making it an independent discipline.

Developments after World War II

Not only did the surgeons' attitude act as a constraint on the development of organized anaesthesia in Germany. A second crucial factor was the isolation of German medicine during two world wars. When, after World War II, information on the state of medicine in foreign countries became available it was soon obvious that anaesthesia had made possible enormous advances in operative medicine by the introduction of endotracheal anaesthesia and muscular relaxation. To link up with these new developments it was essential to find out about innovations in clinical anaesthesia.

Farsighted surgeons sent their assistants to clinics in the USA, Britain, and Scandinavian countries to study modern methods of anaesthesia. Numerous reports were published in medical journals of which that by Hugin (26) is an example. Foreign anaesthetists, too, were invited to provide advanced training in anaesthesia techniques. Jan Henley from New York, for example, having come on a visit to Europe in spring 1949, working for two years in several German hospitals, assisting in setting up anaesthesia services (27). At the suggestion of F. Bernhard, director of the Department of Surgery at the University Hospital of Giessen, she wrote a short handbook entitled 'Introduction to the practice of modern inhalation anaesthesia', which was published in German in 1950 (28).

At the same time articles appeared discussing anaesthesia as a medical specialty. Killian repeated his memorandum of 1939/41 (29), and several other authors made their proposals (30,31).

In 1950, the German Society of Surgery nominated an anaesthesia committee comprising two surgeons and two pharmacologists. In the very same year, to improve the field of anaesthesia, the committee suggested a two-year training for anaesthetists at large clinics performing thoracic surgery, including a one-year turn of surgery, and another year of pharmacology. Furthermore, the anaesthetist was to be assigned to the director of the clinic, and university lecturers for 'general and local analgesia' were to be appointed. Special lectures for students of medicine and dentistry were to be introduced (32).

While practical anaesthesia made rapid progress due to the need of German surgeons to catch up on international developments, the organizational structures took longer to emerge. Many surgeons could not imagine having their own independent anaesthetist as in Britain or the USA, as the eminent surgeon W. Nissen from Basel had advocated (33). At the annual meeting of the German Society of Surgery in 1952 even such a great supporter of anaesthesia as the Heidelberg surgeon K. H. Bauer could present views on the relationship between general surgery and surgical specialties (the 'all-under-one-roof-principle') which were basically in accordance with those of Goetze (34). Following this, Bauer had arranged a special session on 'Modern Anaesthesia' as part of the scientific programme of his congress. This was to be a regular feature of the annual programme of the congress until congresses specially devoted to anaesthesia were started.

Finally, in 1952, Frey, Hügin, and Mayrhofer succeeded in publishing a new German anaesthesia journal entitled *'Der Anaesthesist'* (35).

On the occasion of the First Austrian Congress of Anaesthesiology, 9 September, 1952, 23 participants from Germany founded a 'German Study Group for Anaesthesiology', followed by the foundation of the 'German Society of Anaesthesia' on 4 April, 1953 (35,36).

By now anaesthesiology in Germany had gathered such momentum that the inclusion of a 'specialist in anaesthesia' as part of German medical training requirements was inevitable. On 19 September, 1953, the Council of German Physicians at Lindau, Lake Constance, passed a resolution endorsing this policy, although in the previous year this had not been possible (37).

Even the German Society of Surgery could no longer avoid the issue, and its delegate 'urgently seconded' the motion. He explained that it was no longer feasible in the context of modern surgery for the operating surgeon to take upon himself responsibility for anaesthesia too: 'The anaesthetist must have equal rights alongside the surgeon accepting full responsibility for his actions and decisions'. This he could only do on the basis of adequate training, including theoretical knowledge in fields the surgeon was unfamiliar with, such as pharmacology. Furthermore, he stressed there was no choice but to take this step 'to link up with world-wide medicine' (37).

Anaesthesiology had thus become an independent specialty. It was to take many more years, of course, before every hospital in Germany had its anaesthetist, before all medical faculties had established professorships in anaesthesiology, and before the anaesthetist as a colleague with equal rights had become a reality.

References

(1) Betcher AM, Ciliberti BJ, Wood PM, Wright LH. Fifty years of organized anaesthesiology. *JAMA* 1955; **159**: 766–70.
(2) Fink BR. Leaves and needles: Introduction of surgical local anesthesia. *Anesthesiology* 1985; **63**: 77–83.
(3) Nolte H. The first thirty years of regional anaesthesia in Germany (1884–1914). *Regional-Anaesthesie* 1985; **8**: 63–6.
(4) Sweeney B. Franz Kuhn. His contribution to anaesthesia. *Anaesthesia* 1985; **40**: 1000–5.
(5) Whitacre RJ, Dumitru AP. Development of anaesthesia in Germany in the early years of the twentieth century. *J History Med* 1946; **1**: 618–34.
(6) Lewerenz-Steinsiepe M. Fritz Ludwig Dumont: ein moderner Anaesthetist. *Anaesthesist* 1982; **31**: 302–5.
(7) Klimpel V. Zur ärztlich ausgeführten Narkose in der Frühgeschichte der modernen Anaesthesiologie. *Anaesthesiol Reanimat* 1986; **11**: 241–5.
(8) von der Porten E. Die Frage des Narkotikums. *Zentralbl Chir* 1922; **49**: 830–3.
(9) Tschöp M. Ernst von der Porten 1884–1940 in *der Geschichte der deutschen Anästhesiologie*. Berlin: Springer, 1986: 25.

(10) Gauß CJ, Wieland H, von der Porten E. Zur Einführung. *Der Schmerz* 1928; 1: 1–4.

(11) Cohen HM. Geleitwort. *Der Schmerz* 1928; 1: 5–6.

(12) McMechan FH. Amerikanisches Geleitwort. *Der Schmerz* 1928; 1: 169–70.

(13) Anonymous. Zur Tageschichte. *Der Schmerz* 1928; 2: 144–5.

(14) Killian H. Plan zur Neuordnung des Narkosewesens in Deutschland. *Schmerz Narkose Anaesth* 1941; 14: 73–87.

(15) Schmidt H. Inhalation or injection narcosis? The development of the specialty of anesthesia in Germany. *Curr Res Anesth Analg* 1929; 8(1): 20–4.

(16) McMechan FH. Germany on the way to organized professional anesthesia. *Curr Res Anesth Analg* 1928; 7(4): 195–6.

(17) Killian H. Über amerikanische Narkoseverhältnisse. *Narkose Anaesth* 1928: 1: 448–63.

(18) Schmidt H. Gruß an Hans Killian. In: Frey R, Bonica JJ, Foldes FF *et al.*, eds. *Erlebte Geschichte der Anaesthesie*. Mainz: 1972: 23–26.

(19) Schmidt H. Die Gasnarkose vom Standpunkt des amerikanischen Narkosespezialisten. *Narkose Anaesth* 1928; 1: 530–40.

(20) Anonymous. Zur 90. Versammlung deutscher Naturforscher und Ärzte, Hamburg, September, 1928. *Narkose Anaesth* 1928; 1: 529–30.

(21) Trendelenburg P. Theorie des Narkotisierens mit Gasen. *Narkose Anaesth* 1929; 2: 1–12.

(22) Killian H. Reminiscences of the First German Anaesthesia Congress in Hamburg (1927) and Rolf Frey's Departure to Mainz. In: Ruprhecht J, van Lieburg MJ, Lee JA, Erdmann W, eds. *Anaesthesia. Essays on its history*. Berlin: Springer, 1985: 279–83.

(23) Killian H. 40 Jahre Narkoseforschung. Tübingen: *Verlag der Deutschen Hochschullehrer-Zeitung*, 1964: 211.

(24) Anonymous. Reichsärzteordnung. Berlin: *Reichsgesundheitsverlag* 1944: 140.

(25) Goetze O. Allgemeinchirurgie und Spezialfach. *Langenbecks Arch* 1939; 196: 129–33.

(26) Hügin W. Über moderne Anästhesiemethoden. Beobachtungen in USA. *Deutsch med Wochenschr* 1947; 72: 695–700.

(27) Frey R, Gray C, Lüder M. Anaesthesia: Past and Future. In: Rügheimer E, Zindler M, eds. *Anaesthesiology*. Amsterdam: Excerpta Medica, 1981: 1023–6.

(28) Henley J. Einführung in *die Praxis der modernen Inhalationsnarkose*. Berlin: de Gruyter, 1950.

(29) Killian H. Reorganisation des Narkosewesens. *Krankenhausarzt* 1949; 22(9): 15–9.

(30) Neidermayer F. Der Narkosearzt. *Krankenhausarzt* 1949; 22(9): 20–2.

(31) Hesse F. Das Aufgabengebiet des Facharztes für Narkose und Anästhesie. *Med Welt* 1951; 20: 356–8.

(32) Anonymous. Fachnachrichten und Kongreßkalender. *Anaesthesist* 1952; 1: 32.

(33) Nissen R. Entwicklung von Anästhesie und Anästhesiologie und beider Einfluß auf den Fortschritt in der Chirurgie. *Bull schweiz Akad med Wiss* 1953; 9: 1–10.

(34) Bauer KH. Zur geistigen Situation unseres Faches. *Langenbecks Arch* 1953; 273: 9–14.

(35) Frey R. Die Gründung der Deutschen Gesellschaft für Anästhesie 1953. *Anästh Intensivmed* 1978; 19: 373–6.

(36) Lehmann C. Die Deutsche Gesellschaft für Anästhesie und Wiederbelebung. Gründung und Entwicklung. *Anaesthesist* 1967; 16: 259–68.

(37) Bundesärztekammer. *Stenografischer Wortbericht des Ärztetages* vom 15. bis 20 September 1953 in Lindau. Köln: Ärzte-Verlag, 1953: 22–24.

8.5   Was this certificate the first certification in anaesthesia?

A. B. BAKER
Otago University, Dunedin, New Zealand

On 27 July, 1891, Dr Millen Coughtrey then the Sub-Dean of the Faculty of Medicine at Otago University gave notice of a motion which he would bring to the next meeting of the Faculty.

> *'That it is desirable that a special course of instruction in Anaesthetics, theoretical and practical, should be instituted, and that an examination in this subject followed by a special certificate be given.'* (1)

On 31 August, this motion was passed and a sub-committee (consisting of Drs Coughtrey, J. Macdonald, Jeffcoat and Barnett) was set up to investigate how this should be achieved. (1)
At the meeting of 27 June, 1892, it was

> *'resolved that steps be at once taken to give to senior students instruction in the administration of anaesthetics, and that the Dean and Subdean be empowered to make the necessary arrangements'* (1);

and in the Minutes for 31 October, 1892

> *'Church, Ross, Little, Campbell, Torrance and McAdam received instruction in the administration of Anaesthetics, and were reported by the House Surgeon as qualified to receive the certificate.'* (1)

The status of the Faculty of Medicine in 1892

These are the bare bones of the facts from the Faculty Minute book of the era written in copperplate handwriting by the Dean John Halliday Scott, Professor of Anatomy and Physiology—no secretaries for the fledgling Faculty! The Faculty of Medicine had been instituted earlier that year on 28 April, 1892, with the appointment of the first Dean John Halliday Scott. Prior to this time, from the inception of the Medical School (New Zealand's first) in 1874, there had been no formal Faculty of Medicine and all matters had been referred through the Senate or the Vice-Chancellor of the University. The very first medical Professor at the University in 1874 had been Dr Coughtrey who had been appointed from a field of 18 applicants which included the then undergraduate D. J. Cunningham later of Edinburgh anatomy fame. Following Dr Coughtrey's resignation, the appointment of his replacement Professor John Halliday Scott was also from a large field of 25 which again included D. J. Cunningham, by this time a graduate. The opinion from Britain was that Scott should be appointed:

> *'After a comparative examination of the qualifications of these candidates we have formed the opinion that Mr J. Halliday Scott, M.B., C.M., Demonstrator of Anatomy in the University of Edinburgh, is the one who in our judgement has the strongest claims for the appointment. The grounds on which we base this opinion are his distinguished career as a student, the experience he has acquired since his graduation in the methods of anatomical work and teaching and the high testimony which is borne to his personal character.'* (2)

and Cunningham was free to take Edinburgh!

Anaesthesia at the University of Otago in the late nineteenth century

Thus almost from the very beginning of the Faculty of Medicine, it was only the third meeting, there was debate about the teaching of anaesthetics. At that time because of the close links with Edinburgh and because of Australasian practice, the common form of anaesthesia in

Dunedin was with chloroform. It was not until the first appointment of Dr Russel Ritchie as anaesthetist to Dunedin Hospital in 1904 that ether was much used (2). That ether was used from time to time, however, is demonstrated by the first Australasian book on anaesthesia which was published from Dunedin in 1879 by John Wilkins *Some Remarks on a New Ether Rebreathing Apparatus* (3). Also operations were performed without anaesthesia in some cases, as is told by Dr Wm John Mullin:

> '*In the late eighties tonsils were removed in the hospital by Mackenzie's guillotine without anaesthesia, the patient sitting in a chair.*' (4)

Other Australian certificates in anaesthesia

Why where was this insistence on the teaching of anaesthesia so early in the life of the Faculty is uncertain, but there had been the First and Second Hyderabad Chloroform Commissions in 1888–89 and this may have led to an increased public awareness of problems with anaesthesia. There was obviously an interest more widespread than just in the University of Otago as 'in 1888 new by-laws for the Faculty of Medicine at the University of Sydney required students to produce a certificate of proficiency in the administration of anaesthetics before admission to the final examination' (5); and in February, 1889 Dr Todd was appointed the first Tutor in Anaesthetics to the University of Sydney only to resign in August, 1889 (5). Later, in 1892, the University of Sydney agreed on a new curriculum which included a requirement for 'a certificate from each candidate for the final examination showing that he had administered six anaesthetics under the supervision of a qualified medical practitioner.' (5)

Later on, in 1894, Embley introduced certification in anaesthesia in the University of Melbourne shortly after his appointment as the first anaesthetist to the Royal Melbourne Hospital; and later still in 1905 the University of Adelaide followed.

Perhaps also the Intercolonial Congresses of Medicine which started in 1887 were a contributory factor though there were very few papers on anaesthesia.

Notes on the recipients of the certificates

The students did not flock to gain the Otago certificate as there were only a few who were mentioned each year (1): (October, 1892: 6; August, 1894: 1; November, 1895: 3; May, 1896: 1; November, 1896: 2; November, 1897: 8; October, 1898: 4; October, 1899: 5; April, 1901: 7; November, 1901: 16).

Each year there were more graduates than these few so there was obviously no compulsion in Otago as appears to have been the case in Sydney. Also the students were able to take the certificate in any of their final three years, and some rare individuals even gained the certificate twice!

Of the first six students to gain the certificate the first on the list and the first to graduate (in 1892) was Dr Robert Church. He had two medical sons one of whom (Dr J. S. Church) became a Founding Fellow of the Faculty of Anaesthetists, Royal Australasian College of Surgeons. Another one of the first six certificate holders, Dr Kenneth McAdam, later in 1895 became the senior House Surgeon to Dunedin Hospital and thus responsible for ensuring that those students who wished to obtain certification in Anaesthesia were instructed accordingly.

Conclusion

The answer to the query in the heading of this paper is, therefore, 'no'. The Otago certificate was beaten by the Sydney one in Australasia, though the uses to which the certificates were put may well have been different. The Otago certificate was obviously voluntary in comparison to the compulsory nature of that at Sydney.

Otago University continued to be concerned that students should be taught in anaesthesia and the Medical Faculty in November/December, 1901, proposed, on a motion by the Dean, and passed new regulations for the teaching of anaesthesia which then made it compulsory.

'Regulations as to certificates etc. as at present with the following additions:

(1)   Certificate of having received practical instruction in the administration of anaesthetics.' (1)

Seventy years later Otago University was again to follow Sydney University in the undergraduate teaching of anaesthetics with the formation of the second independent University Department of Anaesthesia in Australasia.

References

(1) Faculty of Medicine, University of Otago, *Minute Book No. 1* 28 August 1891–14 August 1902.
(2) Hercus C, Bell G. *The Otago Medical School under the first three Deans*. London: Livingstone, 1964.
(3) Wilkins J. *Some Remarks on a new Ether Re-breathing Apparatus: Also on Ether its Practical Uses, Mode of Administration, and Advantages over Chloroform*. Dunedin: Mackay, Bracken, 1879.
(4) Barnett LE. The evolution of the Dunedin Hospital and Medical School: a brief history. *Aust NZ J Surg* 1934; **3**: 307–17.
(5) Personal communication from Dr Gwen Wilson, Australia.

8.6   Pictorial progress of Canadian anaesthesia (1954 to 1986)*

J. R. MALTBY
University of Calgary, Alberta, Canada

In any given period an empirical assessment of anaesthetic practice may be made from contemporary drug advertisements. During the past fifty years the drugs which have led to significant changes in anaesthetic practice are thiopentone, halothane, lignocaine, and curare (1). Despite the established popularity of these drugs before the Canadian Anaesthetists' Society Journal (CASJ) was born, manufacturers continued to advertise them for many years. Other drugs were promoted with initial enthusiasm but few achieved the anticipated market penetration, and many of these no longer appear among the advertisements. Some drugs were advertised for a few years but lost popularity when better alternatives became available (gallamine and d-tubocurarine were superseded by pancuronium). Others never became popular and were withdrawn (ethyl vinyl ether). Non-brand name or non-patented drugs, such as nitrous oxide and morphine, despite their widespread use and effectiveness were rarely advertised. Others, such as ketamine, found a small but useful place which apparently did not justify the continuation of advertising.

The CASJ which started publication in 1954, was used to gain an impression of changing clinical practice in Canada from then until 1986.

Intravenous induction agents

In 1954 intravenous induction agents had been in clinical use for twenty years. Thiopentone advertisements appeared in 20 of the CASJ's 33 years (Fig. 1) sometimes missing a year or two

---

*The Editors regret that it has not proved possible to include all the very interesting photographs of advertisements which accompanied the presentation of this paper.

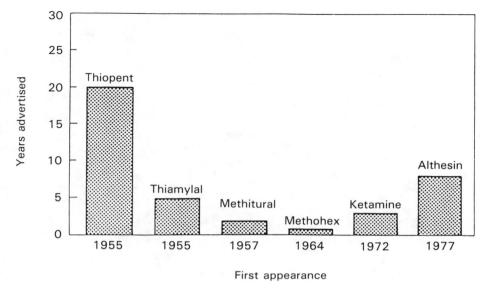

Figure 1   Intravenous induction agents 1954–86. Abbreviations: thiopent—thiopentone, methohex—
methohexitone.

but always reappearing. One of the earliest advertisements in this period (Fig. 2) mentioned
thipentone's 20 years of effective use and its 2150 published reports.

The following year, 1956, saw the first of several advertisements for rectal thiopentone in
children (Fig. 3). These imaginative advertisements drew attention to an alternative to 'the
nightmare of fear', and 'the terrifying fight to breathe as the mask is lowered over the face'
of an anxious child.

The only other intravenous induction agent to be advertised for more than five years was
Althesin, but the extent of its use in Canada never threatened thiopentone. Its advertisements,
which emphasized rapid and complete awakening appeared consistently from 1977 until its
worldwide withdrawal in 1984.

Some intravenous induction agents, including ketamine and methohexitone, although
maintaining a small share of the market were rarely advertised. Others, including propanidid,
etomidate, midazolam, and di-isopropyl phenol, which have been widely used in some countries,
were not available in Canada.

Volatile agents

In the period 1955–59 more inhalational agents were advertised than during any subsequent
five year period (Fig. 4). This suggests that no one agent was outstanding. Divinyl
ether, first used clinically in Edmonton, Alberta in 1932(2), was the one most frequently
advertised.

The entire July, 1957, issue of the CASJ was devoted to a new agent, halothane, and for
nearly a quarter of a century halothane dominated the volatile agent advertisements. Its
promotion and use were maintained in competition with methoxyflurane during the 1960s and
enflurane during the 1970s. The later halothane advertisements emphasized the anaesthetist's
familiarity with an established agent. However, since the release of isoflurane in Canada in
1981, the use of halothane has fallen dramatically and its last advertisement appeared in 1984.

Methoxyflurane's consistent appearance between 1962 and 1974 reflected its moderate
popularity until its rapid demise, following proof of its nephrotoxicity in 1972 (3). In one unusual
advertisement, the manufacturer acknowledged the slow induction characteristic of this agent
by simultaneously advocating the use of thiopentone.

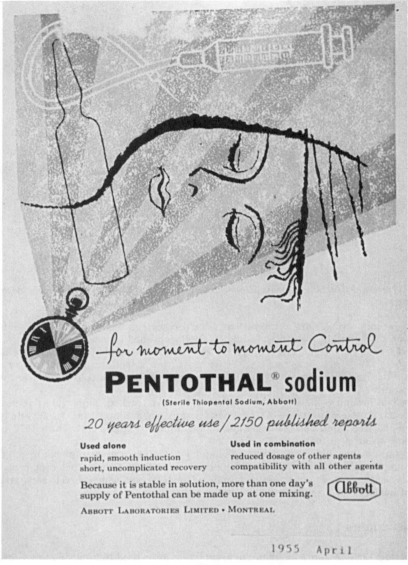

Figure 2   1955 Thiopentone.

Enflurane was released in 1974 and proved to be a useful alternative to halothane. It has been advertised in almost every year since then despite the popularity of isoflurane since 1981.

Local anaesthetic drugs

Lignocaine and bupivacaine stand out above all other local anaesthetic drugs (Fig. 5). Lignocaine is unique in being the only drug that has been advertised in every full year of the CASJ's publication. The early advertisements mentioned its use in infiltration anaesthesia, spinal anaesthesia, major nerve blocks, and topical anaesthesia. Lignocaine CO_2, not available in many countries, was released in Canada in 1973 and has been advertised in eight of the years

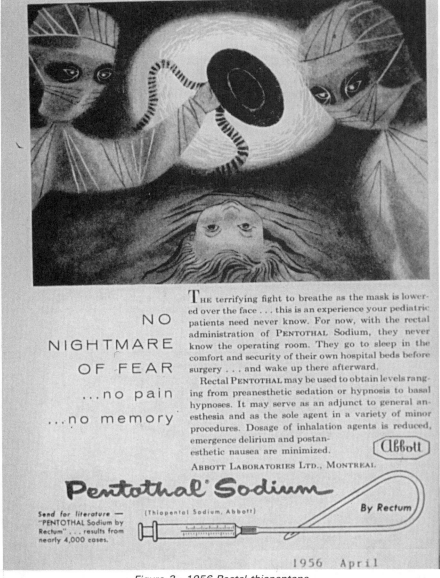

Figure 3   1956 Rectal thiopentone.

since then. In 1975 the convenience of prefilled syringes of lignocaine for the treatment of cardiac arrhythmias was advertised.

The only other local anaesthetic drug to achieve comparable popularity was bupivacaine. Since 1973 it has been advertised every year, with emphasis on the usefulness of its prolonged action in obstetrical analgesia.

Muscle relaxants

The advertisements for muscle relaxants are more difficult to interpret (Fig. 6). For many years Squibb and, later, Burroughs Wellcome advertised succinylcholine (suxamethonium),

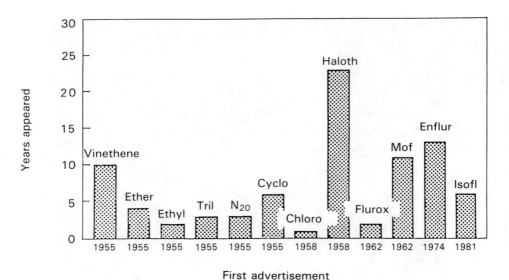

Figure 4   Volatile anaesthetics 1954–86.
Vinethene—divinyl ether. Abbreviations: ethyl—ethyl vinyl ether, tril—trichloroethylene, cyclo—cyclopropane, chloro—chloroform, haloth—halothane, flurox—fluroxene, MOF—methoxyflurane, enflur—enflurane, isofl—isoflurane.

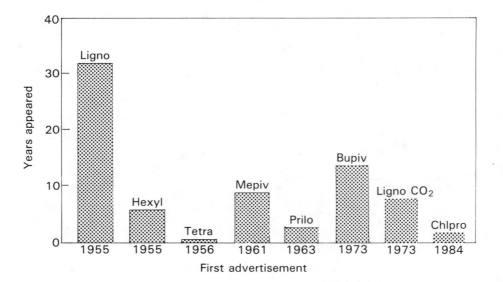

Figure 5   Local anaesthetics 1954–86.
Abbreviations: ligno—lignocaine, hexyl—hexylcaine, tetra—tetracaine (amethocaine), mepiv—mepivacaine, bupiv—bupivacaine, ligno CO_2—lignocaine hydrocarbonate, chlpro—chloroprocaine.

tubocurarine, and decamethonium together. Suxamethonium continued alone after advertisements for curare and decamethonium ceased.

Since the introduction of pancuronium into Canada in 1973, this drug has been the dominant non-depolarizing muscle relaxant, both in advertisements and in clinical use.

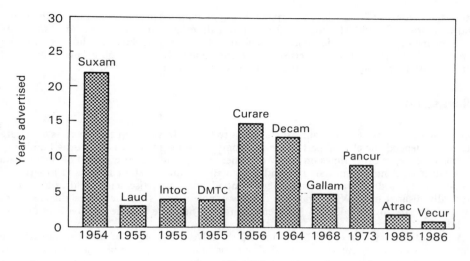

Figure 6   Muscle relaxants 1954–86.
Abbreviations: suxam—suxamethonium, laud—laudexium, intoc—Intocostrin, dmtc—dimethyl tubocurarine, decam—decamethonium, gallam—gallamine, pancur—pancuronium, atrac—atracurium, vecur—vecuronium.

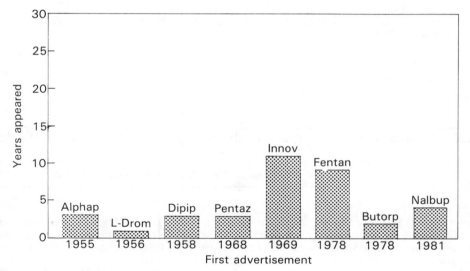

Figure 7   Narcotic analgesics 1954–86.
Abbreviations: alphap—alphaprodine, L-drom—levorphanol, dipip—dipipanone, pentaz—pentazocine, innov—Innovar, fentan—fentanyl, butorp—butorphanol, nalbup—nalbuphine.

Laudexium, gallamine, and dimethyl tubocurarine were occasionally advertised in earlier years. Alcuronium and fazadinium were not released in Canada.

Narcotics

The infrequency of advertisements for narcotic analgesics from 1954 to 1969 (Fig. 7) draws attention to a significant change in anaesthetic practice since that time. Attempts to promote the agonist-antagonists pentazocine, butorphanol, and nalbuphine in anaesthesia met with limited and temporary success. Morphine and pethidine, although commonly used for many years as supplements to nitrous oxide-relaxant anaesthesia, were not advertised. The breakthrough came with fentanyl which was advertised as a component of Innovar (fentanyl and droperidol) for 11 years from 1969, and as fentanyl alone in every year since 1978.

Discussion

Advertisements introduce new anaesthetic drugs to the profession, but their success or failure ultimately depends on clinical performance. Promotion sometimes focuses on drug familiarity or convenience, at other times on safety or patient acceptance. Over a period of thirty years drug advertisements in the CASJ provided vignettes of anaesthetic change and progress in Canada. If a new drug proved to be a significant advance, advertisements for the older drugs gradually disappeared. When the new drug was not clearly superior the established ones continued to be advertised and advertisements for the new one became less frequent or were withdrawn.

A part of history is irretrievably lost when the advertising pages of medical journals are removed before library copies are bound. Some anaesthetists keep unbound journals for many years in their attics or basements; other sources are uncommon. It is in those unbound volumes that there exists a pictorial history of progress in the pharmacology, equipment, and monitoring devices of our specialty.

Acknowledgments

The author thanks the Canadian Anaesthetists' Society for the loan of early unbound copies of its Journal, 1954–1961.

8.7   The continuing progress in the teaching of modern anaesthesia

S. KURIMOTO
Osaka Medical School, Takatsuki, Osaka, Japan

John Snow (1847) used the ether inhaler of copper and defined five stages of etherization in relation to the dose, time and clinical signs (1). These principles were applied in his book *On the inhalation of Chloroform and other Anaesthetics* (2,3). Later anaesthetic apparatus was designed to administer a mixture of gas and vapour by Hewitt (4).

Noci-ceptive spinal reflexes were thought of in terms of tenderness, rigidity and referred phenomena and studied in relation to the philosophy of the nervous irritability by Sherrington (5) and Mackenzie (6). George Crile (7) in 1914 proposed the concept of 'anoci-association' in anaesthesia and surgery (morphine injection and procaine regional anaesthesia were given and nitrous oxide-oxygen anaesthesia was skilfully and sparingly administered).

Ralph Waters (1883–1979) is described by Lucien Morris (8) as the first professor and pioneer educator and investigator of anaesthesia. He was responsible for many developments including the closed system for carbon dioxide absorption and controlled respiration (8). Morris (9) developed the vernier vaporizer 'copper kettle' in 1952 and has continued to refine closed system anaesthesia (10). Since the nineteen-fifties Morris has taught the importance of adequate ventilation in anaesthesia with nitrous oxide-oxygen inhalation after scopolamine premedication—i.e. the concept of controlled respiration using apnoeic threshold, interposed with the diaphragmatic respiratory effort (11).

Further progress was made when nitrous oxide-oxygen inhalation was supplemented with analgesics, the practice of regional anaesthesia was taught especially by Macintosh and Mushin (12), the analysis of the function of the respiratory circuits was advanced by Mapleson (1954), and Mushin and Jones (1987), and the respiratory neuron was investigated by Robson (15).

At the beginning of anaesthetist training the concept of controlled respiration is usefully taught in anaesthesia for general surgical ambulatory and emergency operations. Then, understanding the respiratory signs influenced by physiological factors and pharmacological effects, the anaesthetist can extend his experiences to apply the principles to anaesthesia for cardiac, neurosurgical, paediatric and geriatric patients.

Conclusion

The medical profession has played an important part in this modern age, as has the specialty of anaesthesia. The importance of a career in anaesthesia must be recognized. Progress in this direction, and in the education of anaesthetists, would not have been possible without the leadership of the Faculties of the British Royal Colleges.

Acknowledgments

The author wishes to thank his teachers and friends for the instruction he has received. In chronological order they were: Dr A. Doughty, Professor W. W. Mushin, Professor W. W. Mapleson, Professor L. E. Morris, Professor Sir Gordon Robson and Professor J. G. Whitwam. My acknowledgments are also due to the British Council and Japan–US Educational Commission.

References

(1) Snow J. *On the inhalation of the vapour of ether in surgical operations*. London: Churchill, 1847.
(2) Snow J. *On chloroform and other anaesthetics: action and administration*. London: Churchill, 1858.
(3) Ringer S. *A handbook of therapeutics*, 12th Ed, 1890.
(4) Hewitt F. *Anaesthetics and their administration*, 5th Ed, 1922.
(5) Sherrington C. *The integrative action of the nervous system*. 1906.
(6) Mackenzie J. *Symptoms and their interpretation*. 1909.
(7) Crile G, Lower WE. *Anoci-Association*. Philadelphia: Saunders, 1914.
(8) Morris LE. *Anaesthesia . . . essays on its history*, 1985: 32.
(9) Morris LE. New vaporizer for liquid anaesthetic agents. *Anesthesiology* 1952; **13**: 587.
(10) Linton RAF (Associate Editor). In Churchill-Davidson, ed. Wylie and Churchill-Davidson's *A practice of anaesthesia*, 5th Ed. Lloyd-Luke (Medical Books), 1984: 81.
(11) Morris LE. Concept of adequate ventilation using the apnoeic threshold during curare and nitrous oxide anaesthesia. *Br J Anaesth* 1963; **35**: 35.
(12) Macintosh RR, Mushin WW. Observations on the epidural space. *Anaesthesia* 1947; **2**: 100.
(13) Mapleson WW. Elimination of rebreathing in various semi-closed anaesthetic systems. *Br J Anaesth* 1954; **26**: 323.
(14) Mushin WW, Jones PL (original authors Macintosh, Mushin, Epstein). *Physics for the anaesthetist*, 4th Ed. Oxford: Blackwell Scientific Publications, 1987: 364.
(15) Robson JG. *Modern trends in anaesthesia*, 3, 1967: 42.

8.8   Anaesthetic literature of 1887

C. N. ADAMS
West Suffolk Hospital, Bury St Edmunds, Suffolk, UK

The population of the United Kingdom in 1887 was 36 707 418 and there were 22 316 registered medical practitioners (1). This was the year of Queen Victoria's Golden Jubilee. The postage rate for inland letters remained at one penny.

Examination of the job vacancies for medical practitioners in the *British Medical Journal* yield a post as 'Examiner in Physiology' at the University of Edinburgh with a salary of £75 per annum and one of 'Resident Medical Officer' at the North London Hospital for Consumption for a salary of £40 per annum (2).

Gentlemen reading the *Times* of 23 July, 1887, would be much concerned about the reports of the death of H. M. Stanley. Indeed this very matter was raised in the House of Commons, where Sir J. Fergusson stated that he had no official confirmation (3), which was not surprising as Stanley did not, in fact, die until 1904. The issue of compulsory vaccination was also debated in the House of Commons where Mr A. O'Connor spoke against the idea and Dr Farquharson spoke in favour (3).

1887 was the year of the first recorded electrocardiogram by August Desire Waller (4,5). There was no separate literature for anaesthesia on either side of the Atlantic.

Drumine

On the 1 January, 1887, a short report was given in the *British Medical Journal* of the work of Dr John Reid of Port Germein, South Australia on the new local Anaesthetic, Drumine (6). A full text appeared in March (7). This substance was obtained from the plant *Euphorbia Drummondii*. Sheep, cattle, and horses were said to die in great numbers as a consequence of having eaten the plant. A 4% solution of drumine rendered the cat conjunctiva insensitive to touch.

Professor Ogston, Professor of Surgery at Aberdeen University received 40 grains (1 Grain = 60 mg) of drumine from Dr Reid and reported on his experiences with this drug (8).

He prepared a 4% solution of the drug in alcohol and water and injected it hypodermally into two patients. One was undergoing gouging of tuberculous cervical glands, and the other scraping of a chronic cervical abscess. The injections were made in the 'immediate neighbourhood of the diseased parts'. Upon incision, Ogston noted that 'no anaesthesia was observable'.

He then injected 4 minims (1 minim = 0.06 ml) subdermally upon himself and upon a medical student, a Mr Middleton. Neither observed any diminution of sensation though the medical student did note that he felt 'as if under the influence of a small dose of morphine'.

The next day a further test was made by the two investigators by injecting 6 minims (0.36 ml) of the drug into each other's forearms. Again there was no anaesthetic effect, but the investigators experienced a sharp pain, which lasted a day, in their forearms. The site of injection remained tender and swollen for weeks.

Their final experiment was to compare drumine with 'cucaine' ('cucaine' is a variant spelling of cocaine but is the same drug). 5 minims (0.3 ml) of a 10% solution of cucaine were injected hypodermically into the back of their left forearms and following a surgical incision made in this region they proceeded to suture each other's wounds without discomfort. They concluded that drumine had little if any local anaesthetic effect.

Looking at this paper in 1987, I must note the very small volumes of local anaesthetic solution that these investigators used.

A report about Drumine appeared in the American Medical press in September 1887. They hoped that an addition to their meagre list of vegetable local anaesthetics would not prove a disappointment (9).

Drumine never came into common use in the United Kingdom, and was never marketed here.

Local anaesthesia

The successful painless extraction of teeth by the injection of the gums with a solution of 3% carbolic acid and about one grain of cocaine was reported in the *Boston Medical and Surgical Journal* (10) from an original article in *Bulletin Gen. de Therapeutique* by Larange in December of the previous year (1886).

A method of producing local anaesthesia of the skin by the use of electricity in combination with cocaine was reported by Reynolds to the American Medical Association (11). He felt that cocaine had no practical use topically on the skin and so attempted to overcome this by using electricity. He saturated the positive electrode of an 18 Cell McIntosh battery with a 5% solution of cocaine and applied it to the skin. He placed the negative electrode a short distance away and then switched on a 'moderate current' for 5 to 10 minutes. His results were in general good except where the skin was very sensitive so that the current gave discomfort, for example on the face. Reynolds made no comment about burns as a result of this technique.

In the ensuing discussion of the paper Dr Smith of Iowa and Dr McCaskey of Indiana stated their use of hypodermic injection of cocaine as an alternative to electricity.

Pupil size and chloroform anaesthesia

Dr Neilson, in an abstract from his MD thesis, discusses pupillary size in assessing when a patient is sufficiently under the influence of chloroform to begin surgery (12) in the *British Medical Journal*. He concludes:

1. That chloroform at first causes the pupil to dilate, varying in degree and duration; then to contract as the narcosis becomes profound; then to dilate as sensibility returns. If chloroform administration continues whilst the pupil is strongly contracted, then the pupil will dilate, coincident with a state from which it will be difficult or impossible to resuscitate the patient.

2. If the pupil dilates in response to excitation, for example by pinching, then the patient is not sufficiently narcotized for the operation to proceed.

3. When the pupil becomes strongly contracted and immobile, no more chloroform should be given until it begins to dilate.

4. The occurrence of vomiting also causes the pupil to dilate, but vomiting helps to awaken the patient.

Neilson proposed that the pupil is a better marker of depth of anaesthesia than conjunctival insensitivity. He also noted the constant relation he found between blood pressure and pupil size. He emphasizes the importance of observing respiration and pulse in the administration of safe anaesthesia.

It is interesting that Neilson quotes references from the current literature in support of his work.

Stages of anaesthesia?

Dr Packard of Philadelphia was also concerned about the stages of anaesthesia (13). He had noticed that administering ether to full insensibility required time and furthermore produced a long period to recovery. However, if ether was administered only until an arm held up by the patient dropped, then sufficient anaesthesia was produced for a short procedure (such as lancing an abscess, reducing a dislocation, or even reducing a hernia). The recovery with this method was then as rapid as though the patient had had a nitrous oxide anaesthetic.

Incidentally, in 1887, Arthur Guedel was four years old.

Anaesthesia and obstetrics

In a paper primarily discussing the risks of post-partum haemorrhage following the use of anaesthesia for pain relief in labour, Dr Barker of New York continued the debate of the relative merits of chloroform and ether for this purpose (14). He preferred chloroform as it had a more rapid onset, a more agreeable 'odour' and it was easier to control depth of anaesthesia.

He affirmed that when either chloroform or ether were used to produce profound narcosis, temporary paralysis of the uterus resulted, thereby failing to 'close the open mouths of the utero-placental vessels'. He believed that the use of chloroform also shortened the labour, hence removing the risk of 'uterine exhaustion' caused by prolonged labour. Barker argued that there was no increased risk of post-partum haemorrhage with the use of anaesthetics during parturition. He said that only one death had occurred with many 'hundred thousand' administrations of chloroform in labour.

In Shanklin, Dr George H. Roque Dabbs (15) reported on his use of a 4% solution of cucaine soaked on a cotton wool plug and applied to the cervix uteri to promote analgesia and dilatation of the cervix. He also commented on the use of ergot, given hypodermically in combination with his technique.

This method of inserting cocaine vaginally was noted in America that year by Dr Blodgett (16). He also condemned the use of a 'saturated ether sponge' because of the risk of development of ether habituation. (It is assumed the 'saturated ether sponge' was used via the face.)

Anaesthesia for neurosurgery

Horsley, the Assistant-Surgeon at University College Hospital discussed 10 consecutive cases of operations upon the brain (17) on patients aged 4 to 38 years. These operations included those for space occupying lesions, for the relief of epilepsy, and for removal of scar from a depressed skull fracture.

The anaesthetics were given by Drs Wilson and Stedman. The method was early administration of morphine followed by chloroform. Horsley was impressed by the rapidity with which the level of anaesthesia could be altered, especially when the patient was awakened during surgery.

The Hewitt nitrous oxide/ether apparatus

Frederick Hewitt, who presented himself as 'Instructor in Anaesthetics at the London Hospital; Administrator of Anaesthetics at Charing Cross Hospital and the Dental Hospital of London' described his apparatus for administering nitrous oxide and ether either in combination or succession (18).

Hewitt said that the induction with nitrous oxide was pleasant but was worried that, to produce its full effects, under normal atmospheric pressure, the gas must be given in the absence of air. He said that the total exclusion of air throughout an administration of an anaesthetic was inadmissible, except for a brief space of time. Also he found the apparatus currently available for the administration of nitrous oxide cumbersome.

His objections to ether were its pungent taste and odour, the length of time it took to induce anaesthesia in a patient, and the excitement and struggling during induction. Hewitt made the point that prior administration of nitrous oxide without air, followed by etherization, circumvents the problems of both gases used alone. It would be desirable for an apparatus to obtain either (a) an anaesthesia partly due to nitrous oxide and partly due to ether or (b) an anaesthesia due entirely to ether, the nitrous oxide in this case having only been used as a preliminary anaesthetic to obviate the drawbacks of ether.

The parts of the inhaler were shown on the paper's original diagrams (Fig. 1 & 2) as a simple face piece (F); a valvular stopcock (V); Clover's ether chamber (E); and the gas bag. Hewitt did not comment in this paper on the volume of the gas bag, though he did use a 1¼ gallon bag (5.68 litres) as a reservoir when using nitrous oxide alone (19).

To administer an anaesthetic by method (a) the apparatus was set up as shown in Fig. 1. The arrows on the diagram show the route of air through the apparatus, and by rotating the valve (T), nitrous oxide could be admitted instead of air (note that Hewitt had not at this stage allowed for air to be admitted in combination with nitrous oxide). With a nitrous oxide administration in progress, ether could be added by using the Clover's inhaler. Hewitt suggested that this was done after first giving a nitrous oxide anaesthetic. Although this would be nearly

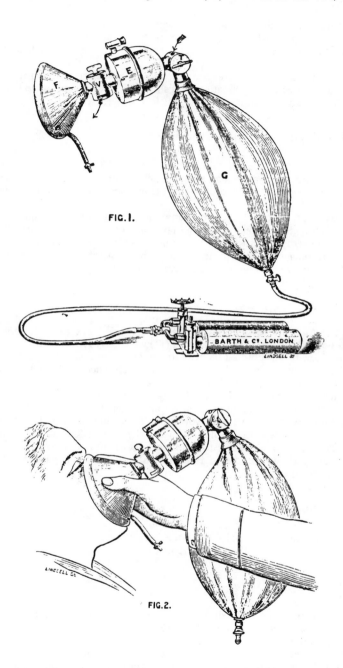

FIG. I.

FIG. 2.

100% nitrous oxide, it is assumed that there could be air from the lungs in the circuit, if rebreathing into the bag occurred. If (V) is set to allow expiration to the air, then no rebreathing would occur.

If method (b) was employed (Fig. 2), Hewitt used the bag as a reservoir for nitrous oxide, and at first allowed expiration to escape to the atmosphere via the valvular stopcock (V). He then turned (V) and (T) to allow rebreathing into the bag whilst the ether was gradually turned on. It is possible to admit air via (T). Hewitt does advise that air should be admitted when cyanosis develops or when there were epileptiform movements. As shown in Fig. 2, the apparatus became portable. The apparatus was made by Messrs Barth and Company of London.

A paper published in 1887 by Kreutzmann, of San Francisco (20), on the administration of chloroform and oxygen in combination, was shown to Hewitt and this led him to experiment with nitrous oxide and oxygen in combination in later years.

Single handed operator/anaesthetist?

A letter (21) to the *British Medical Journal* under the pseudonym 'Tory' asked 'When called two miles into the country to see a man with crushed fingers, and I find it necessary to remove one digit, am I legally justified in chloroforming the man and operating without another surgeon being present?'

The reply given in the journal, though anonymous (articles in the journals at this time were often unsigned), suggested that, whilst the law did not fix any rules regarding the use of chloroform, there were risks attendant to the use of chloroform, and that by proceeding on his own, a practitioner may be held negligent in the event of mishap. Further, in the event of death, a full Coroner's inquest would have to be held.

Discussion

In reviewing the Anaesthetic Literature of 1887 I have seen the early development of ideas still accepted today. Neilson (12) and Packard (11) were early reporters of the stages and signs of anaesthesia. Hewitt (18) pointed the way to combining anaesthetic agents and techniques. Reynolds (11), Neilson (12) and Barker (14) quoted references, showing the beginning of a rational scientific approach, to their work.

Though a varied group of people seemed to have given anaesthetics in 1887, it is interesting that Dr Hewitt was already calling himself an anaesthetist.

Communications seem to have been good in 1887 in that news of Drumine spread from Australia to the United States of America and to the United Kingdom within five months.

Even 100 years ago, the medical establishment was obviously concerned about the single-handed operator/anaesthetist, considering such a situation as negligent. This debate has continued until recent times.

Acknowledgment

The author would like to thank the Editor of the *British Medical Journal* for his kind permission to reproduce the diagrams of the Hewitt Apparatus.

References

(1) The relative proportion of medical men to the population of the United Kingdom and of Australia. *Br Med J* 1887; **i**: 34.
(2) Medical appointments. *Br Med J* 1887; **i**: 46.
(3) Parliamentary intelligence. *The Times* 1887 July 23: (col 1).
(4) Waller AD. A demonstration on man of electromotive changes accompanying the heart's beat. *J Physiol* 1887; **8**: 229–34.
(5) Sykes AH. A. D. Waller and the electrocardiogram. *Br Med J* 1987; **294**: 1396–8.
(6) Anonymous. Drumine: A new local anaesthetic. *Br Med J* 1887; **i**: 30.
(7) Reid J. Drumine. *Br Med J* 1887; **i**: 674–5.
(8) Ogston A. Experiences with Drumine as a local anaesthetic. *Br Med J* 1887; **i**: 451–2.
(9) Anonymous. The new local anaesthetic. *JAMA* 1887; **10**: 374–6.

(10) Anonymous. Local anaesthesia in dental surgery. *Boston Med Surg J* 1887; **116**: 98.
(11) Reynolds HJ. A new method of producing local anaesthesia of the skin. *JAMA* 1887; **10**: 235–7.
(12) Neilson HJ. On the observation of the pupil as a guide in the administration of chloroform. *Br Med J* 1887; **ii**: 234–5.
(13) Packard JH. The primary anaesthetic stage of ether. *Boston Med Surg J* 1887; **116**: 537.
(14) Barker F. Is the danger from post-partum haemorrhage increased by the use of anaesthetics during parturition? *Boston Med Surg J* 1887; **116**: 125–7.
(15) Dabbs GHR. Cucaine in labour and gynaecological cases. *Br Med J* 1887; **i**: 927–8.
(16) Kingman. Anaesthesia in normal labour—second paper. *Boston Med Surg J* 1887; **116**: 457–8.
(17) Horsley V. Ten consecutive operations upon the brain and cranial cavity to illustrate the details and safety of the method employed. *Br Med J* 1887; **i**: 863–5.
(18) Hewitt F. The administration of nitrous oxide and ether in combination or succession. *Br Med J* 1887; **ii**: 452–4.
(19) Smith WDA. *Under the influence, a history of nitrous oxide and oxygen anaesthesia.* 1st Ed. London and Basingstoke: Macmillan, 1982: xxii.
(20) Kruetzmann H. Anaesthesia by chloroform and oxygen combined. *Pacific Med Surg J* 1887; **30**: 462.
(21) "Tory" Anaesthetics. *Br Med J* 1887; **ii**: 1406.

Chapter 9

MILITARY ANAESTHESIA AND THE TRANSPORT OF CASUALTIES

9.1 Anaesthetics in British military practice 1914–18

J. RESTALL
Cambridge Military Hospital, Aldershot, Hampshire, UK

Although Sigmund Freud was an ardent pacifist, there can be few who would disagree with him when he wrote in 1933 of World War I 'We are constrained to believe that never has any event been destructive of so much that is valuable in the common wealth of humanity nor so misleading to many of the clearest intelligence, nor so debasing to the highest that we know' (1). In his Mitchiner Lecture of 1983, entitled 'Another Side of Mars' Professor Cecil Gray appreciated that some good, sociological, technological and medical, does accrue from war. He investigated the significant advances made in anaesthetic practice by medical officers in the armed services or by civilian physicians working under the stimulus of wartime extingency. He concluded that up to the Boer War anaesthesia had not been advanced in any way by war and it was possible that, on occasion, it may have delayed the progress (2). It would seem that the Great War of 1914–18 produced some of the first major advances.

Casualties and personnel

The Casualty Clearing Stations (CCS) were mobile units, generally situated seven to 50 miles behind the front line. Officially they had 800 beds but were capable of major expansion. An average complement of staff was seven medical officers, nine nursing sisters, 180 orderlies and three chaplains. Surgical teams, consisting of one surgeon, one trained orderly who acted as an assistant, one sister and one anaesthetist would be sent to supplement the CCSs in the event of a major offensive. At times the influx of casualties was overwhelming. In September, 1916, during the latter part of the Battle of the Somme, No. 36 CCS received 17 000 stretcher cases and suffered 700 deaths. During one push, it received 5000 casualties in five days. It was in this environment that anaesthesia by experts came into its own. No longer could anaesthetics be given by just any doctor. The day of the anaesthetic specialist had dawned.

Patients and standard equipment

When the War started anaesthesia had advanced only little beyond the open administration of ether and chloroform. This was the situation here in Britain, on the Continent and in the United States. Throughout the war there was little else available for the administration of anaesthetics in the front line, forward of the casualty clearing stations. Captain Heddy (3) of the Middlesex Hospital, writing in 1918, classified the cases requiring the administration of an anaesthetic before being evacuated to a casualty clearing station into three main groups:

Group 1. Cases where it was desirable to dress an extensive wound or to immobilize a fracture.

Group 2. Cases where it was considered necessary to perform an immediate operation for the relief of some urgent symptom.

Group 3. Cases of wounds or injuries accompanied by shell-shock of an acute maniacal type.

The most important items of the anaesthetic equipment were contained in the field surgical pannier No. 1 and included '3 lbs' (1400 ml) chloroform in sealed glass tubes, two drop-bottles, a hypodermic case with the essential drugs and an excellent saline infusion apparatus. He wrote further than an 'outfit' containing a mouth-gag, tongue forceps, and a Skinner's mask had been recently added. Ether was now available, and should the administration of oxygen be urgently indicated, even this commodity would frequently be at hand, but that it was there for another purpose and should be used only in cases of grave emergency. There were tracheotomy instruments, good hot water bottles, improvised stomach tubes and plenty of lint and gauze. Thus it was evident that, from an anaesthetist's point of view, the equipment at a field ambulance 'left nothing to be desired'.

Nitrous oxide, oxygen and ether

At the beginning of the War the technique of 'gas' (nitrous oxide) and oxygen anaesthesia was in its infancy. Most progress was made in the United States and the important advance was the development of the water sight feed, the bubble bottle, for measuring the flow rate of the gases at the Boston City Hospital, by Cotton and Boothby (4). The idea was seized upon by James Taylor Gwathmey, one of the great American pioneers, who incorporated it in his machine.

J. Blomfield (5), in the 4th edition of his book *Anaesthetics—a practical handbook* (1917) has what I believe to be the first chapter specifically devoted to anaesthetics in military practice. He discourages the use of chloroform stating that the anaesthetist is sacrificing safety for convenience. He advocated that, although open ether might prove inadequate, the routine use of chloroform 2 parts/ether 3 parts for induction, followed by open ether for long, and closed ether from a Clover inhaler for short cases, would be found to give very satisfactory results.

Captain Geoffrey Marshall, later Sir Geoffrey Marshall, the eminent physician at Guy's Hospital was posted, early in 1915, to No. 17 CCS in France having served as a medical officer with No. 2 Ambulance Barge Flotilla for six months (6). Sir Anthony Bowlby knew that Marshall had worked on the physiology of anaesthesia before the war and he was tasked with reducing the large number of deaths in the forward hospitals from shock. Soldiers often lay for many hours on the battlefield after being hit, getting cold and damp. If they had shattered limbs that had to be amputated the mortality was appalling—about 90% for lower third of the thigh. Marshall did haemoglobin concentrations on these casualties. He found that the blood was very concentrated in shock and that if they were given chloroform or ether, or a mixture of the two, the blood got more and more concentrated, the blood pressure fell and they died.

Initially he tried intravenous 5% ether and intravenous alcohol but it was no good for shock and appeared to drown the patients. He started to experiment with make-shift machines he made himself for giving gas and oxygen by inhalation. He gave continuous gas and added oxygen via a tube to a mask that he made himself and judged the patient's condition by the colour. Eventually Marshall got a tinsmith in France to make a machine and subsequently brought drawings home and got Coxeter to make a machine for him. This machine had a bottle sight feed as suggested by Gwathmey and another bubble bottle for the vaporization of ether. The machine was put into production by Coxeters and became the standard machine used by the RAMC. But Marshall did not write it up until after the war in 1920 (7).

Henry Edmund Gaskin Boyle of St Bartholomew's Hospital was 39 years old at the outbreak of war. He was commissioned into the RAMC and served throughout the war with the 1st London General Hospital at Camberwell (8). He imported a Gwathmey gas–oxygen–ether machine into this country in 1916. These machines developed mechanical defects, the chief of these being leakage at the gas unions. The early pattern was clumsy—a heavy wooden box with two metal cross bars from which hung the four cylinders. The 'bubble bottle' and the ether container were just above them. An early difficulty was caused by the tendency for the nitrous oxide to freeze up at the valve. This was prevented by the addition of a small metal spirit lamp hung upon one of the bars so that its open flame could play upon the valve in use—this, in spite of the fact that the ether container was but a few inches away.

Captain Boyle has described how he personally gave 2000 gas and oxygen and ether anaesthetics, and a Captain Trewby and the residents had given a further 1600. He acknowledged the help that he had had with its design from Geoffrey Marshall when he published his 'new invention' in the Lancet in 1919 (9). It must be stated that the machines described by Gwathmey, Marshall and Boyle offered little real advance on the original concept of Cotton and Boothby in the Boston City Hospital.

Marshall, despite his interest in gas and oxygen recommended that ether, given by Shipway's warmed ether apparatus was the most suitable technique for patients who had suffered abdominal injuries. He stated that the contra-indication for the administration of ether were cases in which the projectile had penetrated the chest as well as the abdomen; in these cases chloroform should be used.

Tracheal intubation

Perhaps the most significant advance in anaesthetic practice attributable to the Great War was the development of endotracheal intubation. Major (later Sir) Harold Gillies had established a plastic surgical unit at the Military Hospital, Sidcup. Two returning Regimental Medical Officers were drafted to give anaesthetics to the evacuated war casualties. These two anaesthetic recruits were Ivan Magill and Stanley Rowbotham. Their work was carried out after 1918 and therefore consideration of it is not within the scope of this presentation. Two papers about the life and work of Sir Ivan Magill have been delivered at this Symposium.

Marshall and shock

Marshall was very·interested in the physiology of shock and was nearer to understanding the mechanisms than some of his contemporaries (10). In the treatment of surgical shock he stressed the importance of external warmth. Fluids were given by mouth or rectum. He appreciated that sub-cutaneous saline delivered into the axillary folds was not absorbed. Marshall believed that the intravenous administration of saline was of little use before the operation because it produced a temporary rise in blood pressure and slowing of the pulse rate but did not render the patient less susceptible to further shock—the blood pressure falling as soon as the operation began. Transfusion was used at the end of the operation—hypertonic saline producing better results than the normal solution. Transfusion of blood gave the best results but was difficult to perform since not infrequently it had to be direct from donor to recipient. Much interest was shown by Marshall in the new artificial viscous fluids—in particular the 6% solution of gum acacia as suggested by Professor W. M. Bayliss (11). Bayliss recommended gum acacia because it had a suitable viscosity to be a blood replacement and because it exerted an osmotic pressure. Hogan and Fisher recommended the use of 2% gelatin in saline for intravenous infusion. These workers all realized that colloid infusion should be started early as soon as signs of wound shock appeared. Delay could be dangerous, and, in any case, these solutions were more readily available and cheaper than blood. They appreciated that the maintenance of circulating blood volume was imperative.

Geoffrey Marshall stated that local anaesthesia could be employed in only a small number of cases, on account of the multiplicity of wounds and their lacerated and soiled condition. Anaesthetists of the time were urged to use spinal anaesthesia but Marshall appreciated that spinals using Stovaine (amlyocaine hydrochloride) produced profound hypotension. Not only did the patients succumb on the operating table or shortly after leaving it, but it was found that there was a greater likelihood of gas gangrene appearing in their wounds within the next few days.

Conclusion

It was Charles Saint, Professor of Surgery at the University of Capetown who wrote in 1920; 'one of the greatest aids in the treatment of shocked patients during the latter part of the war was the advent of gas and oxygen and ether as an anaesthetic; its introduction into general use was one of the most important and beneficial events of the campaign' (12). Notwithstanding 'Dulce bellum inexpertis'—('War is pleasant to those who have not tried it') some good can come out of the evil of war.

References

(1) Rickman J. *Sigmund Freud. Civilisation, war and death*. Psychoanalytical Epitomes 4. London: The Hogarth Press, 1953: 82.

(2) Gray TC. Mitchiner Memorial Lecture. Another side of Mars. *J R Army Med Corps* 1984; **130**: 3–11.

(3) Heddy WRH. Anaesthetics in the field. *J R Army Med Corps* 1918; **31**: 76–9.

(4) Cotton FG, Boothby WM, Gwathmey JT. *Anaesthesia*. New York and London: Appleton and Co., 1914: 161.

(5) Blomfield F. *Anaesthetics. A practical handbook*. 4th Ed. London: Ballière, Tindall and Cox, 1917.

(6) Evans B. A doctor in the Great War—an interview with Sir Geoffrey Marshall. *Br Med J* 1982; **285**: 1780–3.

(7) Marshall G. Two types of portable gas–oxygen apparatus. *Proc Roy Soc Med* 1920; **13**: 16–9.

(8) Hadfield CF. Eminent anaesthetists. H. Edmund, G. Boyle. *Br J Anaesth* 1950; **22**: 107–17.

(9) Boyle HEG. Nitrous–oxide–oxygen–ether outfit. *Lancet* 1919; i: 226 (v also Annotation, 232).

(10) Marshall G. The administration of anaesthetics at the front. *Br Med J* 1917; **1**: 722–5.

(11) Bayliss WM. Intravenous injections in wound shock. London: Longmans, Green and Co., 1918.

(12) Saint CFM. The influence of the Great War on modern surgery. *Lancet* 1920; ii: 1130–4.

9.2   Flying intensive care

C. A. B. McLAREN
Princess Alexandra Royal Air Force Hospital, Wroughton, UK

The great numbers of sick and wounded transported safely by air during the Second World War and in the later conflicts proved conclusively that it was possible to transport the sick and wounded in safety sometimes over considerable distances.

There is of course nothing new in this world (1). The first 'Flying Ambulance' made its appearance on the battlefields of the Rhine Valley in 1792. It was a light horse drawn vehicle designed by Baron Dominique Jean Larrey, Surgeon to Napoleon's Imperial Guard. This removed the wounded from the battlefield before they could be wounded for a second time and so that rapid amputation could be effected (2).

Although the first flight by the Wright Brothers did not take place until 1903 interest in aerial transport of the sick and wounded was maintained throughout the 19th century in many countries, especially in Holland, where Surgeon General de Mooy had many revolutionary ideas in the use of balloons and airships to move casualties (3).

The first intensive care/respiratory care units did not become established until the 1950s, but prior to this date there had been attempts to move paralysed patients by air to Respiratory Units.

Air transport of patients in tank respirators

The first recorded attempt was made in Michigan in 1940, a small child being flown in a home made tank respirator to the unit. The second flight ended in disaster. Without any equipment other than an oxygen supply, an Army patient was moved, only to die 15 hours after the flight (4). At this time the only available equipment was the 'Tank Respirator' which had been rediscovered in 1929. The initial description of a machine designed to apply negative and positive pressure to the body was described by Dalziel in 1833. He described the construction of an airtight box, with the patient's head and neck exposed. The patient was maintained in the sitting position as the air was removed from the interior of the box, 'so that the external air which the patient breathed, rushed into the air passages without effort' (5). Although there were some enthusiastic supporters of the device it did not become popular.

Drinker and Shaw produced their tank respirator in 1929 and after many modifications it became generally used to ventilate respiratory cripples (6). Although the tank respirator was ideal for negative pressure ventilation in respiratory units, it was much too cumbersome for in-flight use (the weight of version in use in the 1940s being 1000 lb (455 kg) and it was eight feet (2.44 m) long. A further problem was the incompatibility of the aircraft power supplies with the requirements of the machine. It is of course essential to secure everyone and everything that is taken on board an aircraft. There were obviously no problems with the respirator, but it was impossible to safely secure the patient, since it was not possible to fit the normal stretcher harness. The only anchorage point was the stiff rubber neck seal and rigid fixation at this point could prove fatal in very turbulent conditions. The aircraft types in use at that time were in the main unpressurized and so could not fly much above 10 000 feet (3000 metres) and so were subject to all the weather conditions often found at that sort of height (7).

The likely in-flight problems were first addressed in 1945 during the transfer by air from the Azores of a patient with poliomyelitis. There had been a severe epidemic of 36 cases there in 1944 with 100% mortality which led to the provision of a Both respirator. It was therefore thought prudent to use the equipment to transfer the patient. Unfortunately there was no compatibility between the power supplies of the only available aircraft, a B17 (Flying Fortress) and the machine. It was therefore necessary to hand pump the patient throughout the ten hour flight to the United Kingdom (8).

A suitable pump was developed and there are records of two further air transfers using the tank respirator with successful results, despite the problems of an overnight stop (the 'lung' and all the medical equipment had to be offloaded, necessitating the doubtful pleasure of reloading the next morning). The night stops were necessary at this time because of the aircraft types in use. It was obvious that there was an urgent need for some better means of in-flight ventilation.

The cuirass respirator

In 1880 Waldenburg, a German physician had introduced the first cuirass respirator which covered only the chest and trunk of the patient (9), but nothing more was heard of this obviously more suitable piece of equipment until 1947 when the Council on Physical Medicine of the American Medical Association issued the draft specification of a cuirass type respirator (10).

The Monaghan Portable respirator was approved in 1949. Although on testing it was obviously not as efficient as the tank equivalent, it was considered to provide adequate air exchange and be useful for patient transfer, as it offered the advantages of access for nursing care (11). There were several problems inherent in the use of this equipment for transfer by air including the difficulty in weaning the patient from the tank respirator. It was necessary for the patient to accept the cuirass for the duration of the flight but, at the overnight stop, the patient would usually spend the night in a tank respirator. Despite the presence of an inflatable seal around the margins of shell it was sometimes difficult to get a good seal. The patients complained of a feeling of being underventilated despite not being hypoxic and having a normal carbon dioxide tension. The negative pressure exerted by the shell was up to a maximum of 20 cm H_2O and this produced a tidal volume of around 400 ml which was found to be adequate in most circumstances. The shells were produced in differing sizes for the different age groups. The Monaghan cuirass ventilator was first used by the Royal Air Force in 1950 to effect the transfer of a child suffering from spinal poliomyelitis from Ceylon to the United Kingdom, and continued to give valuable service for many years.

Positive pressure ventilation

The Copenhagen poliomyelitis epidemic in 1952, produced so many cases that there were obviously not enough tank respirators available in Denmark to treat them all. This led to the development by Lassen and his colleagues of the technique of intermittent positive pressure ventilation (IPPV) to treat respiratory insufficiency, patients being hand ventilated via a tracheostomy or endotracheal tube (12).

The excellent results obtained during the epidemic resulted in the development of positive pressure ventilators to replace negative pressure equipment but it was soon realized that during IPPV apparatus was required for securing adequate humidification of the bronchial tree and for clearing secretions from the chest.

The first reports of using IPPV for in-flight ventilation were made in 1954 by Crampton Smith. In 1955 Harries and Lawes reported the successful air transfer of three polio patients using the Radcliffe respiration pump operated from a 12 volt battery (13).

The American developments for IPPV resulted in the introduction of the Bird respirator which was gas driven. It was therefore necessary for a choice to be made in 1955 between gas and electric power operated ventilators.

Oxygen or air cylinders used to drive the ventilators are both heavy and bulky. In view of the long distance over which aeromedical flights were already by then being made, electrically operated equipment was selected. The effect of this decision has been that all medical equipment used from that time has had to be modified to work from 28 volts DC from the aircraft supplies.

Developments in equipment

The original IPPV equipment consisted of the Radcliffe pump and a heated water humidifier with lagged tubing designed to keep the water vaporized in the inspired gas, and the Stott flutter one-way valve at the tracheostomy tube. The efficiency of the humidifier was such that there was a heavy water deposition around the valve, necessitating changing the valve approximately every 20 minutes, for drying and cleaning. There was at that time only very minimal patient monitoring other than inflation pressure measurement. Although much lighter than the 'tank Respirator', this equipment was still quite cumbersome during the off-loading for the overnight stops but, as the aircraft types available improved, from piston engined, through turboprops to pure jets, the transit times back to the United Kingdom were drastically reduced, and overnight stops were no longer necessary—even if arrival in the United Kingdom was often at strange hours of the night. However the transfer of the patient on arrival in the United Kingdom still gave some problems due to size and weight and difficulty in handling. This was especially the case when helicopters began to be used for the final stage of transfer as it was not possible to move the patient, the equipment and the medical staff in one lift because of the weight penalty. It was therefore necessary to develop light weight respiratory equipment for use in the helicopters. As has already been noted oxygen cylinders are bulky and heavy but, despite this a development of the high altitude escape oxygen systems used by the Luftwaffe was evaluated and gave good results although it, in its turn, produced problems. This equipment consisted of 30 feet (9.1 m) of coiled steel tube, filled with oxygen at 1600 p.s.i. (110 bar); it was very lightweight and ideal to provide the gas source for the East Freeman mini-ventilator. A condenser humidifier was plugged into the circuit and gave adequate humidification during the transfer (14,15). The East Radcliffe ventilator was adequate down to tidal volumes of 150 ml but it was necessary to use other ventilators of the occluding thumb variety to ventilate inflight, neonates and small children.

Postscript

The passage of time changes medical practice and disease so it is of interest to note that during a twenty year period from 1950–1969 in a series of forty air transfers, there were 38 cases of poliomyelitis. In the last twenty year period there have been no cases of the disease moved by the Royal Air Force.

References

(1) Ecclesiastes 1 verse 8.
(2) Richardson AG. *Larrey: Surgeon to Napoleon's Imperial Guard.* London: John Murray, 1974.
(3) Vincent A. *Le Transport des Blesses par Avions International Croix Rouge,* 1924; **6**: 720-3.
(4) Anonymous. Simple workable respirator. Council on Physical Medicine *JAMA* 1942; **118**: 535.
(5) Dalziel J. 'On sleep, and an apparatus for promoting artificial respiration'. *British Association for the Advancement of Science,* 1838; **2**: 127.
(6) Drinker P, McKhann. The use of a new apparatus for prolonged administration of artificial respiration. *JAMA* 1930; **95**: 1249.
(7) Merrifield AJ. Air transport of patients with respiratory paralysis; experience in the Royal Air Force. *Aerospace Medicine* 1965; **36**: 374-5.
(8) Anonymous. *History of the Second World War Royal Air Force Medical Services Coastal Command.* London: HMSO 1955; 320-2.
(9) Waldenburg L. *Die Pneumatische Behandlung der Respirations und Circulationskrankheiten im Anschluss an die Pneumatometrie und Spirometrie,* Berlin: Hirschwald, 1880.
(10) Anonymous. Tentative requirements for acceptance of respirators of the cuirass type. Council on Physical Medicine. *JAMA* 1947; **135**: 715.
(11) Anonymous. Monaghan Portable Respirator Acceptable. Report of the Council on Physical Medicine. *JAMA* 1949; **139**: 1273.
(12) Lassen HCA. A preliminary report on the 1952 epidemic of poliomyelitis in Copenhagen with special reference to the treatment of acute respiratory insufficiency *Lancet* 1953; **i**: 37.
(13) Harries JR, Lawes WE. Intermittent positive pressure respiration in Bulbo spinal Poliomyelitis . . . use of the Radcliffe Respiration Pump. *Br Med J* 1955; **1**: 448-54.
(14) Collis JM, Bethune DW, Tobias MA. Miniature ventilators, an assessment. *Anaesthesia* 1969; **24**: 81-9.
(15) Mapleson WW. Assessment of condenser humidifiers, with special reference to a multiple gauze model. *Br Med J* 1963; **i**: 300.

PART III

THE HISTORY OF ANAESTHETIC AGENTS

Chapter 10
INHALATIONAL AGENTS

10.1   The origins of the first gaseous agents

W. D. A. SMITH, O.B.E.
University of Leeds, Yorkshire, UK

The first gaseous agents—carbon dioxide, nitrous oxide, oxygen, air—have material and conceptual origins. Their ultimate origin dates from the 'Creation' of matter. Subsequent evolution of atmospheric gases has been outlined by Nunn (1). This paper begins at the beginning; then glances at selected developments towards our understanding of the existence and nature of air and other gases; and ends at the dawn of anaesthesia with some questions.

Early physical concepts of air, atmosphere and vacuum

Prehistoric folk surely linked life with breath and apnoea with death. Perhaps they took for granted that fanned embers flamed and that, although unsupported objects usually fell to the ground, birds flew and hovered without visible support. Aware of the vagaries of weather they probably thought more of wind than air, but when, within the limits of language and imagination, they pondered experience, wind entered mythology—said the Bushmen: 'The Wind . . . formerly a person . . . became a bird.' (2).

Earliest comprehension of a material fluid supporting flight is undated, but Anaximenes in the 6th century BC conceived a Primary Mist: invisible when uniform; generating winds when dense, forming clouds and rain; when denser still, snow or hail. In the 5th century BC, Empedocles perceived invisible air through water not filling an immersed clepsydra unless air escaped or emptying unless air entered. Leucippus and Democritus thought matter comprised atoms within a void, as did Epicurus in the 4th century BC and Lucretius in the 1st century BC. Aristotle, denied the void, explaining transmission of light by media transparency rather than by an unobstructing void; and unweighed Air was an element presumed to have weight. Although Lucretius was rediscovered in the 15th century, Aristotlean orthodoxy prevailed into mid-17th century when philosophers began to investigate air (3–6).

In Italy, Balliani believed the atmosphere's lower levels were compressed by those above. Beekman, in Holland, conceived the analogy of an immense sponge, its lower part packed tightest. In 1638, five years after Galileo, threatened by torture, recanted his belief in a central sun, his *Discorsi* upheld the possibility of an inter-atomic void, and described how he had balanced against fine sand the weight of air compressed by syringe in a glass bottle. Balliani pondered the failure of Florentine well-diggers to raise water by suction more than 18 cubits, which Galileo attributed to water's lack of cohesiveness (7–10).

Around 1640, Berti and friends in Rome tried to create a vacuum. They used an eleven metre vertical lead pipe up the side of a building. It had a brass tap at its lower end which was immersed in water. A glass vessel surmounted by a plug was cemented to the top. They filled the system with water, replaced the plug, and opened the tap. The glass vessel emptied and it impeded neither light nor magnetism. Upon closing the tap and removing the plug, air rushed in.

A depth-sound showed the water level 18 cubits above the reservoir. In another experiment water from a raised reservoir was admitted to the presumed vacuum, but it incompletely filled the vessel which rendered the experiment inconclusive. Further trials may have been discouraged by their unorthodoxy and Berti died in 1643 (7,9).

In 1644, Torricelli proposed, and Viviani performed, similar experiments using mercury which was supported to a height of 29 inches. Lifting the tube's lower end into water floated on the mercury in the reservoir, the mercury in the tube and the space above it were completely replaced by water. Torricelli accepted that there had been a vacuum, and that the mercury was supported by atmospheric pressure which, he predicted, should support a 32 foot column of wine (7,8).

Torricelli and Ricci communicated these experiments to Mersenne in France where discussion was freer. By 1648, they were being discussed in England. In 1646, Petit and Pascal repeated Torricelli's experiment and confirmed his prediction. Pascal got his brother-in-law, Perier, living in Clermont, to repeat Toricelli's experiment near the foot and summit of the Puy-de-Dome. The mercury column was indeed three inches shorter at the summit, 500 fathoms above Clermont. Roberval demonstrated distension of a near-empty swim-bladder in a Torricellian vacuum. Reduced pressure allowed expansion of the normally compressed and resilient air contained in the bladder (7-9).

Jean Pecquet added a description of these studies to his work on lymphatics. Its English translation of 1653 probably influenced Henry Power of Halifax (then at Cambridge and also interested in lymphatics), his friend Richard Towneley of Burnley, and Robert Boyle. Power repeated the experiments, including an 800 ft version of the Puy-de-Dome experiment on Halifax Hill (8,11).

Meanwhile Von Guericke of Magdeburg experimented with vacua, pumping water from a sealed cask (which leaked) and from a hollow copper sphere (which collapsed). He developed an air pump and by 1654 had evacuated the space between matching hollow hemispheres and explored the force required to part them. Sixteen horses failed to do so (12,13).

Air, atmosphere, fire and life

Boyle learned of the pump and Robert Hooke made for him an improved 'Pneumatical Engine'. Boyle's *New Experiments Physico-Mechanical Touching the Spring of Air* (1660), reported the extinction, *in vacuo*, of flame and life, and re-kindled Towneley and Power's interest. An appendix to the 2nd edition, 1662, described an experiment using an asymmetrical U-tube. In the short closed limb a parcel of air was progressively compressed by adding increments of mercury to the long open limb. He found 'the spring' of air proportional to its density, results which were 'consistent with the hypothesis that the pressures and expansions were in reciprocal proportion.' Boyle acknowledged discussions with Towneley who 'had endeavoured to reduce to a precise estimate how much air dilated, itself loses of its elastical force, according to the measure of its dilatation.' Webster interpreted this as acknowledgment that Boyle's findings, compressing air, also applied to Towneley's, expanding it (8, 13-16).

Boyle also described 'fermentations' and 'corrosions' producing 'factitious airs' which extinguished flame and life. He reported enclosed mice living longer if their air was compressed; and he suspected 'that there may be dispersed through . . . the atmosphere . . . some odd substance . . . on whose account the Air is so necessary to the subsistence of flame.' He noted an effect of temperature on volume, but it was one hundred and twenty-five years before Charles' Law emerged, from the race to be airborne, between the Montgolfier Brothers, using hot air, and Jaques Charles who used Hydrogen (17). 1987 is the year of the first hot air balloon across the Atlantic, the bicentenary of Charles' Law and, to remind us of the relevance of gravity, the tercentenary of Newton's *Principia*.

Returning to mid-17th century, the word 'gas' was coined by Van Helmont, in Belgium. Without devising apparatus for collecting gases he distinguished between them. Some were identical and some well known. Choke damp, for example, was discussed by Francis Bacon. Van Helmont suspected 'something in air' which was 'anihilated by fire'. Leonardo made similar comment: 'Fire constantly destroys the part of air that nourishes it . . . when air cannot support flame nothing else can live in it.' Van Helmont's works were not translated into English until 1662 (13,18,19).

In 1654, Bathurst's *Lectures on Respiration* in Oxford, as published much later, referred to 'nitrous spirit entering in respiration and tempering blood.' Partington suggested that the idea of 'nitrous spirit' was floating in the Oxford air. Thomas Willis, who was assisted by Lower in Oxford, referred to 'The heat of blood being due to combustion by nitrous particles present in the air . . .' and to blood changing to scarlet 'by admixture of nitrous particles . . .' (18).

In 1663, Robert Hooke excised a dog's ribs and diaphragm, pricked holes in its lungs and maintained life by pumping air into the trachea. A window excised in the lung revealed free circulation of blood even when ventilation was temporarily withheld. Hooke concluded that the function of respiratory movement was to provide fresh air. In a similarly treated dog Richard Lower injected venous blood into a pulmonary artery. Blood in the pulmonary veins remained red, provided ventilation was maintained, so the florid colour seemed due to something brought to the lungs in the air. In 1674, John Mayow, identified the something as nitro-aerial particles. He also confirmed that combustion in a closed space was self-limiting and found it associated with a small volume reduction; but a century later, Scheele found the contraction due to a temperature artefact, and that the air consumed was replaced by an aerial acid. Burning hydrogen, however, Scheele did find a one-fifth contraction (19–21).

Mayow imagined nitro-aerial particles extracted from the air by respiration, carried by blood throughout the body, involved in heating it, in the action of brain and nerves and in muscle activity. Focus on nitrous spirits and particles related to nitre's ability to burn without air. Robert Hooke suggested, in 1665, that combustion in air probably relied upon 'a substance inherent, and mixt with the Air, that is like, if not the very same, with that which is fixt in nitre.' These workers seemed on the scent of oxygen, until masked by Phlogiston, emanating from George Ernst Stahl in Germany (18,20,22).

Phlogiston

Stahl said that substances were rich in Phlogiston according to their flammability. Burning released it. Metals were made of calx (now oxide) and phlogiston. Burning metal released phlogiston leaving calx. Carbon heated with Calx donated phlogiston producing metal Phlogiston saturating closed spaces extinguished flame. Plants scavanged Phlogiston from the atmosphere. Priestley and Scheele believed it all, Lavoisier did not (13,18,19,23).

Stephen Hales showed that 'air' was obtainable from some solids and absorbed by others. He devised apparatus for its collection which others improved. His 'airs' were distinguished by their 'parent substances and yields', although he did report red fumes from Walton Pyrites and nitric acid (13,18,19,24).

Carbon dioxide

Joseph Black presented his classic series of experiments in 1754 for his MD dissertation about Magnesia Alba as an antacid (magnesium carbonate). Magnesia Alba dissolved in acids with violent effervescence. The salts had specific properties. On heating Magnesia Alba, the residual calcined magnesia weighed only 5/12ths of the original weight. It dissolved in the same acids, producing exactly similar salts but, without effervescence. The amount of acid required to dissolve 2 drams (7.8 g) of Magnesia Alba equalled that required to dissolve the calcined magnesia obtained from the same weight of magnesia alba; the former with effervescence, the latter without. Magnesia Alba, 3 ounces, lost more than half its weight upon distillation, but only 5 drams of whitish water collected, accounting for only 17% of the weight lost—so the volatile matter was mostly 'air'. He again calcined 2 drams (7.8 g) of Magnesia Alba. To the resulting calcined magnesia he added sufficient sulphuric acid to dissolve it. Then he added alkali. The washed and dried precipitate weighed 1 dram 50 grains (7.1 g), a 90% recovery of weight. The precipitate effervesced with acids, so at least part of the weight was regained as 'air'. Black presumed that the acid forced 'air' from the alkali into the magnesia. The crude Magnesia Alba differed from the calcined chiefly in containing a considerable quantity of 'air'. Its action on lime water identified it as the same air as that produced by respiration, fermentation and the burning of charcoal. He called it 'fixed air' (25–27).

Priestley experimented with 'fixed air' in 1767, in a Leeds brewery, exposing frogs till comatose, reviving them in fresh air. In 1771, a sprig of his sunlit mint rendered wholesome air in which a candle had burned. He investigated Hales's red fumes, dissolving metals in nitric acid instead of pyrites. The invisible gas generated (i.e. nitric oxide which he called nitrous air) produced red fumes when mixed with common air, its volume contracting according to what he called the 'goodness' of the air. This he had previously assessed by the survival time of mice, but thenceforth by the diminution of two measures of common air by one measure of nitrous air (28,29).

Nitrous oxide

In 1772, knowing that moist iron filings and brimstone reacted with common air, he exposed nitrous air to this mixture over water. A vigorous reaction produced heat, effervescence and considerable reduction in volume: but he identified the residual gas as phlogisticated air, i.e. nitrogen. In late 1773 or early 1774, knowing that fixed air and water dissolved iron, and wondering whether fixed air alone would do the same, he exposed fixed air to iron nails over mercury, and while he was at it set up a similar experiment with nitric oxide. Two months later the fixed air was unchanged but the nitric oxide had 'diminished by one fourth'. The residual gas killed animals and paradoxically allowed a candle to burn, sometimes with an enlarged flame. Water destroyed this property. He had discovered what we call nitrous oxide. He called it Dephlogisticated Nitrous Air. (Nitrous Air was presumed loaded with phlogiston.) He repeated the 1772 experiment, taking serial gas samples which supported combustion during the last stages of the reaction, but only before water had time to act. In 1772, Priestley lost the nitrous oxide into solution, which explains the considerable volume reduction (30,31).

Oxygen

On 1 August, 1774, using a burning lens, he heated mercurius calcinatus *per se* over mercury and readily obtained an air which was insoluble in water ('per se' refers to mercuric oxide obtained directly by prolonged heating in air rather than indirectly through salts) '. . . what surprised me . . .' he wrote, 'was, that a candle burned in this air with a remarkably vigorous flame, very much like that . . . with which a candle burns in nitrous air exposed to iron . . . but as . . . I knew no nitrous acid was used in the preparation of mercurius calcinatus, I was utterly at a loss how to account for it.' Visiting Paris in October, Priestley met Lavoisier and told him about it. Lavoisier already attributed weight gained on calcination to 'air' fixed in the calces and he had wondered whether this was Black's fixed air. He also knew that Bayen had heated mercurius calcinatus and obtained mercury and an 'air'. What greatly surprised him about Priestley's 'air' from mercurius calcinatus, and from red lead, was its support of combustion. He used this clue in unravelling the mysteries of combustion and calcination, and to support his arguments against the phlogiston theory. Priestley went on to find that this new air retained its properties despite vigorous exposure to water; that it produced red fumes with nitrous air and was diminished by it; that a full grown mouse survived in it for an hour instead of the expected 15 minutes; and, in March, 1775, that his test for the 'goodness' of air showed it four or five times as good as common air. He called it dephlogisticated air. Two years later Lavoisier renamed it oxygen (31,32).

When Priestley published his first volume on *Different Kinds of Air*, Scheele had already discovered oxygen, but delay of publication until 1777 (32), reduced the impact of his contribution (21).

Back in the 17th century, Glauber prepared his secret fiery sal ammoniac, which was nitrum flammans or ammonium nitrate. Around 1767, Joseph Black may have unknowingly produced nitrous oxide by heating ammonium nitrate. In 1775, Bryan Higgins, by heating ammonium nitrate, got an air which supported combustion. In 1785, while investigating ammonia, Berthollet heated ammonium nitrate and got nitrous oxide, and so did the Dutch Chemists in 1793 who, the following year prepared ethylene. Carefully heating ammonium nitrate was Davy's preferred method of preparing the gas, as minutely detailed in his *Researches Chemical and Philosophical* and this became the generally accepted method (26,31,33).

Gaseous medicine and laughing gas

Before the joys of laughing gas spread beyond the Pneumatic Institution in Bristol, Davy wrote in a footnote: 'A pound of nitrate of ammonia costs 5s.10d. This . . . produces rather more than 34 doses . . . so . . . the expense of a dose is about 2d . . .' His *Researches* recorded three ways of making ammonium nitrate (from ammoniacal solution and nitric acid; from ammonium carbonate and nitric acid; and from nitre and ammonium sulphate) but as he did not cost individual ingredients it seems likely that it was also bought ready made. But if ammonium nitrate was available at 5s.10d. per pound, for what uses would it have been stocked in 1800? In the context of anaesthesia the question becomes even more relevant in the 1840s (36).

Fourcroy's *Encyclopedia* published in 1808, said there was no natural source of ammonium nitrate and that its only use was for chemical experiments. Although the English Chemists, Davy and Beddoes, recommended breathing it, this was disfavoured in Paris because subjects became asphyxiated, pale and even green. Rees's *Cyclopaedia* of 1819, said subjects became livid and purple, and: 'During the rage for gaseous medicine, it was held up as promising great advantage in certain diseases. This idea has been some time abandoned with little hope of its revival.' (37,38).

In 1819, Michael Faraday reported on impurities in 'ammonium nitrate of commerce', suggesting that at least by then ammonium nitrate was a commercial commodity; but did this reflect the activities of laughing gas pushers and pullers, or serious scientific pursuit? (39).

Frederick Accum's *System of Theoretical and Practical Chemistry*, 2nd edition, 1807, listed chemicals, 'prepared and sold in as pure a state as possible by Frederick Accum. . . .' Ammonium nitrate was not included, but Accum was prepared 'to supply every . . . article not in general demand. Apparatus and instruments supplied, included 'Improved gazometers, with glass bells . . . stop-cocks . . . &c. for collecting, measuring, breathing, transferring gases &c. In 1814, Richard Reece published *The Chemical Guide or Complete Companion to the Portable Chest of Chemistry* which briefly indicated how to make ammonium nitrate. The Chest included nitric acid, ammonium carbonate and pure ammonia solution, and mentioned the preparation and effects of breathing gaseous oxide of azote. In 1823, Griffin published the second edition of *Chemical Recreations* which gave fuller instructions for making ammonium nitrate from nitric acid and ammonium carbonate, priced at 3d and 2d per ounce respectively (40–42).

Recently Averley (43) drew attention to the late 18th and early 19th century chemical societies, often small, private, ephemeral groups. They were sometimes associated with individuals having skills and facilities. Higgins and Accum were involved. I wonder how significant these societies were in keeping the image of laughing gas alive and I come back to the question; what were the demands for ammonium nitrate over this period and how were they met?

References

(1) Nunn JF. *The gaseous environment: an inaugural lecture* Leeds: Leeds University Press, 1966.
(2) Lang A. Mythology. *Encyclopaedia Britannica* 13th Ed. vol. 19, 1926.
(3) Burn AR. *The Pelican history of Greece* Harmondsworth: Pelican Books, 1966.
(4) Partington JR. *A history of chemistry*, vol 1. London: Macmillan, 1970.
(5) Last H. Empedokles and his klepsydra again. *Class Quart* 1924; **18**: 169.
(6) Farrington JR. *Greek science*. Nottingham: Spokesman, 1980.
(7) Middleton WEK. *The history of the barometer*. Baltimore: Johns Hopkins, 1964.
(8) Webster C. The discovery of Boyle's Law, and the concept of the elasticity of air in the seventeenth century. *Arch Exact Sci* 1965; **2**: 441–502.
(9) Waard Cde. *L'experience barometrique ses antecedent et ses explications: etude historique* Thouars, 1936.
(10) Galileo G. *Discorsi e dimostrazioni matematiche intorno a due nuoue scienze* Leyden, 1638. Trans. Crew H, Salvio Ade. *Dialogues concerning two new sciences* London: Macmillan, 1940.
(11) Pecqueti J. *Diepoei experimenta nova anatomica*. Paris, 1651.

(12) Dannemann F. *Otto von Guericke's neue "Magdeburgische" versuche uber den leeren Raum (1672).* Ostwald's Klassiker Der Exacten Wissenschaften Nr. 59. Leipzig: Engelmann, 1894.

(13) Astrup P. Severinghaus JW. *The history of blood gases, acids and bases.* Copenhagen: Munskgaard, 1986.

(14) Boyle R. *New experiments physico-mechanicall, touching the spring of air and its effects. (Made for the most part in a new pneumatical engine.)* Oxford: Tho. Robinson, 1660.

(15) Boyle R. *A defence of the doctrine touching the spring and weight of the air proposed by Mr R. Boyle in his new physico-mechanicall experiments: against the objections of Franciscus Linus.* London: Thos. Robinson, 1662.

(16) Boyle R. *The Works of the Honourable Robert Boyle in six volumes too which is prefixed a life of the author.* London: Russington, 1772.

(17) Scott AF. The invention of the balloon and the birth of modern chemistry. *Scientific American* 1984; **250**: 102–11.

(18) Partington JR. *A history of chemistry* vol 2. London: Macmillan, 1961.

(19) Perkins JF. Historical Development of Respiratory Physiology. In: Fenn WO, Rahn H, eds. *Handbook of physiology: respiration.* Washington: American Physiological Society, 1964.

(20) Mayow J. *Medico-Physical Works being a translation of Tractus Quinque Medico-Physici (1674).* Alembic Club Reprint No 17 Edinburgh: Alembic Club 1907.

(21) Scheele CW. *The discovery of oxygen (1777).* Alembic Club Reprint No 8. Edinburgh: Clay 1894.

(22) Lysaght DJ. Hooke's theory of combustion. *Ambix* 1937; **1**: 93–108.

(23) McKie D. The phlogiston theory. *Endeavour* 1959; **18**: 144–7.

(24) Hales. S. *Vegetable staticks (1727),* Facsimile. London: Macdonald, 1969.

(25) Black J. *Experiments upon Magnesia Alba, Quick-lime, and other Alcaline Substances (1856).* Alembic Club Reprint No 1. Edinburgh: Clay 1893.

(26) Partington JR. *A history of chemistry* Vol 3. London: Macmillan, 1962.

(27) McKie D, ed. *Notes from Doctor Black's lectures on chemistry 1767/8.* Cheshire: Imperial Chemical Industries Limited, 1966.

(28) Priestley J. Experiments and observations on different kinds of air. *Phil Trans* 1772; **62**: 216.

(29) Priestley J. *Experiments and observations on different kinds of air.* Vol 1. London: J. Johnson, 1774.

(30) Priestley J. *Experiments and observations on different kinds of air.* Vol 3. London: J. Johnson, 1777.

(31) Smith WDA. *Under the influence: a history of nitrous oxide and oxygen anaesthesia.* London: Macmillan, 1982.

(32) Priestley J. *The discovery of oxygen (1775).* Alembic Club Reprint No 7. Edinburgh: Clay, 1894.

(33) Perrin CE. Prelude to Lavoisier's theory of calcination; some observations in mercurius calcinatus per se. *Ambix* 1969; **16**: 140–51.

(34) McKie D. Some early work on combustion, respiration and calcination. *Ambix* 1938; **1**: 143–65.

(35) Robison J, ed. *Lectures on the elements of chemistry delivered in the University of Edinburgh by the late Joseph Black MD.* Edinburgh: Longman Rees, 1803.

(36) Davy H. *Researches, chemical and philosophical; chiefly concerning nitrous oxide, or dephlogisticated nitrous air, and its preparation.* London: J. Johnson, 1800.

(37) Fourcroy M. *Encyclopedie methodique, chimie et metallurgie* Vol 15. Paris, 1808.

(38) Rees A. *The Cyclopaedia; or universal dictionary of arts, sciences and literature.* Vol 2. London: Longman, Rees, Orme and Browne, 1819.

(39) Faraday M. Miscellanea. 8: nitrous oxide. *J Science Arts* 1819; **6**: 361.

(40) Accum F. *System of theoretical and practical chemistry.* 2nd Ed. London, 1807.

(41) Reece R. *The chemical guide or complete companion to the portable chest of chemistry* 2nd Ed. London: Longman, Hurst, Rees, Orme and Brown. 1814.

(42) Griffin R. *Chemical recreations: a series of amusing and instructive experiments to which are prefixed first lines of chemistry.* Glasgow, 1823.

(43) Averley G. The 'social chemists': English chemical societies in the eighteenth and early nineteenth centuries. *Ambix* 1986; **33**: 99–128.

10.2	Volatile agents and vaporisers

I. McLELLAN
University of Leicester, Leicester, UK

Since the day when Morton demonstrated satisfactory ether anaesthesia in Boston, exploration and examination of chemical compounds has gone on in an effort to find a better anaesthetic agent. This communication will review some of those agents used mainly in Great Britain and the apparatus designed or adapted for their administration. Dr Richard Ellis has investigated fully the story of the first usage of ether in this country. The vaporizer itself was adapted from apparatus for making carbonated water as were several others described both here and in Europe at the same time. It was a common 19th century practice to inhale from volatile liquids, for fun, for their odours, or whatever, and continuing throughout this period inhalers were made which bore a striking resemblence to anaesthetic vaporizers but were not in actual fact for anaesthesia. These first few years produced a large variety of different apparatus and really in terms of today's prices were very expensive because in 1847 the type of vaporizer used by Robinson was on sale for £3 to £4. Of course the number of vaporizers developed were enormous.

Early agents and vaporizers

The well-known ether inhaler of Snow was further developed after the introduction of chloroform by James Young Simpson in 1847, though some different methods were used, for example, just a handkerchief. In the United States, as we know from Dr Barbara Duncum's book, a move was made against complicated inhalers, the handkerchief technique being preferred perhaps due to feelings resulting from Morton's desire to patent ether. John Snow is said to have used the technique with a handkerchief for administering chloroform to Queen Victoria for the birth of Prince Leopold. During the 19th century two names particularly come up in the search for further anaesthetic agents. One is Sir Benjamin Ward Richardson whose name constantly recurs in anaesthetic literature in the next 50 years. He was a medically qualified scientist, interested in many aspects of medicine and he tested a large number of agents both for general as well as local anaesthesia. Another person who also investigated substances for anaesthetic properties was Thomas Nunnelly of Leeds. He published in 1849 a whole series of papers on anaesthetic agents and a variety of agents were investigated at that time (Table 1).

This communication cannot describe all the different volatile agents and their vaporizers, only some pieces of apparatus and agents which the author finds of interest.

The problem and prevention of chloroform mortality was in the mind of the anaesthetic community for a period of 70/80 years. Snow's first technique of vaporizing chloroform was to use it vaporized in a bag, generally at a concentration of 4%. This technique was rather cumbersome and he went on to develop his well-known chloroform vaporizer. However, of course, this technique of using chloroform vapour was not lost because after Snow's death the technique was taken up by Joseph Clover who took over his anaesthetic practice. (Benjamin Ward Richardson who had been involved in administering anaesthetics with John Snow was first offered the practice and turned it down.) There are photographs of Clover preparing and administering chloroform vapour in this way but one of the problems with this technique was

Table 1

Volatile Agents

Ether
Chloroform
Ethyl bromide
Amylene
Dichloroethane
Acetone
Benzene
Carbon tetrachloride
Ethidene dichloride
Ethyl nitrate
Carbon disulphide
Tribromomethane
Methylene bichloride
Ethyl chloride

that there was a limited volume of chloroform vapour available. In the latter decade of the 19th century, Robert Marston, a dentist, invented an apparatus, based on Snow and Clover's bag, in which the chloroform was vaporized in a metal tank under pressure which increased the volume of the chloroform vapour available. He increased the effective capacity even further by using a very high concentration of chloroform vapour in the tank and having a variable orifice injector between the tank and the patient so that the chloroform vapour could be diluted with known air flow resulting in a lower and variable known concentration of chloroform vapour given to the patient. This apparatus, although it was rather cumbersome was used in his dental practice and manufactured by his own firm. Marston also made a more portable apparatus. Later the technique changed, using nitrous oxide with or without a volatile agent, and it was still in use in the Midlands until the late 1930s, and perhaps also in London.

Now what about the agents? Benjamin Ward Richardson worked with Snow and other anaesthetists throughout the latter half of the 19th century. Some of the volatile agents used have been noted. The gaseous agents have not been referred to, but it is interesting that under the carbon dioxide entry in Richardson's Journal, Hickman's work is not mentioned. Of the agents other than chloroform and ether the most important was ethyl bromide. This continued in widespread use for at least 50 years. It is of interest that ethyl chloride was investigated in 1849 by Nunnelly and introduced by him at that time. It was also tested by John Snow and Richardson in 1852 but was too volatile and was not re-introduced until the turn of the century. Of the others, amylene seemed to be a reasonable agent when introduced in November, 1856. However, two deaths occurred in the next 8 months in 238 administrations and it was then not used any more in anaesthetic practice in this country but continued in use in Europe, particularly Germany, in dental practice. It should be pointed out that the drug used in obstetrics rectally with the trade name Avertin, tribromethanol, is in fact a mixture of tribromethanol 1 g plus amylene hydrate 0.5 g in each cc so perhaps amylene has been used since. Of course at this period a large number of mixtures were made partly to deal with the problems of chloroform and partly to deal with the problems of induction with ether. Some of the most famous ones are the ACE, the Vienna mixture, which was made up of 8 parts of ether with one part chloroform in hot weather and six parts of ether and two parts of chloroform in cold weather. This was so much approved, in practice, that in 1856 a local law was passed that this was to be the only anaesthetic agent employed. It had been administered 33 000 times without a fatality, although, as with ether, severe vomiting was the major problem. Mixtures of course continued with vinesthene anaesthetic mixture (VAM) and the halothane ether azeotrope in this century.

One of the things that is not realized is that, even in the first quarter of this century, most operations took a short time. Therefore, early apparatus had to be easily portable. Not only were they used for a short time on each administration, but as operating lists were infrequent there was a need for the anaesthetist to travel from hospital to hospital. This must have provoked the simplicity of the Junker's apparatus, the Vernon Harcourt apparatus and the simple Waller's wick inhaler which was introduced at the same time as his balance. Other than the Schimmelbusch mask the two most long-lasting were the Junkers apparatus and the Clover ether apparatus, as Hewitts modification. The Junkers apparatus originally devised for 'bichloride of methylene' and used mainly with chloroform or chloroform and ether mixtures underwent several adaptations, mainly concerned with safety to obviate the possibility of squirting neat anaesthetic agent onto or into the patient if it was connected up incorrectly or if splashing occurred. It was used originally with a mask and with nasal prongs for oral work. It was the vapour under pressure which made it obviously an ideal apparatus for use with endotracheal insufflation apparatus and formed the basis of many pieces of apparatus specially developed for this purpose and, as seen in illustrations, a coaxial circuit was used. It continued in use into the late 1950s with one of the Leicester anaesthetists and the bottle on her model was in fact an old pickle jar. Three years ago a Junkers apparatus was found all ready for use in an anaesthetic room of a major county hospital. The Clovers ether apparatus was again widely used throughout the first half of this century either with or without nitrous oxide and oxygen. It vanished from the catalogues in the 1960s but until recently a similar apparatus, the Ombredanne, could be obtained from manufacturers in Europe.

The 20th century

What about agents introduced in this century? I have mentioned the reintroduction of ethyl chloride. The standard anaesthesia machine, was developed, with the bottle vaporizers adapted during the First World War and used by Boyle. The next full step was the introduction of trichloroethylene, whose anaesthetic properties described in 1917 by Plessner, and which was used in 1935 by Jackson, and then re-popularized by Hewer and Hadfield in England at St Bartholomew's Hospital in 1939. Although divinyl ether had been described in 1930, its use was limited. Since then we have seen fluroxene introduced into clinical use in 1953, ethyl vinyl ether introduced in the 1950s, halothane, methoxyflurane first available in 1962, then methyl propyl ether (metopryl) briefly and now of course enflurane and isoflurane.

Although this paper must be brief reference must be made to the development of a vaporizer in the comparative recent past as it is important in the evolution of such apparatus. The simple drawn-over analgesia or anaesthesia vaporizer described by Marrett in 1942 underwent a further development into a vaporizer within the closed circuit during the Second World War. The first prototype is in the Association of Anaesthetists' Museum at 9 Bedford Square and this was further modified after the war and eventually developed into the Marrett apparatus used eventually with halothane.

10.3   Faith against science. The ethanesal mystery

DAVID ZUCK
Chase Farm Hospital, Enfield, UK

On 10 April, 1917, at a meeting of the Academy of Medicine, Toronto, Canada, a paper was read by Dr J. H. Cotton reported that he had prepared, by a process of his own, a perfectly pure ether, free from aldehydes and alcohols. The minute of the meeting continues—'To this is added CO_2 and he obtains an anaesthetic which produces analgesia without of necessity narcosis. Two cats were anaesthetized—one with ordinary ether and the other with Dr Cotton's anaesthetic and it was evident that the second cat went under more rapidly and easily and recovered much more quickly. A patient was then given a sufficient amount of the ether and Dr Bothwell extracted a number of teeth. The demonstration was most convincing and the rapid return of the patient to normal without nausea remarkable.'

'Narcotics' and 'Analgesics'

In a more detailed report (1), Cotton explained that this work had been initiated two years earlier by the observation that certain cans of commercial ether emitted an unusual odour. Investigation had revealed the presence of impurities, aldehydes, alcohols, methyl-ethers, and acetones. Some of these were irritant, and Cotton speculated that they might have something to do with ether pneumonia.

He went on to assert that the constituents of commercial anaesthetic ether could be divided into two groups. Firstly, narcotics, producing peripheral congestion and drunkenness; and secondly, analgesics, producing loss of sensation and peripheral vasomotor spasm. Pure ether, or, as he calls it, absolute di-ethyl ether, falls into the first class. '. . . ethyl ether, with which we are so familiar, is not an anaesthetic, and the analgesia which comes from the administration of commercial ether, is not due to ether, but rather to the impurities occurring in it.' The administration of absolute ether, he continues, 'produces peripheral congestion and drunkenness. . . . As much as twenty ounces has been administered to one patient with only this effect. If, however, a small amount of carbon-dioxide be present, the peripheral congestion is relieved, and the patient enters the natural anaesthetic and analgesic stages. In order, therefore, to obtain anaesthesia proper, we must have acting a narcotic such as di-ethyl ether, together with an analgesic such as carbon-dioxide.' We may be prepared to regard this as a very early statement of the concept of 'balanced' anaesthesia.

Cotton's ether

Cotton designed an apparatus with which to administer this carbonated ether. He described it as 'a can capable of acting as a syphon-soda bottle . . . the carbon-dioxide being injected into the ether under high pressure.'

Continuing his researches, Cotton prepared an ether that possessed 'remarkable analgesic qualities. With it almost major operations were performed with the patient able to articulate clearly, without pain, and not at all sleepy. Its odour was found to be slightly sweeter than that of ordinary pure ether. . . . The results obtained were so peculiar that men refused to believe them even on the word of our highest medical authorities unless they were witnesses. The symptoms were carefully studied in over two hundred cases.' Cotton was describing the phenomenon of ether analgesia, popularized by Artusio in the 1950s (2).

Analysis of this remarkable ether disclosed the presence of ethylene, which, Cotton postulated, must have developed during the process of preparation. He went on to prepare an ether with added carbon dioxide and 2% ethylene, which, he claimed, had the property of inducing anaesthesia smoothly and rapidly, with no stage of excitement, and no nausea postoperatively. This preparation was manufactured by Dupont and marketed in North America as 'Cotton process ether' or 'Cotton's ether'. He read a further paper in 1919 (3), elaborating the theory, and describing improved apparatus. Cotton was a thinking anaesthetist, and introduced ideas ahead of his time.

In a paper read before the American Association of Anaesthetists in 1920 (4), an independent witness, Lumbard, confirmed that 99.8% pure ether 'acted on trial like a very weak ether' while Cotton process ether 'certainly acts like a stronger ether.' It was less irritating during induction, recovery was less disturbed, and there was greater stability of the pulse rate and the blood pressure. However, he thought there was more of a tendency to cyanosis. During the discussion that followed, several speakers confirmed that Cotton process ether was, clinically speaking, a 'superior ether'. One compared it to chloroform, and another wondered, prophetically, why ethylene alone could not be used as an anaesthetic agent. But there were also one or two speakers who, while they evidently did not wish to swim against the current, were not entirely convinced.

Ethanesal

Meanwhile, at St Bartholomew's Hospital in London, England, the chemical pathologist, Dr Mackenzie Wallis, continuing the work he had begun in India, had quite independently pursued a similar line, preparing a very pure ether by distillation of the commercial product with potassium permanganate. In the residues, which were evil smelling, highly irritant, and extremely poisonous, he identified a mixture of impurities which included alcohol, water, acetone, mercaptans, thioethers, aldehydes, peroxides, and acids. At this point he was approached by his anaesthetist colleague, Dr Langton Hewer, with a sample of unpleasantly smelling ether that had been used on two patients, both of whom had stopped breathing soon after the start of induction. He identified the presence of mercaptans, and supplied Dr Hewer with his own highly purified ether. This was found to be incapable of producing anaesthesia, and it was decided that he had removed the active compound or compounds. At this point his attention was drawn to the work of Dr Cotton.

Wallis then prepared a pure ether to which he added carbon dioxide and ethylene. This was non-irritant and sweet-smelling, and after animal trials it was used to anaesthetize 100 patients. All this work by Wallis and Hewer was described in detail in a paper read before the Anaesthetics Section of the Royal Society of Medicine on 1 April, 1921, and published in *The Lancet* three months later (5). In a very obscure passage, Wallis goes on to describe how a residue containing ketones was tested, and it was proved that ketones were the essential element in the production of good and safe anaesthesia. But these were very potent, and it was necessary to use a volatile solvent. For this solvent, ether was chosen. The anaesthetic action was enhanced by the addition of carbon dioxide and ethylene. Wallis described this as, 'The discovery of a compound possessing powerful anaesthetic properties, which has no relation chemically to either chloroform or ether . . .' Commercial preparation of this anaesthetic, in which it was claimed that ether was only the vehicle, was undertaken by the long-established pharmaceutical chemists Savory and Moore, who put it on the market under the name, 'Ethanesal'.

The second part of this paper consisted of a thorough analysis of the clinical effects of Ethanesal by Dr Hewer. He reported on 200 cases, but had since anaesthetized a total of 500. Ethanesal had been administered by Clover's inhaler, open mask, and Boyle's machine with nitrous oxide and oxygen. The age of the patients ranged from eight hours to 70 years, the duration of the operations from three minutes to two hours 45 minutes, and the magnitude from cystoscopy to partial oesophagectomy. For open chest operations the insufflation technique was used.

The main advantages claimed were that it was less irritant, that salivation was less, that respiration was usually quieter, and that post-anaesthetic vomiting was less than with ether or chloroform. The effects on the blood pressure and pulse rate were demonstrated graphically, the effect being intermediate between ether and chloroform. These illustrations are 'graphs' rather than 'charts' because, as Dr Hewer explains, 'They were obtained by calculating the averages of a number of cases whose operations were of approximately the same severity.' The study of blood pressure charts in early anaesthetics publications is a subject in itself. It is an indication of the practical problems that beset the single-handed anaesthetist in the years before endotracheal intubation became common that Dr Hewer found it necessary to conclude by expressing his thanks both to his assistant and to those surgeons who afforded him the opportunity to take blood pressure readings.

The same issue of *The Lancet* contains an Editorial (6) in which it is asserted that, as regards ether, 'the myth of anaesthetic action is apparently finally laid, ether becoming merely a convenient vehicle . . .' The author goes on to suggest that a number of other drugs, particularly organic chemicals, might owe their actions to the impurities they contain. Salvarsan and salicylates are mentioned as examples; Dr Wallis had opened up a wide field for investigation.

In June, 1921, Dr Edmund Boyle, Anaesthetist at St Bartholomew's, attended the Joint Meeting of the Canadian and New York Anaesthetists at Niagara Falls, as the official representative of the Royal Society of Medicine. A welcoming editorial in the *American Journal of Surgery* (7) described him as 'a very splendid and delightful type of English gentleman.'

In his address as Honorary Chairman of the Joint Meeting (8) Boyle spoke at length about Ethanesal, and asserted also that, 'Many hypnotics and analgesics owe their specific action to the ketones they contain.' He stated, perhaps rather revealingly, that for certain types of major surgery he used nitrous oxide, oxygen, and a mixture of equal parts of Ethanesal and chloroform.

Surprisingly quickly, Ethanesal got into the textbooks. It is mentioned with bemused approval in Blomfield's (9) major textbook of 1922; in his experience it was a distinctly weaker anaesthetic than ether, but produced less nausea and vomiting. Ross, (10) in the second edition of his textbook, provided a factual summary of the publications of Cotton, and Wallis and Hewer, but seemed not to have used the agent himself; and it is mentioned in the third edition of Boyle, of which Hewer was co-editor. In his book *Anaesthesia in Children*, of 1923, (11) which may well be the first monograph ever published on paediatric anaesthesia, Hewer devoted a whole chapter to it. He describes it as containing 3% of mixed ketones in a purified ether saturated with ethylene and carbon dioxide. He illustrates a drip-feed apparatus that he had designed to facilitate its use. Ethanesal, and Hewer's apparatus, are also described in the 1922 edition of the *Medical Annual*, in an article by Blomfield (12).

Interest was widespread. In South Africa an anaesthetist manufactured his own version of Ethanesal (13) and found that it fulfilled all his expectations. But the following year a review article by Webster (14) described Cotton process ether used by the open method as disappointing. If used by a semi-closed method, the time to the regaining of consciousness, and the incidence of postoperative vomiting, were about the same as with ordinary ethers. Ethanesal was found to be more satisfactory. Webster mentioned that when Cotton ether was poured into a vaporizer bottle, 'bubbles of carbon dioxide gas could be seen rising, very much as from a good brand of champaigne.' But Cassidy, a dental surgeon, (15) pointed out that even in a reasonably closed vaporizer the concentration of ethylene, also, fell off rapidly. He therefore had devised a closed transfer apparatus to obviate this, and a vaporizer that sounds like the precursor in one respect of the copper kettle.

Dale and others have doubts

In anaesthetics terms, whether the proponents realized it or not, acceptance of Wallis's assertions was equivalent to joining the flat-earthers. It implied, for example, the throwing overboard of the Meyer-Overton theory of the mode of action of anaesthetics; and it was such theoretical implications as much as the practical problems that stimulated the first truly scientific enquiry into the anaesthetic action of pure ether. In a paper (16) that investigated and exploded the claims made for Cotton process ether and Ethanesal, Hewer's own colleague at St Bartholomew's Hospital, Charles Hadfield, is to be found sandwiched between the 'A' Team of British pharmacology and its associated chemistry, Henry Dale and Harold King.

Dale points out that acceptance of Wallis's and Cotton's arguments entail, 'a wholesale revision of laboratory data on which current theories of anaesthesia have been founded, and the abandonment of all theories relating anaesthetic action to physical properties.'

He goes on to describe in detail the preparation in his laboratory, based on the criteria established in the classic, Gwathmey-inspired series of papers by Baskerville and Hamor, (17) of an extremely pure ether, and the demonstration, first on a number of cats and then by Dr Hadfield on eight patients, that, 'chemically pure ether is an anaesthetic at least as satisfactory and effective as the best ethers usually sold for that purpose.'

Dale and his team also examined Ethanesal, buying a number of different samples of different batches on the open market. Now since, according to Goodman and Gilman, (18) a 90 volumes per cent concentration of ethylene in oxygen is required for the induction of surgical anaesthesia, it is difficult enough to account for the enthusiasm with which Ethanesal was welcomed by the action of the initial and rapidly diminishing 3% ethylene and the even more evanescent carbon dioxide content. But Dale's team's findings increase the mystification even further. They describe these samples as containing 95.5% ether, 4% n-butyl alcohol, and 0.5% mixture of ethyl alcohol and an aldehyde. They were unable to detect any ethylene, nor any ketones, which were claimed to be the active constituent, and should have been present to the extent of 5%. They had approached the manufacturers, who were unable to explain the discrepancy, and Dale concluded by stating that contrary to the claims they were investigating, the purest ether makes the best anaesthetic. In Canada, Dale's conclusions were supported by Stehle and Bourne (19).

A second paper on the subject was read before the Anaesthetic Section of the Royal Society of Medicine on 7 March, 1924, by Professor W. Storm van Leeuwen, a pharmacologist at the University of Leyden (20). He explained his involvement in the subject. The first rumours of the non-activity of ether had reached Holland at a time when the manfacturers were doing all they could to produce a very pure anaesthetic ether, because the German ether, which was in use before the War, was no longer available. Consequently there arose the unfortunate position that the surgeons had 'lost their faith,' a very revealing phrase, in the purest ether, and the manufacturers, whose ether had reached a high degree of purity, were at a loss as to how to proceed. Consequently he had been asked by the largest ether manufacturer in Holland to investigate the matter.

He had set out to answer two questions: firstly, has pure ethyl ether a narcotic action; and secondly, is it possible to increase the narcotic action by adding 'impurities' or other constitutents?

Preliminary tests showed that a number of commercially available ethers, including both Cotton's and Ethanesal, apart from the deliberately added impurities, already reached a very high standard of purity. Since these ethers had been used satisfactorily thousands and thousands of times, he argued, Cotton and Mackenzie Wallis must have made a mistake. However, more direct proof was necessary.

He therefore devised a method whereby absolutely pure ether, purer even than that of Dale and King, was prepared by crystallization with benzidine. This ether was found, both in animals and man, to be perfectly active as an anaesthetic. Cats were anaesthetized to respiratory arrest, and the blood level of ether determined. This was found to be the same for the pure ether of crystallization, Ethanesal, and commercial anaesthetic ether.

When 5% methylethyl ketone was added to this pure ether, thus rendering it equivalent to Ethanesal, it was noted that induction went very smoothly, there was less salivation, and less agent was required. However, the addition of methylethyl ketone to ether made it very toxic. Cats anaesthetized every second day with this mixture died of liver failure and multiple haemorrhages after the third anaesthetic. To use such an ether on man would be criminal.

Fortunately his analysis of Ethanesal agreed with that of Dale; although the reaction for ethylene was slightly positive, no ketones had been found—through a fortunate mistake of the manufacturers. His conclusion was that anaesthetic ether should be of the highest purity possible, and should contain a stabilizing agent.

Dale spoke next, repeating in public an offer that he said had already been made in private. 'If Dr Mackenzie Wallis and Dr Hewer obtained another sample of pure ether which was not anaesthetic, he begged them to communicate with him, so that, either in his own laboratory or at St Bartholomew's, they might arrange to make a joint observation, and endeavour to find the cause of the discrepancy. Meanwhile, it was useless to argue about a direct contradiction of experimental fact.'

He went on to deal with Wallis's suggestion that the manufacturer had substituted butyl alcohol for the ketone for reasons of cost. He regarded this as an extraordinary suggestion. Methylethyl ketone was not, as Dr Wallis seemed to imagine, a costly and rare material, but a common solvent, obtainable in any quantity, and cheaper than good ether itself.

During the discussion that followed Wallis repudiated responsibility for the manufacturer's product; but Hadfield thought this was unfair. He had found it impossible to discover the correct formula for Ethanesal, because Wallis kept changing his mind. Dr Hewer and Dr Boyle also spoke, conducting a rearguard action in damage limitation. Boyle showed two slides to illustrate his satisfaction with the results of 10 000 administrations of Ethanesal. But that was not the point. No one questioned that Ethanesal worked; it did, though for the 'wrong' reason. The question was why it was thought that pure ether did not.

Discussion

Anaesthetists must have observed individual variations in the response of patients to anaesthetic agents on many occasions, but because this phenomenon had not yet been conceptualized it did not enter into academic discussion. But even so, from the published material it is difficult to explain why Hewer, presented with a sample of what he was told was pure ether, and which did not work, was prepared to disregard his years of experience and question the anaesthetic potency of pure ether in general rather than the contents of that particular bottle.

While both Cotton and Wallis mentioned animal experiments in passing, the only trials that are described are on three cats and three patients by Cotton, and 'several children' and a girl of nineteen by Hewer. One of Cotton's cats served as its own control, naively accepting Cotton's ether on the first occasion, but half an hour later, no doubt sadder and wiser, objecting strongly to 'absolute' ether. Although Hewer states that 'In all the foregoing experiments, the bottles were numbered, some being pure ether, and others controls of ordinary ether, and thus all bias was eliminated', it is difficult to conclude that either author conformed to the criteria for scientific investigation even of his own times. Neither study could be described as blind, both involved very small numbers, and there is no indication of how the patients were selected. There was no way of standardizing or monitoring the inspired ether concentration, and none of the ineffective ethers was analysed afterwards; although Baskerville and Hamor (14) had pointed out the changes which appear in ether during storage, and had drawn attention to the hygroscopic nature of ether, whereby significant quantities of water could be absorbed from the atmosphere during as short an exposure as half an hour. In fact both reports have all the characteristics of a demonstration of an expected outcome.

Medawar (21) has claimed that the published paper conceals as much as it reveals: '. . . all scientific work of an experimental or exploratory character starts with some expectations about the outcome . . .' So we may wonder to what extent Wallis and Hewer's publication '. . . misrepresents the process of thought that accompanied or gave rise to the work that is described . . .' Was Hewer's mind '. . . a virgin receptacle, an empty vessel . . .'? At the least, Hewer's reaction, or over-reaction as we might say today, argues an existing dissatisfaction with ether; but it also appears that he was acquainted with Cotton's work and had told Wallis about it. So it may well be that his mind was already conditioned to the possibility, or even the expectation, that pure ether would not work.

Popper (22) has directed attention to the asymmetry which results from the logical form of universal statements. These are never derivable from singular statements, but can be contradicted by singular statements. Thus, against the evidence of a million white swans, the refutation of the statement, 'All swans are white', requires only one black one. The Renaissance philosopher Lodovico Vives (23) went so far as to deny that any generalization was ever valid; universal propositions are derived from particular observations, and since these are infinite in number, if only one is missing the universal is not established. Or as Kuhn (24) more moderately, has expressed it, 'A scientific theory cannot be shown to apply successfully to all its possible instances, but it can be shown to be unsuccessful in particular applications.'

In the present instance a very small number of observations were allowed to dictate a sweeping generalization about pure ether, rather than the more appropriate one that *it is not possible on all occasions to induce anaesthesia quickly and smoothly with pure ether administered by the perhalational method*; something that was difficult enough to achieve in the best of circumstances, (25) and in which, of course, it was no different from commercial ether. Instead, there was a loss, or transfer, of faith; and new drugs, like new beliefs honestly introduced, are introduced by those with faith; and it is a common observation that they seem to work better in the hands of their proponents. Why this should be, whether because the enthusiasts are less observant or less critical, or because of a reflexive placebo effect, or some other irrational thing that is not known of in our pharmacology, is beyond the scope of this enquiry.

Ross, (26) in the third edition of his textbook, states conclusively that, 'The theory advanced some eight years ago that ether in a state of purity was not capable of producing anaesthesia has been convincingly disproved by the work of Dale, King, and van Leeuven, and care should be taken that ether used for anaesthesia should be as free from impurities as possible.' But from the first (27) to the seventh edition of *Recent Advances in Anaesthesia*, Hewer opened the chapter on the ethers with the statement, 'It is not proposed to enter into the somewhat prolonged discussion as to whether absolutely pure freshly prepared di-ethyl ether does or does not possess anaesthetic properties', as if there was still any doubt in the matter; and, strangely, although he includes Van Leeuwen in his references, he does not mention Dale.

But even more strangely, unless the minute is incorrect, Cotton appears to have started off with a perfectly pure ether, which worked perfectly well.

Acknowledgments

I am grateful to Mrs E. Swanson, librarian, and my brother, Dr J. Zuck, for the copy of the minute of the Academy of Medicine, Toronto; to Mrs M. Butler, medical librarian, and Martin Moor, medical photographer, Chase Farm Hospital, Enfield; and my secretary, Miss E. Massen.

References

(1) Cotton JH. Anaesthesia from commercial ether administration and what it is due to. *Can Med Assoc J* 1917; **7**: 769–77.
(2) Artusio JF, Jr. Ether analgesia during major surgery. *JAMA* 1955; **157**: 33–6.
(3) Cotton JH. Cotton process ether and ether analgesia. *Am J Surg (Anesth Suppl)* 1919; **33**: 34–43.
(4) Lumbard JE. Remarks on Cotton process ether from personal experience and the reports of other observers. *Am J Surg (Anesth Suppl)* 1920; **34**: 118–21.
(5) Wallis RLM, Hewer CL. A new general anaesthetic: its theory and practice. *Lancet* 1921; **i**: 1173–8.
(6) Editorial. Potent impurities in anaesthetics. *Lancet* 1921; **i**; 1194–5.
(7) Editorial. Anesthesia singularly honored. *Am J Surg (Anesth Suppl)* 1921; **35**: 91–2.
(8) Boyle HEG. Gas–oxygen–ethanesal–chloroform combined anesthesia for nose and throat and abdominal surgery. *Am J Surg (Anesth Suppl)* 1922; **36**: 17–21.
(9) Blomfield J. *Anaesthetics in practice and theory: a textbook for practitioners and students.* London: Heinemann, 1922: 32–3, 156–7.
(10) Ross JS. *Handbook of anaesthetics.* 2nd Ed. Edinburgh: Livingstone, 1923: 115–6.
(11) Hewer CL. *Anaesthesia in children.* London: HK Lewis, 1923: 36–53.
(12) Blomfield J. Ethanesal. In: Coombs CF, Short AR (eds). *The Medical Annual.* Bristol: Wright, 1923: 27–8.
(13) Hall TG. A short note on an ether representing Ethanesal. *Med J South Africa* 1921; **17**: 191–2.
(14) Webster W. Some new anesthetic ethers. *Am J Surg (Anesth Suppl)* 1922; **36**: 71–3.
(15) Cassidy P. Experimental and clinical observations on Cotton process ether. *Am J Surg (Anesth Suppl)* 1922; **36**: 73–5.
(16) Dale HH, Hadfield CF, King H. The anaesthetic action of pure ether. *Lancet* 1923; **i**: 424–9.
(17) Baskerville C, Hamor WA. The chemistry of anaesthetics, I: ethyl ether. *J Ind Eng Chem* 1911; **3**: 301–317 and 378–398.
(18) Goodman LS, Gilman A. *The pharmacological basis of therapeutics.* 2nd Ed. New York: Macmillan, 1958: 80–2.
(19) Stehle RL, Bourne W. The anesthetic properties of pure ether. *JAMA* 1922; **79**: 375–6.
(20) van Leeuwen WS. On the narcotic action of purest ether. *Proc Roy Soc Med* 1924; **17**: 17–34.
(21) Medawar PB. Is the scientific paper a fraud? *The Listener* 1963 Sept 12: 377–8.
(22) Popper K. *The logic of scientific discovery.* London: Hutchinson, 1959 (1977): 41–2.
(23) Blake RM, Ducasse CJ, Madden EH. *Theories of scientific method: the renaissance through the nineteenth century.* Seattle: University Washington Press, 1966: 7–9.
(24) Kuhn TS. *The essential tension: studies in scientific tradition and change.* Chicago: University Chicago Press, 1977: 280.
(25) Ross JS. *Handbook of anaesthetics.* 1st Ed. Edinburgh: Livingstone, 1919: 83–9.
(26) Ross JS. *Handbook of anaesthetics.* 3rd Ed. Edinburgh: Livingstone, 1929: 118.
(27) Hewer CL. *Recent advances in anaesthesia and analgesia.* 1st Ed. London: Churchill, 1932: 40.

10.4 The first use of divinyl ether as an anaesthetic agent in humans

ROY M. HUMBLE

University of Alberta, Edmonton, Alberta, Canada

In Chauncey Leake's *Letheon: The Cadenced Story of Anesthesia*, the following lines occur, referring to the introduction of divinyl ether into anaesthetic practice.

> '. . . *divinyl ether is as prophesied a rapid acting useful drug for anesthesia. Here at last had science triumphed in predicting what a new drug might do on living things before it had existence.*' (1)

This is not a novel concept for us today, but it was in 1930. Two of the anaesthetic agents which were in widespread use at that time were diethyl ether and ethylene, diethyl ether from the birth of modern anaesthesia in the 1840s, and the gas ethylene from 1923 (although as olefiant gas ethylene had originally been tried as an anaesthetic by Thomas Nunneley in 1848) (2). The introduction of divinyl ether stemmed from a general consideration of the properties of these two agents.

Leake and Chen predicted in 1930 that the lower members of a series of unsaturated ethers combining the chemical characteristics of diethyl ether and ethylene might be found to be satisfactory inhalational anaesthetic substances. Using an impure sample of divinyl ether on mice they then found, as predicted, that it had anaesthetic properties equal or superior to diethyl ether. They concluded their article with the words 'further study of this interesting series of agents is justified, and cordially invited' (3).

Doctors Samuel Gelfan and Irving Bell at the University of Alberta were attracted by that report and invitation. They tried unsuccessfully to prepare pure divinyl ether in their own laboratory, but were encouraged by the promising results of continuing experimental studies with the agent on dogs which were being carried on at the University of California, and which were communicated to them by Chauncey Leake. When the pure drug became available in 1931 (4), they determined to use it for the first time in the human subject.

The first experimental administrations to man

Open drop divinyl oxide, so called to avoid confusion with the ordinary diethyl ether, was administered by Bell to his co-worker Gelfan for a period of ten minutes. Bell described the induction as smooth, prompt, and even, with no signs of excitement or struggling. Two minutes after removal of the mask, Gelfan had fully recovered, and was able to converse intelligently. Several days later he again received the anaesthetic, this time for eighteen minutes. The effects on respiration, pulse, blood pressure, eye reflexes and pupillary activity were recorded throughout. Blood pressure varied by no more than 5–10% from preinduction levels, and the pulse did not vary significantly. A fair degree of relaxation of the abdominal muscles was obtained, and the presence of complete analgesia confirmed by the application of strong tetanising currents to the foot and leg. There was again a rapid recovery with complete absence of nausea and vomiting.

After two such administrations, Gelfan obviously wished to see the anaesthetic in a more objective way. A member of the Zoology Department, Dr Winifred Hughes, happened to be walking in the corridor outside their laboratory at the time (5), and was invited (? cajoled) into being a volunteer for the third successful administration of the agent. It is noteworthy that all three trials were made within two and three hours of a meal, and both subjects were stated to have found no difficulty in continuing their teaching duties shortly after the anaesthesia. The rapid induction and recovery with absence of nausea and vomiting, which these early workers found, were to be the hallmarks of anaesthesia with divinyl ether.

The reports by Gelfan and Bell (6) and animal studies from the University of California (7) were both published in the same journal in January, 1933, Gelfan and Bell's article concluding with the words 'on the basis of the experiments performed by Leake and his associates and our tests of the anaesthetic in the human we feel that divinyl oxide is worthy of clinical trial and evaluation.'

The first administration for clinical surgical anaesthesia

The first successful administration of divinyl ether for a surgical case was carried out later in 1933 by Dr Dorothy Wood at the University of California, and a large series of cases subsequently reported by Goldschmidt and his colleagues from the University of Pennsylvania (8). Divinyl ether retained a place in the anaesthetic armamentarium for over four decades, with a high safety record as either an induction agent, or as the sole anaesthetic for short surgical procedures. Its use in such cases was well described by Dr Bill McConnell in the 'Lest We Forget' series of the Section of Anaesthetics of the Royal Society of Medicine in 1974.

Discussion

Gelfan and Bell's work was a brief practical study, typical of the uninhibited work of many of the anaesthetic pioneers, who continually used themselves as initial guinea pigs in their researches. Although primarily an internist, with a joint appointment in therapeutics and pharmacology at the University of Alberta, Dr Bell administered anaesthetics at two major Edmonton hospitals for many years, up to the start of World War II. He was subsequently elected to honorary membership of the Canadian Anaesthetists Society. He died in Edmonton in 1953. Dr Gelfan was Assistant Professor in Physiology and Pharmacology at the University of Alberta from 1930–1932, and went on to become Professor and later Emeritus Professor of Neurophysiology at the New York Medical College. He died in New York in 1975.

Their work was carried out in the then conjoined Departments of Physiology and Pharmacology at the University of Alberta in what is now known as The Old Medical Building. Two years after Dr Bell's death the Alberta Anaesthetists Society erected a plaque in the foyer of that building to commemorate this first use of divinyl ether in humans, a second visual landmark in a structure which had earlier been the site of the first isolation of parathyroid hormone.

Chauncey Leake's use of the phrase 'before it had existence' in his 1947 Letheon verses is open to question. Thirteen years earlier he had also stated that the compound 'did not exist, although theoretically known to chemists' (10), despite being aware (7) of the work of Frederich Semmler in Germany in the latter part of the 19th century in isolating a small quantity of impure divinyl ether (9). It is to Semmler that the actual discovery must be credited (11), but it is to Leake and his colleagues, and to the subsequent pioneering trial carried out by Gelfan and Bell which they stimulated, that the credit for the introduction of divinyl ether into anaesthesia must jointly go. That introduction forms a small but unique chapter in our anaesthetic history.

References

(1) Leake CD. *Letheon: The cadenced story of anesthesia.* Austin: University Texas Press, 1947: 60.

(2) Nunneley T. On anaesthesia and anaesthetic substances. *Trans Prov Med Surg Assoc* London 1849; **16**: 228–30; 330–1.

(3) Leake CD, Chen MY. The anesthetic properties of certain unsaturated ethers. *Proc Soc Exper Biol Med* 1930; **28**: 151.

(4) Ruigh WL, Major RT. Preparation and properties of pure divinyl ether. *J Am Chem Soc* 1931; **53**: 2662.

(5) Cameron T. *Personal communication*, 1987.

(6) Gelfan S, Bell IR. The anesthetic action of divinyl oxide on humans. *J Pharmacol Exp Ther* 1933; **47**: 1.

(7) Leake CD, Knoefel PK, Guedel AE. The anesthetic action of divinyl oxide in animals. *J Pharmacol Exp Ther* 1933; **47**: 5.

(8) Goldschmidt S, Ravdin IS, Lucke B, Muller GP, Johnston CG, Ruigh WL. Divinyl ether: experimental and clinical studies. *JAMA* 1934; **102**: 121.

(9) Semmler FW. Vinyl ether: the ethereal oil of Allium Ursinum. *Ann Chemie* 1887; **241**: 90–116.

(10) Leake CD. The role of pharmacology in the development of ideal anesthesia. *JAMA* 1934; **102**: 1, 1.

(11) Faulconer A, Keys TE. *Foundations of anesthesiology*. Springfield: Thomas, 1965: 571.

10.5 　 Cyclopropane and the development of controlled ventilation

RICHARD BODMAN
Dartmouth, Nova Scotia, Canada

Cyclopropane had a short life in the mainstream of anaesthesia, but its importance proved to be out of proportion to its brevity. It was introduced in 1934 (1) and its demise was heralded by the introduction of curare in 1942. But during this time and with its use the principles of controlled ventilation were established, greatly facilitating the progress of thoracic and abdominal surgery. As the potential of curare was exploited, cyclopropane lost its importance in providing quiet relaxation and was gradually relegated to special situations such as obstetrics and paediatrics.

Ethylene and closed apparatus

More than any previous agent in anaesthesia, cyclopropane depended on the development of appropriate apparatus for its use. Its high cost and high risk of explosion required a closed system for its administration. In this respect the development of its precursor, ethylene, paved the way. It is not surprising that both were the progeny of the same stables—Wisconsin and Montreal. Brown (2) introduced ethylene in Canada in 1923 and Ralph Waters (3) described his 'to-and-fro' closed system in 1924, at first advocating it for nitrous oxide and ethyl chloride. Harold Griffith adopted it for ethylene. The first circle absorber system for anaesthesia was described by Brian Sword in 1930 (4).

Experimental work

Meanwhile Canadian workers continued to explore the hydrocarbons for more powerful anaesthetic properties, with the result that Lucas and Henderson (5) in 1929 proposed a new agent, cyclopropane, which they tried on themselves.

Early clinical use

Stiles, Neff, Rovenstine and Waters (5) in Wisconsin published their experiences with this new agent in 1934 and Griffin (6) in Toronto published his results in the same year.

Ronald Jarman (7) in 1933 in the United Kingdom had pioneered the use of intravenous barbiturates with 'Evipan' (hexobarbitone) and Lundy (8) introduced 'Pentothal' (thiopentone) at the Mayo Clinic in 1934. We are not concerned with these intravenous agents on this occasion, except to note that the stage was set by 1934 for a quantum leap forward in the practice of anaesthesia. This year can be said to have seen the birth of modern anaesthesia. In the early accounts of the use of cyclopropane—always in a closed system—no mention is made of assisting or controlling respiration. Anaesthetists were accustomed to using ether for major surgery, an agent which stimulates respiration by virtue of its irritant properties. It was not until a deep level of anaesthesia was reached—the third plane of the third stage of anaesthesia in the terminology then used—that respiration began to quieten and only in even deeper levels was there evidence of depression of respiration, as judged by diminished movement of the chest and abdomen. Consequently it rarely appeared to be necessary to interfere with the natural processes of respiration under ether anaesthesia. The picture changed with the introduction of cyclopropane. This gas was not unpleasant to smell nor was it irritating to breathe, as soon as administrators realized that concentrations of 15 to 20%—low compared to the 80 or 90% used with ethylene or nitrous oxide—were adequate for surgical anaesthesia. Quite contrary to the experience with ether, cyclopropane tended to depress respiration at an early stage in the anaesthesia; while this greatly improved operating conditions for the surgeon, there was a critical limit to this depression beyond which carbon dioxide built up, with a consequent increase in blood pressure, pulse rate and capillary oozing. The idea of actually controlling the respiration by squeezing the bag was viewed with alarm, for fear of losing the principle indicator of the depth of anaesthesia.

Here we may briefly review the status of anaesthesia in the United States and the United Kingdom. Such generalities are patently superficial, but serve to remind us that our specialty was in its infancy in the 1930s. With few notable exceptions in the United States anaesthetics were given by nurses, employed by hospitals and directed by surgeons. In the United Kingdom anaesthetics for the most part were given by general practitioners with less training and little more expertise than the nurses in the States. I quote our distinguished colleague Dr Eckenhoff (9), long associated with Dr Dripps in the establishment of that prestigious centre of anaesthetic excellence in Philadelphia:

> *'in 1938 the first anaesthesiologist at the University of Pennsylvania was appointed. By then, nurses had administered most of the inhalational anesthetics for the previous 30 years. Surgeons gave all spinal anesthetics . . . the chief nurse anesthetist resigned shortly after . . .'*

Dr C. S. Williams (10) of New Zealand reported on a visit to the United States in 1937:

> *'The gaseous anaesthetics, nitrous oxide and cyclopropane, were used almost universally . . . ether being relegated to a position of less importance.' . . . 'The use of ethylene is being discarded rapidly, and in some hospitals is forbidden.'*

By contrast cyclopropane made slow progress in the United Kingdom, probably on account of its high cost and the fact that the teaching hospitals, which were supported by voluntary contributions, by 1939 were in a parlous state financially.

It is interesting to note the comments of Dr W. L. Garth (11) of San Diego in *Some observations of anaesthesia abroad* published in 1938. He visited Florence, Vienna, Geneva, Munich, Heidelberg, Wiesbaden and Paris before arriving in London, where he met Dr Nosworthy and Dr Ronald Jarman and visited the Westminster and St Thomas's Hospitals:

> *'In England the picture is very different. Anesthesia there was never turned over to technicians, as in our country, so their personnel set-up is much better than our own . . . As a result they have been the leaders in the art of anesthesia. However, their ingrained conservatism is such that they have fallen behind in the present forward surge of anesthesia progress . . . they failed to accept ethylene when it was brought out by Luckhardt in 1923, and are now just as staunchly refusing to try cyclopropane.'*

Though cyclopropane was being widely used in the States at this time, it was chiefly in the hands of nurses and technicians. Dr Flagg (12) in the 6th edition of his popular textbook in 1939 remarks:

> *'. . . this new agent has been popularized by less conservative groups to a degree out of keeping with its safety and value.'*

So it was only in a few relatively isolated centres in North America and the United Kingdom that real developments in anaesthetics and techniques were occurring. For instance, at my medical school until the end of the Second World War all anaesthetics were given by general practitioners and students were taught to use ethyl chloride or chloroform for induction, followed by ether by open drop on a Schimmelbusch mask. The only exception was Dr Bradbeer who became the first full-time anaesthetic specialist in Bristol when he gave up general practice in 1935. The cyclopropane cylinder was kept under lock and key and would be produced only when Dr Bradbeer requested it.

In spite of Dr Garth's comments, cyclopropane was being used in the United Kingdom in a limited number of centres, notably in London by Dr Langton Hewer at St Bartholomew's Hospital and Dr Ivan Magill and Dr Nosworthy at the Brompton and the Westminster Hospitals. As early as 1936 Magill (13) reporting on 128 thoracic operations (23 done under spinal anaesthesia) commented:

'. . . *the choice of anaesthetic at present lies between nitrous oxide and oxygen . . . with chloroform as an adjuvant—and cyclopropane*

depending on whether the surgeon wanted to use the diathermy in the chest.

Controlled ventilation

If we now turn our attention to the technique of controlled ventilation, as early as 1934 Guedel and Treweek (14) had described 'ether apnoea':

'. . . *increase the ether tension by rhythmic manual compression of the breathing bag, synchronous with inspiration . . .*'.

But it was by no means accepted that controlled ventilation was either necessary or desirable. Dr Beecher (15), already an eminent professor of anaesthesiology in Boston, speaking to the American Association for Thoracic Surgery in 1940 commented:

'*the deliberate production of respiratory failure (sic) in patients under anaesthesia removes the greatest safeguard against overdosage . . . puts ether in the position of being at least as good and perhaps better than cyclopropane . . .*'.

Of the five thoracic surgeons for all over the States whose comments are recorded at this meeting, the general opinion was that they had not been impelled to employ 'controlled' ventilation, which they considered a potentially dangerous procedure.

Meanwhile, Nosworthy had visited Waters at Wisconsin and Guedel in Los Angeles in 1939. He adopted the former's apparatus and the latter's technique but, although he had been to Sweden to visit the famous thoracic surgeon Professor Crafoord, who with an engineer Dr Frenckner, had developed a mechanical ventilator—the Spiropulsator—Nosworthy never adopted mechanical ventilators, preferring to use his own hands. By 1941 he had also gained considerable experience of war wounds at the Horton Chest Unit, having anaesthetized 200 patients with thoracic wounds, following the Dunkirk evacuation. Of these 12 died, six from multiple injuries and six from gross infection—this was before the introduction of penicillin. This was a very creditable performance when we consider Crafoord's (16) published figures for the previous year:

'. . . *ninety four intrathoracic operations in which we have used rhythmic ventilation in connection with inhalation anesthesia . . . there have been twenty seven deaths, two of which occurred during operation.*'

On 4 April, 1941, Dr Nosworthy (17), at the Anaesthetic Section of the Royal Society of Medicine, presented his classic paper 'Anaesthesia in chest surgery, with special reference to controlled respiration and cyclopropane'. This proved to be the definitive description of the principles of anaesthesia for thoracic surgery as we know them today. Nosworthy's method required pre-medication with an opiate, induction with thiopentone, mild hyperventilation with cyclopropane and controlled respiration. He thus established the technique which is now universally used for all major thoracic and abdominal surgery, though we now substitute nitrous oxide and curare for cyclopropane. He described the problems of mediastinal shift and paradoxical respiration, arguing the superiority of controlled respiration over 'positive pressure respiration' as advocated by Beecher and which we would today call 'continuous positive airway pressure' (CPAP).

Dr Langton Hewer at this same meeting reiterated that producing apnoea with high concentrations of cyclopropane and controlled respiration left the anaesthetist with no indications of the depth of anaesthesia or the concentration of carbon dioxide in the blood, echoing the comments made by Beecher. Nosworthy countered these criticisms by explaining that a number of manoeuvres could quickly establish the depth of anaesthesia. Stopping ventilation, removing the soda-lime or adding ether would encourage spontaneous respiration and the time this took to return would be an indication of the depth of anaesthesia. In abdominal surgery with the chest closed simply the tightness of the bag in the hand gave an indication of the degree of relaxation and so of the depth of anaesthesia. Finally, it was common practice to smell the contents of the reservoir bag—it was not difficult to tell the difference between 15 and 50% (the practice of 'sniffing' later fell into disrepute when it was abused!)

A large part of Nosworthy's paper concerns the problems of the 'wet lung'. The change in morbidity effected by the introduction of antibiotics has effaced the memory of the gross infections which were so pervasive. Breast abscess, paronychia, Bartholin's abscess, acute mastoiditis were the common daily inventory of a Casualty department. Chronic chest infections seemed to be endemic. Of the ordinary civilian sick requiring chest surgery Nosworthy observes

> *'Many of these however are more or less chronic invalids. They may have had prolonged toxaemia and be suffering from amyloid disease.'*

The commonest chest operations would be for empyema, done under local anaesthesia, and thoracoplasty, often done with paravertebral block with or without light nitrous oxide anaesthesia. Operations within the pleura, for lung abscess, bronchiectasis or bronchial carcinoma, would require general anaesthesia with intubation.

The conventional position for chest surgery was the lateral; this would be dictated by the surgeon. The problem was that the lung to be operated on was uppermost and its contents would run down the main bronchus or be displaced by handling to reach the carina and cross into the 'good' side. Many manoeuvres and devices were proposed to prevent this happening, such as endobronchial tubes and bronchial blockers, or a 45 degree head-down tilt advocated by Beecher. The necessity for many of these has been obviated by the introduction of antibiotics and double-lumen endotracheal tubes. While the principles enunciated by Nosworthy were accepted whole-heartedly, alternative techniques were used by a group who preferred the circle absorption to Waters' 'to-and-fro' system and the prone position to the lateral.

We have mentioned the financial plight of the voluntary hospitals in the 1930s. We will briefly note what could be called the alternative system. In 1931 the Poor Law Institutions in UK were taken over by the County Councils and the more progressive and wealthier councils converted these to general hospitals. Middlesex took advantage of this law to expand their institutions and provide special units, for instance a neurosurgical unit at the Central Middlesex Hospital, a plastic surgery unit at the West Middlesex and a thoracic surgery unit at Hillingdon; at the same time a new tuberculosis sanatorium was built at Harefield, nearby. These hospitals were staffed by whole-time salaried doctors. These developments were not confined to the London area; for instance in Bristol, Southmead Hospital was taken over and an obstetric unit was established and later with the advent of the war the National Blood Bank was set up there; the hospital at Frenchay was built by the county and on completion was occupied by a US army hospital for the duration of the war. In 1948 all the hospitals in the country were taken over by the central government with the establishment of the National Health Service.

The principals in the thoracic unit at Hillingdon were Mr L. Fatti the surgeon and Dr H. J. V. Morton the anaesthetist. They were both active and progressive. In 1939 they had been the first in the country to tie a patent ductus. In 1944 Fatti and Morton (18) published a paper on 600 bronchoscopies—a phenomenal number in those days. In 1942 (19) Morton presented his MD thesis on the effect of smoking on post-operative pulmonary complications. Morton had been a colleague of Nosworthy's at St Thomas's Hospital. He readily adopted the latters principle of controlled respiration for thoracic surgery, but he rejected the Waters apparatus, preferring to use a circle anaesthetic system. He observed that the Waters 'to-and-fro' system, with the soda-lime so close to the patient's face, rendered the inspired gases very hot and allowed fine dust from the soda lime to enter the trachea. Having experimented on himself by breathing through a soda lime canister for 15 minutes at a time, he came to the conclusion that this could contribute to postoperative pulmonary complications.

Mr Fatti, while visiting the United States, had been impressed with the Connell anaesthetic machine and brought two back to be installed at Hillingdon and Harefield. Bryn Thomas (20) has described this machine, it was the first apparatus designed for closed circuit use and not simply as an attachment to an existing gas machine. All the copper piping was welded within the apparatus, the only detachable parts being the corrugated tubing, which being of rubber provided a leak-proof connection to the inspiratory and expiratory ports. A pressure of 20 cm of water could be maintained in the circuit for 60 seconds without the loss of any gas. The importance of this facility lay in the evanescent effect of cyclopropane, such that loss of gas mixture made it difficult for the administrator to maintain a steady depth of anaesthesia. By using a completely closed circuit and the concertina reservoir bag Morton (21) was able to record tidal volumes and study the patterns of spontaneous respiration.

Morton was also fortunate in that Fatti agreed to adopt the Overholt position for operations on the lung: the patient lying prone, with a six inch block under the sternum and a wedge under the pelvis. The surgeon was seated and on opening the chest the 'wet' lung hung down (forward anatomically) providing an unobstructed view of the hilum, with no danger of the contents of the lung entering the trachea. There was little or no mediastinal shift or paradoxical respiration with ventilation and bronchial blockers and endobronchial tubes were not necessary. When doing a lobectomy the remaining good lung would tend to collapse owing to the absorption of cyclopropane and oxygen, aided by the assistant's retractor. It was then the practice to halt the surgery every 15–20 minutes in order to reflate the offending lobe. If this were not done a lobe could collapse completely and would require a dangerously high pressure to reflate it at the end of the procedure.

The exploitation of curare in clinical anaesthesia and the pervasive use of the diathermy were the principle reasons for the relegation of cyclopropane to a minor role in clinical practice. But, during its short period of popularity cyclopropane provided the opportunity for man to control a vital physiological function—respiration: a significant step in transforming anaesthesia from an art to a science.

References

(1) Stiles JA, Neff WB, Rovenstine EA, Waters RM. Cyclopropane as an anaesthetic agent. *Curr Res Anesth Analg* 1934; **13**: 56–60.

(2) Brown WE. Preliminary report: Experiments with ethylene as a general anaesthetic. *Can Med Assoc J* 1923; **13**: 210.

(3) Waters RM. Clinical scope and utility of carbon dioxide filtration in inhalation anesthesia. *Curr Res Anesth Analg* 1924; **3**: 20–2.

(4) Sword BC. The closed circle method of administration of gas anaesthesia. *Curr Res Anesth Analg* 1930; **9**: 198–202.

(5) Lucas GHW, Henderson VE. A new anaesthetic gas: cyclopropane. *Can Med Assoc J* 1929; **21**: 173–5.

(6) Griffith HR. Cyclopropane anaesthesia: a clinical record of 350 administrations. *Can Med Assoc J* 1934; **31**: 157–60.

(7) Jarman R, Abel L. Evipan: an intravenous anaesthetic. *Lancet* 1933; **ii**: 18–20.

(8) Lundy JS, Tovell RM. Some of the newer local and general anesthetic agents: methods of their administration. *Northwest Med J* 1934; **33**: 308–11.

(9) Eckenhoff JE. *Anesthesia from colonial times: a history of anesthesia at the University of Pennsylvania*. Philadelphia: JB Lippincott, 1966.

(10) Williams CS. Cyclopropane: a new anaesthetic agent. *NZ Med J* 1937; **36**: 193.

(11) Garth WL. Some observations of anesthesia abroad. *Curr Res Anesth Analg* 1938; **17**: 292–7.

(12) Flagg PJ. *Cyclopropane in the art of anesthesia*. 6th Ed. Philadelphia: JB Lippincott, 1939: 420–7.

(13) Magill IW. Anaesthesia in thoracic surgery with special reference to lobectomy. *Proc Roy Soc Med* 1936; **29**: 643.

(14) Guedel AE, Treweek DN. Ether apnoeas. *Curr Res Anesth Analg* 1934; **13**: 263–4.

(15) Beecher HK. Some controversial matters of anesthesia for thoracic surgery. *J Thorac Surg* 1940; **10**: 202–19.

(16) Crafoord C. Pulmonary ventilation and anaesthesia in major chest surgery. *J Thorac Surg* 1940; **9**: 237–53.

(17) Nosworthy MD. Anaesthesia in chest surgery, with special reference to controlled respiration and cyclopropane. *Proc Roy Soc Med* 1941; **34**: 480–506.

(18) Fatti L, Morton HJV. Pentothal anaesthesia in bronchoscopy. *Lancet* 1944; i: 597–8.

(19) Morton HJV. Tobacco smoking and pulmonary complications after operation. *Lancet* 1944; i: 368–70.

(20) Thomas K Bryn. *The development of anaesthetic apparatus.* Oxford: Blackwell Scientific Publications 1975: 168–71.

(21) Morton HJV. Respiratory patterns during surgical anaesthesia. *Anaesthesia* 1950; **5**: 112–28.

10.6   Introduction of halothane to the USA

C. RONALD STEPHEN, C.M. and LEONARD W. FABIAN
Washington University School of Medicine, St Louis, Missouri, USA

Following the Second World War and the burgeoning of anaesthesiology as a medical specialty, there was intense interest generated in finding an inhalational drug which was potent, nonflammable, nonexplosive and physiologically safe. As it turned out, the work of Dr C. W. Suckling of the United Kingdom in synthesizing a series of fluorinated hydrocarbons would prove a landmark in medical history. There probably have been more papers and volumes written concerning the pharmacology and applications of halothane than any other anaesthetic compound. In North America our early introduction to halothane was based perhaps more on happenstance than anything else.

One morning early in 1956, while at Duke University Medical School in North Carolina, a telephone call was received from Dr John J. Jewell, a medical school classmate of the author from McGill University in Montreal, Canada. At the time Dr Jewell was Medical Director of Ayerst Laboratories in New York and we had done some investigations with him on trichloroethylene. Would we be interested in looking at a new fluorinated compound, Fluothane, about which he had been contacted by Imperial Chemical Industries (Pharmaceuticals) in England? The author, being young and full of vim, vigour and vitality, the answer was obvious. So, in February Dr Jewell travelled to North Carolina, carrying with him the first and only pound of the drug in the United States, along with some preliminary physical and pharmacological data available from England. The experiments of Dr J. Raventos were encouraging, as was the information that Dr Michael Johnstone had successfully anaesthetized a few patients with the drug.

Preliminary laboratory investigations

We went first to the laboratory and at once ascertained that it was indeed a potent drug, at least in the dog. Increasing depth of anaesthesia was rapidly achieved because of its non-irritability, and was matched by progressive hypotension. In a few weeks supplies became more available and progress was made in determining some of the pharmacological properties of the drug, particularly its arrhythmic potential by sensitization of the conduction system of the heart.

A matter of concern associated with clinical administration related to the possibility of hepatic damage. To this end, seven dogs and two monkeys were exposed to anaesthetic concentrations of the drug for a total of 24 hours over a period of six days. Histological studies revealed pallor about the centralobular veins, but no evidence of cellular destruction.

The development of clinical technique

Armed with data and information gleaned in the laboratory, we approached the problems of clinical administration. Using the open-drop technique turned out to be a fiasco. The potency of the drug negated the establishment of a safe, even plane of anaesthesia. Apart from the 'ether copper kettle', with which very few of our anaesthetic machines were equipped, we had no vaporizers which could be calibrated with any degree of accuracy. We soon learned that the standard 'in circuit' ether vaporizer could be hazardous because increasing the minute ventilation by assisting the ventilation could markedly increase the plane of anaesthesia to dangerous depths. Using non-rebreathing circuits were much safer, but except in children these were not feasible because of the limited supplies of the drug available. Moreover, American anaesthesiologists were firmly entrenched in using the 'circle' system. It became clear that an accurately calibrated vaporizer placed in an 'out of circuit' position was the safest way to proceed. To this end we used the Goldman divinyl ether vaporizer with a modicum of success, but its accuracy was limited. With the help of an engineer, Mr George Newton, the F-N-S vaporizer was designed which allowed concentrations of zero to 4.4% to be delivered at a flow rate of four litres per minute from the anaesthetic machine. It possessed inherent inaccuracies, but always on the safe side because it was not temperature-compensated. It remained for Mr Fraser Sweatman (United Kingdom) to devise the 'Fluotec', which became a standard means of safe vaporization.

In addition to monitoring the physiological changes associated with the administration of this new, potent anaesthetic, we grossly looked at changes in liver function in 18 patients as monitored by the bromsulfalein test: fourteen showed a retention of 8% to 39% within 24 hours, but none had significant retention in five days. These results were similar to those found in a comparable group of patients anaesthetized with ether.

The first reports

The first report of our preliminary laboratory and clinical experiences in 145 patients was presented at the Annual Meeting of the American Society of Anaesthesiologists in Kansas City in October, 1956 (1). Almost simultaneously Michael Johnstone's landmark paper appeared (2), along with the lucid pharmacologic data by J. Raventos (3). Little did we realize at that time what a profound influence halothane would have on future developments in anaesthesia.

References

(1) Stephen CR, Bourgeois-Gavardin M, Fabian LW, Grosskreutz DC, Dent S, Coughlin J. Fluothane—a preliminary report. *Anesthesiology* 1957; **18**: 174–5.
(2) Johnstone M. The human cardiovascular reponse to Fluothane anaesthesia. *Br J Anaesth* 1956; **28**: 392–410.
(3) Raventos J. The action of Fluothane—a new volatile anaesthetic. *Br J Pharmacol* 1956; **11**: 394–410.

10.7	The historic misuse of anaesthetic and related agents

ALBERT M. BETCHER
Mount Sinai School of Medicine, New York, USA

Long before the discovery of anaesthesia there were therapeutic uses for ether. It had been on the pharmacist's shelf as a medicinal agent since 1743 (1). It was prescribed in wine for various complaints, and later was applied to a bit of linen rag and stuffed up a nostril. The inhalation of ether vapour was advocated for patients with tuberculosis in 1795 (2). The wife of a British Admiral was treated for her asthma by inhaling the vapour from two teaspoonfuls of ether poured into a saucer and placed on her lap with a shawl over her head. She reported a delightful sense of tranquility (3). Soon, other patients for whom ether inhalation was prescribed also appreciated the extra dividends of experiencing pleasurable properties. They believed it was a less immoral and vulgar method of getting intoxicated than by means of common spirits. Men were known to recommend its use on wives to keep them quiet.

Intoxication and the introduction of inhalation anaesthesia

In the chemistry lectures at universities the professor would pour a little ether into a bladder of air during his lecture upon it, and allow some of the students to inhale the vapour. This led to the so-called 'ether frolics' of the 19th century in which students were interested in the antics that were performed by those inhaling the vapour.

About this time, the same effect being produced by the inhalation of nitrous oxide led to its utilization as an entertainment device. The entertainer informed the public that 'gas would be administered only to gentlemen of the first respectability. The object was to make the entertainment in every respect, a genteel affair' (4). Sometimes there occurred near tragedies. In 1821 a druggist came to Oneida County, New York to exhibit the effects of the inhalation of nitrous oxide. After the exhibition while many were standing around talking over what they had witnessed a young man was found lying on the floor close by the gasometer entirely senseless. After a long and anxious suspense he awoke unharmed (5).

In the Fall of 1839, some young people in Athens, Georgia, attended a quilting and followed it with an ether frolic. One of them noticed a negro boy at the door who seemed to be enjoying the sport. He invited the boy to inhale the ether. When he refused, the other boys grabbed him and held him while one poured ether upon a handkerchief and pressed it firmly over his nose and mouth. Finally, the negro boy lay quiet and they were surprised that he didn't move. One was sent on horseback to get a doctor. The doctor (Crawford Long) on his arrival, began to restore the boy to consciousness by throwing water in his face, shaking him and pricking him until he awoke (6).

Chloroform produced in 1831 remained a curiosity until Sir James Simpson of Edinburgh was told about it by a pharmacist. On the evening of 4 November, 1847, Simpson brought out a bottle of chloroform after dinner and he and his two assistants all inhaled simultaneously. Within minutes all three were under the table. Fortunately they required no resuscitation (7).

Tales of South American arrow poisons were reported as early as the 15th century, by the Spaniards in their expeditions in the 16th century and well into the 18th century when found to be curare (8,9).

Following the independent discoveries of Wells, Long and Morton it was not too long before it was realized that these drugs could be used in ways other than for producing anaesthesia.

Addiction

The greatest misuse of these agents was in the area of addiction. The first drugs which became popular were nitrous oxide and morphine. Originally taken to relieve the stress of their daily tasks the agents were soon taken for their pleasurable sensations. Addicted dentists favoured the use of nitrous oxide and, physicians morphine sulphate. The nonmedical use of narcotics increased with ease of availability and through illegal entry.

Nitrous oxide

Originally the use of nitrous oxide for relief or pleasure was limited to dentists, physicians and allied health personnel who had access to anaesthetic machines and gas cylinders but it has more recently become easily available to the general public through its use as an industrial agent, particularly in the food industry (10). Because it is non-inflammable and bacteriostatic, and has a neutral flavour when added to food, it is used as a propellant in whipped cream dispensers. It is also readily available as an additive for automobile engines (11). Apparently there is a possible association between the effects of nitrous oxide and the endogenous opioid system (12).

In 1985 Gillman reviewed the literature and found 32 cases of nitrous oxide abuse many of whom developed myeloneuropathy. Four cases died following inhalation of 100% nitrous oxide, one developed a pneumomediastinum as a result of inhaling nitrous oxide without reducing valves (10). Unlike the amnesic drugs, the inhalation of nitrous oxide can produce sensations which are attractive to those who indulge in sniffing (13).

Trichloroethylene

There has been an increase in sniffing solvent material which contains trichloroethylene. The agent was originally studied during World War II as a non-explosive safe substitute for chloroform and initially used on casualties during the London bombing attacks (14), and has continued in use by a minority of anaesthetists in the United Kingdom. It is present in cleaning agents and paint thinners and has been inhaled from a piece of cloth or from a balloon or a bag over the head. It is used mostly by young teenagers with problems (15). Where death resulted trichloroethylene was most likely used in conjunction with alcohol and/or hypnotics, resulting in sudden sniffing death (SSD) syndrome.

The illicit use of anaesthetic agents in recent years

Bass, a forensic pathologist, reported in 1970 on 110 SSDs without plastic bag suffocation (16). Subjects sprayed the contents of the aerosol can into a paperbag, tin can, rag or inflated balloon then took several deep inhalations, collapsed and died. 'Chloroform parties' also were reported in Wisconsin in 1973 where a bottle of chloroform was passed around and each one inhaled the vapours from a saturated cloth. Some of them also drank small amounts of the chloroform in addition to inhaling it (17). A 21-year-old male was admitted to a hospital in California after injecting 5 ml of chloroform in his left antecubital vein (18). He also admitted having inhaled chloroform for a 'high' on several occasions. Also in the seventies, ketamine and its chemical derivative was a major component of street drug preparations. In liquid form it was sprayed on marihuana and sold as 'angel dust'. The abuse of these compounds was generally unrecognized (19).

Criminal users—fact and fiction

Throughout history, in novels, and newspapers there are accounts of drugging prospective victims to facilitate robbery, rape and kidnapping. Masson described many accounts which were reported during the 19th century (20,21). Chloroform was the drug most often claimed as the offending substance. The advent of anaesthesia had introduced a new dimension with the fear that unconsciousness could be produced instantly and at will. It was believed that London robbers put their victims to sleep before they relieved their pockets (21). The recording of such muggings gained great publicity in the newspapers particularly in 1850 causing John Snow to write to the *London Medical Gazette*. He claimed it impossible to force a victim to inhale the chloroform. In short he wrote 'it is most unlikely that it was anything more than the ingenious invention of the reporter' (20). Nevertheless, many trials were held which resulted in severe sentences being meted out. And so strange accounts continued into the 20th century. As late as 1975 the *London Times* reported that passengers on the *Orient Express* were being robbed by sleeping car gangs equipped with a new high technology weapon, the chloroform aerosol can (20).

The advent of anaesthetic agents also led to stories of its use in kidnapping (abduction) for love, for involuntary servitude and for political reasons, which found their way into novels. Worse, however, were the charges of rape or sexual assault of women, some real, and mostly imaginary (21). Sometimes even the presence of a third person will not prevent a woman on awakening from believing she had not been sexually assaulted. Masson told of a young lady, accompanied by her fiance, who could hardly be convinced that the dentist had not made an assault on her chastity (21). A report quoted from the *Philadelphia Medical Times* (1881) told of a dentist who had been murdered by the husband of a woman allegedly raped by him while she was under the influence of chloroform. In a March 1987 television programme in the USA called '60 Minutes' a family practitioner was accused by a half dozen women of having been sexually assaulted by him in his examining room over a period of years. Incredibly, they continued to return and one woman even sent her daughter to him. Nor are doctors and dentists the only ones accused of these events. Accusations have been made of women being attacked with chloroform soaked pads and sexually assaulted; of young boys being indecently assaulted after being invited to inhale chloroform; of a suitor administering chloroform to a woman, kidnapping her and locking her in his apartment until she consented to marry him. The most sensational story was about a neurologist in Turin, Italy, who admitted anaesthetizing his female patients and photographing them naked in indecent positions. When he was caught with the negatives he admitted taking the pictures but claimed it was 'a new Freudian treatment for cases of slight nervous exhaustion' (21).

Use for suicide

The incidence of suicide and attempted suicide with anaesthetic and related drugs has increased three times in relation to other means which have remained stationary (22). The route depends upon the availability of the drug and the person's occupation. The barbiturates remain the most popular, accounting for 75% of attempted suicides as against 2.5% for the tranquillizers (23). There is the possibility of some fatal and non-fatal cases of barbiturate poisoning being due to accidental overdose (24). Sometimes, the individual will take a non-fatal barbiturate dose, not with the intention of committing suicide but rather to frighten a spouse or lover.

Persons who have access to special drugs or agents can use any route. Veterinarians and animal laboratory technicians use veterinary euthanasia drugs as suicide agents. One preparation called 'Fatal' contains a large concentrated solution of pentobarbital, propylene glycol, and alcohol. Another preparation called 'T-61' contains tetracaine, embitramide (a general anaesthetic), and mebezonium (a curare derivative). Both preparations are commonly used in the USA for killing animals in the laboratory. Some took the preparations orally or intravenously by syringe (25–27). Anaesthetists who attempt suicide appear to favour the intravenous route by infusion. The ultra short-acting barbiturates in parenteral form, are available to operating room personnel and used by all categories (28). In one report, a middle-aged anaesthetist used a plastic intravenous catheter with a 10 ml syringe attached and inserted in a downward direction in a vein above the medial malleolus of the right ankle (29). At least two anaesthetists, one who served with the author in World War II and the other an associate at another hospital, simply made up an infusion of pentothal and inserted it into their own left arm. The latter case closeted himself in his apartment on a Friday afternoon and was only missed when he failed to report on Monday morning. Three cases of self-poisoning with intravenous halothane were reported in which only one survived (30). A student nurse anaesthetist treated herself for cold sores on her lower lip by putting enflurane on topically. She was seen applying the drug from a full 250 ml bottle and three hours later when she was found unconscious the bottle was empty; cardiopulmonary resuscitation was unsuccessful (31).

Fifty-two-year-old male twins were found dead in the bathroom of their home with an empty bottle of chloroform by their side. They used a towel impregnated with the chloroform and a plastic bag over their heads (32). In Pittsburg there appeared a newspaper account of 10-year-old twin brothers who after being scolded attempted suicide by taking rat poison and inhaling ether from an aerosol can used to start cars in cold weather (33).

Homicide with anaesthetic agents

Murder is usually done for money or love and occasionally anaesthetic and related drugs are used. Drugs have been injected also into patients with the idea of creating a problem for others. When death occurs in patients who have been ill for some time it usually arouses no suspicion. Even when sudden death occurs in a previously healthy person the attending doctor will rarely suspect criminal poisoning until a relative or acquaintance questions the circumstances. Maltby of Canada collected several of these cases (34).

In 1892 a New York physician was accused by a friend of his wife of killing his new spouse with morphine. He was arrested, tried, found guilty and electrocuted. In 1950 another physician who held an anaesthetic appointment in Eastbourne, England, was tried also for morphine poisoning. Despite the fact that he gave up to 30 mg of morphine and heroin each during the last few days of the patient's life, and the testimony by a nurse who saw him inject morphine while the patient was unconscious, he was acquitted. In 1886 the wife of a deceased in Merton, England, accused of murdering her husband with chloroform, was acquitted because the jury did not think there was sufficient evidence to show how, or by whom, the drug was administered. In 1910 a physician in London was found guilty and hanged for murdering his wife with a lethal hyoscine in a dose several hundred times that normally required for sedation.

There were two incidents of unintentional death involving sodium thiopentone. In 1955 a male scrub nurse in a Bronx New York hospital, in order to help a friend whose girlfriend was pregnant, performed an abortion in their apartment under thiopentone drip infusion. He was both surgeon and anaesthetist and allowed a full litre of the solution to go into the patient with disastrous consequences. In the second incident in 1972 an English physician, a heavy drinker, became involved with one of his patients. In one of their drinking episodes, the woman asked the doctor to take some erotic pictures, but she wanted to be unconscious beforehand. The doctor then injected rectally 2 g of thiopentone and two hours later another dose. After that, intramuscular injections of morphine, pethidine and chlorpromazine were added. In both incidents the administrator was found guilty of manslaughter.

In the 1960s there occurred a series of deaths caused by muscle relaxant drugs, although not realized at the time. An anaesthetist was found guilty by a Florida court of injecting suxamethonium into his physician wife and causing her death (35). Close on the heels of this case a surgeon was accused of putting a muscle relaxant drug into the infusions of postoperative patients of other surgeons. The trial went on for 34 weeks, at the end of which he was acquitted (36). In 1975 there was a bizarre series of respiratory failures in a Veterans Hospital in Ann Arbor, Michigan. All of the cardiorespiratory arrests occurred on the 4 pm to 1 am hospital shift, and all were being given solutions intravenously when they went into arrest. One of the solutions was found to contain pancuronium. Two nurses of Filipino extraction admitted their guilt in court. Their explanation was overwork and the drug was only given to very sick patients. Because of a legal technicality they went free and are practising in another state (37). In 1986, a nurse in a Texas paediatrician's office was convicted of causing respiratory arrest and death in six children with suxamethonium in order to show the need for a paediatric intensive unit at the local hospital (38). Robin Cook, physician author of the book *Godplayer*, used the theme in which the cardiac surgeon put a muscle relaxant into postoperative infusions of other surgeons' patients (39).

Capital punishment

Fifteen states have enacted statutes prescribing lethal injection of drugs as a method of carrying out the death penalty. The usual drugs given are a mixture of sodium thiopentone and suxamethonium or similar derivatives. Sometimes potassium is added (40). The American Medical Association, the British Medical Association and other professional societies have all passed resolutions declaring that physicians should not participate. Texas and Oklahoma use volunteer medical technicians to administer the injection. This means often that unskilled people can't find veins or inadvertently inject into tissues resulting in unduly long executions (41). This description in a newspaper indicates that the technique is faultless when done properly:

> '*The injection began at 12:13 am. Mr Moreno, who appeared happy and almost cheerful, gasped three times. He was pronounced dead six minutes later*' (42).

Euthanasia

Over the years there are occasional reports of a physician or a member of a family using these agents to help a terminally ill or incurable patient end their life, called mercy killing. There have been attempts in the USA to permit voluntary euthanasia but only the Netherlands to date allow it. An estimated 5000 cases of voluntary euthanasias occur each year. The use of euthenasia threatens to increase because AIDS victims in unbearable pain have been requesting this form of relief. The doctors administer a combination of barbiturates and curare to produce a peaceful death (43).

The misuse of cocaine

Although the natives of Peru knew about the local anaesthetic qualities of the coca plant earlier than the 19th century it was not until Carl Koller, working in the same hospital as Sigmund Freud, proved its effectiveness as a local analgesic agent (44). Freud studied the coca plant to find out whether the characteristic euphoria was justified or illusory (45). He tried the effect of a small dose of cocaine and found it turned the bad mood he was in into cheerfulness and gave him the feeling of having dined well (46).

One of the first surgeons in the United States to use cocaine as a local analgesic agent was William Halsted in 1884. He and his three associates, after experimenting with cocaine, performed over a thousand operations using it. Their published paper was confused and incomplete due to his unrecognized addiction and that of his associates (47). He was treated for the withdrawal symptoms by his good friend, Welch, of Johns Hopkins (48). The three associates never recovered from their addiction (49). After Halsted's 'cure' he took to morphine (50). He once alluded to his experience with cocaine as follows: 'only those who have experienced the distress which follows so promptly the brief period of exhilaration can at all comprehend it' (51).

Through the years that followed cocaine was used sporadically and mostly by more highly intellectual people. Heroin and marijuana grabbed the headlines after World War II. Then in 1985 a new phenomenon in drug traffic appeared, the use of crack, in which sodium bicarbonate is used to powder cocaine into smokable crack. As crack has replaced heroin as the preferred drug of addiction, the inner cities are seeing a rising number of homicides and violent unpredictable behaviour among drug users, where before heroin maintained people on an even keel (52).

The condition called cocaine psychosis was first described by Freud in 1884, in which a patient given cocaine over weeks described swirling white snakes, the sounds of voices and intense paranoia (53). The psychotic symptoms are caused by the effect of cocaine on dopamine mechanisms, producing sudden rises in dopamine levels with a profound sense of euphoria. After repeated rises in blood levels the user tends to be agitated, prone to violence and psychosis. This is true only with crack, particularly when smoked in day long binges. Thus during the first years of widespread cocaine use in the United States in the late 1970s, relatively few people experienced addiction or psychotic symptoms, and some experts even believed the drug to be harmless. Freud and other authorities in the 1890s stated that cocaine addiction occurred only in individuals already addicted to morphine, cocaine having no habit forming qualities of its own and the Surgeon General compared its importance as equivalent to that of coffee drinks (51).

But now, with the rise of crack over the past 18 months, reports of crime and psychiatric difficulties associated with cocaine addiction have risen dramatically. This has become one of the best examples of misuse of a superior local analgesic agent.

References

(1) Armstrong-Davison MH. The discovery of ether. *Anaesthesia* 1949; **4**: 188.

(2) Slatter EM. The evolution of anaesthesia. 1. Ether in medicine before anaesthesia. *Br J Anaesth* 1960; **32**: 31.

(3) Gardner HB. *A manual of surgical anaesthesia*, 2nd Ed. New York: William Wood & Co, 1916: 7.

(4) Mushin WW. Triumph over pain. *Br J Anaesth* 1955; **27**: 449.

(5) Hubbard OP. A case of anaesthesia by the inhalation of nitrous oxide. Supposed to be the first on record. *Tr. NY State Med Assoc* 1888; **5**: 32.

(6) Nevius GW. *The discovery of modern anaesthesia. By whom was it made?* New York: Cooper Institute, 1854: 9–11.

(7) Hadfield CF. *Practical anaesthetics*. New York: William Wood & Co, 1923: 7.

(8) McIntyre AR. *Curare: Its history, nature and clinical use*. Chicago: University of Chicago Press, 1947: 17.

(9) Hammond WA, Mitchell SW. Experimental researches relative to Corroval and VAO— two new varieties of Woorari, the South American arrow poison. *Am J Med Sci* 1859; **38**: 13–60.

(10) Gillman MA. Nitrous oxide, an opioid addictive agent. Review of the evidence. *Am J Med* 1986; **81**: 97–102.

(11) Messina FV, Wynne JW. Nitrous oxide: No laughing matter. *Ann Intern Med* 1982; **96**: 333–4.

(12) Berkowitz BA, Finck AD, Ngai SH. Nitrous oxide analgesia: Reversal by naloxone and development of tolerance. *J Pharmacol Exp Ther* 1977; **203**: 539–47.

(13) Barber DN. Nitrous oxide analgesia—possible addiction. *SAAD Digest* 1975; **2**: 242.

(14) Dripps RD, Eckenhoff JE, Vandam LD. *Introduction to anesthesia. The principles of safe practice*. Second Ed. Philadelphia: WB Saunders, 1961: 82–83.

(15) Alla A, Korte T, Tenho M. Solvent sniffing death. *J Legal Med.* 1973; **72**: 299–305.

(16) Bass M. Sudden sniffing death. *JAMA* 1970; **212**: 2075–9.

(17) Storms WW. Chloroform parties. *JAMA* 1973; **225**: 160.

(18) Timms RM, Moser KM. Toxicity secondary to intravenously administered chloroform in humans. *Arch Intern Med* 1975; **135**: 1601–3.

(19) Rainey JM, Crowder MK. Ketamine or phencyclidine. *JAMA* 1974; **130**: 824.

(20) Masson AH. Crime and anaesthesia—robbery. *Hist Med* 1980; **8**: 18–9, 32.

(21) Masson AH. Crime and anaesthesia—rape and abduction. *Hist Med* 1981. **9**: 8, 25.

(22) Berger FM. Drugs and suicide in the United States. *Clin Pharmacol Ther* 1967; **8**: 219–23.

(23) Weddige RL, Steinhilber RM. Attempted suicide by drug overdose. *Post Grad Med* 1971; **49**: 184–6.

(24) Dorpar TL. Drug automatism, barbiturate poisoning, and suicidal behavior. *Arch Gen Psychiatry* 1974; **31**: 216–20.

(25) Poklis A, Hameli AZ. Two unusual barbiturate deaths. *Arch Toxicol* 1975; **34**: 77–86.

(26) Clark MA, Jones JW. Suicide by intravenous injection of a veterinary euthanasia agent: Report of a case and toxicologic studies. *J Forensic Sci* 1979; **24**: 762–7.

(27) Cordell WH, Curry SC, Furbee RB, Mitchell-Flynn DL. Veterinary euthanasia drugs as suicide agents. *Ann Emerg Med* 1986; **15**: 939–43.

(28) Backer RC, Caplan YH, Duncan CE. Thiopental suicide—case report. *Clin Toxicol* 1975; **8**: 283–7.

(29) Bruce AM, Oliver JS, Smith H. A suicide by thiopental injection. *Forensic Sci* 1977; **9**: 205–7.

(30) Berman P, Tattersall M. Self-poisoning with intravenous halothane. *Lancet* 1982; **i**: 340.

(31) Lingenfelter RW. Fatal misuse of enflurane. *Anesthesiology* 1981; **55**: 603.

(32) Giusti GV, Chiarotti M. 'Double suicide' by chloroform in a pair of twins. *Med Sci Law* 1981; **21**: 2–3.

(33) Scolded twins, 10, try suicide. *New York Post* 1975. Aug. 26, 3 (Col 4).
(34) Maltby JR. Criminal poisoning with anaesthetic drugs: murder. *Forensic Sci* 1975; **6**: 91–108.
(35) Coppolino v. State, 223 So. 2d. 75 (Fla. app. 1968).
(36) Hall LN, Hirsch RF. Detection of curare in the Jascalevich murder trial. *Analyt Chem* 1979; **8**: 812–9A.
(37) Waldron M. Injections in 15 V.A. patients in Michigan called deliberate. *New York Times* 1975. Aug. 24. 1 (Col 1–6).
(38) Jones v. State of Texas, 716 S.W. 2d 142 (Tex Ct. of App., Aug. 13, 1986). *The Citation* 1987; **54**: 108.
(39) Cook R. *Godplayer*. New York: G. P. Putnam's Sons, 1983: 9–11.
(40) Finks TO. Lethal injection. An uneasy alliance of law and medicine. *J Legal Med* 1983; 4: 383–403.
(41) Stolls M, Heckler v. Chaney: Judicial and administrative regulation of capital punishment by lethal injection. *Am J Law Med* 1985; **11**: 251–77.
(42) Anonymous. Texan who killed 6 in 1983 is executed by lethal injection. *New York Times* 1987. Mar 5: B9 (Col 4).
(43) Clines FX. Dutch fear: AIDS cases' last stop. *New York Times* 1987, Apr 15: 12 (Col 1).
(44) Keys TE. *The history of surgical anesthesia*. New York: Dover Publications, 1945: 40.
(45) Jones E. *The life and work of Sigmund Freud* Vol I. New York: Basic Books, 1953: 54.
(46) *Ibid*. Vol I, Chapter VI. *The cocaine episode 1884–1887*, 1953: 80–1.
(47) Halsted WS. Practical comments on the use and abuse of cocaine; Suggested by its invariably successful employment in more than a thousand minor surgical operations. *NY Med J* 1885; **42**: 294.
(48) Whipple AO. Halsted's New York period. *Surgery* 1952; **32**: 542.
(49) Fulton JF. *Harvey Cushing: A biography*. Springfield, IL: Thomas, 1946: 142–3.
(50) Colp R. Notes on Dr William S. Halsted. *Bull NY Acad Med* 1984; **60**: 879.
(51) Olch PD. William S Halsted and local anaesthesia: Contributions and complications. *Anesthesiology*. 1975; **42**: 482.
(52) Kerr P. New violence seen in users of cocaine: Crack abuse is linked to paranoid behavior. *NY Times* 1987; Mar 7: 29 (Col 6), 32 (Col 5).
(53) Rosecan JS. Chief of cocaine addiction program at Columbia-Presbyterian Medical Center. Personal communication.

Chapter 11
CHLOROFORM

11.1   The first human chloroformization

RICHARD W. PATTERSON
University of California, Los Angeles, California, USA

A small early 19th century military cemetery in upper New York state contains a stone engraved in memory of a private 'who was severely wounded in the discharge of his duty while firing a national salute'. An adjoining cemetery, for the town of Sackets Harbor, contains the grave and memorial to the inventor of reliable devices that would ensure against such disasters; a punch-lock firing device for cannons and the development of percussion caps to replace flintlocks. Additionally this man, Samuel Guthrie, first produced the compound later to be named chloroform.

Benjamin Silliman, first professor of chemistry at Yale College and editor of the leading scientific journal in America in the eighteen-eighties, the *American Journal of Science and Arts*, considered the communications received from this untutored chemist to be 'honorable to the rising chemical arts of this country. I presume it was little suspected that such things were doing in a remote region on the shore of Lake Ontario.'

Accidental inhalation

During the winter of 1830 the product of an experiment, a thick limpid liquid, lay in Guthrie's vats. His children were accustomed to playing in his laboratory when he was experimenting and an event which occurred to his eight year old daughter Cynthia was related in a family letter:

> '*He had large tubs of liquid standing on the floor and she used to stick her fingers in the tub and taste the liquid, one tub she liked to taste, so did often, and he was watching her and one day she got too much and fell over and he ran to her and picked her up and then found that the liquid in this tub put her to sleep, hence his accidental discovery what chloroform would do.*' (1)

It is remarkable that this astonishing event was not recognized there and then to be worthy of further investigation and exploitation for this experimenter was accustomed to capitalizing on his observations. His chemical investigations were not those of a dilettante, but were designed to solve specific needs or problems and frequently led to commercial undertakings which for the time and place were extensive and profitable.

Years later Simpson's introduction of chloroform for the relief of pain was met with opposition from clerics, 'in sorrow thou shall bring forth children', and from fellow physicians, 'Is there not danger in the use of anything that puts into abeyance self consciousness?' However, there is nothing to suggest that the constellation of objections that beset the use of anaesthetics had anything in common with the failure to initially recognize the phenomenon.

Medical philosophy in New England in 1831

At least four days' journey from urban commercial centres such as New York, Boston and Philadelphia, Sackets Harbor following the war of 1812 epitomized the roistering, robust, expansive environment conducive to pragmatic individuals who modified their political philosophy and theology to square with the actuality of the frontier. In turn Dr Guthrie typified the republican farmer-physician formulated by Dr Benjamin Rush as the ideal American practitioner (2). Though his forefathers were staunch Calvinists and he was well read in the

Bible, 'he did not read it as of Divine origin in all its parts. The Deity he worshipped was manifested in all the works of Nature. These he contemplated with the most profound admiration and reverence' (3). Though of locally unrivalled scientific acumen and a practising physician he did not belong to the Jefferson County Medical Society, a very active organization in 1831 having over forty members, allopaths all. His numerous entrepreneurial ventures into diverse fields of agriculture, chemistry, distillery, and powder manufacture served to keep him both aloof from his more prosaic neighbours and impervious to their restrictive comments.

The factors responsible for interfering with the realization of the import of the phenomenon of the witnessed drug induced reversible comatose state are to be found in the 'theory of medicine' common to the medical scientists and practitioners of the time. Medical practice in 1830 was dominated by the dictums of John Brown, William Cullen, and Benjamin Rush—the Solidist tradition that necessarily arose in reaction to the unwieldy impracticality of the complicated 18th century hypotheses of disease causation. The illuminating function of physiological facts on medical practice anticipated to follow from William Harvey's demonstration of the circulatory pathway failed to materialize for several centuries. One hundred and forty years after Harvey's publication Richard Davies, a Cambridge scientist, wrote to Stephen Hale:

> *'The discovery of the circulation has not been followed by so great advancement in the science of medicine as was naturally to be expected from it. The reason of which is, that our theory has not yet advanced much in the knowledge which is naturally founded upon this grand principle'.*

The new physics and mathematical philosophy of the 18th century added little of importance to the theory of medicine concerned with bridging the gap between disease cause and disease effect. For more than a century explanations of causation required the introduction of various imaginary entities and activities, extensive speculation, and complicated hypothetical concepts. Noting the failure of rational consistency in this area Sydenham suggested that attention be focused on the manifestation of disease with a plea for an enlightened empiricism concerning the 'natural history' of disease based on observation; and in line with this he indicated that disease 'should be reduced to definite and certain species . . . with the same care which we see exhibited by botanists in their phytologies.' Following the botanical method of objective description and classification Bossier de Sauvages categorized some 2400 'species' of disease; a complicated nosology devoid of clues or aids to treatment.

It was a relief when John Brown put forth (1780) the notion that there were only 2 classes of disease; sthenic and asthenic. The Brunonian system was quite simple:

> *'The indication for the cure of sthenic diathesis is to diminish, that for the cure of the asthenic diathesis is to increase the excitement, and to continue to increase it . . .'* (4)

John Brown's Elements of Medicine was enthusiastically accepted and widely disseminated in Europe and America. By 1880 translations were available in English, French, Spanish, German, Italian, and Portuguese.

A mainstay of Brunonian therapy was the use of diffusible stimulants. Brunonian influence and concepts were widespread and may be found in the writings of Humphry Davy who noted 'the immediate effects of nitrous oxide upon the living system are analogous to those of diffusible stimuli' (5). This prompted him to suggest combining carbon dioxide which he believed acted as a sedative with nitrous oxide to obtain 'a regular series of exciting and depressing powers applicable to every deviation of the constitution from health'. Citations of Davy's research appeared in the numerous chemical texts and in the chemical and scientific dictionaries in the first 2 decades of the 19th century.

Benjamin Rush was Professor of Medicine at the University of Pennsylvania for 44 years (1769–1813) during which time the institution graduated three-quarters of all the educated physicians in the country. He therefore had an influence on medical therapy lasting into the third quarter of the 19th century. His system was a mixture of the views of his predecessors with some modifications and variations of his own, but again diffusible stimulants occupied a prominent part in his therapeusis.

Samuel Guthrie became a physician in the milieu of that body of medically educated and licensed practitioners known as 'orthodox', 'regular', or allopathic physicians. Together with two brothers he was taught medicine by case study, the preceptor system, in his father's practice and branched out on his own in 1802. Thereafter he was able to attend a winter course at the College of Physicians and Surgeons of New York, later, a month of lectures (meticulously documented in a notebook of 275 closely written pages) at the University of Pennsylvania, both bastions of the traditional medical doctrine derived from the Solidist tradition. In his father's will he had been bequeathed a set of silver catheters and a compendium of orthodox medical dogma, *Rush's Medical Inquiries and Observations* in five volumes. 'Extravagance in the Doctor's view, was almost a crime, but expending money in scientific investigation was like loaning on bond and mortgage' (3) and his penchant 'for buying the best of books made him an easy mark to book men as his splendid and huge library shows' (6). With an avid desire to keep up to date he subscribed to the latest medical and chemical texts.

Chloroform as a diffusible stimulant

In volume II of Silliman's *Yale College Elements of Chemistry* published in February of 1830 Guthrie read that the 'alcoholic solution of chloric ether is a grateful diffusive stimulant and that as it admits of any degree of dilution it may probably be introduced into medicine.' He immediately set to work to produce this diffusive stimulant in a cheap and easy fashion and, as previously mentioned, a new compound had dripped from the water encased 'worm' of his still. By spring he noted

> '*During the last six months, a great number of persons have drunk of the solution of chloric ether in my laboratory. This free use of the article has been permitted in order to ascertain the effect of it in full doses on the healthy subject; and thus to discover, as far as such trials would do, its probable value as a medicine.*'

In the summer of 1831 he sent a description of his method to Silliman for publication (7). In the fall of that year Silliman noted in his Journal, 'I have written to Mr Guthrie . . . having been requested by some of our physicians to obtain a supply for regular use.' Numerous testimonials attested to its usefulness in various disease states without discovering its true potent attribute; as finely put, 'they rested under the shade of the tree, but neglected to test its fruit' (3). Oversight must be ascribed to yet another instance wherein the significance of a pivotal fact was obscured because there was at hand a 'rational' explanation for its occurrence, or to put the matter conversely—experience is accepted only when based upon a recognized theory.

Combining Brunonian concepts with an erroneous chemical concept that the oxygen in nitrous oxide was available for respiration. Davy suggested:

> '*The quickness of the operation of nitrous oxide, will probably render it useful in cases of extreme debility produced by deficiency of common exciting powers. Perhaps it may be advantageously applied mingled with oxygen or common air, to the recovery of persons apparently dead from suffocation by drowning or hanging.*' (5)

By 1800 this use of diffusible stimuli was recommended for resuscitation (8). The occasional observation of temporary or permanent unconsciousness failed to interfere with the predominance of Brunonian thinking, being ascribed to 'fainting' in the former case, and to severity of disease in the latter.

Guthrie's investigations concerned the development of a diffusible stimulant; he was successful and when a personal occasion was afforded for it to be employed in the accustomed manner he used it and obtained the desired and expected result—a well patient. Writing to his eldest daughter he recalled her need to be resuscitated from carbon monoxide poisoning:

> '*Dear Harriot*
> *. . . sweet whiskey which you remember taking when suffocated with charcoal. You see it called chloroform and the newspapers are beginning to give me credit of discovering it. I made the first particle that was ever made and you are the first human being that ever used it in sickness.*' (1)

Conclusion

In 1831 chloroform as a 'diffusible stimulus' could rationally be administered to one daughter who was suffocating; to recognize and ascribe a therapeutic usefulness to the sleep produced in another daughter was unimaginable. By 1846 the use of chloroform for resuscitation was irrational; that chemically induced sleep thwarted pain was proven by experience.

References

(1) Robinson V. Samuel Guthrie. *Medical Life* 1927; **34**: 102–28.
(2) Rush B. Duties of a physician. In: Runes DD ed. *The selected writings of Benjamin Rush.* New York: Philosophical Library, 1947.
(3) Guthrie O. *Memoirs of Dr Samuel Guthrie and the history of the discovery of chloroform.* Chicago: Hazlitt and Co., 1887.
(4) Brown J. *The elements of medicine, or a translation of the Elementa Medicinae Brunonis, with large notes, illustrations, and comments* Vol I. Philadelphia: Wm Spotswood, 1791: 32.
(5) Davy H. *Researches, chemical and philosophical; chiefly concerning nitrous oxide or dephlogisticated nitrous air, and its respiration.* London: J. Johnson, 1800.
(6) Chamberlin TS. *Historical pictures of the discovery of chloroform and percussion powder.* Guthrie File. The Jefferson County Historical Society. Watertown, N.Y.
(7) Guthrie S. New mode of preparing a spirituous solution of chloric ether. *Am J Sci Arts* 1831; **21**: 64–5.
(8) Hancock J. *Observations on the origins and treatment of cholera and other pestilential diseases, and on the gaseous oxide of nitrogen as a remedy in such diseases, as also in cases of asphyxia from suffocation and drowning and against the effects of narcotic poisons.* London: J. Wilson, 1831.

11.2   Chloroform and controversy

ALLEN I. HYMAN
College of Physicians and Surgeons, Columbia University, New York, USA

The late 1840s were a time of upheaval and revolution. In America the abolitionists were demanding an end to slavery, and most of Europe was on the brink of revolution. While reform and repressive movements battled, religious zealots invoked biblical authority to strengthen their respective positions. Whether the issue was slavery, war, capital punishment or class struggle, they presumed God was their ally.

Into this turbulence anaesthesia began in Boston in October 1846; the news reached London on the next boat. James Young Simpson was the central character in an extraordinary drama involving anaesthesia and in one of the first controversies of medical ethics. Simpson, a Churchillian-like character, was argumentative, but with a wonderful facility for teaching. Endowed with enormous energy and a prodigious memory, he became his generation's most famous obstetrician, or as it was called at the time, accoucheur. But undoubtedly, obscurity, what befell many other famous clinicians, would have been his fate were it not for his discovery of chloroform anaesthesia.

Simpson was pugnacious and his career is smattered with quarrels and disputes ranging from priority of discovery, to alleged wrongful treatment. But his most significant battle was his embroilment in the religious controversy concerning the use of anaesthesia for pain relief during childbirth.

Simpson happened to be in London for Christmas in 1846 to receive his appointment to be one of Her Majesty's physicians. He learned that the great renowned surgeon, John Liston, had just performed a leg amputation under ether anaesthesia. Returning to Edinburgh in glory, he, for the first time ever, administered ether for the relief of pain of labour and delivery. In his notes he wrote 'the mission of the physician is twofold: to relieve human suffering and to preserve life.' Now the search to improve methods for pain relief for childbirth became his obsession. He wrote to his brother after receiving the Queen's honorary appointment:

'*I am less interested in flattery from the Queen than having a woman delivered without any pain. Since administering sulphuric ether I can think of naught else.*'

Simpson was driven. Zealously he continued his experiments with ether. His notebook concludes:

'*With many other medical men I have now taken it myself to try its effects. A great secret is giving a large, full and rapid dose of it all at once.*'

He published his first paper on ether that March stating his claim for priority:

'*I am not aware that anyone has hitherto ventured to test its applicability to the practice of midwifery.*'

His paper *On the Use of Ether* opens the debate:

'*I have been repeatedly asked will we ever be justified in using ether to assuage the pains of natural labour. I believe that question will require to be changed, whether on any grounds a man could deem himself justified in not using such safe means.*'

Now the sides were drawn. His critics were not only clerics, but prominent colleagues as well. One argued:

'*Is there not danger in the use of anything that puts into abeyance self consciousness? Would you not produce evils similar to those that result from stupefying narcotics.*'

Simpson responded with a scientific query:

'*Is the mere condition of intoxication as injurious to the body as is generally supposed?*'

Now he sought the answer in his own characteristic way. He asked the Edinburgh police surgeon for his experience on the effects and dangers of drunkedness, knowing full well that the police would have the widest experience with this problem. The police surgeon answered his question:

'*In five years 28,357 individuals were brought to this office in a state of intoxication. Only three have died and it is doubtful that intoxication was the cause of their death.*'

Simpson was gratified and continued his experiments. He wrote in his journal:

'*Lately to avoid some of the inconveniences and objections to ether, particularly its disagreeable smell and irritation to the bronchi, I have tried upon myself the inhalation of other volatile fluids.*'

Around his dining room table chloroform anaesthesia was discovered. The first woman given chloroform for her delivery was Simpson's own niece, only a day after he tried it on himself. The child was born safely and was christened Anaesthesia, and Anaesthesia's photograph was kept on Simpson's desk.

In discussing the qualities of chloroform Simpson credits the three chemists who first synthesized and described the compound. At the same time he raises and diminishes their contribution and makes an appeal (perhaps the first) for the importance of basic research rather than 'practical' or targeted research. Simpson writes of the three chemists:

'*Their only object was the investigation of philosophical chemistry. They laboured for the pure love and extension of knowledge. They had no idea that the substance would be turned to any practical purpose. I mention this to show the argument against philosophical investigations on the ground of no apparent practical benefit has been refuted. A substance which was merely interesting as a scientific curiosity now has been shown as an object by which human suffering and agony may be abetted or abolished.'*

While accolades were pouring forth on Simpson, opposing voices were also raised. Probably most vexing were adversaries who argued chiefly against anaesthesia because it caused the patients loss of their self control. A paper critical of Simpson was read before the Liverpool Medical Society in November 1847 by a surgeon:

'When I was in Edinburgh during the last month I had several conversations with Professor Simpson and found that he advocated most strongly the use of anaesthesia, not as the exception, but as the rule. I contend that we violate the boundaries of our profession when we seduce our fellow creatures for the sake of avoiding pain alone to pass into a state of existence, the secrets of which we know so little. What right have we say to our brother man "sacrifice thy manhood, let go thy hold upon that noble capacity of thought and reason which thy God hath endowed thee and become a trembling coward before the presence of mere bodily pain".'

Another physician wrote:

'I was struck with a remark in Professor Simpson's last pamphlet where it is said our "patients themselves will force this remedy upon us." Now I ask, is not this the mark of a disorder? Are they, the patients to be permitted to decide upon such a subject and are we to be influenced to give up on our judgement? I fear that in the end many patients will take the law into their own hands. And yet another concern, we have had no time to watch the consequences of chloroform, and one I fear in particular. I hesitate to say it. I mean insanity.'

Simpson brought the question to the people. He openly discussed the issues in public forums and deliberately wrote his papers in plain English to be easily understood by the uninitiated. In fact, one complaint against him was he told the public what presumably only the professional should know. Simpson considered himself a Godfearing religious Christian and most hurtful to him were the words from the pulpits of the Scottish Calvinists. Edinburgh was a place where historically science and religion were in combat. To some pietists heresy lurked around every laboratory. Simpson learned of the clergy's criticisms directly from the pulpit and from his patients. He wrote:

'Many of my lady patients have strong religious scruples against anaesthesia. They have been told that their doctor, who promises to save them from the pangs of labour, is a blasphemer and a heretic.'

Circulars were sent from the churches to all physicians in Edinburgh warning them that anaesthesia for childbirth could lead to the direct collapse of society. Central to the church's position and the basis of their religious objection was Genesis 3 verse 16:

'In sorrow thou shall bring forth children.'

One physician wrote:

'The very suffering that a woman undergoes in labour is one of the strongest elements in the love she bears her offspring. I have fears for the moral effect of this discovery both on the patient and on other physicians.'

The religious issue was as important in New England as it was in Scotland. Walter Channing, the outstanding obstetrician from Boston used ether for childbirth almost as early as Simpson. He also examined the biblical text to determine whether the relief of pain was contrary to the will of God. Like Simpson he considered whether the Hebrew word 'Etzebh', translated sometimes as sorrow and other times as pain, implied mental anguish or actual physical pain. Examining the Hebrew text in detail, he consulted Professor G. R. Noyes, the distinguished Hebrew scholar at Harvard. Noyes's opinion did not provide Channing with any reassurance. He reaffirmed that the word 'Etzebh' refers to the pain immediately attendant on pregnancy and delivery. That is, it means physical torment and not mental or emotional anguish. Simpson took another tack. He explored the Hebrew text further and found the word 'Etzebh' was used in several other biblical passages. Justifying his position he wrote:

> '*In other passages the word Etzebh is not used in any respect or employed to designate the sensation of pain. It is generally elsewhere used as effort, or toil or labour. It is nowhere else used for the feeling or perception of excruciating or bodily anguish.*'

To Simpson the word Etzebh signified the muscular efforts and not the pain to which these efforts or uterine contractions give rise and he went further:

> '*To be consistent, if the first admonition towards woman be observed, that is, "in pain you shall bear forth your children", then what about the second against Adam, "by the sweat of thy brow ye shall work". Should that mean that we should not use ploughs or machines or travel by carriage. Weren't we made to enjoy the fruits of our intellect?*'

The religious argument continued and raged for six more years. Might a physician countervene God's will, God's primal curse on women. The tide was finally turned by a woman herself. The woman on the throne. In April, 1853, Queen Victoria's accoucheur, Dr James Clark, recommended chloroform. John Snow was the anaesthetist and the Queen delivered Prince Leopold. Dr Clark wrote to Simpson:

> '*You will be pleased to hear the Queen had chloroform administered to her during her late confinement. Her Majesty was greatly pleased with the effect and she certainly never has had a better recovery.*'

Victoria inhaled the vapours and by her example blew away the religious opposition. Simpson, or the 'chloroform doctor', as he was now called, had completed his victory. Power of the opposition was broken. Criticism from the clerics was stilled and the doctors, many of whom declared pain to be a biological necessity, were now careful to keep a little chloroform in their bags lest they lose their patients to more accomodating rivals.

11.3   Edward Lawrie and the Hyderabad Chloroform Commissions*

ASRIT RAMACHARI and ABHAY PATWARI
E.S.I. Hospital, Sanathnagar, Hyderabad, India

The discovery of ether anaesthesia in 1846 heralded a new era in the history of medicine, but it soon became apparent that ether had disadvantages such as its explosiveness, its irritancy, its relatively slow induction, its marked stage of excitement, and its tendency to produce vomiting. Within a year James Simpson—in Edinburgh—had introduced chloroform and, at first, this new agent seemed to offer an alternative anaesthetic without the disadvantages of ether. Within a few years, however, misgivings were expressed about chloroform's safety, and some became convinced that chloroform was an inherently dangerous agent capable of causing unheralded stoppage of the heart.

Many London anaesthetists held views about chloroform's use which are summed up in the well known illustration of Dr Clover, with his 'chloroform bag' slung over his shoulder,

*This paper was read by Dr R. H. Ellis in the absence of the authors

anaesthetizing an elderly, seated gentleman whose pulse he is feeling. The London school maintained that it should be given by experienced practitioners, that its concentration should be carefully controlled, and that the anaesthetist should monitor the pulse throughout the administration.

The exactly opposite views of the Edinburgh school were spelled out by Professor James Syme in a lecture in 1854. His teaching was that no special apparatus—or training—was required, the amount of chloroform used should not be stinted, and the only worthwhile guide was the patient's respiration. It was important to prevent the tongue from causing stertorous breathing but the circulation should be ignored completely. He declared:

> '*You never see anyone here with his finger on the pulse while chloroform is given.*'

Syme's conclusion was that chloroform may be used judiciously so as to do good without exposing the patient to the risk of evil.

Edward Lawrie

For the next few decades the question of the safety of chloroform, and whether it killed primarily by stopping the heart, or by first stopping the respiration, was discussed and investigated at length but without any convincing result. Then, in the late 1880s Edward Lawrie (1846–1915) entered the argument (1). Lawrie had been a medical student at Edinburgh, and had been James Syme's house surgeon. For the rest of his life he hero-worshipped Syme whom he later described as 'the wisest man I have ever known'.

On leaving Edinburgh Lawrie joined the Indian Medical Service, and in 1885 was appointed as the surgeon to the British Residency in Hyderabad, which was then an independent state in India ruled over the Nizam. Lawrie soon became principal of the Medical School in Hyderabad and also personal physician to the Nizam. He used chloroform anaesthesia in the manner of his teachers in Edinburgh, and gave it to (quite literally) thousands of patients without incident. This, his own remarkable safety record, coupled with his admiration for Syme's teaching led Lawrie to believe that chloroform was absolutely safe provided it was given by the method of the Edinburgh school.

The First Hyderabad Chloroform Commission 1888

Secure in this knowledge Lawrie decided to settle the chloroform question once and for all, and persuaded the Nizam of Hyderabad to pay for a scientific investigation of chloroform's safety. This investigation, which became known as the First Hyderabad Chloroform Commission, was carried out early in 1888. The Commissioners consisted of three of Lawrie's colleagues in Hyderabad. Surgeon Patrick Hehir was in charge and was assisted by two colleagues—Drs Kelly and Chamarette. Their essential conclusion was that:

> '*Chloroform can be given to dogs by inhalation with perfect safety, and without any fear of accidental death if only the respiration—and nothing but the respiration—is carefully attended to throughout.*'

Lawrie lost no time in publicizing this result, but it was received with scepticism. The Editor of the *Lancet* wrote:

> '*Mr Lawrie arrives at conclusions utterly at variance with the experience alike of experiment and practice as carried out in Europe. . . . We require more than the scanty statements of experiments carried out on dogs. . . . Mr Lawrie has never seen a death from chloroform in the initial stages of narcosis but he seems to forget that others whose authority we are bound to accept have done so.*'

On learning of the *Lancet*'s dismissive reaction Lawrie persuaded the Nizam of Hyderabad to pay for a second, more extensive and more authoritative study. On behalf of the Nizam Lawrie invited the *Lancet* to select its own independent, British expert to work with the experimenters in Hyderabad. The *Lancet* agreed, and later—in 1889—the Second Hyderabad Chloroform Commission began its work.

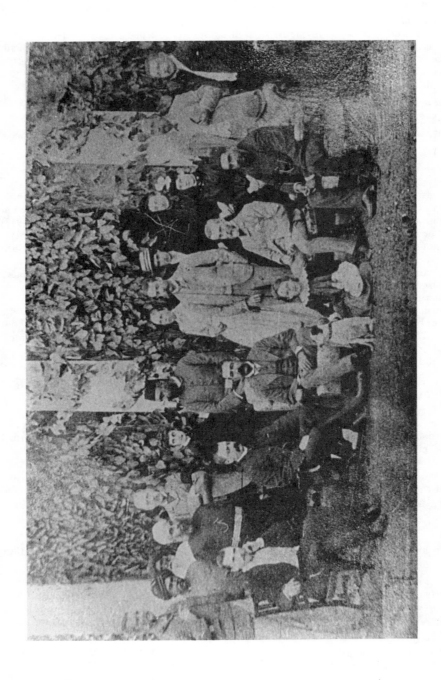

Figure 1   The Second Hyderabad Chloroform Commission 1889. Edward Lawrie (heavy black moustache — centre seated) and Thomas Lauder Brunton (white beard — seated second from right) are easily identifiable. From a photograph in the possession of the late Dr Subba.

The Second Hyderabad Chloroform Commission 1889

The members of the Second Commission were Edward Lawrie himself (who led it as President), Dr (later Sir) Thomas Lauder Brunton (who was the nominated expert retained by the *Lancet*), Surgeon-Major Gerald Bomford (a leading member of the Indian Medical Service) and Dr Rustomji Hakim (who was a member of the Nizam's own Medical Service). All three members of the First Commission also took part (Fig. 1).

For three months the Second Chloroform Commission performed various experiments on some 600 animals. The Commissioners' Report was first published in instalments by the *Lancet* beginning in January, 1890. In 1891 a version of the report was published in India as a single volume (2). The essential conclusion of this Second Commission did not differ from that of the First, and was couched in very similar terms to those used by Syme almost 45 years earlier:

'*The administrator should be guided as to the effect entirely by the respiration. . . Chloroform may be given in any case requiring an operation with perfect ease and absolute safety so as to do good without the risk of evil.*'

The conclusion of the Second Commission provoked numerous adverse comments in England's leading medical journals. Typical of these was that from Leonard Hill, the distinguished physiologist, who said:

'*The doctrine that chloroform kills by paralysing the respiratory centre, propounded by the findings of the two Hyderabad Chloroform Commissions, and the prejudiced enthusiasm of Surgeon-Major Lawrie, is one of the most pernicious and dangerous doctrines ever put before the medical profession.*'

Leonard Hill also found fault with the execution of many of the experiments. In particular he noted that chloroform anaesthesia had begun with the animals in 'induction boxes'. No less than 6% of the animals were found to have died, unobserved, in the boxes during induction with chloroform before any experiments on them had even been set up. Hill wrote:

'*In this the Commission gives away their whole case. They never observed these accidental deaths.*'

He was right. Lawrie, Brunton and their colleagues had ignored these deaths, and had glibly ascribed them to the slip-shod techniques of their unqualified assistants whose task was to render the dogs unconscious prior to the Commissioners' experiments.

Similarly, after publishing the results of the careful researches of Dr E. H. Embley (of Melbourne, Australia), the Editor of the *British Medical Journal* said of the Second Commission that it had:

'*looked upon respiratory failure as the primary cause of death; most other researchers look upon this as secondary to the failure in the circulatory apparatus. The Commission deserves much credit for pointing out the importance of the respiration . . . but from the scientific point of view no impartial observer can maintain that they proved its main contention.*'

Conclusion

Edward Lawrie, strident and didactic, but unconvincing, obstinately replied to all the criticisms of the work of his two Commissioners, and he continued to proclaim, right up until his death in 1915, the infallibility of Syme's (by then) 60-year-old doctrine. Nonetheless, even though the majority of his pronouncements on chloroform were misguided, misleading, cavalier or dangerous his own personal experience of its safety was unique and exemplary. This experience, coupled with his slavish adherence to Syme's teaching, has enabled him to be recognized as one of the most influential participants in anaesthesia's earlier years.

References

(1) Sykes WS, Ellis RH. *Essays on the first hundred years of anaesthesia* Vol III. London: Churchill Livingstone, 1982.
(2) *Report of the Second Hyderabad Chloroform Commission*. Bombay: The Times of India Steam Press, 1891.

11.4 Chloroform for children and the
development of paediatric anaesthesia in Poland

Z. RONDIO
National Research Institute of Mother and Child, Warsaw, Poland

---

In presenting the history of anaesthesia in Poland I would like to discuss a special area of our speciality—anaesthesia in children. It seems worthwhile remembering that:

'even a long time ago, in high-minded efforts to prevent pain in all individuals suffering from physical torment, children—especially infants, were always in the first place.' (1)

Looking at the development of paediatric care, including paediatric anaesthesia, we can assume that the position of the child in community, and the care of poor and ill children in particular, is the expression not only of the culture but of the humanity of the nation, and is perhaps less dependent on civilization.

When chloroform was introduced as a 'sleeping' agent by James Y. Simpson in 1847, one of his first patients was a child five years of age. After chloroform was used by Alexander Le Brun in Warsaw, on the 11 December, 1847, this method of anaesthesia was accepted in our country as the best for children.

Early use of anaesthesia for children in Poland

In 1865 B. Gawlik working at the Jagellonian University in Cracow presented the first clinical report, from this part of Europe, of anaesthetics given to children, describing 36 patients undergoing surgery with chloroform; the youngest one was three years of age (2). There were many different mixtures of inhaled agents (e.g. ether–chloroform–alcohol etc.) used at that time for operations in paediatric patients, but very soon it became clear that anaesthetic death and complications rates were similar to those observed when pure ether or chloroform was administered.

Ludwik Zembrzuski

In 1917 Ludwik Zembrzuski, from the Children's Hospital of Warsaw, in his monograph (3) presented observations of 12 052 chloroform anaesthesias for children of age between one month and 14 years, given in his hospital during the preceding 10 years. There was only one death on the table in a patient with osteomyelitis; it was a boy four years of age in a very bad general condition. There were a few cases of 'syncope', resuscitated successfully after long lasting treatment. Postoperative mortality and morbidity were similar to those observed in other centres of the world. L. Zembrzuski stated that in his hospital chloroform was quite safe, but some contraindications were suggested, mostly in liver and kidney diseases. He recommended light chloroform especially as a supplement to local analgesia, to keep an uncooperative child asleep. Special precautions were stressed to prevent airway obstruction and he started to use peroral intubation according to Kuhn's recommendation. However, at that time it was a very difficult technique. For the open-mask method he suggested a very careful calibration of the drops of chloroform, to prevent overdose. Hedonal or isopral, as sedative agents, were given preoperatively orally. This could be considered an early use of premedication in children.

It seems to us that his *General and Local Anaesthesia in Children* was the first monograph dealing with this problem in central and east Europe. There were many other observations of different methods of anaesthesia reported in the monograph; there was a critique of rectal administration of ether–oil mixture recommended by Pirogow, as useless in children, and presentation of different techniques of local and regional blocks. Zembrzuski's contribution to paediatric care was largely through his clinical study of anaesthetics and mostly through the stimulation of an anaesthesia service exclusively for children.

Children's hospitals in Europe

It is difficult to speak about paediatric anaesthesia at that time without considering the background for this speciality which was evolving in Europe in places where there were well organized hospitals providing care exclusively for sick children.

The children's hospitals originated in the early 19th century and credit for the first has to be given to the Hospital for Sick Children in Paris (1802), followed by those in Dublin, Petersburg, London, Philadelphia, etc. (4).

Originally, Children's hospitals were located in orphan asylums and homes of foundlings which were widely distributed around Europe. The first home of foundlings in Poland was situated close to the cloister in Sandomierz, named The Holy Spirit, in 1222. Then followed other homes in the country in rapid succession. General care of children in those institutions was so good and efficient that King Sigmondus II August proclaimed in 1552 special privileges for them. Children from the homes of foundlings were accepted for all kinds of posts and honour in church and country. One of the institutions in Warsaw, existing since 1732, was rebuilt and reconstructed in 1762 to become the Hospital General named Baby Jesus Hospital, where Dr Le Brun's operations under ether and chloroform anaesthesia were performed in 1847.

The first Chair in Paediatrics of Jagellonian University in Cracow was established in 1833. The oldest children's hospital in Warsaw was opened in 1869 and in 1875 transferred to a new building of more than 100 beds, where it has been working up until the present as the Copernicus Hospital for Children of Warsaw. Thousands of operations in children under different types of anaesthesia were performed there every year. Other children's hospitals were built in Warsaw and all over the country. In 1913 and 1921 paediatric clinics in Warsaw's University had paediatric surgery units, where after World War II paediatric anaesthesia and intensive therapy departments were organized.

From 1918 until 1939 there were 12 regional children's hospitals in Poland with 2351 beds and 5 University paediatrics clinics with paediatric surgery units.

Everyday medical care, teaching and research was developing hand in hand to advance the welfare of children and infants. Chloroform was replaced for a short time by ether and local techniques, until in the second half of the 20th century modern anaesthesia with nitrous oxide and oxygen and relaxants became fully accepted.

In conclusion, one may say that paediatric anaesthesia in Poland has benefited from the long-standing presence of many hospitals for children, where anaesthetists have had a particular interest in children, infants and neonates, and they were ready to accept easily modern ideas coming from world-renowned centres such as those in Liverpool, London and Boston.

References

(1) Zembrzuski L. O znieczulaniu ogólnem i miejscowem u dzieci (General and local anaesthesia in children). In: *Odczyty Kliniczne (Clinical Lectures)*. Warszawa: Gazeta Lekarska, Gebethner i Wolff, 1917: XXI.

(2) Gawlik B. *Chloroform*. Przeglad Lekarski (Physician Review), Warszawa: 1865.
(3) Rondio Z. Nowoczesna anestezjologia i intensywna terapia pediatryczna na tle uwarunkowań
        historycznych (Modern paediatric anaesthesia and intensive therapy and
        historical background). *Proc Symp Hist Anaesthesiol Poland (Historia
        Anestezjologii w Polsce)*; Cracow: Medical Academy, 1986.
(4) Radbill SX. The Children's Hospital of Philadelphia. Philadelphia Medicine. In: *Clinical
        Conference.*, September, 1974.

11.5   Chloroform to a royal family*

OLE SECHER
University Hospital, Copenhagen, Denmark

Not many anaesthetics have gone down in world history and if they have, they have been overshadowed by the importance of the surgical procedure and the tribute has gone to the surgeons.

Queen Victoria

No doubt the most well-known administrations of anaesthesia (or, in reality, analgesia) to have the greatest influence on the development of anaesthesia were the two chloroform inhalations which John Snow (1813–1858) gave to Queen Victoria (1819–1901) for her two last deliveries. They changed the prospect for the delivering woman and counteracted the dogmatism of the church which was strongly against the use of anaesthesia for delivery pains. The differences between the church and James Young Simpson (1810–1871), Edinburgh, had been very bitter (2), but the church had to give in after the acceptance of anaesthesia by Queen Victoria, and 'Chloroform a la reine' became available to all women.

Queen Victoria was married in 1840 to Prince Albert of Saxe-Coburg-Gotha (1819–1861) and they had nine children. In 1850 John Snow was called in for a consultation by Prince Albert about the delivery of the seventh child, Prince Arthur, Duke of Connaught, 1850–1942, but Snow's services were not required on that occasion (1). The eighth delivery took place 7 April, 1853, and Prince Leopold, Duke of Albany (1853–1884) was born and the ninth and last delivery took place at the birth of Princess Beatrice (1857–1944) on 14 April, 1857, who was later married to Prince Henry of Battenberg (1857–1896). In both instances John Snow was called in by Sir James Clark (1788–1870) to give chloroform, and in both cases the obstetrician was Charles Locock (1799–1875) accoucheur to her Majesty (2).

The reason Snow was called upon has been stated by Benjamin Ward Richardson (1829–1898) in his biography of Snow as follows, 'By his earnest labour Dr Snow soon acquired a professional reputation, in relation to his knowledge of the action of anaesthetics, which spread far and wide; and the people, through the profession, looked up to him from all ranks, as the guide to whom to entrust themselves in Lethe's walk' (1).[†]

Shortly after the delivery of Prince Leopold, the issue of *Lancet* of 14, May, 1853 published an article by its well-known editor Thomas Wakley (1795–1862) in which he heavily criticized the use of chloroform for normal deliveries and refused to believe that the Queen had had chloroform as the rumour had it (3). After the delivery of Princess Beatrice the *Lancet* only

---

*Previously published in Danish in *Dansk Medicin historisk Årborg*, 1986, page 107.
[†]Lethe = (Greek) forgetfulness; one of the six rivers in the underworld.

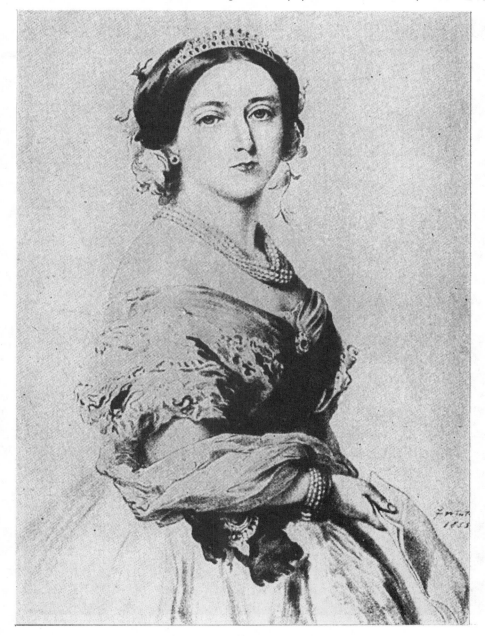

Figure 1   Victoria, Queen of Great Britain (1819–1901).

had a short message that 'Her Majesty was safely delivered of a Princess . . . on Tuesday last'. Dr Snow began to give chloroform at intervals beginning at 11.30 am. This continued for 2½ hours and 'the anaesthetic agent perfectly succeeded in the object desired' (2).

Richardson's biography (13) mentions that Snow in his diary has a note stating that the administration of chloroform to the Queen at the delivery of Prince Leopold lasted 53 minutes 'given on a handkerchief in 15 minims (0.9 ml) doses. The Queen expressed herself as greatly relieved by the administration'. A note in the diary about the delivery of Princess Beatrice

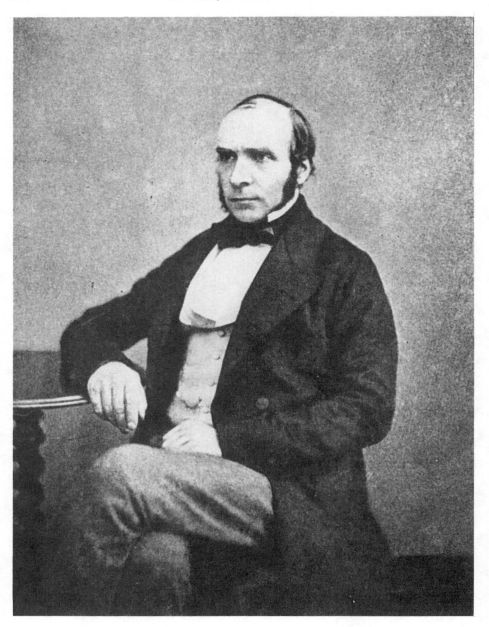

Figure 2   John Snow (1813–1858).

states 'the fact of the second administration of chloroform to Her Majesty' and that 'the chloroform again exerted its beneficial influence; and Her Majesty once more expressed herself as much satisfied with the results'.

Snow's own full entry in his diary for the two deliveries says:

'Thursday 7 April (1853).
Administered chloroform to the Queen in her confinement. Slight pains had been experienced since Sunday. Dr Locock was sent for about nine o'clock this morning,

stronger pains having commenced, and he found the os uteri had commenced to dilate a very little. I received a note from Sir James Clark a little after tea asking me to go to the Palace. I remained in an apartment near that of the Queen along with Sir J. Clark, Dr Fergusson (1808–1877) and (for the most part of the time) Dr Locock till a little a. twelve. At a twenty minutes past twelve by a clock in the Queen's apartment I commenced to give a little chloroform with each pain, by pouring about 15 minims by measure in a folded handkerchief. The first stage of labour was nearly over when the chloroform was commenced. Her Majesty expressed great relief from the application, the pain being very trifling during the uterine contractions, whilst between the periods of contraction there was complete ease. The effect of the chloroform was not at any time carried to the extent of quite removing consciousness. Dr Locock thought the chloroform prolonged the interval between the pains and retarded the labour somewhat. The infant was born at 13 minutes past one by the clock in the room (which was 3 minutes before the right time) consequently the chloroform was inhaled for 53 minutes. The placenta was expelled in a very few minutes, and the Queen appeared very cheerful and well, expressing herself much gratified with the effect of the chloroform.' (4)

Later the same year on 20 October, Snow was called to Lambeth Palace for the confinement of the daughter of the Archbishop of Canterbury and he used chloroform.

Considering the discussion between the church and Simpson, this was an important event (2). For the second delivery Snow has this entry:

Tuesday 14 April (1857)
'Administered chloroform to Her Majesty the Queen in her ninth confinement. The labour occurred about a fortnight later than expected. It commenced about 2 am of this day when the medical men were sent for. The labour was beginning and a little after 10 Dr Locock administered half a drachm of powdered ergot which produced some effect in increasing the pains. At 11 o'clock I began to administer chloroform. Prince Albert had previously administered a very little chloroform on a handkerchief about 9 or ten o'clock. I poured about 10 minims of chloroform on a handkerchief folded in a conical shape for each pain. Her Majesty expressed great relief from the [?]. Another dose of ergot was given about twelve o'clock and the pains increased somewhat about twenty minutes afterwards. The Queen at this time kept asking for more chloroform and complaining that it did not remove the pain. She slept, however, sometimes between the pains. Before one o'clock the head was resting on perineum and Dr Locock [?] the patient to make a bearing down effort, as she said that this would effect the birth. The Queen, however, when not unconscious of what was said, complained that she could not make an effort. The chloroform was left off for 3 or 4 pains and the royal patient made an effort which expelled the head, a little chloroform being given just as the head [?]. There was an interval of several minutes before the child was entirely born, it however cried in the meanwhile. The placenta was expelled about ten minutes afterwards. The Queen's recovery was very favourable.'

When inquisitive patients asked John Snow about these events he always answered: 'Her Majesty is a model patient' (1). Richardson also tells the following story: A woman in labour who was going to have chloroform administered by John Snow, refused to take it before she was told what the Queen said when she was taking it. His answer was: 'Her Majesty asked no questions until she had breathed very much longer than you have; and if you will only go on in loyal imitation, I will tell you everything'. When she woke up Snow had left (1).

Queen Victoria has no references to the administration of chloroform in her letters (2) but the Queen's biographer Elisabeth Longford quoted her as having said after the delivery of Prince Leopold, 'Dr Snow gave the blessed chloroform and the effect was soothing, quieting and delightful beyond measure', which is a quotation from Victoria's diary (5,6).

After the delivery of Prince Leopold Dr Clarke wrote to Dr James Young Simpson (1811–1870) in Edinburgh:

'The Queen had chloroform exhibited to her during her last confinement . . . It was not at any time given so strongly as to render the Queen insensible and an ounce of chloroform was scarcely consumed during the whole time. Her Majesty was greatly pleased with the effect, and she certainly never has had a better recovery.' (5).

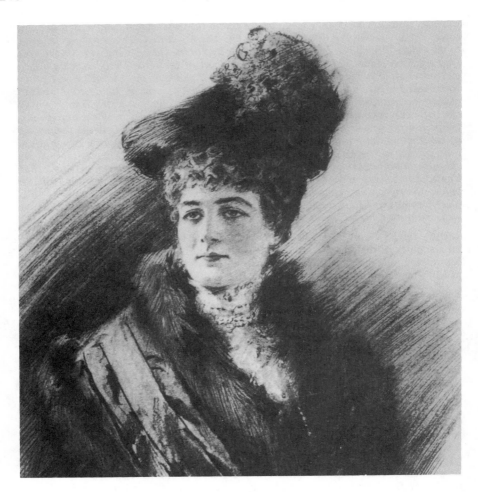

Figure 3   Alexandra, Princess of Wales (1844–1925) was considered as the most beautiful Princess in Europe.

No wonder that she also chose chloroform for the next and last delivery.

These two chloroform inhalations were Queen Victoria's only connection with anaesthetics, she never had an operation, except for the incision of an abscess in the axilla opened by Lord Joseph Lister (1827–1912) without the benefit of anaesthesia. This operation took place at Balmoral Castle in Scotland in 1871 when Lister was Professor of Surgery in Edinburgh. William Jenner (1815–1898) the physician was also present and he operated the bellows of the spray. Lister used a rubber drainage for the first time, a method introduced by Edward P. M. Chassaignac (1804–1879) in Paris (7).

Princess Victoria

Queen Victoria's oldest child Princess Victoria (Vicky) (1840–1901) was married to Prince Friedrich (Fritz) Wilhelm of Prussia, later King of Prussia and Emperor of Germany (1831–1888). He was also called 'Friedrich der Britte' because of his British sympathies and, on the insistence of Queen Victoria, the wedding took place in London in the Royal Chapel, St James's in 1858, and not in Berlin!

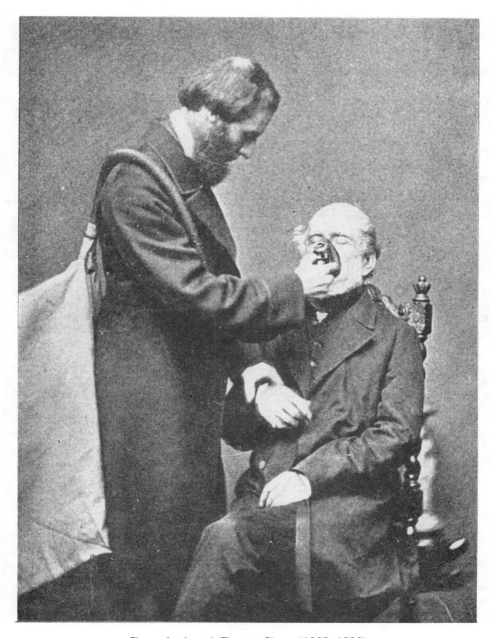

Figure 4   Joseph Thomas Clover (1825–1882).

Princess Victoria's first delivery took place in 1860 when Princess Charlotte (1860–1901), who was later married to Prince Bernhard of Saxe-Meinigen (1858–1928) was born. On this occasion Queen Victoria wrote a letter to Vicky's mother-in-law (Crown Princess Augusta (1811–1890), the wife of Crown Prince Wilhelm, later King of Prussia and Emperor of Germany (1797–1888) in which she said: 'Vicky appears to feel quite as well and to recover herself just as quickly as I always did. What a blessing she had chloroform! Perhaps without it her strength would have suffered very much' (2). This was only 3 years after Queen Victoria's own last delivery in 1857. It is fair to assume that the Princess had chloroform on the recommendation of Queen Victoria for all her eight deliveries.

Alexandra, Princess of Wales

The oldest son of Queen Victoria, Prince Edward, the later King Edward VII (1841–1910), was married to the Danish Princess Alexandra (1844–1925), who was the daughter of King Christian IX (1817–1906) of Denmark and Queen Louise (1817–1898), on the 10 March, 1863. The wedding took place in St Georges Chapel, Windsor Castle, two years after the death of Prince Albert. Queen Victoria was sitting in her box in her mourning and cast gloom on the occasion, the climax of which was the singing of Jenny Lind (1829–1887), the Swedish nightingale.

After the wedding the couple moved into Marlborough House in London. Princess Alexandra had six children and most (possibly all) the deliveries were premature and took place in the home. They were so unexpected that the Princess probably never had a chance to receive chloroform to relieve her labour pains, although Queen Victoria had almost certainly recommended it.

On the 15 February, 1867, Princess Alexandra caught a severe sore throat followed by a severe attack of rheumatic fever. Shortly after on the 21 February, the delivery of Princess Louise (1867–1931) took place. She was later married to the Duke of Fife, Alexander Duff (1849–1912). Before the delivery it was decided by her doctors that chloroform should not be used because of her illness. Among the doctors attending her during this pregnancy were Sir William Jenner, whose special knowledge of fevers, and the surgeon Sir James Pages (1814–1899), but there must have been four more because the day after the unexpected delivery six embarrassed doctors made the Princess laugh when they showed up belatedly.

After a period when it looked as though she was recovering the Princess had another attack of fever with severe pains in the knees. One of the biographies (8) mentions that the pains were so severe that her doctors gave her big doses of chloroform! If this is correct—and it is most likely so—it is a very special indication for the use of chloroform. Is it possible that she had a knee aspiration? Joseph Thomas Clover (1825–1882) was the best known anaesthetist in London at that time. He had taken over the leading position after Snow's death and it was he who was called. Among his patients were some royal persons and among them Princess Alexandra is mentioned (8). In none of the biographies on her or Edward is mentioned that she had an operation. Among the papers of Clover (9), there is a short letter from Prince Edward's secretary General Sir William Thomas Knollys (1797–1883):

> '*Marlborough House—27 April, 1867. General Knollys presents his compliments to Mr Clover and beg to enclose a cheque for £5.50 by device of the Prince of Wales in consideration of his attendance of the Princess of Wales on the 6. Inst.*'

The date fits well with the second rheumatic attack the Princess had in April when her knee pains got specially severe. Clover would probably have used his bag, which gave constant concentrations on this occasion. The payment was for the time a royal one.

The patient recovered quickly and was considered back to good health in the beginning of May. This fitted Prince Edward's plans well and on the 10 May, he went to Paris for the opening of the World Exhibition and other amusements! The Princess had a stiff knee and limped a little the rest of her life as well as becoming increasingly deaf.

Crown Prince Friedrich of Prussia

In January, 1887, Crown Prince Friedrich (Fritz) of Prussia caught a cold and became hoarse. He was treated with the usual remedies by the Deputy Surgeon General Dr Wegner without a satisfactory response. The internist Carl Gerhardt (1833–1903) Berlin, who had interest in throat diseases, was called and he diagnosed a tumour on the left vocal chord, which he tried to remove by several cauterizations. Gerhardt and Wegner became concerned and on 10 May, they called a council consisting of themselves, the surgeon, Professor Ernst von Bergman (1836–1907), and

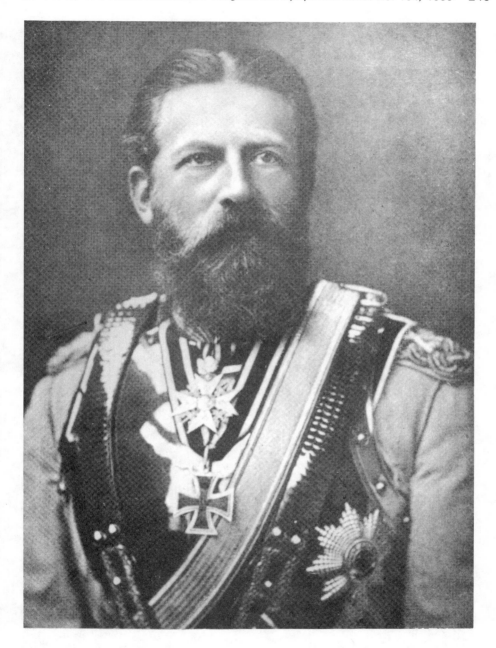

Figure 5   Friedrich, Crown Prince of Prussia (1831–1888) had strong English sympathies. Mackenzie called him 'Friedrich the Noble'.

the laryngologist, Adalbert Tobold (1827–1907), both of Berlin. On 20 May it was decided that a laryngectomy was required, but Otto von Bismarch (1815–1898), the German Chancellor intervened, and on 18 May it was decided to call on the most famous laryngologist of that time, Morell Mackenzie (1837–1892) of London. Crown Princess Victoria also telegraphed Queen Victoria to ask Mackenzie to see her son-in-law, Fritz. This double call caused some

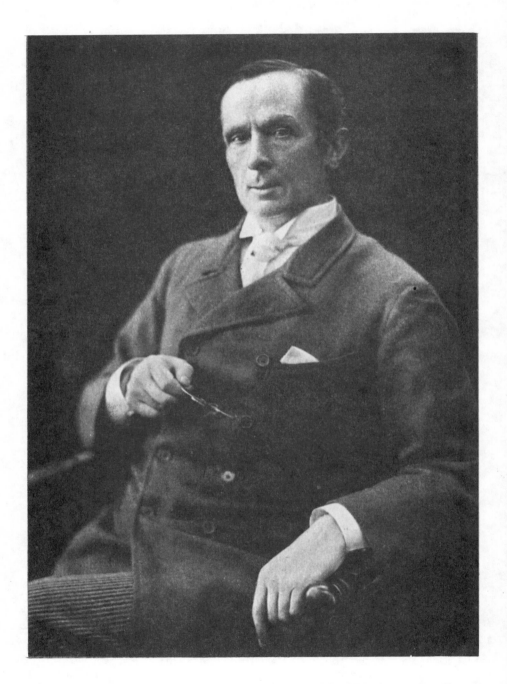

Figure 6   Morell Mackenzie (1837–1898) established in 1865 the world's first hospital for throat diseases: 'The Throat Hospital', Golden Square, London. He was a rather small and delicately built man.

controvery. Mackenzie came and, after examining the patient, pronounced the tumour benign. The tumour was removed in stages and each specimen was examined under the microscope by Rudolf Wirchow (1821–1902), the famous Berlin pathologist. No malignancy was found and further treatment was left to Mackenzie. In June the Crown Prince visited London for Queen Victoria's golden jubilee on 21 June, 1887, and, although tired and hoarse, he made a very good impression riding through London in the Queen's bodyguard of Princes.

On 28 June, Mackenzie removed the last part of the tumour and this was again examined microscopically by Wirchow, who did not find malignant changes.

The Crown Prince left London on 3 September, for recuperation in Toblach in Tyrol together with Dr Wegner and Dr Mark Hovell, an assistant to Mackenzie. At the end of September they went to Venice and in the beginning of November to San Remo in Italy. Mackenzie came to San Remo when the Crown Prince got worse. He diagnosed a malignancy in the larynx below the chords on 6 November, 1887, and called a conference. Professor Leopold von Schrötter (1837–1908) of Vienna, Hermann Krause (1848–1921) of Berlin, Dr Schrader and Prince Wilhelm, later Emperor Wilhelm II (1859–1941), were present. The choice was now between a laryngectomy and a tracheostomy. The patient himself chose the latter.

On 12 December, Mackenzie returned to see the patient and found him better after a potassium–iodine-treatment without informing the patient of the possibility of syphilis. In January the patient coughed a piece of tissue which contained cartilage, but Wirchow again did not diagnose malignancy. By the beginning of February, 1888, the condition of the patient, now short of breath, had deteriorated and Mackenzie was again called to San Remo. Among the many doctors in attendance was Dr Fritz Bramann (1854–1913), who although only 33 years of age, had already performed 400 tracheostomies. He had been sent by Professor Bergmann who could not travel himself. Bramann was not permitted by the other doctors to see the patient or participate in the conferences and this caused great difficulties but, in the end Mackenzie had to give in. Bramann then insisted that the Crown Prince required a tracheostomy before it was too late. On 9 February, 1988, the operation was performed in the living room of the house in San Remo, with the patient lying in his bed near the window for sufficient light.

There was an argument between Mackenzie and Bramann, because Bramann wanted to use chloroform while Mackenzie thought it to be too dangerous. He would have preferred freezing the skin or the use of 'laughing-gas followed by ether', but Bramann got it his way. They also had a discussion whether the operation should be performed on a table, as Bramann wished or in the bed at the request of the Crown Princess (10–12).

Mackenzie has described the operation which took 20 minutes as follows:

> *'The bed was placed opposite one of the windows, so that there was an excellent light. Bramann proceeded to give chloroform, but as soon as the Crown Prince had become unconscious, the administration was continued by Dr Krause; whilst I kept my finger on the pulse at the left wrist. Shortly after Dr Bramann had made the first incision, I noticed that the pulse had become very weak and that the face was blanched; in fact there were evident signs of cardiac weakness. On raising the eyelid the pupil was seen to be widely dilated. The chloroform was suspended for a minute or two, when the pulse became fairly good again, and the operation was proceeded with. After this incident Dr Bramann seemed to become a little flurried, though not to such an extent as to prevent him from operating with skill. In opening the windpipe, however, I noticed that he made his incision a little to the right instead of in the middle line. The deviation appeared to me so slight at the time that I attached no importance to it. After opening the trachea, instead of at once plunging in the canula as is usually done by English surgeons, Bramann held aside the two sides of the wound for a minute or two until the bleeding had ceased, and then inserted a very large and long tube. I will frankly own that the delay in introducing the canula seemed to me an improvement on the ordinary plan of plunging the tube into the windpipe as soon as it is opened—a proceeding which usually sets up a severe spasm and cough.' (13)*

These last remarks on the incision in the trachea and the tube used, later gave rise to controversies and discussion. Bramann also gave a description of the operation in a letter to his chief, Professor von Bergmann, which is very much in accordance with Mackenzie's but shorter (3).

This of course was a narrow escape from a chloroform death. No doubt Dr Bramann had some very unpleasant moments.

The American dentist Thomas Wiltberger Evans (1823–1897) was also present at the insistence of the family as a supportive friend and observer. He also helped to smooth out the medical dispute between the German doctors and Mackenzie and reported directly to Queen Augusta and Crown Princess Victoria. Evans had a prestigious dental practice in Paris. He treated most of the royalty of Europe for their dental troubles and was friendly with a number of them, particularly the Emperor Napoleon III (1803–1873) and Empress Eugenie (1827–1920). Before Evans became a dentist he had been a jeweller. When a cannula was required after the operation to keep the stoma open it was Evans who worked through the night at the local jeweller's workshop in San Remo to make it out of a five-franc silver piece (14). Neither Mackenzie nor Bramann mention that Evans had been present in their descriptions.

The recovery of the patient from the operation went well, and during the continuing discomfort the Crown Prince was very calm and patient accepting it all stoically.

On 9 March, the Emperor Wilhelm I (1797–1888) died and Friedrich, now Wilhelm III, had to leave San Remo for Berlin to be elected Emperor. He developed a tracheo-oesophageal fistula and died on 15 June, 1888. Morell Mackenzie was present at his death. It was the end of a sad story which could have ended earlier in an anaesthetic death.

King Edward VII

When Queen Victoria died at the age of 82 on 26 January, 1901, her eldest son became Edward VII, (1841–1910). He was to be crowned on 26 June, 1902, the first coronation for 62 years. The Boer war had just ended on 31 May, 1902, so the celebration was to be very elaborate. Royalty from Europe and elsewhere as well as representatives from all over the Empire were invited and most arrived in due time.

Twelve days before his coronation on Friday, 13 June, the King felt very fatigued in the evening and retired to his bed. The following morning he complained of abdominal discomfort, and was seen later that day by his Doctor, Sir Francis Henry Laking (1847–1914). In the afternoon he felt much better and went to Aldershot where he attended a dinner with Queen Alexandra (1844–1925) and a tattoo in the evening in inclement weather. On Saturday night he had abdominal pain and felt distended. Upon examination early Sunday morning, Dr Laking recognized that the abdominal troubles might be serious, and called for the internist Sir Thomas Barlow (1845–1945) who stayed for the day.

On Monday 16, the King proceeded in a carriage to Windsor, and felt better in the evening. On Tuesday he stayed at home and on Wednesday he was seen by the surgeon Sir Frederick Treves (1853–1923). His temperature was elevated and there was a swelling and tenderness in the right iliac fossa—a 'perityphlitis' as diagnosed. During Thursday and Friday all the symptoms disappeared. When Sir Fredrick saw the patient the following day the swelling in the iliac region had nearly vanished and the King was feeling much better and was believed to be on the road to recovery. Sunday was uneventful and on Monday the King went by train to London.

A 'perityphlitis' a term implying peritoneal inflammation around the caecum and appendix coined by the Boston surgeon Reginald Heber Fitz (1843–1913) in 1888 was diagnosed. An appendectomy was not a common operation at that time and was still considered serious.

On Monday, 23 June, the King and the Queen gave a magnificent eight course dinner party for some of the coronation guests. This was too much. The King developed considerable abdominal pain and his temperature rose during the night. The doctors Laking, Treves and Barlow became extremely concerned and by 10 o'clock the next morning. Lord Joseph Lister (1827–1912) and Sir Thomas Smith (1833–1909) were consulted, and it was concluded that an operation was necessary. The King's answer to the suggestion was: 'I must keep faith with my people and go to the Abbey'. After arguments Treves said bluntly, 'Then, Sir, you will go in your coffin' (11).

At 12.30 pm the same day the operation was performed. Doctor Fredric Hewitt (1857–1916) gave the anaesthetic and Sir Frederick Treves performed the operation.

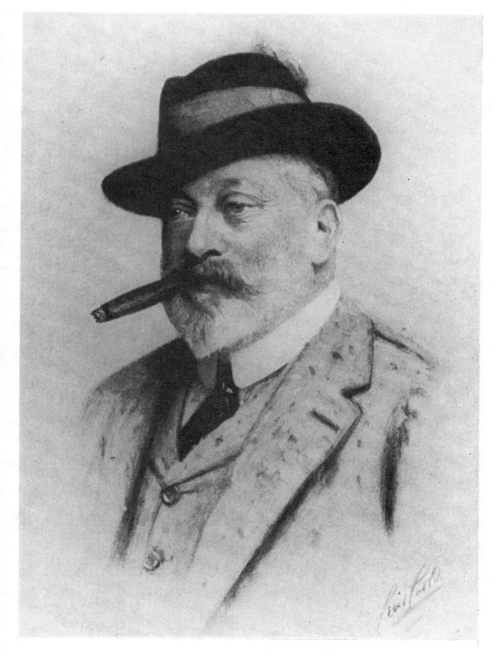

Figure 7   Edward, Prince of Wales (1831–1910). Later King Edward VII. In 1902 he was more stout.

Hewitt started the anaesthetic with a mixture of 2 parts of ether and 3 parts chloroform given in drops on Skinner's mask. Subsequently he changed to ether alone on a Rendle's mask. The King was stout, elderly and plethoric, not a good anaesthetic risk, and soon turned deep purple. Fortunately he had a beard and this was grasped by Dr Hewitt, and the royal head (jaw?) was pulled forward, and the King began to breathe again (15).

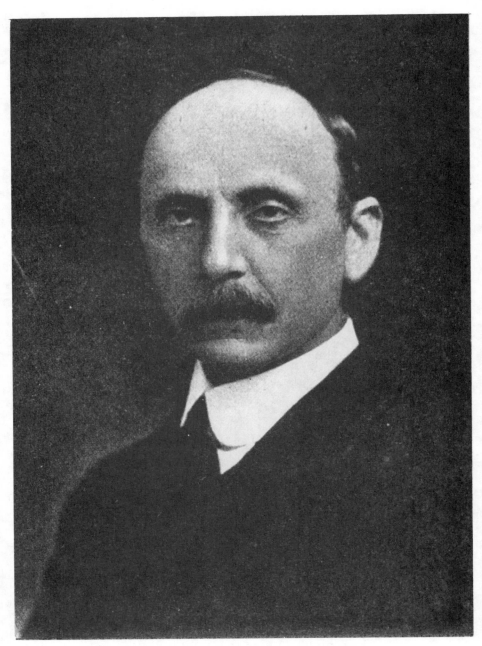

Figure 8   Frederic Hewitt (1857–1916).

While this was going on Dr Treves opened the patient in the usual place and found a large abscess. Pus was found at a depth of 4½ inches and two drainage tubes of wide calibre were inserted surrounded by idoform gauze. The appendix itself was not removed. The operation lasted 40 minutes and everything went well. Present at the operation was Lord Lister and Sir Thomas Smith. When the King woke up after the anaesthetic the first thing he said was 'Where is George?' referring to his oldest son, the later George V (1865–1936) (1).

He recovered quickly from the operation and the coronation took place 9 August, 1902, but attendance was far less.

Thomas Skinner, an obstetrician in Liverpool, described his mask in 1862 (16) and Richard Rendle gave an account of his, which was originally designed for bichloride of methylene in 1869 while he was a surgical registrar at Guy's Hospital (17). Rendle practised surgery in London for some years before going on an emigrant ship to Australia, where he practised in Taringa near Brisbane, Queensland, where he died.

Conclusion

These six events took place within the first 55 years of anaesthesia and all within the same family. When they took place, they were extensively discussed among doctors as well as by the public. The difficulties and dangers of the anaesthetics to two of the patients hardly came to be known. The circumstances under which they took place were special, but due to the importance of the persons involved, they are some of the only well described anaesthetics from that period. No doubt the two anaesthetic (or analgesic) administrations to Queen Victoria were the only ones of importance to the development of the specialty.

Acknowledgments

For information about the different anaesthetics I owe thanks to Professor J. Robertson, Edinburgh on Hewitt's anaesthetic, Dr R. H. Ellis, London on Rendle, Dr R. S. Atkinson, Southend on Sea, UK, on Snow's diaries, Dr R. K. Calverley, San Diego, USA, on Clover's papers, Dr Tom Boulton, Oxford, UK, on apparatus, librarian Lee Perry, Seattle, USA, on Clover's papers and Dr J. Alfred Lee, Southend on Sea, UK, on literature.

References

(1) Richardson JW. *The life of John Snow, M.D.* J. Snow. *On chloroform and other anaesthetics*. London: Churchill, 1858.

(2) Sykes WS. *Essays on the first hundred years of anaesthesia* Vol I. Edinburgh: Livingstone, 1960.

(3) Bramann C. von. Kaiserin Friedrich und die deutschen Ärzte. *Deutsch med J* 1963; **14**: 202–7.

(4) Atkinson RS. The 'lost' diaries of John Snow. *Proc 4th World Congr Anaesth* Rotterdam: Excerpta Medica, 1970, 197–99.

(5) Longford E. *Victoria R.I.* London: Weidenfeld & Nicolson, 1964.

(6) Thomas KB. *The development of anaesthetic apparatus*. Oxford: Blackwell, 1975.

(7) Guthrie D. *A history of medicine*. London: Th. Nelson & Son, 1945.

(8) Tisdall EEP. *Unpredictable Queen*. København: Dansk udgave. C. A. Reitzel Forlag, 1954. Danish edition.

(9) Thomas KB. The Clover/Snow collection. *Anaesthesia* 1972; **27**: 436–49.

(10) Falbe-Hansen J. Strubespejlets opfindelse og en skæbnesvanger følge heraf. (Danish). København 1967.

(11) Stevenson RS. *Famous illnesses in history*. London: Eyre & Spottis, 1962.

(12) Stevenson RS. *Morell Mackenzie*. London: William Heinemann, 1946.

(13) Mackenzie M. *The fatal illness of Friedrich the Noble*. London: Sampson Low, Marston, Searle & Rivington, 1888.

(14) Carson G. *The dentist and the Empress. The adventures of Dr Tom Evans in the gas-lit Paris*. Boston: Houghton Mifflin Co., 1983.

(15) Robertson J. Personal communication, 1985.

(16) Skinner T. Anaesthesia in midwifery with new apparatus for its safer induction by chloroform. *Br Med J* 1862; **II**: 108–10.

(17) Rendle R. On the use of protoxide of nitrogen gas; and on a new mode of producing rapid anaesthesia with bichloride of methylene. *Br Med J* 1869; **I**: 612–3.

Further reading

Bramsen B. *The House of Glücksborg* Vol 1. (Danish). Copenhagen: Forum, 1975.
Duncum B. *The development of inhalation anaesthesia*. Oxford University Press, 1947.
Thornton JL. Royal patients and the popularization of anaesthesia. *Anaesthesia* 1953; **8**: 146–50.
Marston AD. The life and achievements of Joseph Thomas Clover. *Ann Roy Coll Surg Engl* 1949; **4**: 267.

Chapter 12

NEUROMUSCULAR BLOCKING AGENTS

12.1	Development of skeletal muscle relaxants from the curare arrow poisons

R. HUGHES
Wellcome Research Laboratories, Beckenham, Kent, UK

The introduction of skeletal muscle relaxants into clinical anaesthesia was one of the most significant advances made in the speciality. Before their introduction in 1942, when curare was first used, rapid smooth induction of anaesthesia and the maintenance of a state adequate for the surgical procedure was a work of art, accomplished regularly by relatively few practitioners. However, with the use of potent synthetic skeletal muscle relaxants, this is no longer true and their development from the curare arrow poisons is a fascinating story.

Historical background

In 1516 Peter Martyr d'Anghera, an Italian 'gossip columnist' of his time, wrote the first known account of the use of poison arrows by the South American Indians (1). Written in Latin, it contained many references to deadly weapons and the venoms used to poison them. 'The arrows are dipped in juice obtained from certain trees. There are old women skilled in its preparation who, furnished with the necessary materials, are shut in for two days to distil the ointment. When the house is opened if the women are well and not found lying on the ground, half dead from the fumes of the poison, they are severely punished and the ointment is thrown away as valueless. The strength of the poison is such that the mere odour of it during the preparation almost kills its makers.'

The word curare was first used by Marggravius in 1684 (2), and Barrère (3) writing in 1741 related how the Indians coated their arrows with the juice of a tropical creeper. During the 18th century much was written about the effects of curare preparations including works by de la Condamine, Bancroft and Fontana. In 1879 (4) the explorer Charles Waterton, in his 'Wanderings in South America' described the three types of weapons poisoned with curare: darts shot from blow-pipes, poisoned arrows and poisoned spears. 'The arrows were four to five feet in length, with slender tips grooved to contain the curare. The slender points broke off in the prey and the nicely fletched arrow was retrieved and fitted with another point and used again.'

Identification of the plants and their curare alkaloids

From the 19th century efforts were made to identify the plants and their curare alkaloids. Martius (1830) recognized that a number of plants including *Strychnos* were the chief components of some curare preparations (5). The writings of Richard and Robert Schomburgk (1841–1879), the travellers and naturalists, showed that Macusi curare contained an active ingredient prepared from *Strychnos toxifera* (6–8). Rudolf Boehm (1895), a psychiatrist turned pharmacologist, found that there were three kinds of curare commonly available: tube-curare, pot-curare and calabash-curare (9). In fact, curare was prepared from two species of poisonous plants: curare from the forest regions of Ecuador and Peru were derived from several varieties of *Chondodendron* (tube-curare). Whereas those from the more easterly curare producing regions in the Guianas and lower Orinoco contained material from a species of *Strychnos* (calabash-curare). Calabash-curare often contained toxiferin which was several hundred times more potent than the tubocurarine first isolated by Harold King in 1935 from a sample of

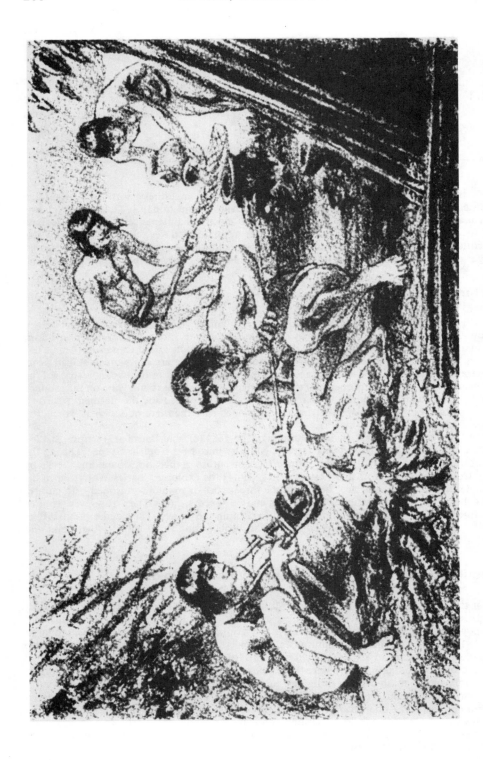

Figure 1   Preparation of the arrow poison by the South American Indians.

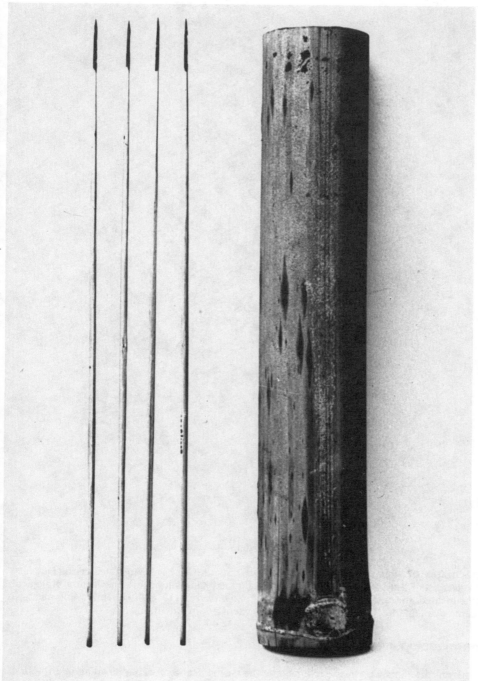

Figure 2   Blowpipe darts tipped with curare, and bamboo quiver.

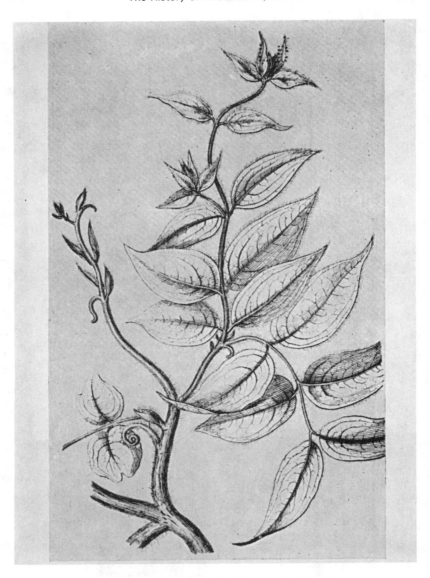

Figure 3   Strychnos toxifera, *a source of curare.*

tube-curare (10). King also elucidated its chemical structure. In 1943 Wintersteiner and Dutcher, two scientists from E. R. Squibb and Sons, obtained King's tubocurarine from a biological authenticated specimen of *Chondodendron tomentosum* (11). Subsequently, this alkaloid became available in sufficient quantities for extensive investigation.

Pharmacological studies

Numerous attempts were made to elucidate the mechanism of curare poisoning and the first significant observation was made by the physician and physiologist Benjamin Brodie in 1812. Brodie found that artificial respiration during paralysis by curare in animals was sufficient to sustain life until spontaneous breathing returned (12). The classical experiments of the French

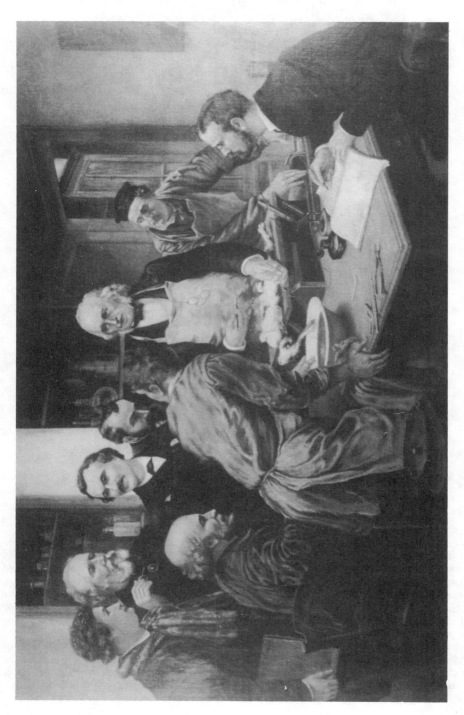

Figure 4   Claude Bernard (1818–1878) with his pupils.

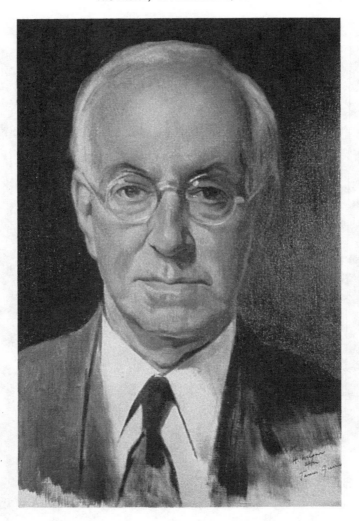

Figure 5   Sir Henry Dale (1875–1968).

physiologist Claude Bernard (1850, 1856, 1864), using calabash curare in frogs, demonstrated that there was no failure of conduction along the nerves, neither was there failure of the ability of muscles to respond to direct stimulation (13–15). Hence, the action of curare was localized at some point between nerve and muscle and not centrally as had previously been supposed. In the following years many theories were proposed but the breakthrough came when the chemical basis of myoneural transmission was established by the researches of Sir Henry Dale and his colleagues in the early nineteen thirties (16,17). They demonstrated that acetylcholine was released from the motor nerve terminals during excitation by nerve volleys and so bridged the gap between nerve ending and muscle. These workers also found that the liberation of acetylcholine was not affected by curare in a dose sufficient to prevent the response of the muscle to excitation by the nerve impulse. The scientific work of William Paton and Eleanor Zaimis (1951–1962) did much to elucidate the action of curiform agents at the neuromuscular junction (18–21). They distinguished between those drugs which acted by competing with acetylcholine for occupancy of receptors on the muscle-end plate and those which caused it to become electrically inexcitable.

Clinical use

The first attempted use of curare as a therapeutic agent in man was in 1858 when two surgeons, Sayres and Burrall, in North America, were unsuccessful in treating two cases of tetanus by applying a curare preparation locally (22). In 1868 Beigel, using partially purified calabash-curarine, was among the first to describe the signs of curarization in man: ocular ptosis, change in voice, difficulty in swallowing and weakness of the neck muscles (23). Further use of crude unstandardized preparations of curare, with their many side effects, for the treatment of tetanus led to disappointment. It was not until 1935 that interest in the therapeutic application of curare was revised when King's isolation of the pure curare alkaloid tubocurarine (10) made the

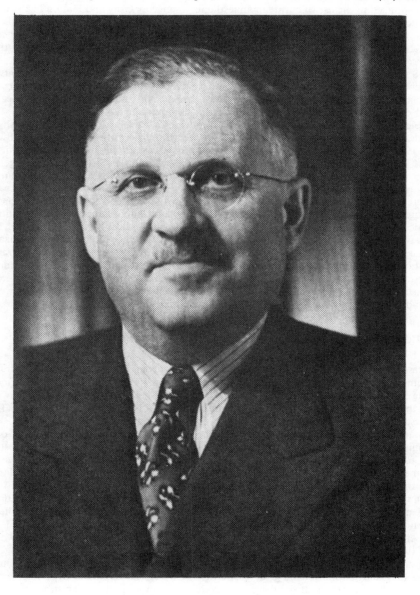

Figure 6   Dr Harold Griffith (1894–1985).

extensive clinical investigations by Ranyard West on paralytic rigidity possible (24). The early curare preparations were standardized in dogs and used by Bennett in 1938, a neuropsychiatrist in Nebraska, for the management of convulsive therapy (25). E. R. Squibb and Sons produced the first commercial preparation of curare under the trade name of Intocostrin which led to its clinical evaluation in anaesthesia.

Dr Lewis Wright, a clinician from Squibb, believed that curare had a potential value in anaesthesia and he persuaded Harold Griffith and Enid Johnson in Montreal to use the drug for the first time as a skeletal muscle relaxant in anaesthesia in 1942 (26). Their results were confirmed by Cross and Cullen a year later in Iowa and these workers also found that ether anaesthesia decreased the amount of curare needed for muscle paralysis (27). British anaesthetists were introduced to the use of curare in anaesthetic practice by Gray and Halton in 1946 when they described a series of over a thousand patients (28). They used the pure crystalline alkaloid synthesized in London by Harold King in 1935 (10) because Intocostrin, the standardized curare preparation used by Griffiths and Johnson (26), was difficult to obtain. Shortly after this in 1946 Prescott, Organe and Rowbotham reported on the use of Intocostrin in 180 cases (29). In 1948 Cecil Gray surveyed the administration of tubocurarine to over 8000 patients and commented that 'anaesthesia had been revolutionized by removing for all time the need for deep anaesthesia' (30). It was the emphasis on the use of light anaesthesia that influenced the clinical development of skeletal muscle relaxation by anaesthetists in Britain.

Ample supplies of *Chondodendron tomentosum* vines became available together with large quantities of crude curare from Ecuador through the efforts of the explorer and adventurer Richard Gill in 1941 (31), which led to its widespread use both in anaesthesia and for the treatment of various spastic states. This material was used by E. R. Squibb and Sons for the large scale production of Intocostrin and the rabbit head drop assay was devised by Varney and his colleagues in 1949 as a convenient and reliable method for standardization (32). It was realized that pure alkaloidal curariform preparations must be controlled for potency because Wintersteiner and Dutcher (1943) had found that pure crystalline tubocurarine contained various quantities of chondocurine dimethochloride (11). These two alkaloids were indistinguishable from each other but the isomers differed markedly in potency, hence the necessity for biological standardization.

The control of potency together with the development of the techniques of endotracheal intubation and pulmonary ventilation enabled curare to be used with safety. Basic principles were established which recommended that curare and similar drugs were used only in those circumstances in which skeletal muscle relaxation was indicated. Thus, these drugs were to be an adjunct to anaesthesia and not a substitute for it.

Synthetic skeletal muscle relaxants

The search for synthetic relaxants began by both pharmacologists and clinicians for drugs to overcome the unwanted side effects of the naturally occurring alkaloids and the difficulties relating to their supply. Gallamine was synthesized by Bovet and his colleagues in 1947 and it was the first synthetic competitive neuromuscular blocking agent to be successful (33). It was first used clinically in Britain by Mushin and his colleagues in 1949 (34).

Preparation of other synthetic substances arose from the work of Barlow and Ing on the methonium compounds in 1948 (35) and, of these, decamethonium was used in anaesthesia in the following year by Organe and his colleagues (36). It was the careful and ingenious experiments of William Paton and Eleanor Zaimis (1951–1953) that revealed the depolarizing action of this group of compounds (19,21,22,37).

Suxamethonium is the most successful of the depolarizing agents by virtue of its unusually short period of action which is particularly suitable in anaesthesia. The drug was synthesized independently by Phillips in 1949 (38) and by Bovet and his colleagues in 1951 (39). Suxamethonium was introduced into anaesthetic practice by Italian (40) and Swedish workers at the International Congress held in London in 1951.

The curare derivative, dimethyl tubocurarine, was isolated by Wintersteiner and Dutcher in 1943 (11) and its pharmacological properties were described in 1948 by Collier and his colleagues who reported that the drug was several times more potent than tubocurarine but with no greater side effects (42).

Diallyl-nor-toxiferine is a semi-synthetic derivative obtained from calabash-curare by Frey and Seeger in 1961 (43). It is now known as alcuronium. Clinical experiences were described by Waser and Harbeck (44) and Lund and Stovner (45) in 1962. The drug is about twice as potent as tubocurarine and perhaps of longer duration, but it causes fewer side-effects.

Pancuronium was synthesized by Savage and his co-workers in 1967 and its design was based on the steroid nucleus (46). Its pharmacology was outlined by Buckett and his colleagues in 1968 (47) and the drug was introduced into anaesthetic practice by Baird and Reid in 1967 (48). Pancuronium is about five to 10 times more potent than tubocurarine. However, unlike tubocurarine, it does not cause ganglion blockade, but tachycardia and hypertension are associated with its vagal blocking properties.

Vecuronium and atracurium are relatively new agents with a duration of action intermediate between that of suxamethonium and pancuronium. Both agents offer a particular advantage in the development of skeletal muscle relaxation. Vecuronium is an analogue of pancuronium and its chemical properties were described by Buckett and his colleagues in 1973 (49) and more recently in 1980 by Savage and his collaborators (50). Durant and his co-workers (1979) showed in animal studies that the drug exhibited pronounced neuromuscular blocking activity coupled with only weak actions at sympathetic ganglia and on the cardiac vagus (51). The first clinical experience was reported by Crul and Booij in 1980 (52). The potency of vecuronium is similar to that of pancuronium but its cardiovascular effects are insignificant. Vecuronium has a low potential for releasing histamine but occasional reactions have been reported.

Atrarcurium represents a new approach to the development of skeletal muscle relaxants. The drug was designed uniquely by Stenlake (1978) to undergo degradation at physiological temperature and pH by a self-destruction mechanism called Hofmann elimination which proceeds independently of renal and hepatic function (53); atracurium also undergoes an enzymic ester hydrolysis. Pharmacological studies by Hughes and Chapple in 1981 demonstrated that atracurium was virtually free from autonomic side-effects and the drug showed little tendency to cumulate when successive doses were administered (54). The first quantitative clinical evaluation of atracurium was reported in 1981 by Payne and Hughes (55). Its neuromuscular blocking potency is similar to that of tubocurarine but the cardiovascular effects of the drug are minimal. Atracurium is a weak histamine liberator with a potency of about one-third that of tubocurarine.

Several new agents are currently undergoing clinical evaluation. Pipecuronium (56) and BW938U (57) have a similar clinical profile to that of pancuronium but appear to be devoid of cardiovascular effects. Another agent, BW 1090U, has a duration of action approximately half that of vecuronium and atracurium (58).

Epilogue

In 1957 Francis Foldes wrote 'the goal of this search will be to find a non-depolarizing skeletal muscle relaxant which will be as short acting and controllable as suxamethonium, its fate in the organism being little affected by pathological changes, its breakdown products having no neuromuscular blocking effect and which will be easily reversible by a harmless antagonist, in the rare instances when an atypical response will make this necessary' (59). Now, thirty years later, despite numerous attempts this goal has not yet been achieved.

However, there is now a greater understanding of the physiology and pharmacology of the neuromuscular junction which in due course may lead to the development of more specific and safer neuromuscular blocking drugs. It is also conceivable that new skeletal muscle relaxants will eventually be designed with a unique mode of action, at present unknown.

Meanwhile, it is commonplace to use neuromuscular relaxation to ease the work of the surgeon during operations, but it still seems incredible that drugs developed from the arrow poisons of the South American Indians are now widely used to paralyse patients during anaesthesia.

Acknowledgment

Figures are reproduced by permission of the Wellcome Institute Library, London.

References

(1) Anghera PM d'. *De Orbe Novo* (1516) translated by MacNutt FA. New York: Putman's Sons, 1912.

(2) Marggravius G. Historiae rerum naturalium Brasiliae libri octo. In: Piso G, ed. *De medicina Brasiliensi libri quatuor*. Leiden: Hackius, 1648: 22.

(3) Barrère P. *Essai sur l'histoire naturelle de la France équinoxiale*. Paris: Piget, 1741: 45.

(4) Waterton C. *Wanderings in South America*. London: Macmillan, 1879: 133–8.

(5) Martius CF von. Ueber die Bereitung des Pfeilgiftes Urari bei den Indianern Juris am Rio Yupura in Nordbrasilien. In: Buchner von, ed. *Repertorium fur die Pharmacie*. Nuremberg, Schrag, 1830; **36**: 337–53.

(6) Schomburgk Robert. On the Urari, the arrow poison of the Indians of Guiana. *Ann & Mag Nat Hist* 1841; **7**: 407–27.

(7) Schomburgk Robert. *Ralegh's discovery of Guiana* London: Hakluyt Society, 1848: 71.

(8) Schomburgk Robert. *On the Urari: the deadly arrow poison of the Macusis, an Indian tribe in British Guiana* Adelaide: Spiller, 1879: 7–9.

(9) Boehm R. Das Südamerikanische Pfeilgift curare in chemischer und pharmakologischer Beziehung. 1 Theil: Das Tubo-curare. *Abh Sächs Akad Wiss* 1895; **22**: 200–238.

(10) King H. Curare alkaloids. I Tubocurarine. *J Chem Soc* 1935: 1381–89.

(11) Wintersteiner O, Dutcher JD. Curare alkaloids from *Chondodendron tomentosum*. *Science (NY)* 1943; **97**: 467–79.

(12) Brodie BC. Further experiments and observations on the action of poison on the animal system. *Phil Trans R Soc* 1812; **102**: 205–27.

(13) Bernard C. Action de curare et de la nicotine sur le système nerveux et sur le système musculaire. *Cr Séanc Soc Biol* 1850; **2**: 195.

(14) Bernard C. Analyse physiologique des propriétés de systemes musculaires et nerveux au moyen du curare. *Cr hebd Seanc Acad Sci Paris* 1856; **43**: 825–9.

(15) Bernard C. Études physiologiques sur quelques poisons Americains: le curare. *Rev d Deux Mondes* 1864; **53**: 164–90.

(16) Dale HH. Chemical transmission of the effects of nerve impulses. *Br Med J* 1934; **1**: 835–41.

(17) Dale HH, Feldberg W, Vogt M. Release of acetylcholine at voluntary motor nerve endings. *J Physiol* 1936; **86**: 353–80.

(18) Burns BD, Paton WDM. Depolarization of the motor-end plate by decamethonium and acetylcholine. *J Physiol* 1951; **115**: 41–73.

(19) Paton WDM, Zaimis EJ. The action of tubocurarine and of decamethonium on respiratory and other muscles in the cat. *Physiol* 1951; **112**: 311–31.

(20) Paton WDM, Zaimis EJ. The methonium compounds. *Pharmac Rev* 1952; **4**: 219–53.

(21) Zaimis EJ. Motor end-plate differences as a determining factor in the mode of action of neuromuscular blocking substances. *J Physiol* 1953; **122**: 238–51.

(22) Sayres LA, Burrall FA. Two cases of traumatic tetanus. *NYJ Med* 1858; **4**: 250–3.

(23) Beigel H. Versuche mit curare und curarin. *Berl Klin Wschr* 1868; **5**: 73–6, 98–101.

(24) West R. The pharmacology and therapeutics of curare and its constituents. *Proc Roy Soc Med* 1935; **28**: 565–78.

(25) Bennett AE. Preventing traumatic complications in convulsive shock therapy by curare. *JAMA* 1940; **114**: 322–4.

(26) Griffith HR, Johnson GE. The use of curare in general anaesthesia. *Anesthesiology* 1942; **3**: 418–20.

(27) Cross ES, Cullen SC. The effects of anesthetic agents on muscular contraction. *J Pharmac Exp Ther* 1943; **78**: 358–65.

(28) Gray TC, Halton J. Milestones in anaesthesia? *Proc Roy Soc Med* 1946; **39**: 400–10.

(29) Prescott F, Organe GSW, Rowbotham S. Tubocurarine chloride as adjunct to anaesthesia. *Lancet* 1946; **ii**: 80–4.

(30) Gray TC. Tubocurarine chloride. *Proc Roy Soc Med* 1948; **41**: 559–68.

(31) Gill RC. *White water and black magic* London: Gollancz, 1941.

(32) Varney RF, Linegar CR, Haladay HA. The assay of curare by the rabbit 'head drop' method. *J Pharmac Exp Ther* 1949; **97**: 72–83.

(33) Bovet D, Depierre F, de Lestrange Y. Proprietes curarisantes des ethers phenoliques a

fonctions ammonium quaternaries. *C.r. hebd Seanc Acad Sci Paris* 1947; **225**: 74–6.

(34) Mushin WW, Wien R, Mason DFJ, Langston GT. Curare-like actions of tri-(diethylamino ethoxy)-benzene triethyl-iodide. *Lancet* 1949; **i**: 726–8.

(35) Barlow RB, Ing HR. Curare-like action of polymethylene bisquaternary ammonium salts. *Br J Pharmac Chemother* 1948; **3**: 289–304.

(36) Organe GSW, Paton WDM, Zaimis EJ. Preliminary trials of bistrimethylammonium decane and pentene diiodide (C10 and C5) in man. *Lancet* 1949; **i**: 21.

(37) Paton WDM. The pharmacology of decamethonium. *Ann NY Acad Sci* 1951; **54**: 347–61.

(38) Phillips AP. Synthetic curare substitutes from aliphatic dicarboxylic acid aminoethyl esters. *J Am Chem Soc* 1949; **71**: 3264.

(39) Bovet D, Bovet-Nitti F, Guarino S, Longo VG, Fusco R. Recherches sur les poisons curarisants de synthese. *Archs Int Pharmacodyn Ther* 1951; **88**: 1–50.

(40) Ottolenghi R, Manni C, Mazzoni P. New short-acting curarizing agent. *Anesth Analg Curr Res* 1952; **31**: 243–50.

(41) Thesleff S, von Dardel O, Holmberg G. Succinylcholine iodide. New muscular relaxant. *Br J Anaesth* 1952; **24**: 238–44.

(42) Collier HOJ, Paris SK, Woolf LI. Pharmacological activities in different rodent species of d-tubocurarine chloride and the dimethyl ether of d-tubocurarine iodide. *Nature (Lond)* 1948; **161**: 817–9.

(43) Frey R, Seeger R. Experimental and clinical experiences with toxiferine (alkaloid of calabash-curare). *Can Anaesth Soc J* 1961; **8**: 99–117.

(44) Waser PG, Harbeck P. Pharmacologie und klinische Anwendung des kurzdauernden Muskelrelaxans. Diallyl-nor-toxiferin. *Anaesthesist* 1962; **11**: 33–7.

(45) Lund I, Stovner J. Experimental and clinical experiences with a new muscle relaxant, Ro4-3816, diallyl-nor-toxiferine. *Acta Anaesth Scand* 1962; **6**: 85–97.

(46) Buckett WR, Howett CL, Savage DS. Potent steroidal neuromuscular blocking agents. *Chimie Therapeutique* 1967; **2**: 186.

(47) Buckett WR, Marjoribanks EB, Marwick FA, Morton MB. The pharmacology of pancuronium bromide (OrgNA97) a new steroidal neuromuscular blocking agent. *Br J Pharmac* 1968; **32**: 671–82.

(48) Baird WLM, Reid AM. The neuromuscular blocking properties of a new steroid compound, pancuronium bromide (a pilot study in man). *Br J Anaesth* 1967; **39**: 775–80.

(49) Buckett WR, Hewett CL, Savage DS. Pancuronium bromide and other steroidal neuromuscular blocking agents containing acetylcholine fragments. *J Med Chem* 1973; **16**: 1116–24.

(50) Savage DS, Sleight T, Carlyle I. The emergence of Org NC45, 1-[2β, 3α, 5α, 16β, 17β)-3,17-bis (acetyloxy)-2-(1-piperidinyl)-androstan-16-yl]-1-methylpiperidinium bromide, from the pancuronium series. *Br J Anaesth* 1980; **52**: 3S–9S.

(51) Durant NN, Marshall IG, Savage DS, Nelson DJ, Sleight T, Carlyle IC. The neuromuscular and autonomic blocking activities of pancuronium, Org NC45 and other pancuronium analogues in the cat. *J Pharm Pharmac* 1979; **31**: 831–6.

(52) Crul JF, Booij LHDJ. First clinical experience of Org NC45. *Br J Anaesth* 1980; **52**: 49S–52S.

(53) Stenlake JB. Biodegradable neuromuscular blocking agents. In: Stoclet JC, ed. *Advances in pharmacology and therapeutics*, Vol 3, *Ions-cyclic nucleotides-cholinergy*. Oxford: Pergamon Press 1978: 303–11.

(54) Hughes R, Chapple DJ. The pharmacology of atracurium: a new competitive neuromuscular blocking agent. *Br J Anaesth* 1981; **53**: 31–44.

(55) Payne JP, Hughes R. Evaluation of atracurium in anaesthetized man. *Br J Anaesth* 1981; **53**: 45–54.

(56) Alánt O, Darvas K, Pulay I. First clinical experience with a new neuromuscular blocker pipecuronium bromide. *Arzneimittelforsch* 1980; **20**: 374–9.

(57) Murray DJ, Mehta MP, Sokoll MD et al. The neuromuscular pharmacology of BW938U during isofluane anesthesia. *Anesth Analg* 1987; **66**: S126.

(58) Basta SJ, Savarese JJ, Ali HH et al. The neuromuscular pharmacology of BW1090U in anesthetized patients. *Anesthesiology* 1985; **63**: A318.

(59) Foldes FF. *Muscle relaxants in anesthesiology*. Springfield, Illinois: Thomas, 1957: 159.

12.2   The rapid onset and short duration of the history of fazadinium

C. E. BLOGG[1] and M. B. TYERS[2]

[1]Nuffield Department of Anaesthetics, Oxford University, and [2]Glaxo Group Research,
Ware Hertfordshire, UK

Neuromuscular blocking drugs were introduced into clinical practice by Griffith and Johnson in 1942 and popularized by Gray and Halton in 1945. In subsequent years other competitive neuromuscular blocking drugs joined d-tubocurarine in the anaesthetist's armamentarium and included gallamine (1940), alcuronium (1961) and pancuronium (1968). All were based on the traditional concept that two quaternary ammonium groups were required, ideally separated by 12–14 Å from each other to fit neatly onto the presumed configuration of the receptor at the neuromuscular junction. Even the most potent, pancuronium, had an onset of action too slow for rapid intubation under emergency conditions. The duration of action of each was too prolonged for use by continuous infusion and so resulted in cumulation and, in some instances, difficulty in reversal with anticholinesterases. It seemed impossible to approach the rapidity of onset and short duration of suxamethonium, which had multiple potential drawbacks. A rapid-acting, competitive agent, with short duration, rapid metabolism or excretion (and inactive metabolites) insignificant cardiovascular effects, no histamine release and no significant placental transfer was required to replace suxamethonium. In addition to the potential for such a drug to be used for rapid and brief neuromuscular block, prolonged block could be produced by infusion.

The search for new, competitive neuromuscular blocking drugs was actively pursued in the 1960s by various organizations including pharmaceutical companies, e.g. Burroughs Welcome (BW 403665), Glaxo (Dimethylconessine), Organon (Dacuronium), and others e.g., DD-188.

The discovery of fazadinium

The intervention of serendipity in drug discovery occurs more often than is sometimes apparent from subsequent rationalizations on molecular design. For fazadinium dibromide (AH8165) there is no doubt that serendipity played a major role in its discovery. As part of the collaborative venture in 1969 between the Chemistry Research Departments at Allen & Hanburys Ltd, Ware (AH), and at Teesside Polytechnic, a student was being sponsored to undertake studies for a PhD. Under arrangements of this type, the student and his supervisor pursue various chemical ideas, usually of their own choosing, and can submit the resulting compounds for biological evaluation at Allen & Hanburys. One such compound, AH7060, a tertiary heterocycle, was evaluated in a general screening procedure designed to detect several types of activity in the central nervous system. The compound appeared to be toxic in mice, but at lower doses, surviving animals had markedly depressed respiratory rate and within a few minutes these animals recovered to normal. The pharmacologist supervising the screening test suspected that AH7060 may have either central muscle relaxant activity or, more likely, a peripheral neuromuscular blocking action. Before the end of the same day, AH7060 had been evaluated in an anaesthetized cat and found, indeed, to have competitive neuromuscular blocking activity with a rapid onset. The mystery was that, for a tertiary heterocycle, this sort of activity was unknown; all previously described neuromuscular blocking drugs had quaternary nitrogen atoms as part of their molecular structure and even d-tubocurarine was only recently recognized to be monoquaternary. However, analysis of the chemical structure at both Teesside and Allen & Hanburys revealed that there had been an error in the initial structure determination and that AH 7060 was a bisquaternary molecule with an interonium distance of 7.48 Å (Fig. 1). Descriptions of the new structures crossed in the post between Ware and Teesside (1).

From the initial observations of experiments in animals, AH7060 appeared to fulfil the criteria of the ideal competitive neuromuscular blocking agent.

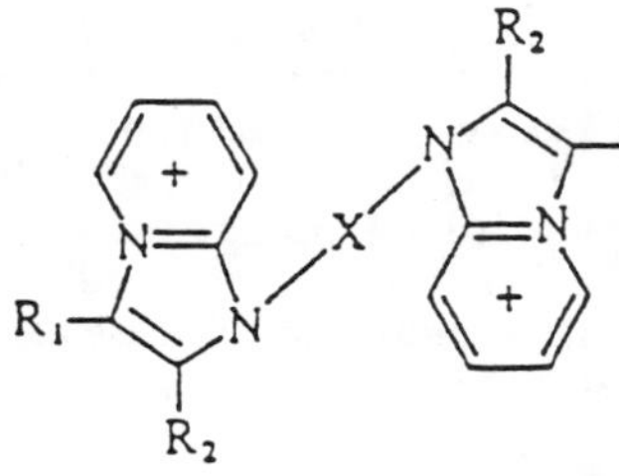

Figure 1   Chemical structure of AH7060
(R_1 = H; R_2 = Ph) and fazadinium (R_1 = CH_3; R_2 = Ph)

The chemists at Allen & Hanburys and Teesside embarked on a programme to synthesize a series of closely related azobisarylimidazo (1,2-a) pyridinium dihaides, chemical analogues of AH7060 (1,2). Pharmacological evaluation in the anaesthetized cat showed that these compounds were competitive neuromuscular blocking drugs which were rapid in onset and of short duration. Furthermore, muscle paralysis could be achieved without adverse changes to blood pressure or heart rate. Because of difficulties in the chemical synthesis of AH7060, a close analogue, AH8165, was chosen for development. This compound underwent exhaustive pharmacological, toxicological and clinical evaluations, and eventually became one of the muscle relaxants available to anaesthetists under the name of fazadinium dibromide (Fazadon).

Pharmacology

The pharmacological properties of fazadinium which lead to its clinical use and eventual demise are described below.

The neuromuscular blocking properties of fazadinium in the anaesthesized rat, cat, dog, cynomolgus monkey and marmoset have been described by several authors (3-9). In contrast to other competitive neuromuscular blocking drugs, the rate of onset of paralysis with fazadinium was particularly rapid even when compared with suxamethonium. Indeed a study carried out in the anaesthetized cat (10) to compare the time course of the circulation of an intravenous bolus of fazadinium with the onset of inhibition of twitches of the tibialis anterior muscle clearly shows that fazadinium achieved maximum neuromuscular block in its first circulation through the muscle.

Species variation in the duration of action of competitive neuromuscular blocking drugs is well known. Fazadinium is no exception, and the duration of paralysis in the cotton-eared marmoset is almost ten times greater than in the anaesthetized cat (3,11). Knowledge of the reasons for the termination of action of neuromuscular blocking drugs has important clinical implications. Renal and hepatic clearance of fazadinium appear not to be important, at least not in single doses, since in the anaesthetized cat with circulation occluded to either the liver or kidneys several single doses of the drug can be given without any indication of accumulation or prolonged paralysis (11). The rate limiting step for the termination of drug action appears not to be related to the rate at which fazadinium is cleared from the plasma but may be dependent on the rate at which fazadinium dissociates from the nicotinic receptors (10,12). Extensive metabolism of fazadinium does not occur (13) and is certainly insufficient to account for the duration of action.

The conclusions from these pharmacological studies were that although the duration of action of fazadinium appeared to be somewhat longer than was originally hoped, the rapid onset of paralysis was considered to be an important property for a new competitive (non-depolarizing) muscle relaxant drug. Such a drug could possibly obviate the use of suxamethonium in circumstances where rapid emergency intubation was indicated. In addition, the scientifically-illogical practice of using pretreating dose of non-depolarizing drug, then a depolarizing agent for intubation followed by a non-depolarizing agent to maintain paralysis may become a practice of the past.

The cardiovascular effects of competitive neuromuscular blocking drugs in anaesthetized animals are variable but generally quite mild. The most obvious changes result either from blockade of sympathetic ganglionic transmission or histamine release. In anaesthetized animals, unlike in man, both sympathetic and parasympathetic resting tone are very low. For fazadinium, experiments to evaluate its effect on sympathetic ganglia showed that, while high doses could block transmission, there was a good separation from those doses required to cause muscular paralysis (3). Plasma measurements of histamine levels in the cat, dog and eventually in man, showed that fazadinium had no propensity to release histamine (14). It is now well known that the vagal inhibitory effects of competitive neuromuscular blocking drugs cause tachycardias in humans as a result of reduced parasympathetic tone (15). The effects of these drugs on parasympathetic transmission can be evaluated against the bradycardias induced by electrical stimulation of the vagus nerve. Such vagolytic activity could be demonstrated for fazadinium in the anaesthetized cat and monkey at doses that produced neuromuscular blockade (3,7). This action is almost certainly by direct antagonism of atrial muscarinic receptors (16,17).

Preliminary studies in humans

The first studies in man were carried out after preliminary animal and toxicological studies on five volunteer anaesthetists from The London Hospital in late 1971. The isolated arm preparation modified by Feldman and Tyrell (18) from the description by Torda and Klonymus was used (19). One tenth of the dose predicted to produce total neuromuscular block was injected intravenously into an arm isolated from the systemic circulation by an arterial tourniquet. The onset of neuromuscular block was observed by recording the adductor pollicis muscle contraction in response to stimulation of the ulnar nerve at the wrist. After three minutes, the cuff was deflated when retrograde spread of the drug into the neuromuscular junction had been achieved. The block persisted when the tourniquet was released, indicating high affinity of the drug for the neuromuscular junction receptors even when the plasma level must have been very low. The only apparent side-effects were transient diplopia in two of the subjects. There was no pain or discomfort on injection and no local adverse effects.

Encouraged by the results of this study, Simpson and colleagues (20), then administered fazadinium to four patients, who had given informed consent, prior to undergoing elective surgery for which neuromuscular block was required.

The results showed a dramatic rapidity of onset of neuromuscular block with peak depression of response achieved in a mean time of 37.1s. Recovery was not as swift as had been predicted from animal studies. The properties of a competitive muscle relaxant (decreased twitch response, fade with tetanic stimulation, post tetanic facilitation and reversal with neostigmine) were confirmed. The cardiovascular system remained stable with no apparent change in blood pressure, cardiac rate or rhythm. Urgent submission of the data resulted in publication of the first study in man in the Lancet in March 1972 (20).

Meanwhile other investigators, notably Dundee and his colleagues in Belfast and Churchill-Davidson at St Thomas' Hospital in London were carrying out preliminary studies. Dundee and Young concentrated on the intubation characteristics of the drug whilst Blogg and colleagues (21) at The London Hospital set out to investigate the whole human pharmacology of fazadinium.

Churchill-Davidson (22) compared different doses of fazadinium on grip strength in conscious volunteers and found that 0.0625 mg/kg had no effect, 0.125 mg/kg produced 50% reduction in grip strength and 0.1825 mg/kg reduced grip strength to 30% of control values. The doses required for tracheal intubation (0.49 mg/kg–1.0 mg/kg) were thought by Churchill-Davidson to be too long acting with a range of 6–45 min. Despite this, others considered the rapidity of onset of AH8165 likely to be of great practical importance and offering advantages over the current competitive agents by approaching the rapidity of onset of paralysis to which anaesthetist who used suxamethonium were accustomed. The clinical studies were then extended, and are summarized.

Neuromuscular blocking potency

The potency of fazadon was compared to d-tubocurarine in cumulative dose-response studies (23). The patients were anaesthetized, intubated and ventilated to normocapnia before repeated small doses of either relaxant were given. The ratios of the mean doses of d-tubocurarine to fazadinium to produce 90% depression of adductor pollicis twitch response were 1.0:1.9 (23). The ratio was constant whether based on body weight, surface area or lean body mass and was subsequently confirmed by Hughes and colleagues (24). Hussain and colleagues (25) found the ratio of d-tubocurarine to fazadinium to be 1:1.25 when ED 80 doses were compared. It is interesting to note that these investigators suggested, from their experience, that the onset of action of d-tubocurarine could be accelerated by the use of divided doses—a concept subsequently propounded as the 'priming principle' (26,27).

Schuh (28) used a different rate of stimulation (0.2 Hz) in patients previously given suxamethonium before tracheal intubation, and also found the dose-response curves to be parallel, and the ratio 3:4, d-tubocurarine to fazadinium.

Onset of action

Onset of action of a neuromuscular blocking drug can be assessed clinically in various ways which have significant drawbacks. For instance, anatomical abnormalities may slow the time to achieving tracheal intubation. The use of peripheral nerve stimulation and measurement of the elicited electromyogram or muscle twitch response, although reproducible and apparently accurate, may provide information of dubious relevance to the needs of clinical anaesthesia.

Coleman *et al* (29) gave fazadinium 1.5 mg/kg through a central venous catheter to remove the influence of varying circulation times on the rapidity of onset of block measured mechanically in the forearm and face; there was complete abolition in 17 s (range 10–24 s) and 11 s (range 9–13 s) respectively. The speed of onset appeared to increase with larger doses and, in retrospect, this may be attributable to the increased cardiac output consequent on the vagolytic action of fazadinium. Hughes *et al* found (24) that the response to an intermittent tetanus indicated onset of action within two minutes with 0.4 mg/kg fazadinium, whereas when a slow twitch response was elicited, larger doses of at least 0.9 mg/kg were required.

Duration of action

The duration of action of fazadinium depends upon many factors, ranging from dose administered to the end point chosen for deciding that full recovery had been achieved. Clinical

Table 1

The duration of the neuromuscular blocking action of various doses of Fazadon in man as measured by return of muscle twitch response.

Parameter measured	Dose of Fazadon (mg/kg)	Mean duration (min)	Reference
Time to first sign of recovery of twitch (0.5 Hz)	0.25	8.7	Ungerer and Erasmus (1974)
	0.50	13.0	
	1.00	30.0	
Time to 10% recovery of twitch (0.5 Hz)	0.25	10.7	Kean (1975)
	0.50	41.6	
	0.75	49.3	
	1.00	79.4	
Time to 20% recovery of twitch (0.5 Hz)	0.25	13.8	Ungerer and Erasmus (1974)
	0.50	26.3	
	1.00	57.0	
Time to 90% recovery of twitch (2 Hz)	0.1	4.0	Schuh (1975)
	0.2	16.0	
	0.4	32.0	
	0.8	113.0	
Time to 100% recovery of twitch (2 Hz)	0.50	25.0	Blogg *et al* (1973)
	0.75	41.7	
	1.00	49.0	

methods lack the objectivity of mechanical or electromyographic measurement of responses to motor nerve stimulation. In Table 1 can be seen that the duration is dose-related and varied between investigators—for instance Schuh (28) found a mean duration to 90% recovery of 113 minutes following 0.8 mg/kg whereas Blogg *et al* (21) reported the duration from a larger dose (1.0 mg/kg) to complete recovery took a mean time of 49.0 minutes.

Reversal of neuromuscular blockade

Comparison of reversibility of neuromuscular blockade carries the same limitations due to variation methods as comparison of onset or duration of block. Blogg and colleagues (21,23) established equivalent neuromuscular block in 19 patients given increments of either fazadinium (nine patients) or d-tubocurarine (10 patients). When the twitch height had been reduced to 10% of control values, a further 25% of the drug was given. Exactly five minutes later, neostigmine 0.05 mg/kg was given intravenously and the recovery of twitch response was followed. The mean times to complete recovery were comparable following either drug (d-tubocurarine 5.3 min (SD 2.36 min), and fazadinium 4.4 min (SD 2.04 min). Schuh (28) used a smaller dose of neostigmine (0.02 mg/kg) and found that the rate of recovery was greater the more spontaneous recovery had already occurred and that reversal was possible within five minutes of the initial dose ranging from 0.1 mg–0.8 mg/g. Coleman *et al* (29) sounded a note of caution when the neuromuscular block in a patient who weighed 94 kg was difficult to reverse and advised that the dose of fazadinium be restricted to the order of 100 mg.

Repeated doses of fazadinium

A neuromuscular blocking agent which does not cumulate on repeated administration would be valuable during prolonged procedures since the duration of action would be predictable, rapidly reversible and it could be administered by continuous infusion. Schuh (28) and Bunodiere *et al* (30) showed that a much reduced second dose (0.14 mg/kg) of fazadinium would produce equivalent neuromuscular block to the initial dose of 0.75 mg/kg, reflecting a combination of cumulation and the effect of the drug occupying sufficient neuromuscular receptors sites to overcome the 'margin of safety' (31).

Cardiovascular effects

When the original study was extended in humans at The London Hospital (20) care was taken to remove the other factors likely to affect the cardiovascular system, so patients who were already anaesthetized, intubated, and in a stable cardiovascular state were given 0.5 mg/kg fazadinium (32) and in a second series (21) given atropine incrementally until the heart rate was restored to resting awake values, before fazadinium was administered. There was an immediate 30% increase in heart rate in the group who were not pre-treated with atropine, but in those to whom atropine had been given, the increase in mean heart rate was only 10%; indicating the vagal blocking effect of fazadinium at neuromuscular blocking doses. A larger dose of fazadinium was investigated (29) under similar conditions and the increase in mean heart rate was more dramatic at 58% and was associated with an increase in cardiac output of 38%.

Hughes *et al* (24) found similar changes in heart rate in a small series of patients and showed that incremental doses of fazadinium resulted in progressive increase in heart rate. They suggested that vagal blockade was occurring at subneuromuscular blocking doses, and subsequently demonstrated this phenomenon in animal experiments (9).

Histamine release

Preliminary studies in man found no clinical signs of histamine release (21), and laboratory measurement of plasma histamine levels by members of the Biochemistry Department of Allen & Hanbuys Ltd showed no consistent pattern of change in histamine values.

Fate in the body

Prior to the investigation of the action of fazadinium, information about the redistribution, metabolism and excretion of competitive muscle relaxants was mainly derived from animal studies. Tritium-labelled fazadinium was used in initial studies in man to elucidate the pharmacokinetics of the drug (21). There was a rapid decline in plasma level followed by a slower elimination phase. The majority of the drug was excreted unchanged in the urine (13). The pharmacokinetic data were confirmed using a fluorimetric method and showed the decrease of the plasma concentration to be more rapid than with other current non-depolarizing muscle relaxants (76 minutes for fazadinium, 132 minutes for pancuronium (33), 128 minutes for gallamine (34)). The amount of fazadinium excreted in the urine was similar to pancuronium, and was principally unchanged fazadinium. This pattern differed markedly from that seen in rats and rabbits in whom metabolism was the main route for excretion of the drug, whereas in man, fazidinium was almost entirely excreted in urine (35). The metabolites appeared more rapidly in animals than in the human, and it is thus possible that rapid metabolism accounted in part for the very brief duration of action in animals.

Duvaldestin and his colleagues (36) studied the pharmacokinetics of fazadinium in 14 patients in renal failure. They found the elimination half-life to be prolonged by 60% compared to patients with normal renal function. Despite this, the degree of prolongation of action of fazadinium was, on theoretical grounds, less than for other non-depolarizing muscle relaxants. There appeared to be a supplementary biliary pathway for excretion of fazadinium, and these factors probably accounted for the lack of prolongation of action of fazadinium in 10 patients in renal failure (37).

Duvaldestin and his colleagues (38) also studied the effects of fazadinium in patients who had either cirrhosis or total biliary obstruction. Little difference was found in the volume of distribution or elimination half-lives in patients with total biliary obstruction. By contrast, in patients suffering from cirrhosis prolongation of the elimination half-life and renal excretion did not compensate for the absence of hepatic excretion. They concluded that liver disease would have only little influence on the duration of fazadinium.

Intubation studies

The principal perceived advantage of fazadinium was its rapidity of onset. For the first time, a competitive drug became available which could produce conditions for emergency or rapid intubation without the hazards and disadvantages of suxamethonium (39). The dose of fazadinium appropriate for easy intubation is controversial. Schuh (28) used 0.4–0.6 mg/kg, Simpson et al (20) and Camu and colleagues (40) gave 0.5 mg/kg and reported no difficulties in intubation. Rowlands (31) used 0.76 mg/kg in an unselected series of 500 patients and found in more than 75% patients that intubating conditions were excellent or satisfactory in less than one minute. Other studies have shown that fazadinium 0.5 mg/kg produced better intubating conditions than pancuronium 0.1 mg/kg during the first 60 s after administration (42).

Hartley and Fidler (43) compared conditions for rapid intubation with fazadinium 1.0 and 1.25 mg/kg and suxamethonium 1 mg/kg and reported that fazadinium did not differ in times for rapid intubation from suxamethonium and may be a useful neuromuscular blocking agent in emergency cases. However, others (44) reported that suxamthonium 100 mg allowed intubation 6 s quicker than fazadinium 1.0 or 1.5 mg/kg and that suxamethonium 100 mg produced better intubating conditions. Arora and colleagues (45) pointed out the disadvantages of using traditional non-depolarizing drugs for rapid intubation since it is not possible to intubate in less than 120 s and found with fazadinium 21 of 26 patients became apnoeic in an average time of 38.8 s and could be intubated in 100 s or less—subsequent studies from Belfast, however, found that fazadinium 1.25 mg/kg was less satisfactory (46).

Duration and reversibility of action

Hopes that fazadinium would have a significantly shorter duration of action than other non-depolarizing muscle relaxants were not fulfilled. The duration was dose-related (20,47).

Doses of 0.5–0.67 mg/kg lasted approximately 30 minutes whereas a higher dose 0.75 mg/kg lasted approximately 40–50 minutes and 1.0 mg/kg persists for at least 60 minutes (21).

Most investigators found that the neuromuscular block from fazadinium was readily reversible with neostigmine, but several (29,44) found that reversal required repeated doses of neostigmine.

Use in obstetrics

Studies in animals showed that no significant placental transfer occurred (8). Placental transfer is unlikely because of the large molecular weight, ionization and lipid insolubility of fazadinium. Blogg and colleagues found in 10 patients undergoing elective Caesarian section that there was no clinically apparent transmission of fazadinium across the placenta and adequate intubation conditions were obtained (48,49). The placental transfer was also studied by estimating the total transfer of 3H—fazadinium to the fetus in early pregnancy when termination hysterectomy was carried out and amounted to approximately 0.008% and 0.005% of the maternal dose (48). The use of fazadinium was studied in patients undergoing emergency Caesarian section (50) and proved to be satisfactory for rapid intubation without adverse effects on the infant, however, a dramatic tachycardia (mean heart rate 29 patients 153 bpm) resulted on induction following 1.0 mg/kg fazadinium. A note of caution was expressed, however, by Jackson (51) about the dangers of failed intubation in obstetric patients when long-lasting neuromuscular block has been produced.

Other uses of fazadinium

Small doses of competitive neuromuscular blocking drugs given before an intubating dose of suxamethonium have been shown to reduce the potential adverse effects of hyperkalaemia, myalgia, increased intragastric or intra-ocular pressures. Fazadinium proved to be ineffective in preventing post-operative muscle pain from suxamethonium (52,53). Others have suggested that fazadinium can satisfactorily be used for ophthalmic anaesthesia without increase in intraocular pressure (54,55).

The recent history of fazadinium

Fazadinium was released for general clinical use in Britain in 1976 prepared as a solution containing 75 mg in a 5 ml ampoule. Although many anaesthetists used it, it disappointed on two main counts—the likely tachycardia and the unpredictability of perfect rapid intubating conditions. Sales slumped.

The advent of the new non-depolarizing neuromuscular blocking agents, atracurium and vecuronium which have an intermediate duration of action and minimal cardiovascular effects satisfied many of the needs of anaesthetists for which fazadinium had been developed. However, it is interesting to note that a derivative of fazadinium, AH10407 (56), was found to produce very rapid, very brief neuromuscular blockade due to rapid breakdown of the drug related to pH and temperature—some years in advance of similar principles being put to use in the design of atracurium!

The place of fazadinium in the history of anaesthesia

Fazadinium provided a major stimulus in interest in the development of neuromuscular blocking drugs in the 1970s, destroyed some of the strongly held concepts (for instance that two quaternary ammonium groups at 12.5 Å were needed and rapid onset of non-depolarizing blockade was impossible). The brief history of fazadinium has left a dynasty of investigators of many aspects of neuromuscular blockade who were poised and practiced ready for the investigation and development of subsequent, more successful drugs.

Acknowledgments

Our gratitude is due Miss R. Vincent for her deep interest in the history and preparation of this manuscript.

References

(1) Glover EE, Yorke M. *J Chem Soc* 1971; (C) 3280.

(2) Bishop DC, Glover EE, Rowbottom KT. 1972 JCS Perkin I, 2927.

(3) Brittain RT, Tyers MB. The pharmacology of AH8165: a rapid-acting, short-lasting, competitive neuromuscular blocking drug. *Br J Anaesth* 1973; **45**: 837–43.

(4) Bolger L, Brittain RT, Jack D *et al*. Short lasting competitive neuromuscular blocking activity in a series of azobisarylimidazo-(1,2-a)-pyridinium dihalides. *Nature* 1972; **338**: 254–5.

(5) Bouyard P, Mesdjian E, Balansard P, Gastant JA, Jadot G. Pharmacologie du dibromure de 1-l'azo'bis-3-methyl-2-phenyl-1H-imidaZo-(1,2-a) pyridinium, AH8165, nouveau curarimimetic. *Ann Anaesthesiol Fr* 1973; **XIV**: 397–403.

(6) Marshall IG. The effects of three short-acting neuromuscular blocking agents on fast and slow-contracting muscles of the cat. *Eur J Pharmacol* 1973; **21**: 299–304.

(7) Marshall IG. The ganglion blocking and vagolytic actions of three short-acting neuromuscular blocking drugs in the cat. *J Pharm Pharmacol* 1973; **25**: 530–6.

(8) Tyers MB. Pharmacological studies on new, short-lasting competitive neuromuscular blocking drugs. PhD thesis (CNAA).

(9) Hughes R, Chapple DJ. Effects of non-depolarising neuromuscular blocking agents on peripheral autonomic mechanisms in cats. *Br J Anaesth* 1976; **48**: 59–68.

(10) Tyers MB. Factors limiting the rate of termination of the neuromuscular blocking action of fazadinium dibromide. *Br J Pharmacol* 1978; **63**: 287–93.

(11) Tyers MB. Fazadinium Dibromide. In *Neuromuscular blocking agents. Handbook of experimental pharmacology*, Berlin: Springer-Verlag, 1986: 629–36.

(12) Hashimoto Y, Shima T, Matsukawa S, Satou M. Neuromuscular blocking potency of fazadinium in man. *Anaesthesia* 1979; **34**: 10–3.

(13) Blogg CE, Simpson BR, Martin LE, Bell JA. Metabolism of 3H-AH8165 in man. *Br J Anaesth* 1973; **45**: 1233–4.

(14) Martin LE, Harrison C. An automated fluorometric method for the determination of histamine in biological samples. *Biochem Med* 1973; **8**: 292–308.

(15) Kelman GR, Kennedy BR. Cardiovascular effects of pancuronium in man. *Br J Anaesth* 1971; **43**: 335–8.

(16) Marshall RJ, Ojewole JAO. Comparison of the autonomic effects of some currently used neuromuscular blocking agents. *Br J Pharmacol* 1979; **66**: 77P.

(17) Dalton D, Tyers MB. The selective muscarinic antagonist actions of pancuronium and alcuronium. *Br J Pharmacol* 1981; **74**: 784P.

(18) Feldman SA, Tyrrell MF. A new theory of the termination of action of the muscle relaxants. *Proc Roy Soc Med* 1970; **63**: 692–5.

(19) Torda TAG, Klonymus DH. The regional use of muscle relaxants. *Anesthesiology* 1966; **27**: 689–90.

(20) Simpson BR, Strunin L, Savege TM *et al*. An azo-bis-arylimidazo-pyridinium derivative: a rapidly acting non-depolarizing muscle relaxant. *Lancet* 1972; **i**: 516–9.

(21) Blogg CE, Savege TM, Simpson JC, Ross LA, Simpson BR. A new muscle relaxant AH8165. *Proc Roy Soc Med* 1973; **66**: 1023–7.

(22) Churchill-Davidson HC. A philosophy of relaxation: 11th Annual Baxter-Travenol Lecture. *Curr Res Anesth Analg* 1973; **52**: 495–501.

(23) Buckley FP, Blogg CE, Simpson BR, Savege TM. A comparison of dose-response curves and reversibility of d-tubocurarine and AH8165. Paper presented at the *IV Eur Cong Anaesthesiologists*, Madrid, 1974.

(24) Hughes R, Payne JP, Sugai N. Studies on fazadinium bromide (AH8165): A new non-depolarizing neuromuscular blocking agent. *Can Anaesth Soc J* 1976; **23**: 36–47.

(25) Hussain SZ, Healy TEJ, Birmingham AT. Comparative potency and speed of onset of fazadinium and d-tubocurarine. *Acta Anaesth Scand* 1979; **23**: 331–5.

(26) Schwartz S, Ilias W, Lackner F, Mayrhofer O, Foldes FF. Rapid tracheal intubation with vecuronium: The priming principle. *Anesthesiology* 1985; **63**: 338–91.

(27) Foldes FF. Rapid tracheal intubation with non-depolarising neuromuscular blocking drugs: The priming principle. *Br J Anaesth* 1984; **56**: 663.

(28) Schuh FT. Clinical neuromuscular pharmacology of AH8165D, an azo-bis-arylimidazo-pyridinium compound. *Anaesthetist* 1975; **24**: 151–6.

(29) Coleman AJ, O'Brien A, Downing JW, Jeal PE, Moyes DG, Leary WP. AH8165: A new non-depolarizing muscle relaxant. *Anaesthesia* 1973; **28**: 262–7.

(30) Bunodiere M, Deligne P, Sicard JF, Goussard D. Etude electromyographique preliminaire d'un nouveau curarisant, derive de l'azo-bis-arylimidazo-(1,2a)-pyridinium (AH8165). *Ann Anesthesiol Fr* 1973; **14**: 418–23.

(31) Waud BE. Kinetic analysis of the AH8165-receptor interaction at the mammalian neuromuscular junction. *Anesthesiology* 1977; **46**: 94–6.

(32) Savege TM, Blogg CE, Ross L, Lang M, Simpson BR. The cardiovascular effects of AH8165, a new non-depolarizing muscle relaxant. *Anaesthesia* 1973; **28**: 253–61.

(33) Somogyi AA, Shanks CA, Triggs EJ. Clinical pharmacokinetics of pancuronium bromide. *Eur J Clin Pharm* 1976; **10**: 367.

(34) Feldman SA, Cohen EN, Golling RC. The excretion of gallamine in the dog. *Anesthesiology* 1969; **30**: 593.

(35) Bell JA, Martin LE. The metabolism of fazadinium bromide. *Proc Brit Pharm Soc* 1979; 443P.

(36) Duvaldestin P, Bertrand JC, Concina D, Henzel D, Lareng L, Desmonts JM. Pharmacokinetics of fazadinium in patients with renal failure. *Br J Anaesth* 1979; **51**: 943–7.

(37) Camu F, D'Hollander A. Neuromuscular blockade of fazadinium bromide (AH8165) in renal failure patients. *Acta Anaesth Scand* 1978; **22**: 221–6.

(38) Duvaldestin P, Sasada J, Henzel D, Saumon G. Fazadinium pharmacokinetics in patients with liver disease. *Br J Anaesth* 1980; **52**: 789–94.

(39) Gibbs DB. Suxamethonium. A review. Part II Neuromuscular blocking properties. *Anaesth Intens Care* 1973; **1**: 183–200.

(40) Camu F, Sanders M, D'Hollander A. A comparative evaluation of neuromuscular blockade and reversibility of AH8165 and pancuronium bromide in man. *Acta Anaesth Belg* 1976; **27** (Suppl): 80–5.

(41) Rowlands DE. Fazadinium in anaesthesia. *Br J Anaesth* 1978; **50**: 289–93.

(42) Corrall IM, Ward ME, Page J, Strunin L. Conditions for tracheal intubation following fazadinium and pancuronium. *Br J Anaesth* 1977; **49**: 615–7.

(43) Hartley JMF, Fidler K. Rapid intubation with fazadinium; a comparison of fazadinium with suxamethonium and alcuronium. *Anaesthesia* 1977; **32**: 14–20.

(44) Mehta S, Lewin K, Fidler K. Rapid intubation with fazadinium and suxamethonium. *Can Anaesth Soc J* 1977; **24**; 270–3.

(45) Arora MV, Clarke, RSJ, Dundee JW, Moore J. Initial clinical experience with AH8165D, a new rapidly acting non-depolarizing muscle relaxant. *Anaesthesia* 1973; **28**: 188–96.

(46) Young HSA, Clarke RSJ, Dundee JW. Intubation conditions with AH8165 and suxamethonium. *Anaesthesia* 1975; **30**: 30–3.

(47) Inoue K, Erdmann W, Stegbauer HP, Frey R. Klinische erfahrungen mit einen neuen muskelelaxans Fazadon-ein azobis-arylimidazo-pyridinium derivatives. *Munch med Wschr* 1974; **116**: 1839–44.

(48) Blogg CE, Simpson BR, Tyers MB, *et al*. Placental transfer of AH8165. *Br J Anaesth* 1973; **45**: 1233–4.

(49) Blogg CE, Simpson BR, Tyers MB, Martini LE, Bell JA. Human placental transfer of AH8165. *Anaesthesia* 1975; **30**: 23–9.
(50) Cane RD, Sinclair DM. The use of AH8165 for Caesarian section. *Anaesthesia* 1976; **31**: 313–4.
(51) Jackson DM. Rapid intubation with fazadinium. *Anaesthesia* 1977; **32**: 668.
(52) Bennetts FE, Khalil KI. Reduction of post-suxamethonium pain by pretreatment with four non-depolarizing agents. *Br J Anaesth* 1981; **53**: 531–6.
(53) Budd AJ, Scott RPF, Blogg CE, Goat VA. Adverse effects of suxamethonium. Failure of prevention by atracurium or fazadinium. *Anaesthesia* 1985; **40**: 642–6.
(54) Couch JA, Eltringham RJ, Margauran DM. The effect of thiopentone and fazadinium on intraocular pressure. *Anaesthesia* 1979; **34**: 586–90.
(55) Tattersall MP, Manus NJ, Jackson DM. The effect of atracurium or fazadinium on intraocular pressure. A comparative study during induction of general anaesthesia. *Anaesthesia* 1985; **40**: 805–7.
(56) Blogg CE, Brittain RT, Simpson BR, Tyers MB. AH10407—A novel, short-acting, competitive neuromuscular blocking drug in animals and man. *Br J Pharm* 1975; **53**: 446P.

13.1   Cocaine intoxication

JOHN E. STEINHAUS

Emory University, Atlanta, Georgia, USA

The highly publicized death due to cocaine abuse of a very talented young basketball player in Maryland this past year revealed a serious lack of medical and scientific knowledge, as well as reminding us of the significantly ambivalent feelings exhibited by the medical profession in addressing the adverse and injurious reaction of our favourite drugs or treatments. Toxicity from drug abuse and that from clinical usage is often compartmentalized as though dealing with different drugs. It even extends to medical specialties as illustrated in adoption of lignocaine by cardiologists as an antiarrhythmic with little or no consideration of the accumulated knowledge of this drug by anaesthetists.

Coca leaf chewing by South American Indians for the extraction of cocaine and its resultant central nervous system effects is reputed to be 5000 years old (1). Its early introduction into Europe in the 16th century produced limited interest due, in part, to the loss of potency of the cocaine in the drying and transport of the coca leaves. With isolation and characterization of the active principle cocaine in 1859 by Nieman, cocaine joined the growing groups of natural alkaloids that were applied empirically as therapeutic principles to many conditions and diseases. An excellent account of the introduction of cocaine as a local analgesic has been published by Fink (2), but it is of interest that no mention is made of the down side of the therapeutic equation (toxicity) for this drug. In the last half of the 19th century pharmacology was a newly developing biomedical science, in France under Magendi and his famous pupil Bernard, and in Germany under Buchheim and his famous pupil Schmiedeberg (3).

Notwithstanding these developments, much medical therapy was highly and uncritically empirical. Warner (4) describes changes in therapeutics during the 19th century from a holistic approach which attempted to restore the natural balance of nature to one based on the correction of an abnormal physiological process. In the list of therapies at the Massachusetts General Hospital for the year 1880, the most common treatment was morphine (or an opium containing medicine) with substantial use of ethyl alcohol, bromides, quinine and salicylates. Also listed but showing steady decrease from earlier decades were cupping, leeching and venesection. Older physicians still exhorted their colleagues to 'observe the patient' instead of being concerned by 'some unseen germ' or 'chemical or physiological speculations'.

Mortimer's monograph 1901

In 1901, a book of some 600 pages by Mortimer (5) was published in New York entitled *History of Coca—The Divine Plant of the Incas* which cited over 700 references. He reports that the library of the Surgeon General of the United States Army catalogued over 2000 publications on cocaine between 1885–1898. This author claims that the central nervous system stimulation of the drug is due to a direct action on cells which stimulate the cell, setting free energy which builds new tissue and protoplasm. It was also stated that cocaine has the property of freeing blood from wastes. The stimulation which was thought to generate 'vital force', was recommended for heart failure (replacing digitalis), as well as the treatment of opium addiction, eczema, herpes, dropsy, and debilitating fever. One concluding statement, 'Coca simply makes better blood and a healthy blood makes healthy tissue' illustrates a common medical opinion of cocaine at the turn of the century.

Although Mortimer's (5) monograph extols the beneficial action of cocaine and depreciates its toxic effects with a statement 'coca poisoning and addiction often sensationally reported are open to grave doubts', he further reports the toxic and lethal reactions of cocaine as convulsions, prostration, dyspnoea and rigor mortis of respiratory muscles.

For the treatment for cocaine toxicity he suggests stimulants may be needed including amyl nitrite, ammonia, and hypodermic ether. It is further recommended that chloroform or chloral may be given to treat the spasm of respiratory muscles and 'even artificial respiration may be indicated'. After severe symptoms were passed, chloral and morphine were considered to be effective antagonists of cocaine.

In Koller's (7) historical notes published some 40 years after his first usage of cocaine as a topical local analgesic, he is greatly impressed with cocaine's merits, but makes only a brief note of its occasional poisonous effects. William Halsted, the noted Baltimore surgeon, is usually credited with the first use of cocaine for nerve block. In Halsted's (8) early paper, he finds no contraindication to its use nor gives any precaution.

Coca Cola—a connection with Crawford Long

An interesting side note by Wilson (6) is the account of cocaine and Coca Cola. Joseph Jacobs was an apprentice pharmacist in Crawford W. Long's pharmacy in Athens, Georgia, where one of his duties was the preparation of soda water for the new fountain with its several 'tonics'. Some years later in Atlanta, a pharmacist, Dr John Penberton, created a tonic consisting of the extracts of coca leaf and Kola nut. The fountain in Jacob's store was leased to Willie Venable, a relative of James Venable, Crawford W. Long's first patient. The new tonic was carbonated at the suggestion of Venable in an arrangement with Pemberton. The commercial success of Coca Cola occurred after Asa Candler, another Atlanta pharmacist, purchased control of this carbonated beverage and changed the Kola to Cola and hence, the highly successful trade name Coca Cola. Cocaine was removed from the base syrup in 1906 but many natives continued to refer to a 'dope' instead of a Coke. In its early days, Coke was strictly an item from the soda fountain at the pharmacy and not clearly differentiated from tonics and medicinals.

Early scientific studies

Basic medical science was developing rapidly in the latter half of the 19th century. Anrep studied the effect of cocaine on respiration in 1880. This study, and numerous studies which followed, showed the depressant action of local anaesthetics on both circulation and respiration (9). In their review, Hirschfelder and Bieter (10) give an extensive account of the early studies which clearly characterize the systemic actions of cocaine and other local analgesic agents. Allowing for species variation, the serious depressant action on respiration and circulation for large doses of local analgesic drugs were consistently identified. Mortimer (5) reported these adverse effects but did not give proper emphasis to these deleterious pharmacological effects.

Investigations of abuse, misuse and toxicity

Parallel to medical use of cocaine was its increasing abuse as a mind altering drug. The first decade of the 20th century saw a culmination of public reaction to the abuse and overuse of narcotics and cocaine and led to the passage of the Harrison Narcotic Act in the US in 1914.

Medical usage of anaesthetic drugs never expands independently but follows, in part, the demand created by the growth of surgical procedures. In 1901, there were some 300 surgical procedures carried out at the Massachusetts General Hospital. The great development of the basic sciences in the late 19th century were followed in the 20th century by the rapid growth and expansion of surgery. Demand of pain relief led to a rapid increase in the use of anaesthetic drugs including cocaine. Knowledge and judicious use of potent drugs was found in only a few physicians; consequently, the opportunities for errors and fatal reaction were magnified. In the US, Flexner had conducted his study of some 500 medical schools in this first decade. Only a few of these schools, less than 75, provided a reasonable medical education at that time. Hence, the education of many physicians was substandard.

Eggleston and Hatcher (11), pharmacologists in New York, investigated the pharmacology of cocaine because of the increasing number of serious and fatal episodes in man. As a consequence of their studies, they emphasized the importance of absorption and elimination, of the local analgesic drug as it relates to toxicity and the use of adrenaline to reduce spread and systemic uptake. They also reported the value of artificial respiration in the treatment of these episodes. In Sollmann's (12) section on local analgesics in his *Manual of Pharmacology* in 1920, he points out the uncertainty about rate of absorption as a cause of toxicity for local analgesics; however, his recommendations for the treatment of toxic reactions included caffeine, ammonia and sinapism, treatments without medical merit. Artificial respiration is mentioned but not given any emphasis.

As pharmacologists showed increasing interest in the toxic or untoward actions of drugs, in this case, cocaine, the concept of Therapeutic Coefficient instituted by Ehrlich became a point of interest. Toxicity became a serious component in the measure of a drug's usefulness. The original concept was a comparison of the minimal doses producing therapeutic action to the minimal dose producing toxic effects. Later it was pointed out that only the mid point of a distribution curve of doses could be defined with accuracy (13), consequently, the introduction of the ED_{50} and the LD_{50}.

The recognition by the American medical community of a growing crisis due to the fatalities from cocaine and other local analgesic reactions led to the formation of a Therapeutic Research Committee of Council of Pharmacy and Chemistry of the American Medical Association for the study of those toxic reactions (14). Under the leadership of Dr Sollmann, the Section on Laryngology, Otology and Rhinology collected reports of some 48 deaths. These cases were analysed by the special committee chaired by Dr Emil Mayer consisting of both clinicians and pharmacologists, including Dr Robert Hatcher. Reports of 43 fatalities were studied in detail and it was concluded that 40 were due to the local analgesic drugs. Although cocaine was the offending agent in over 50% of the cases, all local analgesics were reported to be involved with deaths. In a series of some 20 fatalities in surgery for tonsillectomy, cocaine was used in concentrations of 10–20% applied topically often with additional local drug injected. The dosage of cocaine utilized was seldom recorded with any accuracy. Cocaine paste, a mixture of cocaine powder and adrenaline was implicated in two of the cases.

Treatment of toxicity

The committee concluded that morphine and ether had no place in the treatment of these toxic episodes. Calcium was considered as a treatment but it was not recommended. Cardiac massage and artificial respiration were recommended as probably the best means of treatment. The use of intracardiac adrenaline, or digitalis preparations were thought to be of limited use.

The pharmacologists, who recommended artificial respiration in earlier studies, usually had animals with cannulas in their tracheas for recording respiration and consequently had no difficulty in providing artificial respiration. In this study of 43 fatalities, artificial respiration was applied to 11 patients and the pulmotor to four. The level of understanding and practice of artificial respiration during the 1920s leads to significant doubts as to the likelihood of successful ventilation. Likewise, cardiac massage in an animal is a very different therapy from cardiac massage in man. It should be noted that internal cardiac massage did not appear commonly in medicine until after World War II and external massage even later. Here again is a correct but unlikely practical therapy at that time.

It is also interesting to note that in the discussion of the deaths of patients, status thymicolymphaticus was considered to be a serious factor. An additional point of interest was that *no cases* were attributed to allergy or hypersensitivity. The 'caine reaction' had not yet been raised as a serious contender as the cause of these reactions. Discussion regarding dosage and its related problems of high concentration were suggested to be a serious problem but the committee in 1924 made no definite recommendation as to dosage or its control.

The report of the Mayer committee further raised the level of medical attention to toxic reactions to local analgesic drugs. One of their specific recommendations, that cocaine be not injected subcutaneously is not supported by their case reports since only 5 cases out of 43 were listed as involving injections and two of these had gross overdose due to mistakes.

Nonetheless, this recommendation carried great weight and cocaine essentially disappeared as an injectable local drug. A series of some 30 000 cocaine administrations for tonsillectomy, including injection, with only 3 deaths were reported from the University of Michigan (15), which suggests that careful usage of cocaine is reasonably safe and that cocaine was probably 'tarred' with the brush of bad usage.

The concern and interest in the problem of cocaine 'toxicity' in the 1920s led to a number of pharmacological studies directed toward both treatment and prevention. Tatum and coworkers (16) reported that artificial respiration markedly increased the minimal fatal dose of cocaine in rabbits but not in dogs. The unusual enzymes possessed by the rabbit hydrolyzes cocaine and illustrates a difficulty in the direct transfer of the results from animal studies to a given drug effect in man. These workers also utilized dogs and later monkeys to minimize the species difference. Tatum and coworkers (17) later reported that fatal doses of cocaine could be increased (decreased toxicity) in both animal species if barbitone was given in amounts sufficient to control the convulsions. This research led to the common practice of treating toxic reactions with barbiturates. A further extension of this therapy was the administration of preanaesthetic doses of barbitone and phenobaritone to prevent toxic reactions to cocaine and other local agents. The above studies by Tatum did not address this point but even so the practice of barbiturates for local analgesia premedication became standard. Later research from his laboratory (18) showed no benefit from these smaller doses.

New agents

The other approach to reducing the problem of cocaine toxicity was the introduction of numerous new local drugs almost all of which were claimed to have lower toxicity than cocaine. Unfortunately, deaths continued to occur with these new drugs and some of the more potent local analgesic agents such as cinchocaine (Nupercaine, Dibucaine) were considerably more toxic than cocaine. There is much evidence to suggest that the inherent toxicity of cocaine contributed less to the serious reactions and deaths than the misuse and ignorance attending cocaine's administration. New local analgesic drugs usually have the advantages of the experience, learned the hard way, that was accumulated from the errors and omissions occurring with the use of the first local agent.

Studies of possible allergy

The increasing awareness of the toxic reaction of local analgesic drugs led to an association with a parallel medical problem that was attracting much attention, namely allergy or hypersensitivity. In the second and third decades, there was increasing investigation and study of this troublesome immune response. Among allergens noted were some drugs. The sudden and unexpected nature of local analgesic toxic reaction, at least to the physician using these drugs, together with the lack of accurate data as to dosage or technique attracted the attention of allergists to this problem. Waldbott's (19) early publication in 1935 reported both local and general agents, namely cocaine and ether, as the cause of allergic shock or 'hives of the lung'. He further speculated that spinal analgesia would also provide allergic reaction including vascular collapse and respiratory arrest. Based on case reports of variable types and less than solid information, the problem of allergic reaction to local analgesic drugs persists in the literature (20) without solid evidence. Even so, many hospitals today use special markings on patients' charts having a 'caine reaction'. A similar equally doubtful practice today is that of associating nausea and vomiting as an allergic manifestation of codeine and its related drugs. On the other hand, millions of patients have received local analgesia in the last 50 years and there are almost no instances of repeatable and verifiable allergic reactions except for skin reactions in dentists. In contrast, there are serious problems with the antibiotics and lesser but well documented allergic phenomena with anaesthetic drugs such as narcotics, muscle relaxants, and even thiopentone.

As mentioned previously, the 1924 study of local analgesic drugs did not mention allergy as a cause. It did, however, list status thymicolymphaticus as an explanation of death, a term that has just about disappeared in recent years. Sudden deaths that are unexpected usually occur without good circumstances for collecting data. The concern and guilt of the medical personnel makes recollection a questionable source of reliable data. The pressure on physicians to meet present standards of practice make it difficult for all but the most courageous to admit error, mistakes or lack of knowledge as the cause of serious mishaps. Consequently, the physician is comfortable in explaining the episode with drugs as a sensitivity, hypersensitivity, allergy or idiosyncracy. On the other hand, although we have increasing knowledge and understanding of therapy and treatment today, we still encounter episodes that cannot be explained with certainty based on the data available, even by our most experienced and knowledgeable physicians.

Present day attitudes to toxicity

As the specialty of anaesthesiology grew after the Second World War, anaesthetists became especially interested in the problem of toxic reactions to local analgesic drugs. It was recognized the type of the toxic reaction varied and that this could be related to dose, rate of absorption, distribution and elimination of the drugs (21,22,23). The unintentional intravenous injection of local agents provided the best explanation of the sudden reaction. Dosage related to the size of patient and the vascularity of the absorbing bed became recognized as critical features in production of high blood level concentrations of these drugs. The intravenous use of lignocaine as an antiarrhythmic led to pharmaco-dynamic studies and knowledge that made rational explanations of toxic reactions common place.

It is of interest that the more recent reports of bupivacaine toxicity have caused so much discussion. Basic to the problem is the tendency to conclude that new drugs are more effective and less toxic than they really are. It appears that as physicians we emphasize the positive and depreciate the negative until experience teaches us that the truth lies somewhere below our hopes and expectations.

History repeats itself

Although drug abuse problems of cocaine has been mentioned only in passing in this discourse, the epidemic of cocaine abuse and the consequent deaths suggest that we have come full circle (24,25). Whether cocaine is given as a topical analgesic for nasal surgery and bronchoscopy or abused by smoking crack or snorting powder, the drug action in central nervous and circulatory systems are the same for a given blood concentration. The drug abuse problem is complicated by various adulterating chemicals and other drugs (often lignocaine), or the abuse combinations including narcotics or other depressants. Despite the medical examiner's report of fatal heart attack in the Baltimore case, the more complete evidence indicates a familiar story of convulsions, respiratory depression, obstruction and death. History does repeat itself and we in medicine are not exempt.

REFERENCES

(1) Van Dyke C, Byck R. Cocaine. *Scientific American* 1982; **246**: 128–141.
(2) Fink BR. Leaves and needles: the introduction of surgical local anaesthesia. *Anesthesiology* 1985; **63**: 77–83.
(3) Leake CD. *An historical account of pharmacology to the twentieth century.* Springfield, Illinois: Thomas, 1975: 140–70.
(4) Warner JH. *Therapeutic perspective* Cambridge: Harvard Press, 1986: 120–35.
(5) Mortimer WG. *Peru, history of coca.* New York: JH Vail & Company, 1901: 400–35.
(6) Wilson RC. *Drugs and pharmacy in life of Georgia.* Atlanta: Foote & Davis, 1959: 219–29.
(7) Koller C. Historical notes on the beginning of local anesthesia. 1928: *JAMA* **90** 1742–3.
(8) Halstead WS. Practical comments on the abuse of cocaine. *NY Med J* 1885; **42**: 294–5.

(9) Mannheim PU. Ueber das Cocain und seine Gefahren in physiologischer, toxikologischer und therapeutischer Beziehung. *Zeit F Klin Med* 1891; **18**: 380–416.

(10) Hirschfelder AD, Bieter RN. Local anesthetics. *Physiol Rev* 1932; **12**: 190–280.

(11) Eggleston C, Hatcher RA. A further contribution to the pharmacology of the local anesthetics. *J Pharmacol Exp Ther* 1916; **13**: 433.

(12) Sollman T. *Manual of pharmacology*. Philadelphia: W B Saunders, 1920.

(13) Wilson A, Schild HO. *Clark's applied pharmacology*. Philadelphia: Blakiston, 1952: 573–4.

(14) Mayer E. The toxic effects following the use of local anesthetics. *JAMA* 1928; **82**: 876–85.

(15) Furstenburg AC, Wood LA, Magielski JE, McMahon GF. An evaluation of cocaine anesthesia. *Tr Am Acad Ophth* 1951; **55**: 643–50.

(16) Tatum AL, Atkinson AJ, Collins KH. Acute cocaine poisoning, its prophylaxis and treatment in laboratory animals. *J Pharmacol Exp Ther* 1925; **26**: 325–35.

(17) Tatum AL, Collins KH. Acute cocaine poisoning and its treatment in the monkey (Macacus Rhesus). *Arch Intern Med* 1926; **38**: 405–409.

(18) Steinhaus JE, Tatum AL. An experimental study of cocaine intoxication and its treatment. *J Pharmacol Exp Ther* 1950; **100**: 351–61.

(19) Waldbott GL. Allergic shock from local and general anesthetics. *Anesth Analg* 1935; **14**: 199–205.

(20) Criep LH, Ribeiro C. Allergy to procaine hydrochloride with three fatalities. *JAMA* 1953; **151**: 1185–87.

(21) Steinhaus JE. A comparative study of the experimental toxicity of local anesthetic agents. *Anesthesiology* 1952; **13**: 577–86.

(22) Steinhaus JE. Local anesthetic toxicity: a pharmacological re-evaluation. *Anesthesiology* 1957; **18**: 275–81.

(23) Campbell D, Adriani J. Absorption of local anesthetics. *JAMA* 1958; **168**: 873–7.

(24) Wetli CV, Wright RK. Death caused by recreational cocaine use. *JAMA* 1979; **241**: 2519–22.

(25) Musto DF. Lessons of the first cocaine epidemic. *Wall Street Journal*, 1986, June 11.

13.2   The history of morphine analysis

K. G. QUINN and G. R. PARK
Addenbrookes Hospital, University of Cambridge, UK

The biotransformation of morphine has been unravelled in man in the past 10–15 years as the result of the advent of more sensitive analytical techniques. The basic principles of chromatography were clearly stated by Martin and Synge in 1941 (1). This led to the development in the early 1950s of the first gas chromatograph. Gas chromatography as a technique for the analysis of morphine only became possible with the development of capillary columns and more sensitive detectors, e.g. electron-capture detector (ECD).

The technique of high performance liquid chromatography (HPLC) was introduced by Horvath and Lipsky, Huber and Kirkland (2) who developed high pressure systems using small particle pellicular packing materials with constant monitoring of the eluate. This allowed the measurement of drugs in biological fluids (Table 1).

Radioimmunoassay

Radioimmunoassay (RIA), as its name implies, is an analytical method that invokes the combined disciplines of both chemistry and immunology. Since the first radioimmunoassay,

Table 1

Important events in the history of morphine analysis

Investigator	Event	Year
Martin and James	Theory of partition chromatography	1941
Martin, James and Synge	Development of GLC	1951
Yallow and Berson	Development of RIA	1957
Horvath, Huber, Lipsky and Kirkland	Development of HPLC	1967
Spector *et al.*	First RIA for morphine	1971
Dahlstrom *et al.*	GLC for morphine	1975
Rane, Sawe and Svensson	HPLC for morphine and its glucuronides	1984

for insulin, was reported in 1957, the technique has been used to measure a wide variety of both endogeneous and exogenous compounds in biological fluids in low concentrations (pgs/ml).

The ability to monitor morphine concentrations at pharmacological doses (e.g. 0.14 mg/kg) in man has been a recent event since the RIA was introduced for morphine analysis by Spector *et al.* in 1971 (3). Assays with sufficient sensitivity to determine therapeutic concentrations of morphine (at ng/ml) in biological fluids use RIA (3), spectrofluorometric (19,20), HPLC (21–25), GLC (26–30) and TLC (31) techniques.

RIA techniques are exquisitely sensitive (50 pgs) but suffer from lack of specificity by measuring metabolites and morphine analogues. Dependant upon the site of conjugation with bovine serum albumin to make morphine immunogenic, the major metabolite morphine-3-glucuronide can have a potency of between 1% to 100% of the parent compound in displacing radiolabelled ligand from the antibody binding site.

GLC assays with detection limits low enough for pharmacokinetic investigations, where only a few mg/ml of morphine are to be detected are only possible with mass spectrometry (28,29) or with electron-capture detection (26,27,30,31). In order to reduce the polarity of morphine and related compounds, and to increase the sensitivity for ECD, acylation with fluorinated anhydrides and N-heptafluorobutyrylimadazole have been used.

HPLC methods require no derivitization step for either the chromatographic separation or the detection of morphine. However, methods utilizing ultra-violet (UV) detection are not sensitive enough so far. Alternatively, HPLC methods utilizing amperometric detection (HPLC-ED) increase the sensitivity for morphine by 100-fold over UV detection techniques. By this method, morphine was quantified by HPLC with electrochemical detection (23–25). The method described by Owen and Sitar (25) used a somewhat simpler extraction method which makes it more suitable for routine measurements. In addition, the HPLC-ED assay was compared with GLC-ECD, which was a modification of an earlier method described by Dahlstrom *et al.* (26). In GLC, N-ethylmorphine was used as an internal standard. The HPLC-ED analysis or HPLC-UV analysis of morphine presents several advantages over GLC-EC because HPLC combines the increased sensitivity for morphine quantification with a simplified extraction procedure of smaller (0.5 ml) samples and the absence of a derivatization process. In addition, under the right extraction conditions with solid-phase cartridges, the possibility of measuring morphine and its metabolites by HPLC is feasible.

Conclusion

To date, controversy still exists over the inter-laboratory analysis of morphine samples, resulting from clinical studies. It is hoped that the newer sensitive and specific assays for morphine will resolve these difficulties and result in a better understanding of the pharmacokinetics and pharmacodynamics of morphine.

References

(1) Martin AJP, Synge RLM. *Biochem J* 1941; **35**: 1358.

(2) Horvath CG, Preiss BA, Lipsky SR. *Anal Chim Acta* 1967; **39**: 1422.

(3) Spector S, Vessel ES. Disposition of morphine in man. *Science* 1971; **174**: 421-2.

(4) Catlin DH. Pharmacokinetics of morphine by radioimmunoassay: The influence of immunochemical factors. *J Pharmacol Exp Ther* 1977; **200**: 224-35.

(5) Brunke SF, Delle M. Morphine metabolism in man. *Clin Pharmacol Ther* 1974; **16**: 51-7.

(6) Murphy MR, Hug CC Jr. Pharmacokinetics of intravenous morphine in patients anaesthetised with enflurane-nitrous oxide. *Anesthesiology* 1981; **54**: 187-92.

(7) Dahlstrom B, Paalzow LK. Pharmacokinetic interpretation of the enterhepatic recirculation and first pass elimination of morphine in the rat. *J Pharmacokinet Biopharm* 1978; **6**: 505-19.

(8) Garrett ER, Gurkan T. Pharmacokinetics of morphine and its surrogates. I. Comparison of sensitive assays of morphine in biological fluids and application to morphine pharmacokinetics in the dog. *J Pharm Sci* 1978; **67**: 1512-7.

(9) Holt V, Teschemacher HJ. Hydrophobic interactions responsible for unspecific binding of morphine-like drugs. *Naunyn-Schmiedeberg's Arch Pharmacol* 1975; **288**: 163-77.

(10) Montgomery MR, Holtzman JL. Determination of serum morphine by the spin-label technique. *Drug Metab Dispos* 1974; **2**: 391-5.

(11) Olsen GD. Morphine binding to human plasma proteins. *Clin Pharmacol Ther* 1975; **17**: 31-5.

(12) Olsen GD, Chan EM, Riker WK. Binding of d-tubocurarine di(methyl^{14}C)ethyl iodide and other amines to cartilage, chondroitin sulphate and human plasma proteins. *J Pharmacol Exp Ther* 1975; **195**: 242-50.

(13) Garrett ER, Jackson AJ. Pharmacokinetics of morphine and its surrogates III. Morphine and morphine-3-glucuronide pharmacokinetics in the dog as a function of dose. *J Pharm Sci* 1979; **68**: 753-71.

(14) Nishitateno I, Ngai HS, Finck AD et al. Pharmacokinetics of morphine: Concentrations in serum and brain of the dog during hyperventilation. *Anesthesiology* 1979; **50**: 520-3.

(15) Kaufman JJ, Sano NM, Koski WS. Microelectromagnetic filtration measurements of the pka's and partition and drug distribution coefficients of narcotics and narcotic antagonists and their pH and temperature dependence. *J Med Chem* 1975; **18**: 647-55.

(16) Benson DW, Kaufman JC, Koski WS. Theoretic significance of pH dependence of narcotics and narcotic antagonists in clinical anaesthesia. *Anaesth Analg* 1976; **55**: 253-6.

(17) Davis ME, Michendale MH. Absence of metabolism of morphine during accumulation by isolated perfused rabbit lung. *Drug Metab Dispos* 1979; **7**: 425-8.

(18) Herz A, Teschemacher H-J. Activities and sites of antinociceptive action of morphine-like analgesics and kinetics of distribution following intravenous, intracerebral and intraventricular application. In: Harper NJ, Simmonds AB eds. *Advances in drug research* Vol 6. New York: Academic Press, 1971: 79-119.

(19) Mule SJ, Hushin PL. *Anal Chem* 1971; **43**: 708.

(20) Loh HH, Ho IK, Cho TM, Lipscomb W. *J Chromatogr* 1973; **76**: 505.

(21) White MW. *J Chromatogr* 1979; **178**: 229.

(22) Jane I, Taylor JF. *J Chromatogr* 1975; **109**: 37.

(23) Wallace JE, Harris SC, Peek MW. *Anal Chem* 1980; **52**: 1328.

(24) Peterson RG, Rumack BH, Sullivan JB Jr, Makowski A. *J Chromatogr* 1980; **188**: 1328.

(25) Owen JA, Sitar DS. *J Chromatogr* 1983; **276**: 202.

(26) Dahlstrom B, Paalzow L, Edlund PO. *Acta Pharmacol Toxicol* 1977; **41**: 273.

(27) Christophersen AS, Rasmussen KE. *J Chromatogr* 1979; **168**: 216.

(28) Eppinghausen WOR, Mowat JH, Stearns H, Vestergaard P. *Biomed Mass Spectrom* 1974; **1**: 305.

(29) Gudzinowicz BJ, Gudzinowicz MJ. *Analysis of drugs and metabolites by gas chromatography—mass spectrometry* Vol 5. New York, Basel: Marcel Dekker, 1978: 334.

(30) Edlund PO. *J Chromatogr* 1981; **206**: 109.

(31) Garrett ER, Gurkan T. *J Pharm Sci* 1978; **67**: 1512.
(32) Hess R, Stiebler G, Herz A. *Eur J Clin Pharmacol* 1972; **4**: 137.
(33) Lehmann KA, Moseler G, Daub D. *Anaesthetist* 1981; **30**: 461.
(34) Lehmann KA, Hunger L, Brandt K, Daub D. *Anaesthetist* 1983; **32**: 165.
(35) Henderson G, Frincke J, Leung CY, Torten M, Benjamini E. *Proc West Pharmacol Soc* 1974; **17**: 64.
(36) Michiels M, Hendriks R, Heykants J. *Eur J Clin Pharmacol* 1977; **12**: 153.
(37) Schleimer R, Benjamini E, Eisele J, Henderson G. *Clin Pharmacol Ther* 1978; **23**: 188.

13.3   The origins of intravenous anaesthesia

T. M. SAVEGE
The London Hospital, UK

Published by title only. Neither text nor abstract available.

PART IV

THE HISTORY OF ANAESTHETIC APPARATUS

Chapter 14
ANAESTHETIC MACHINES

14.1	The Zaaijer nitrous oxide anaesthetic apparatus

M. VAN WIJHE[1] and H. BEUKERS[2]
[1]*Streekziekenhuis Midden Twente, Hengelo,*
[2]*State University of Leiden, The Netherlands*

From the beginning of this century up to and following the Second World War, general anaesthesia in the Netherlands was administered by general practitioners or nurses. The open mask (Schimmelbusch) method, usually in combination with ether, was most commonly used. Prof. J. H. Zaaijer (1876–1932), appointed to the chair of Surgery at the Leiden University Hospital in 1914, was one of the first to use nitrous oxide as a general anaesthetic for major operations. The dangers of anaesthesia, and his wish to perform intrathoracic surgery, led him to investigate the use of the gas. He developed an apparatus, inspired by the examples of H. E. G. Boyle, G. Marshall and F. Sauerbruch, which he introduced for general use in December 1923. Remarkable for that time was the expulsion of waste gases through a specially made hole in the floor of the operating theatre. According to present day standards the apparatus functioned inefficiently, carbon dioxide was retained and the ether concentration within the system was poorly controlled.

Historical background

Joseph Priestley isolated and recognized nitrous oxide and oxygen between 1772 and 1777, when he was experimenting with 'different kinds of air'. After exposing nitric oxide to a mixture of iron filings, sulphur and water, a different gas of smaller volume was produced, identified as nitrous oxide. The 'airs' were kept in bell jars with a mercury or water seal and put into oiled silk bags for experiments (1). Humphry Davy described the analgesic effects of nitrous oxide in 1800 in his book *Researches, chemical and philosophical, chiefly concerning nitrous oxide and its' respiration*. London, 1800 (2,3). He had extensively researched the properties of nitrous oxide in his capacity as superintendent of the Bristol Pneumatic Institute. At this institution the cure of various ailments was sought through the inhalation of vapours and gases. Davy described the effect of the gas on his aching wisdom tooth and suggested its use in surgical operations. However, society was not ready for analgesia in relation to surgery. The idea seemed absurd to 18th and early 19th century people; pain was part of disease and was an unavoidable heavenly punishment (4). Nitrous oxide was to remain unused for half a century, and the abatement of the pain of all operations was to take much longer.

After 1844 many dentists in the United States followed Horace Wells's example, using nitrous oxide for reducing the pain of tooth extractions. The gas was made in the dental office by heating ammonium nitrate; it was then collected in a large reservoir at atmospheric pressure. Patients breathed it pure, unconsciousness set in within the minute, and the tooth was then quickly extracted.

The regular use of nitrous oxide in dentistry in London dates from 1868 when T. W. Evans, an American dentist working in Paris, gave several demonstrations (5).

Nitrous oxide became available, compressed to liquid in metal cylinders, in 1868 (6). It was used as an anaesthetic for very short procedures. An authoritative Dutch professor of Pharmacology, B. J. Stokvis, stated in 1870 that the action of nitrous oxide was based upon asphyxia. He based his opinion on the work of L. Hermann of Zurich, who assumed that nitrous oxide destroyed the erythrocytes by the irreversible fixation of haemoglobin. Stokvis was to correct this mistake thirty years later, but he had effectively discouraged the use of nitrous oxide in the Netherlands in the meantime (7). The famous French physiologist Paul Bert worked on the mechanism of its action from 1878 to 1885. He proved that nitrous oxide had anaesthetic properties by demonstrating its effectiveness as a 50% mixture with oxygen in a high pressure chamber. This disproved the theory that asphyxia could be the mechanism of action of nitrous oxide in anaesthesia. His fundamental achievement was his understanding that the action of an anaesthetic gas or vapour was related to its concentration in the inhaled gas mixture. It took years before the implications of Paul Bert's work were generally understood, appreciated and applied (8).

Nitrous oxide in the Netherlands

When Professor Zaaijer was appointed at Leiden in 1914, the methods of anaesthesia available comprised ether, chloroform, or mixtures thereof, dropped on an open gauze-covered mask, sometimes following an induction of ethylchloride on the same mask; rectal ether-oil mixture, local analgesic infiltration, intramuscular morphine and scopolamine, and nitrous oxide.

The Dutch textbook of anaesthesia of the time, (*Leerboek der Narcose* by T. Hammes 1874–1951) in its third edition in 1919 (the first had been in 1906), described nitrous oxide as safe for short procedures, having little effect on the circulatory system, but not worth the trouble. The author himself, did not use it at all (8). Hammes, who had received his anaesthetic training in London, was the Dutch authority on anaesthesia. He was one of the very few medical practitioners in private anaesthetic practice. In 1903 he had written a paper with the aim of rehabilitating nitrous oxide, reporting his experience with 700 anaesthetics given at the National Dental Hospital in London (7) but he was apparently unsuccessful in rousing any enthusiasm for its use.

In 1867 C. L. G. Becht included in his thesis, *Local anaesthesia and its use*, the following statement:

> '*It is desirable that nitrous oxide be used more as a general anaesthetic . . .*'.

Unfortunately Becht did not elaborate on this theme (9).

J. W. R. Tilanus, an Amsterdam surgeon, presented the use of 'protoxydum azoti' (nitrous oxide) for operations of short duration at a meeting of the Dutch Medical Association in 1870. This met with the strong opposition of the pharmacologist and toxicologist Stokvis (10).

From 1911 nitrous oxide and oxygen anaesthesia apparatus was developed by E. I. McKesson and F. J. Cotton in the United States, while H. E. G. Boyle worked along similar lines in the United Kingdom. During the First World War G. W. Crile stated that a 'silent revolution' had taken place: a nitrous oxide and oxygen anaesthetic, preceded by an opiate premedication and accompanied by local analgesic infiltration was much safer than the hitherto used monoaesthetics. It was in this spirit and along these lines that Zaaijer, in approximately 1910, set to work, developing his own apparatus.

The Dutch weekly medical journal, *Het Nederlandsch Tijdschrift voor Geneeskunde*, contained many translated excerpts from foreign medical journals, often with a reviewer's comment. The publicity given to anaesthetic mishaps in the British journals was available to Dutch practitioners with very little delay. Chloroform was accused of causing unnecessary death in 0.5–2.0% of the patients to whom it was administered. As these were generally healthy young people, these cases were very distressing (11,12). 'Heliophobia' is the word used by Hammes to describe the reluctance of Dutch (and other Continental) doctors to report anaesthetic mishaps in the journals. At a meeting in 1906, Hammes said that he personally knew of five cases of death under chloroform anaesthesia in Amsterdam alone, and that these had not been published (13). Hammes continued, however, to use chloroform and his textbook on anaesthesia in its' 1919 edition, concerning 530 references, does not mention Goodman Levy's experiments, nor does it mention the conclusions on the effects of chloroform and adrenaline on the heart published in 1911 and 1912 (8,14,15). In 1928 the Leiden University Hospital Pharmacy issued 43 kg of chloroform for anaesthetic use (16).

The cautious beginning of intrathoracic surgery and the associated pneumothorax problem provided yet another reason for desiring a change in anaesthetic technique. It was proving difficult to operate in the thorax and to keep the patient alive at the same time. 'Overpressure' anaesthesia as described by Sauerbruch made thoracic surgery possible by keeping the lungs inflated and functioning.

Reports of mishaps were not published. However surgeons' operation reports provide an idea of these occurrences. An example is described by Bolsius (1915) (17). A nine-year-old girl had been kicked by a horse, sustaining a fractured shaft of femur. During reposition under open ether anaesthesia the pulse became 'poor' and the subsequent necessary resuscitation was to no avail. At necropsy the organs were anaemic and there were no signs of fat embolus. The case was a bit of a mystery.

Development of apparatus

Apparatus developed along parallel lines in the US, in the UK and on the continent. Compressed gases were brought to atmospheric pressure, led through a bubble bottle to assess flow, through an anaesthestic vaporizing bottle, and to the face mask. The inspiration tube contained a reservoir bag. Expiration took place through a valve at the mask, or, typical for the continental apparatus, through a variable water lock, for obtaining overpressure (6). Technical hurdles to be taken were a nonfreezing reducing valve for the compressed nitrous oxide, the precise proportioning of the mixed gases, and the control of the concentration of an inhalation anaesthetic, if added. The gases were humidified and heated in the earlier versions of most apparatus.

The American, a French and Sauerbruch's German apparatus were known to Zaaijer. As there was no importer in the Netherlands and as the foreign apparatus was, in his opinion, too complicated, he preferred to manufacture his own. He had only to import the cylinders of nitrous oxide from London (18,19). Van Deene, an instrument maker in Leiden, made and sold the apparatus.

The Zaaijer apparatus

After Zaaijer's preliminary personal work on nitrous oxide, in which he demonstrated that thoracic operations were possible, two of his pupils continued to develop and improve the apparatus (20–22). The theses of W. C. Meiss (23) and T. Mansoer (24) tell us how operations were performed and how nitrous oxide anaesthesia was given from the beginning of anaesthesia in Leiden. The way the apparatus functioned is shown in Fig. 1. The nitrous oxide and oxygen gas enter the water filled bottle (C) where the rate of flow is estimated by the bubbling. They are mixed, humidified and heated. The gases then partially flow through an ether vaporizer (J) into the reservoir bag. The patient inhaled through the firmly applied mask attached to this bag and then attempted to exhale through a water lock (R).

Meiss (1925) defined the properties of a perfect anaesthetic agent. He stated that it should provide, for the patient, complete analgesia and unconsciousness without damage; for the surgeon, complete relaxation of the muscles, and for the anaesthetist, simplicity in administration. He admitted that the agents then used did not satisfy all these conditions.

In the 1920s, one hour of nitrous oxide and oxygen anaesthesia cost Dfl 1.10 (40 pence UK), one hour of ether anaesthesia Dfl 2.50 (90 pence UK). Today exactly the opposite applies: in the developing countries the use of ether in air is advocated because of the simplicity of the technique and because of the high price of nitrous oxide cylinders.

Conduct of anaesthesia in the nineteen twenties

The standard practice at Leiden at that time was as follows. The patient was examined with special attention given to the heart, to the lungs and to the analysis of the urine. The oral

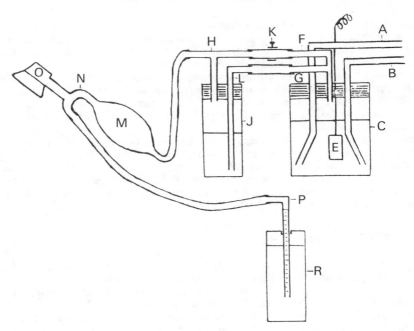

Figure 1   Drawing from Meiss' thesis on nitrous oxide anaesthesia, to demonstrate the working
of the nitrous oxide anaesthetic apparatus.
A, B: oxygen and nitrous oxide from the cylinders.
C: 'bubble bottle' for assessing flow of gases, mixing, humidifying and heating them.
E: heating element.
F: valve controlled tube bypassing vaporizer.
G: tube to ether vaporizing bottle.
H: tube from ether vaporizing bottle.
J: ether vaporizing bottle.
K: valve determining amount of gas flow through the ether vaporizing bottle.
M: reservoir bag in inspiratory tubing.
N: 'Y' piece, where in- and expiratory gases mix.
O: face mask.
P: graded plunger of the waterlock, for determining the amount of expiratory resistance.
R: expiratory resistance waterlock bottle.
note: the exhaust of the bottle 'R' has been omitted (23).

cavity, especially the (remains of) the teeth, was scrupulously cleaned. This was done in an
attempt to avoid postoperative pneumonia. The stomach, and if necessary, the intestines were
kept or made empty. To sedate the patient, to make induction smoother, to reduce the amount
of anaesthetic agent needed and to reduce salivation, a morphine and scopolamine premedication
was given intramuscularly one hour prior to surgery.

The patient was then brought to the operating theatre, where up to 150 onlookers could
silently observe the proceedings. The induction of anaesthesia was often carried out in an
adjacent preparation room due to the time needed before the patient could actually undergo
surgery (25). In the early years, the induction was with pure nitrous oxide with 3–10% oxygen
being added when cyanosis was detected. The percentages were approximations as 'read' from
the bubbling in the mixing bottle. The proper gas ratio was based primarily upon the patient's
clinical signs. The amount of expiratory resistance was slowly increased to 10 cm water in the
first fifteen minutes. This was accomplished by pushing down the expiration gas plunger to
the appropriate depth in the waterlock bottle. An adult's respiratory rate would then be about
30 per minute. Local analgesic (procaine) was injected subcutaneously by the surgeon at the
site of the incision; most patients still reacted to this stimulus. Approximately twenty minutes

after the beginning of anaesthesia, the skin incision could be made. Most patients did not then respond to this stimulus. If muscle relaxation at this time was insufficient, ether vapour was added to the inspired gases but it must have taken quite some time before its effects could be appreciated by the surgeon. The expiratory resistance at this stage would typically be 4 cm H_2O. The closing of a laparotomy wound was not always easy due to insufficient relaxation of the abdominal wall. Most patients responded to commands five to ten minutes after the end of the procedure (24).

Problems

Although considered safer than inhalational anaesthesia with a single agent there were many serious problems during and after the administration of nitrous oxide and oxygen anaesthesia using the Zaaijer apparatus. Zaaijer was confronted with apnoea at the commencement of induction, possibly the result of the tendency of the patient to hold their breath. The solution was to wait until the patient began to breathe spontaneously. If that took too long the thorax was compressed to stimulate the patient.

Vomiting posed another problem and, although it occurred in half the patients, it was considered the anaesthetist's fault. If vomiting occurred, the patient's head was held to the side and the table tilted slightly head downwards, so that the vomitus could run off freely. Many patients became what was considered too cyanotic or they remained cyanosed too long.

Pollution of nitrous oxide in the cylinder with carbon monoxide posed a very serious potential problem. The bright red colouration of the blood belied the resulting hypoxia, deceiving the anaesthetist with disastrous results. Although descriptions of such cases are scarce, the possibility must have been unnerving. Yet another concern of the nitrous oxide method was the poor relaxation of the muscles; only the later application of muscle relaxant drugs would solve this problem.

The impairment of venous return by the overpressure was one of the drawbacks of this method (19). Problems only partly recognized at the time included the lack of control over the airway, leading among other complications, to poor ventilation, an uncontrollable degree of cyanosis and aspiration pneumonia. Lack of support to the circulatory system formed another partially recognized problem. Blood pressure was not measured in the operating theatre as this could cause unrest and upset the surgeon's inner harmony. There was doubt also as to whether a drop in blood pressure actually preceded the clinical syndrome of shock.

The giving of intravenous fluids was considered of doubtful use and led only to more undesirable unrest in the theatre. The third edition of Hammes's textbook (1919) does not mention intravenous fluid therapy at all. In evident cases of circulatory collapse, acacia gum solution was administered intravenously. Acacia gum solution fell into disfavour following several deaths attributed to allergic reactions to it (26). In the UK 0.9% saline solutions came into use after the First World War. Fluids were often given hypodermically, perhaps due to the difficulty of procuring a vein in a shocked patient.

Mansoer stated in his thesis of 1928 that after two thousand anaesthetics administered in a five year period, there were no deaths attributable to the anaesthetic. Unfortunately he did not define the term 'anaesthetic death'; he meant 'death on the table'. With our present understanding and the definitions of anaesthetic mortality and morbidity, the results would undoubtedly be much less favourable.

Discussion

If one judges Zaaijer's apparatus according to the requirements of the time, as defined by McKesson, who owned a factory producing anaesthetic apparatus, the results are not bad (6). The apparatus was reliable and solidly built. The gases were properly mixed before going to the patient. The pressure of the inflowing gases was under complete control. Not properly controlled, however, was the degree of 'rebreathing' which was allowed to occur. Rebreathing had been recognized almost since the beginning of anaesthesia, but the importance given to it varied greatly. Zaaijer effectively paid no attention to it.

FE CO$_2$
(mm HG)

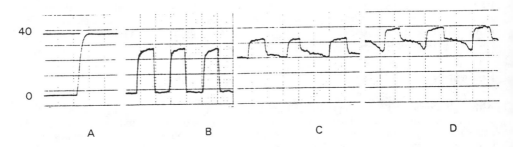

Figure 2   Capnograph display of a normal person breathing through a replica of the Zaaijer nitrous oxide anaesthetic apparatus.
A: calibration
B: subject breathing through the mask only
C: subject breathing through the Zaaijer apparatus
D: the same after 10 minutes of breathing through the Zaaijer apparatus.

What if one were to judge the apparatus according to today's requirements? A predictable and precise percentage of anaesthetic would have to be delivered. The oxygen percentage would likewise have to be predictable and correct. Adequate elimination of expired carbon dioxide is considered necessary. All of the above would have to be verifiable. Zaaijer's apparatus would fail on all counts. In the context of the 1920s, however, it was quite appropriate.

Meiss mentioned rebreathing in his thesis, stating that it meant economic profit with conservation of humidity and of temperature, which is undoubtedly correct. He noted that the respiration rate was related to the degree of rebreathing, and he warned that both the oxygen level and the ether concentration had to be considered, especially in operations of long duration. Unfortunately, he had no way of determining these variables. The importance of the expulsion of carbon dioxide and the physiological effects of hypercarbia went, with the exception of the tachypnoea, unmentioned.

Recent experiments with a replica of the Zaaijer apparatus had the following results. Expiratory carbon dioxide levels as measured with a capnograph rose steadily to 150% of normal levels within 15 minutes. Dead space estimated from the capnogram increased considerably, see Fig. 2. The inspiration:expiration ratio, normally 1:2, also rapidly decreased, becoming 1:1 as the frequency rose. The work of breathing increased.

As the University Hospital surgeons had their private practices in the two other local hospitals, they were the only ones ever to adopt this anaesthetic technique. It is obvious that the nitrous oxide and oxygen technique required considerably more skill on the part of the anaesthetist than the skill required to drop fluid from a bottle onto the gauze mask. The advantage of the 'overpressure' technique for thoracic surgery, mitigating the problem of the open pneumothorax, is obvious.

The question remains, if Zaaijer wished to adopt a new and more laborious anaesthetic technique for all surgical patients based on the grounds of increasing patient safety, why was he the only one wishing to do so? Was the reason for not adopting supposedly safer techniques the perception that anaesthetic safety was sufficient, or the fact that most hospitals had no one capable of administering anything more complicated than mask anaesthesia? Presumably a combination of both was the case. The integration of pathophysiological insights in the practice of anaesthesia at Leiden, as well as in the rest of the Netherlands, lagged behind comparable institutions in Great Britain and in the United States. Endotracheal intubation, the development of thoracic surgery, intravenous fluid therapy as circulatory support, and the development of anaesthesia as a profession were virtually nonexistent in the Netherlands. The Netherlands at the time was scientifically oriented to the European continent, dominated by Germany. A. Delingat has described the comparatively late development of anaesthesia in Germany (27)

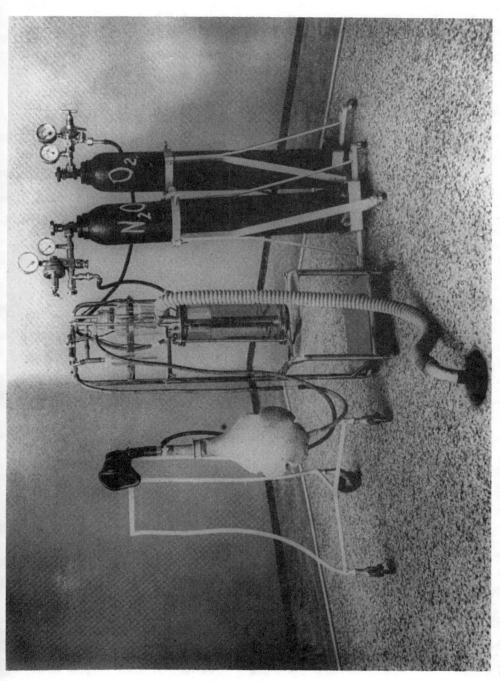

Figure 3   The construction of the modified Zaaijer nitrous oxide anaesthetic apparatus around 1927. The inspiratory reserve bag has been enlarged, and the waste gas disposal tubing is prominently visible, leading to a hole in the theatre floor (24).

which she ascribes to several factors; these surgeons were unwilling to share responsibility for their patient at the operating table, the rivalry between the different specialties and the difficulty of establishing a new specialty, especially one of very low respectability. Tracheal intubation, for example, was not practised in Germany or the Netherlands in the 1930s.

Reports of anaesthetic sequelae at the University of Marburg cover a very important transition period and provide the following information. In 1949–50 ether open mask anaesthesia was still in use but this changed to nitrous oxide and tracheal intubation in 1951–52. In the latter period five times as many intrathoracic operations were performed but despite this increase, post-operative mortality dropped dramatically from 2.6% to 0.6% (15,27,28).

Zaaijer's initiative to remove the waste gas from the operating theatre, as can be seen in Fig. 3, was remarkable. During the Second World War nitrous oxide had been unobtainable and medical conditions in the Netherlands became primitive. After the war, the purpose of the holes in the floor of the theatres had been forgotten. Concern regarding theatre pollution and its effects on the health of theatre personnel led to waste gas removal systems being installed everywhere in the 1960s.

Conclusion

In 1923 Professor J. H. Zaaijer of the Leiden University Hospital was the first to introduce nitrous oxide and oxygen anaesthesia for routine use in the Netherlands. This represented a true improvement in anaesthetic care, although it did not reach the level of some overseas centres. Zaaijer's contribution was an innovative one, which was not followed by other hospitals in the Netherlands.

Acknowledgment

The authors wish to thank Mrs M. E. van Wijhe-Wheeler, who corrected the English.

References

(1) Smith WDA. A history of nitrous oxide and oxygen anaesthesia. Part I: Joseph Priestley to Humphrey Davy. *Br J Anaesth* 1965; **37**: 790–8.
(2) Smith WDA. A history of nitrous oxide and oxygen anaesthesia. Part Ia: The discovery of nitrous oxide and of oxygen. *Br J Anaesth* 1972; **44**: 297–304.
(3) Smith WDA. A history of nitrous oxide and oxygen anaesthesia. Part II: Davy's researches in relation to inhalation anaesthesia. *Br J Anaesth* 1965; **37**: 871–82.
(4) Pernick MS. *A calculus of suffering.* New York: Columbia University Press, 1985.
(5) Duncum BM. *The development of inhalation anaesthesia.* London: Oxford University Press, 1947.
(6) Bryn Thomas K. *The development of anaesthetic apparatus.* Oxford: Blackwell Scientific Publications, 1975.
(7) Hammes T. Iets over lachgasnarcose. *Ned Tijdschr Geneeskd* 1903; **39**; 652–9.
(8) Hammes T. *Leerboek der narcose.* 3rd Ed. Amsterdam: Scheltema & Holkema, 1919.
(9) Becht CLG. *Over de plaatselijke anaesthesie en hare aanwending.* Leiden [Dissertation] 1867.
(10) Tilanus JWR. Handelingen 21ste Algemene Vergadering van de Nederlandse Maatschappij ter Bevordering van de Geneeskunst. *Ned Tijdschr Geneeskd* 1870; **6**: 240.
(11) Sykes WS. *Essays on the first hundred years of anaesthesia I.* Edinburgh: Churchill Livingstone, 1960.
(12) Hammes T. Over chloroform syncope. *Ned Tijdschr Geneeskd* 1904; **40**: 1444–52.
(13) Hammes T. Wetenschappelijke vergadering Koninklijke Maatschappij ter Bevordering der Geneeskunst. *Ned Tijdschr Geneeskd* 1906; **42**: 655.
(14) Sykes WS. *Essays on the first hundred years of anaesthesia II.* Edinburgh: Churchill Livingstone, 1960.

(15) Hammes T. Syncope door shock of door chloroform. *Ned Tijdschr Geneeskd* 1908; **52**: 838–40.

(16) Leiden University Hospital. *Annual Report* 1928.

(17) Bolsius DHJM. *Verslag van de Chirurgische Kliniek der RijksUniversiteit te Leiden '14– '15 met resultaten na twee jaar.* Leiden [Dissertation], 1920.

(18) Patterson RW. The forgotten foundations of modern closed-circuit anaesthetic technique. In: Rupreht J, van Lieburg MJ, Lee JA, Erdmann W eds. *Anaesthesia, essays on its history.* Berlin: Springer, 1985.

(19) Rendell-Baker L. History of thoracic anaesthesia. In: Mushin WW ed. *Thoracic anaesthesia.* Oxford: Blackwell, 1963.

(20) Zaaijer JH. Experimentale oesophagus en cardia resectie. *Handelingen van het 13e Nederlandsch Natuur en Geneeskundig Congres.* Haarlem: Kleynenberg, 1911.

(21) Zaaijer JH. Intrathoracale oesofagus operaties. *Handelingen van het 14e Nederlandsch Natuur- en Geneeskundig Congres.* Haarlem: Kleynenberg, 1913.

(22) Zaaijer JH. Lachgas narcose. *Ned Tijdschr Geneeskd* 1924; **68**: 1449.

(23) Meiss WC. *De Lachgas narcose in de Heelkunde.* Leiden [Dissertation] 1925.

(24) Mansoer T. *De Lachgas narcose in de Heelkunde.* Leiden [Dissertation] 1928.

(25) Van Iterson JE. *De Nieuwe operatiekamer in het Rijks-ziekenhuis te Leiden.* Leiden oration 1893.

(26) Jenkins MTP. History of fluid administration during anaesthesia and operation. In: Rupreht J, van Lieburg MJ, Lee JA, Erdmann W eds. *Anaesthesia, essays on its history.* Berlin: Springer, 1985.

(27) Delingat A. *Die Geschichte der Anaesthesiologie in Deutschland.* Koln, [Dissertation] 1975.

(28) Sweeney B. Franz Kuhn. *Anaesthesia* 1985; **40**: 1000–5.

14.2   Self administered inhalation analgesia in obstetrics

T. A. THOMAS
Bristol Maternity Hospital, Bristol, UK

Self administered inhalational analgesia during labour has been a method of pain relief peculiar to the British Isles for just over 50 years. The agent initially chosen for this purpose was nitrous oxide, the analgesic properties of which had been noted originally by Sir Humphry Davy and first exhibited, unsuccessfully, by Horace Wells in 1845.

The prototype apparatus for use during labour was constructed by Dr Ralph Minnitt and Mr A. Charles King in response to an invitation issued in October 1932, by the Clinical Investigation Sub-Committee of the Medical Board of the Liverpool Maternity Hospital. The original Minnitt apparatus was adapted from a McKesson anaesthetic apparatus and is illustrated in Dr Minnitt's book, *Gas and Air Analgesia* (1).

Investigations into the use of the method were carried out during 1934 and 1935 by the British (now Royal) College of Obstetricians and Gynaecologists. Their report (January 1936) resulted in the Central Midwives Board (CMB) recommendations as to the use of the method by midwives and the production in 1936 of the Queen Charlotte's Gas–Air Analgesia Apparatus by the British Oxygen Company.

The subsequent Minnitt Gas–Air Analgesia Apparatus of 1943, comprising the Walton–Minnitt bag-type of machine and incorporated in the Queen Charlotte case became the standard midwife's equipment for home deliveries and remained in use for a further 21 years. In the

Minnitt apparatus nitrous oxide is supplied from a 50 or 100 gallon cylinder via an Adams reducing valve which maintains a pressure of approximately 4lb per square inch. Air is entrained through five small holes in the body of the 'check valve' contained within the closed compartment of the Charlotte's case. The resulting mixture which is delivered on demand by the patient was claimed to contain 45% nitrous oxide. By inference it contained 11% oxygen and this latter feature was its greatest drawback. The apparatus was approved by the CMB, for use by midwives working alone, in 1936; approval was finally withdrawn in 1970.

Nitrous oxide and oxygen

Later design modifications of the Minnitt apparatus overcame the problem of hypoxia by mixing nitrous oxide and oxygen. This version of the apparatus was not widely used and few examples of it survive. Its lack of success can probably be ascribed to competition from the Lucy Baldwin variant of the Walton V dental anaesthetic and, more significantly, Entonox.

The Lucy Baldwin apparatus is an interesting anachronism. It takes its name from a generous benefactor to maternal welfare and first appeared in 1962. It facilitated the self administration by the mother of varying concentrations of nitrous oxide and oxygen, the proportions of which were reciprocally adjusted by means of a single sliding lever arm moving over the percentage scale from 100% oxygen down to a minimum concentration of 30% oxygen. The use of concentrations outside this range was made possible by the operation of a stop key, which it was intended could only be operated by a midwife or doctor so qualified. The machine never obtained CMB approval in England, Wales or Scotland but approval was obtained on 3 May, 1966, for its use in Northern Ireland where it is still occasionally used today.

Entonox, premixed 50% oxygen and nitrous oxide, and demand valve apparatus for its use became available a year later in 1963 and rendered the Lucy Baldwin and Minnitt apparatus obsolete.

The production of Entonox mixture was feasible because of the Poynting effect which was originally described in the late 19th century. The Poynting effect explained the means by which one gas (nitrous oxide) can dissolve in another (oxygen) when at high pressure without being compressed to a liquid. This is the basis of Entonox 50/50 nitrous oxide and oxygen which can be stored in a single cylinder and be safely self administered in a manner somewhat similar to the Minnitt apparatus. It combines the well-known pain relieving properties of the latter with the benefit of higher inspired oxygen concentrations, thus giving double benefit to both mother and baby, particularly in the event of a difficult delivery or fetal distress.

Entonox for self administration was introduced following work by Tunstall (2) in conjunction with engineers at British Oxygen Company.

It is interesting to note that this method of pain relief is now widely available in the United Kingdom not only in midwifery but to all patients exposed to sudden or acute pain associated with road accidents or heart attacks etc. The safety record of this gas is such that it can, with very few exceptions, be self administered in the presence of ambulancemen and paramedical personnel. Such initiatives and early pioneering work was undertaken in Bristol and Gloucestershire in the early 1970s.

Analgesia with volatile vapours

Nitrous oxide was not the only inhalational agent to have been used to ameliorate labour pain during this time. Between 1943 and 1984 both trichloroethylene (Trilene) and less commonly methoxyflurane were used with considerable effect.

Trichloroethylene (Trilene) is well known for its solvent and cleaning properties. It produces good analgesia in concentrations of 0.35–0.5% w/v in air. Administration of 0.5% for periods greater than three hours produces a high incidence of drowsiness and reduction of the concentration to 0.35% is necessary.

Self administered trichloroethylene and air analgesia was used by unsupervised midwives from 1955 when CMB approval was conferred on the Emotril and Tecota inhalers. This method of analgesia for pain relief in labour was made possible when, in 1952, the Medical Research

Council (MRC) defined the standard for such an inhaler. The CMB accepted these standards for providing analgesia from an inhaler being used by an unsupervised midwife conducting home deliveries. The MRC 1952 standards stated that:

1. The concentration of trichloroethylene vapour delivered should be 0.5% volume/volume in air with a permissible variation of ±20%. If possible, there should be available also a weaker setting, delivering 0.35% of trichloroethylene, to allow for the increased susceptibility of some patients after prolonged inhalation.
2. The concentration of trichloroethylene vapour should remain within these limits with variations of room temperature from 12.5°C to 35°C (55°F to 95°F); a respiratory rate of 12–30 per minute; a tidal volume of 250–1000 ml; and a minute volume of 7–10 litres.
3. Where the respiratory minute volume falls to 7 litres or less, the concentration of vapour should also fall.
4. The resistance to air drawn through the apparatus should be not more than 1.25 cm (0.5 inch) of water at a flow of 30 litres a minute.
5. The weight and bulk of the apparatus should be as small as possible. It should weigh not more than 6.1 kg (15lb), should hold 60 ml of liquid trichloroethylene, and should be sufficiently robust to stand up to reasonable wear and tear.
6. The apparatus must comply with these specifications in all working positions and after shaking and inversion. It must not be possible for liquid trichloroethylene to leak out.

The CMB regulations further demand that each inhaler must be tested and certified by the National Physics Laboratory at 12 monthly intervals to ensure accuracy under the stated conditions.

The two most widely used inhalers for this purpose were the Tecota MK6 and the Emotril Automatic Inhalers.

The Emotril 'draw-over' inhaler, designed by Epstein and Macintosh in 1949, fulfilled the MRC standards and was accepted by the CMB for use by unsupervised midwives in 1952.

Early models were not 'automatic'; lacking a thermostatic auto regulation bellows. Compensation for the effect of temperature change was achieved by the operator varying the size of the chamber exit port in accordance with the position of the pointer of the thermometer incorporated in the first version.

Temperature compensation was achieved subsequently by means of a small bellows thermostat which varied the size of the chamber exit port in response to changes in temperature. The automatic Emotril delivered 0.5% trichloroethylene in air with the mixture control set at 'normal'. Changing the setting to 'weak' opened a second bypass port and produced a 0.35% mixture. These concentrations were maintained between 12°C and 37°C and temperature variation of the trichloroethylene liquid was minimized by a water jacket incorporated in the outer wall of the vaporizer. Manufacture of the Emotril ceased in 1984 when CMB servicing and testing were discontinued and approval was finally withdrawn.

The Tecota 'draw-over' inhaler was derived from the Cyprane 'Tec' range of low resistance, temperature compensated vaporizers. Like the Emotril it met the MRC 1952 standards. The MK6 was the eventual outcome of visually dissimilar models. Concentrations of 0.5% and 0.35% trichloroethylene in air were achieved, the settings in this case being Max and Min.

Temperature compensation was achieved with the 'Tec type' bimetallic strip which automatically varied the size of the chamber egress port in response to temperature changes. Manufacture began in 1952 and ceased in 1984 when the CMB discontinued their certification/maintenance scheme, begun in 1955 when CMB approval was first given to the Tecota MK6.

Conclusion

In spite of the great advances in analgesia since the 1930s it is salutory to note Dr Ralph Minnitt's comments made in 1933:

> *'What has been done is not a terminus. It is a thoroughfare to greater possibilities for painless labour. So may there dawn renewed hope in the hearts of women.'*

Although the agents and methods have changed, Minnitt's sentiments are still apposite today.

References

(1) Minnitt RJ. *Gas and air analgesia* London: Baillière Tindall and Cox, 1938.
(2) Tunstall ME. Use of a fixed nitrous oxide and oxygen mixture from one cylinder. *Lancet* 1961; **ii**, 964.

14.3	The house of Dräger

PETER W. THOMPSON
University of Wales, Cardiff, UK

Today the name of Dräger is a household word not only on the Continent but also in this country and North America. This paper will draw attention to a few of the Dräger developments which have left an imprint on anaesthetic apparatus design to this day. Some of them were developed well ahead of their time but lost sight of temporarily—and then redeveloped.

The first decade of this century deserves particular emphasis. This was a decade in which, in Germany particularly, so many startling developments occurred. In this connection the names of Kirstein, Kuhn, Killian, Bier and Sellheim are five which might be mentioned.

The author is deeply indebted to the Company of Drägerwerk of Lubeck, for providing him with a great deal of information and material from their archives, and in particular to Herr Joseph Haupt of Dräger's, who is not only a great archivist and historian of the Dräger Group but has also reconstructed several of their original models for exhibition purposes.

Gas, beer, reducing valves and gauges

The house of Dräger was not founded primarily as a medical enterprise. It was in the 1880s that technology succeeded in storing pure oxygen (prepared by the newly developed Lind process) in steel cylinders at high pressure. It was a prerequisite for the utilization of compressed gases stored in this way that there should be a serviceable and efficient means of controlling both the flow and the pressure of the released gas. The founders of Drägerwerk, Heinrich Dräger (1847–1917) and his son Bernhard Dräger (1870–1928) became involved with compressed gas engineering while it was still in its infancy.

It must be emphasized here that accurate translation—especially of idiom—is of great importance. The phrase, 'noch in den Kinderschuhen stechenden', which occurs in an early history of the Dräger Company, would appear to imply that originally the Company was involved in the manufacture of children's shoes. However, since Drägerwerk were unable to confirm this information, I thought perhaps I had better look up 'Kinderschuhen' in the dictionary and found that this is, in fact, an idiom comparable to our 'still wet behind the ears' i.e. 'in its infancy'. In fact, the Drägers were acting as agents for equipment used in connection with compressed gas pressurizing of beer barrels etc. They felt that the reducing valves for which they were agents were not very satisfactory, and, having tried others of various origins and considerable unreliability, they decided that their first step should be to develop an 'excellent and efficient' pressure reducing valve. They offered this valve to the manufacturers for whom they were agents but their offer was declined and they therefore set up a business on their own. It is clear that this was the foundation of the Drägerwerk Company as such.

From this 'inventive self-help step' the first clearly recognizable result was their Bierdruck Automat, a mechanism for the automatic control of carbon dioxide pressure in beer pumps.

(It is not possible to deny that the Drägers had their priorities right). The original reducing valve was followed almost immediately by the development of an effective control valve for cylinders. The combination of these two allowed an even flow of gas to be drawn from a cylinder with accuracy, regardless of whether the pressure in the cylinder was low or high. At the same time they developed a range of pressure gauges and injectors as basic elements in pressurized gas techniques.

Oxygen inhalation apparatus

In 1902 the Company built its first oxygen inhalation apparatus. Before that time oxygen therapy had been difficult, the oxygen being supplied by pharmacists in large rubber bags from which the patient could inhale. This apparatus stood the test of time and was further developed by Dräger after the First World War by the addition of a simple humidifier.

The first Dräger anaesthetic apparatus

The 'automatic oxygen dispenser' (as they called it) was combined with an injector which had previously been developed as part of a welding torch, to form the basis for the construction of an anaesthetic apparatus in the first year of manufacture (1902). It is not certain whether the initiative for building an anaesthetic apparatus came from the engineers, the Dräger father and son, or from the physicians but it is known that there was close co-operation in the early 1900s between Dr Roth, the Chief Physician at the German Hospital in Lubeck and the Drägers, and that Roth tried out the resulting apparatus clinically.

This apparatus allowed an accurate measurement of drops of chloroform to be combined with oxygen from the storage cylinder. Roth demonstrated this apparatus at the German Congress of Surgeons in Berlin in 1902 and published a report of it in November the same year. In this apparatus the oxygen from the cylinder was used to operate two injectors which sucked in and vaporized drops of ether and/or chloroform from separate reservoirs. The resultant mixture was inhaled from a reservoir bag through somewhat narrow bore tubing and a facemask. This apparatus performed so well that production was started in 1903, and it was sold throughout the world under the title 'Roth–Dräger mixed anaesthesia apparatus'. It was shown in 1904 during the universal exposition in St Louis in the United States, and the Company was awarded a diploma for it. By 1913 more than one and a half thousand had been sold.

'Over-pressure' and the pneumothorax problem

Another problem which was exercising the minds of surgeons at this time was the open chest. The problem of the open thorax was becoming more and more acute as surgeons became more and more eager to embark on surgery within the chest. It was generally thought that the most important thing, to eliminate the ill-effects of opening the chest, was simply to keep the lung expanded. To this end the main thrust of development was to produce an 'over-pressure' during respiration to prevent the lung from collapsing, relatively little attention being paid to the ventilatory exchange. A number of test apparatuses were developed, one being the result of cooperation between Professor Brauer and the Drägers. Eventually the Roth Dräger apparatus was developed as an over-pressure apparatus known as the Roth/Dräger Kronig apparatus of 1907. Again the fundamental effect was achieved by an oxygen injector. This was the first anaesthetic apparatus, designed specifically for thoracic surgery, to go into series production.

An early ventilator

In the same decade (1900–1910) other remarkable developments took place. In 1907 Heinrich Dräger invented the Pulmotor. This unit was driven by compressed oxygen the positive pressure of which inflated the lungs; this alternated with the generation, again through an injector, of suction which was effective during the expiratory phase. The pressure valves were permanently set, and the control of the valves which determined the changeover from the inspiratory to the expiratory phase and vice versa, was by a spring motor.

Carbon dioxide absorption

Finally another development which was going on at this time was of carbon dioxide absorption apparatus. On 6 March, 1852, in a Belgian coalmine, a fall caused the death of 80 miners and as an immediate result some five or six weeks later, the Ministry of Public Works offered a special prize for a practical means of allowing people to remain underground in the presence of harmful gases. This led Theodore Schwann to develop his carbon dioxide absorption mine rescue apparatus which, not surprisingly was the forerunner of many commercial models; as might be expected, the name Dräger was soon featuring in this field.

Kuhn in 1906, adapted the absorption canisters of a Dräger mine rescue apparatus for anaesthetic use in his positive pressure apparatus. However, the dead space was so large that it proved unsatisfactory and moreover, since chloroform (which was used as the main anaesthetic agent of that time) decomposed in the absorption chamber, experiments were discontinued.

Summary

Thus by 1910 Dräger had played a leading part in the development of equipment for the control of compressed gases and of anaesthetic apparatus with accurate dispensing of the agents used, experimental work on carbon dioxide absorption, and the development of an exceedingly effective ventilator. All these ideas came together in 1911 in the form of the Dräger Combination Anaesthesia Apparatus which became known affectionately as 'The Combi'.

Chapter 15
BREATHING SYSTEMS

15.1	The development and function of anaesthesia breathing systems

LESLIE RENDELL-BAKER

Loma Linda University, California, USA

To appreciate the reasons for the various breathing systems in use today some knowledge of their development is helpful (1).

Early anaesthesia breathing systems

The first nitrous oxide and oxygen anaesthesia apparatus were designed for dentistry. Dr (later Sir) Frederic Hewitt of London from 1885 (2) experimented with various premixed proportions of oxygen in nitrous oxide and found that provided the mixture was delivered under a slight positive pressure, 12.5% oxygen (O_2) with 87.5% nitrous oxide (N_2O) provided a rapid induction of anaesthesia in an average time of 126 seconds and gave an average of 44 seconds of anaesthesia for the dentist after the face mask was removed. His apparatus had separate bags for nitrous oxide and oxygen with a control to provide from 1 to 13% oxygen in nitrous oxide with a non-rebreathing system (see Figs. 1, 2, and 3) (3,5). However, Hewitt pointed out that the actual oxygen percentage delivered would vary with the relative pressures in the two bags (4). Hewitt's *Anaesthetics and Their Administration* (1893), which described his methods, became the standard anaesthetic text (3).

However, by 1897, when Hewitt published his book on nitrous oxide and oxygen anaesthesia for dental operations, he had concluded that:

> 'the best results will be obtained by starting the inhalation with from 2 to 4 percent of oxygen and then progressively increasing this proportion to 8 or 9 percent.' (4)

This percentage might have been ample for brief dental operations where the face mask had to be removed for the operation but it is unlikely that Hewitt envisaged this would be adopted for surgical operations lasting an hour or more (6). This practice inevitably led to anoxic deaths with the result the method was by 1916 condemned as 'Nitrous oxide–oxygen, the most dangerous anesthetic' (6).

When Dr S. S. White's Dental Manufacturing Company of Philadelphia produced the first American gas and oxygen apparatus, (Fig. 4) it followed Hewitt's plan with separate bags for nitrous oxide and oxygen, and a similar control on the O_2 reservoir calibrated from 1 to 10% of O_2 (6,7). (The user was again cautioned that the exact percentage would vary.) This apparatus had a non-rebreathing system with an inspiratory check valve on the mixing chamber and an expiratory valve on the mask. Once anaesthesia was achieved the face mask was removed and the teeth were extracted during the 50 or so seconds the anaesthesia lasted. A gas-tight breathing system able to exert some positive pressure was the main requirement.

The dentist Charles K. Teter of Cleveland introduced his apparatus in 1903. It too had separate N_2O and O_2 bags. However, only the O_2 bag had a check valve so that rebreathing into the N_2O bag could occur (6). Teter did much to popularize N_2O/O_2 anaesthesia for all types of surgery (8,9,10). He so convinced George W. Crile, the famous surgeon, (and later founder of the Cleveland Clinic) of nitrous oxide-oxygen's superiority (11) that Crile and Lower with their nurse anaesthetist, Miss Agatha Hodgins, in 1914 wrote the first book on 'balanced anaesthesia'. Their method, which they called Anoci Association, consisted of narcotic premedication with N_2O/O_2 and a local field block for added analgesia and muscle relaxation (12). However, the high flows of gas used by Teter's apparatus made the method so expensive that any system using less gas was attractive.

301

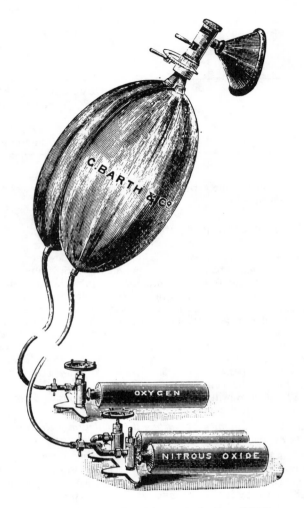

Figure 1   Hewitt's nitrous oxide–oxygen apparatus ready for use (1893).
There was a single partition wall between the two bags. This was intended to balance the supply pressures of the two gases but Hewitt found that 'considerable practice was necessary to keep both bags equal in size throughout' (5).
From Hewitt FW(3) p. 124.

Dr Willis D. Gatch of Johns Hopkins Hospital in Baltimore in 1910 introduced the method of rebreathing of the gas mixture as a simple, cheap and effective means of reducing the cost of nitrous oxide/oxygen anaesthesia (13). His apparatus (Fig. 4) had one bag connected by a tube to the face piece which had valves permitting non-rebreathing or total rebreathing. Once anaesthesia was induced with 100% nitrous oxide using non-rebreathing, 'a small puff of oxygen was admitted to the bag, just enough to restore the natural color to the face.' The gas flow was then stopped and the valves changed to total rebreathing. The patient then rebreathed the eight litres of gas mixture in the bag for 16 breaths before it was emptied and refilled with a fresh mixture. Gatch calculated that the inspired CO_2 did not exceed 4%, below which the physiologist Haldane had found that volunteers showed no ill effects. With rebreathing Gatch reported that 'the respiration becomes deep and full and the pulse rate usually falls and the blood pressure rises.' The noted American physiologist Yandell Henderson had just postulated that surgical shock was due to loss of CO_2 so Gatch felt that in addition to economy in use

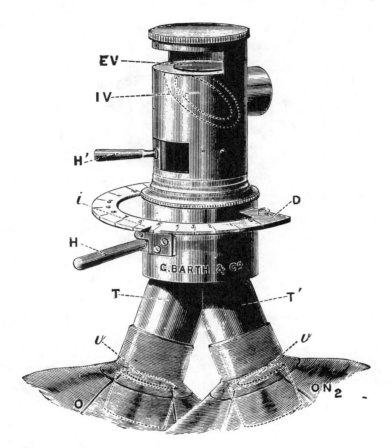

Figure 2   The control on Hewitt's (1893) apparatus for the addition of oxygen to the nitrous oxide. The nitrous oxide flowed from the righthand bag (ON₂) through the check valve (V) and tube T' to the central passage T' of the mixture control. 'To permit free escape of each expiration, two flap valves, one an expiratory (EV) and one an inspiratory (IV) were provided', making this a non-rebreathing system. Oxygen from the lefthand bag (O) passed through its check valve (V) and tube T which above was expanded to surround the nitrous oxide channel T'. From Hewitt FW (3).

of nitrous oxide, conservation of the patient's expired CO_2 was an added benefit of his method. Most apparatus introduced after Gatch's and Yandell Henderson's reports included means for rebreathing of expired gas.

McKesson's intermittent flow apparatus 1911

With his 1911 apparatus Dr E. I. McKesson of Toledo, Ohio introduced two new principles for economy of gas consumption (Fig. 4). The first principle was that of intermittent gas flow, in which gas flowed from the N_2O and O_2 reservoir bags only during the patient's inspiration. The second principle was that of fractional rebreathing, in which only the dead space gas was conserved while the rest of the expired gas was vented from the system (14,15). The breathing tube in this system thus separated both the dead space gas and fresh gas, in the reservoir bag and contiguous tubing, from the CO_2 containing alveolar gas, at the patient end of the tubing, thus making it an efficient CO_2 removal system. This method of fractional rebreathing of dead space gas was re-emphasized by Kain and Nunn in 1968 (16) (Fig. 7).

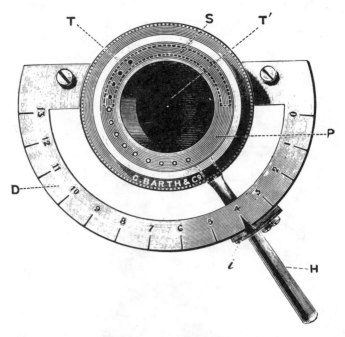

Figure 3 The control on Hewitt's (1893) apparatus for the addition of oxygen to the nitrous oxide. The proportion of oxygen added to the nitrous oxide was controlled by the number of the 13 holes opened by rotation of the control plate (P) by the handle (H). From Hewitt FW (3).

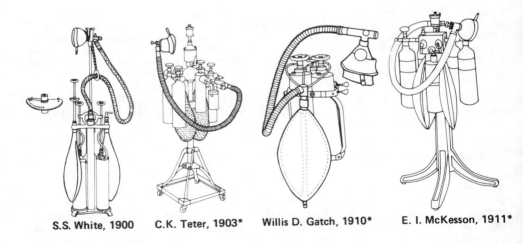

S.S. White, 1900   C.K. Teter, 1903*   Willis D. Gatch, 1910*   E. I. McKesson, 1911*

*Mapleson Type A Breathing Systems

Figure 4.

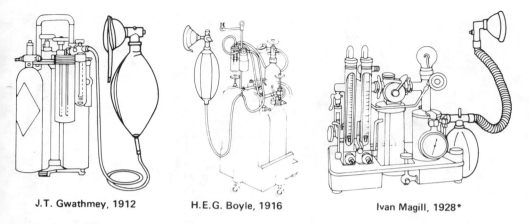

J.T. Gwathmey, 1912   H.E.G. Boyle, 1916   Ivan Magill, 1928*

*Mapleson Type A Breathing Systems

Figure 5.

Gwathmey, Boyle and Magill

Drs James T. Gwathmey and W. C. Woolsey's 1912 apparatus (17), built in New York originally by Langsdorf (10) and after 1915 by Richard Foregger, incorporated an improved version of Boothby and Cotton's bubble flowmeters (18,10), thus providing a more accurate estimation of the gas mixture being delivered (Fig. 5). This apparatus is important because it was the prototype for the British Boyle machine. Unfortunately, unlike Teter, Gatch, and McKesson, Gwathmey eliminated the breathing tubing and attached the breathing bag to the facemask. As a result the expired and fresh gas became mixed.

The Gwathmey apparatus with its inefficient breathing system came to be adopted in Britain as a result of the fortuitous meeting of Dr H. E. G. Boyle in London in 1913* with Gwathmey, Teter, and Crile (19) at the 17th International Congress of Medicine symposium on nitrous oxide/oxygen anaesthesia. Boyle (20–22) was favourably impressed with Gwathmey's methods and apparatus and in 1914 imported a Gwathmey apparatus which he used with success on World War I casualties in London (15,22).

At the Lakeside Unit of the American Ambulance, Neuilly, Paris in 1914 Agatha Hodgins and Crile gave a convincing demonstration of the superiority of their nitrous oxide–oxygen method to Col. Berkley Moynihan, the Consultant Surgeon to the British Expeditionary Forces in France (9) (Fig. 6). It was following this and the success reported by Boyle in London (20–23) and Captain Geoffrey Marshall, RAMC in France, who also designed a similar apparatus for nitrous oxide-oxygen anaesthesia (24,25), that the British Army ordered a large number of 'Boyle machines' for use in France. This was a Gwathmey apparatus (20) adapted to British cylinders by Boyle and with it came Gwathmey's inefficient arrangement of the breathing system. The descendents of the machine are still called Boyle machines.

As it was unsatisfactory to have the breathing bag near to the patient's face in maxillofacial surgery, Ivan W. Magill in 1928 (27) attached the bag to the machine once more and used a length of corrugated tubing to connect it to the tracheal tube connector and the expiratory valve (Fig. 5). Magill thus reintroduced the breathing system used earlier by Teter, Gatch and McKesson. This has been known as the Mapleson A system since 1954 when W. W. Mapleson of Cardiff, Wales published his mathematical analysis of the fresh gas flows necessary for the elimination of rebreathing in various semi-closed anaesthetic systems (30). Mapleson's

*The 17th International Congress of Medicine at which Teter, Gwathmey and Crile spoke on nitrous oxide-oxygen anaesthesia and Boyle read a paper on 'Ether anaesthesia by intra-tracheal insufflation', was held in London in 1913 (17), rather than 1912, as Boyle later recounted (24).

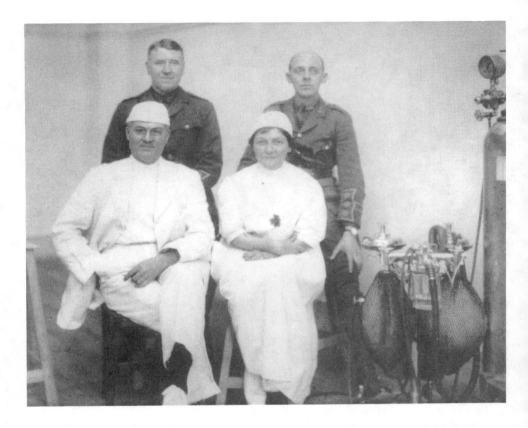

Figure 6   The noted surgeon George W. Crile (later founder of the Cleveland Clinic) with his nurse anesthetist Miss Agatha Hodgins and their Ohio Monovalve nitrous oxide–oxygen apparatus at the Lakeside Unit of the American Ambulance, Neuilly, Paris, France 1914.
The visiting Consultant Surgeon to the British Army in France, Colonel Berkeley Moynihan (left rear) and Captain Leonard Braithwaite (right rear), had just witnessed a convincing demonstration of the superiority, in poor risk casualties of 'Anoci Association', Crile's term for 'balanced anesthesia' with morphine—N_2O/O_2 and local block. Miss Hodgins later trained in their methods Col. Moynihan's American nurse, a Miss Colton, who took over as anaesthetist to the Unit when Miss Hodgins returned to Cleveland in 1915 (8). Reproduced in 1960 by kind permission from a photograph in the Crile family album.

calculations showed that the A system was the most economical for it only required a fresh gas flow at least equal to the patient's minute volume to eliminate rebreathing. However, Kain and Nunn in 1968 (16) found that it was even more economical (Fig. 7). They used fresh gas flows equal to the patient's *alveolar* minute volume—(70 ml/kg/min) and 'in no case was rebreathing evident at a fresh gas flow rate of more than 3.6 litres/min'.

Though it is efficient with spontaneous respiration the Magill system does not work efficiently with manually controlled respiration. That the Mapleson A breathing system could be used efficiently with controlled respiration was proved by an apparatus designed by Rendell-Baker and Chalmers Goodyear in 1971 and built for Mount Sinai Hospital of New York (Fig. 8). In this design a Bird nitrous oxide–oxygen Blender provided the anaesthetic gas mixture and the 50 psi (3.5 bar) pressure gas supply for the Bird Mark II ventilator's jet. The jet and the venturi entrained gas mixture from the breathing system to deliver the patient's tidal volume. The negative pressure developed by the venturi held the lightly spring loaded expiratory valve closed during inspiration.

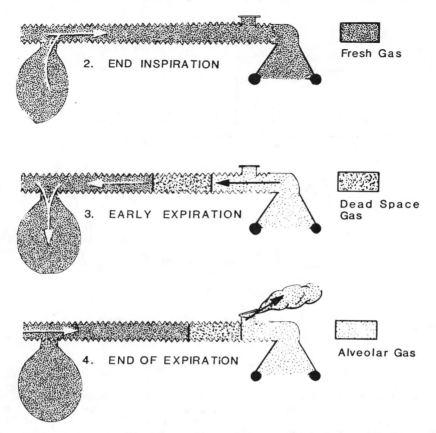

Figure 7   Sequence of events during a respiratory cycle in the Magill system with spontaneous respiration: 'In 2 inspiration has been completed and the system is filled with fresh gas. 3. During the early part of expiration dead space gas, followed by alveolar gas, passes into the tubing until the reservoir bag is full and the relief valve opens. 4. During the latter part of expiration further exhaled alveolar gas passes through the relief valve. Gas in the tube is purged by fresh gas which cannot enter the reservoir bag. Maximum economy is attained when all the alveolar gas is vented but the patient's dead space gas is retained'. From Kain & Nunn (16).

When the reservoir bag filled in expiration the remainder of the expired alveolar gas escaped via the expiratory valve. Like the Magill system the APL valve in this system was inconveniently placed for scavenging of surplus anaesthetic gases when this later became essential. However, a similar jet ventilator could work efficiently with the Lack modification of the Mapleson A and similar breathing systems.

T-piece systems

The T-piece system (Fig. 9) was introduced in 1937 (28) by Phillip Ayre of Newcastle upon Tyne after repeated unsatisfactory attempts to use N_2O/O_2 anaesthesia with the Magill system for facial and cranial surgery in babies. He found babies did not tolerate any hypoxia or the increased dead space and resistance imposed by this rebreathing system. Ayre reported that a flow of 1.5 to 3 litres/min of oxygen and ether with the T-piece gave excellent results.

In 1950 Gordon Jackson Rees of Liverpool (29) lengthened the T-piece tubing and added an open tailed bag to facilitate manually controlled respiration when using muscle relaxants in babies. He used a fresh gas flow rate of 3–4 litres/min for neonates.

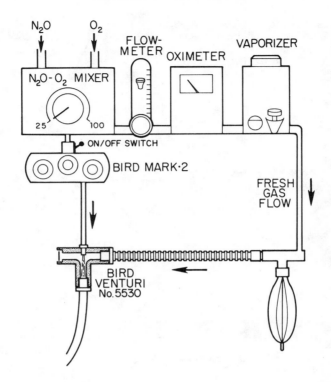

Figure 8   Mapleson A breathing system designed by L. Rendell-Baker, MD and Chalmers Goodyear in 1971 to work efficiently with controlled ventilation. The Bird Blender provided the N_2O/O_2 anaesthetic gas mixture and the 50 psi supply to drive the Bird Mark II ventilator's jet. The jet's passage through the venturi creates a negative pressure which holds the APL valve closed and entrains gas mixture from the breathing to provide the patient's tidal volume. When the reservoir bag fills during expiration the pressure rises in the breathing system, opening the APL valve releasing the alveolar gas from the system.

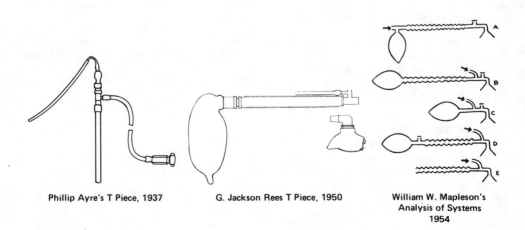

Phillip Ayre's T Piece, 1937   G. Jackson Rees T Piece, 1950   William W. Mapleson's
                                                                              Analysis of Systems
                                                                              1954

Figure 9.

Mapleson D

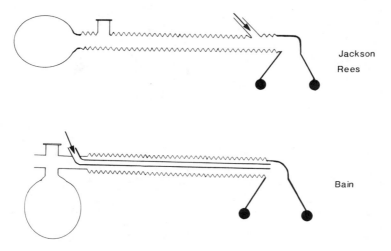

Jackson Rees

Bain

Figure 10.

William W. Mapleson, of Cardiff, in his 1954 mathematical analysis of these breathing systems (30), referred to this arrangement as the D system. He calculated that slightly more than twice the patient's minute volume would be needed to eliminate rebreathing. In later experiments Mapleson (31) used the letter F to distinguish the original Jackson Rees system which used an open tailed bag in place of the expiratory valve shown in Mapleson's original D system. These experiments, on conscious volunteers, confirmed his earlier recommendations.

Coaxial systems

In 1972 Bain and Spoerel of London Ontario (32) took the Mapleson D system and enclosed the gas supply tubing within the corrugated one, to provide a more compact 'coaxial' breathing system (Fig. 10). Bain and Spoerel recommended a fresh gas flow of 100 ml/kg/min with their system but others have advised that 150 ml/kg/min be used (33). Mapleson pointed out that a 'peaky' respiratory wave form with its faster inspiratory and expiratory flow rates as may be seen during halothane anaesthesia will require a higher fresh gas inflow. On the other hand, lower fresh gas inflows may be adequate in enflurane anaesthesia where lower inspiratory and expiratory flows combined with an expiratory pause provide time for the fresh gas to flush out the alveolar gas from the system (34).

Using the Mapleson D system Meakin and Coates (35) found that, with patients breathing spontaneously, the depressant effect of anaesthesia reduced peak respiratory flows and prolonged the expiratory time. This permitted fresh gas flows approaching the patient's estimated minute volume when conscious to be used, without significant rebreathing.

Lindahl *et al.* (36) found that the minute volume varied greatly in infants and children and did not correlate with their weight but that the tidal volume of 6 ml/kg did correlate with their weight. This figure multiplied by the respiratory frequency (f) gave the minute volume (i.e. $6 \times kg \times f$). Thus Mapleson's recommended fresh gas flow for the D system is given by: $2.5 \times 6 \times kg \times f$.

In recent years there has been considerable work on coaxial breathing systems in Britain and South Africa. In 1976 Lack of Salisbury, UK (37) converted the Magill to a coaxial system so that the expiratory valve could be mounted on the machine for more convenient gas scavenging (Fig. 11). The tubes were wider in bore than in the Bain system. The inner tube had an inside diameter (ID) of 12 mm and the outer one had an ID of 28 mm in place of the

Mapleson A

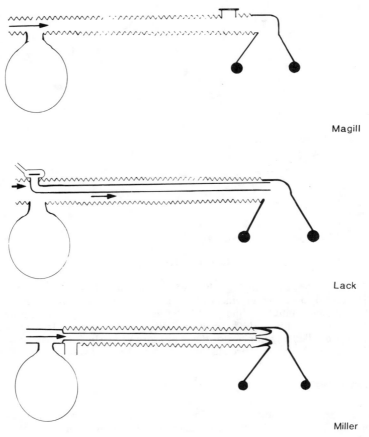

Magill

Lack

Miller

Figure 11.

usual 20 mm. This system proved to be more efficient than the Magill requiring a fresh gas flow of 51 ml/kg/min for adequate CO_2 elimination. This was 30% less than required for the Magill system (38).

In 1980, Miller and Couper of Capetown, South Africa (39) described the Preferential Flow System which had a 19 mm ID central fresh gas tube which offered less resistance to gas flow than the 30 mm ID outer exhalation tube (Fig. 11). Unlike the Bain system the reservoir bag was connected to the central fresh gas pathway. The system had no valves, but used a jet to direct the flow of expired gas preferentially into the central fresh gas tubing until the pressure within the central tube rose as the bag filled. The expired gas then left the system via the outer tubing, through the open expiratory port to the scavenging system. Thus, as in the Magill system, the dead space gas is retained and the alveolar gas is eliminated. Like the Magill system, it requires a fresh gas flow equal to or greater than the alveolar minute volume for CO_2 removal.

Also in 1980, David Humphrey and colleagues of Durban, South Africa (40) described the ADE coaxial system as a universal system which could be arranged from spontaneous breathing as a Mapleson A, for controlled respiration as a Mapleson D, or for minimal resistance with paediatric patients as an E or A system without valves (Fig 12a,b&c). Again, the tubes were wider in bore than in the Bain system. Like the Lack system the inner tube had a 12 mm ID and the outer one a 28 mm ID. Dixon, Chakrabarti and Morgan (41) tested the ADE system in the Mapleson A mode. They found that 'in anaesthetised patients the fresh gas flow at which

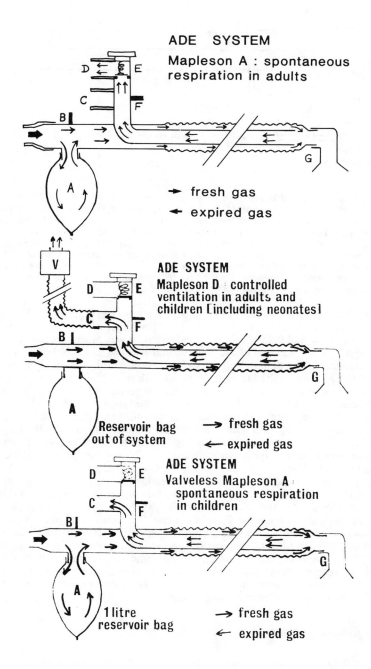

Figure 12   Humphrey's ADE Breathing Systems 1980 (40). This system may easily be changed into (Fig. 12a) a Mapleson A system with the expiratory valve on the gas machine like a Lack system, (Fig. 12b) a Mapleson D system for controlled ventilation, or (Fig. 12c) a Mapleson A system without valves.

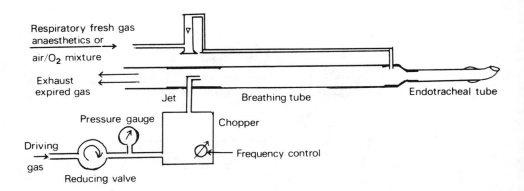

Figure 13   Chakrabarti and Whitwam's valveless jet ventilator 1983 (42,43). This used an open Mapleson E T-piece breathing system. The 1.5 m long breathing tube separated the high pressure air or oxygen delivered by the jet to the machine end of the tube from the humidified respiratory fresh gas mixture delivered close to the patient. During weaning this open system permitted the patient to take breaths, out of phase, without 'fighting' the ventilator. As the humidifier was located within the narrow bore gas supply tubing rather than in the breathing system the latter had a low compressible volume as well as a low resistance to gas glow. As a result the ventilator worked efficiently at respiratory frequencies from 10 to 100 breaths/min. The maximum airway pressure exerted by the jet was from 30 cm H_2O to 100 cm H_2O.

rebreathing occurred in the ADE system (45.6 ml/kg/min) was highly significantly lower than in the Magill system' (56.5 ml/kg/min). Also the resistance of the ADE system at 0.15 kPa at 30 litres/min flow and 0.25 kPa at 60 litres/min flow was much less than the resistance in the Magill system which was 0.32 kPa at 30 litres/min and 0.48 kPa at 60 litres/min. Humphrey's earlier studies had shown that normal arterial carbon dioxide levels could be maintained with *spontaneous respiration* in the Mapleson A mode with fresh gas flows down to 51 ml/kg/min (which was the same as for Lack's system). This compared with fresh gas flow requirements with spontaneous respiration of 72 ml/kg/min for the Magill system and 153 ml/kg/min for the Bain system. In the Mapleson D mode with controlled ventilation the minimum fresh gas requirement was 70 ml/kg/min with a ventilation minute volume of 140 ml/kg/min (37).

A Mapleson E breathing system was used by Whitwam, Charabarti and colleagues in 1983 to provide an open breathing system with low compressible volume for their valveless all purpose jet ventilator (42,43) (Fig. 13). In this system the humidified gas mixture for the patient was delivered to the patient-end of the 1.5 m long breathing tube. The jet of high pressure air or oxygen was delivered to the machine-end of this tube to produce the desired tidal exchange. As the internal volume of the tube exceeded the patient's tidal volume the gas from the jet did not reach the patient's airway. The patient could breathe out of phase without 'fighting' the ventilator. As the humidifier was within the separate small bore fresh gas system it did not contribute the compressible volume of the breathing system.

Thus all these Mapleson systems effectively eliminate expired carbon dioxide without using absorbent, at fresh gas flows commonly used with circle absorption systems. As a result of these studies and developments, the Mapleson A and D breathing systems continue to be widely used in Britain and other Commonwealth countries.

Carbon dioxide absorption methods

Using a different approach to lower the cost of nitrous oxide-oxygen anaesthesia, the pharmacologist Dennis E. Jackson of St Louis (44,45) in 1915 introduced apparatus for circle and 'to and fro' CO_2 absorption and in 1927 he introduced a combined CO_2 absorption apparatus and mechanical ventilator (46). He was 'light years' ahead of his clinical colleagues who showed no interest in his absorption apparatus or his ventilator. After he had successfully

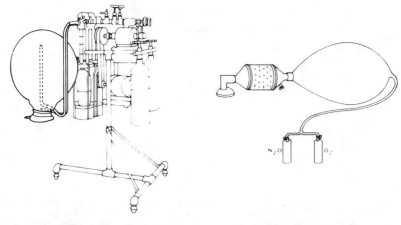

Dennis Jackson, 1915   Ralph Waters, 1924

Figure 14   CO$_2$ absorption breathing systems I.

maintained artificial respiration for 22 hours with his ventilator in an 18-year-old young man apnoeic from a cerebral abscess he regretfully concluded that 'it would appear, however, that the interval of time required for artificial respiration in the dog to evolute into artificial respiration in man may be almost as great as that required for an animal comparable to the dog to evolute into a man. It is in the hope that this long wait may be diminished, even if ever so little, that this article is published' (47). As a result only the dogs in his laboratory benefited from his advanced equipment (Fig. 14).

In 1924, Ralph M. Waters of Sioux City, Iowa (48) introduced a 'to and fro' CO$_2$ absorber for use with N$_2$O/O$_2$-ether anaesthesia based on Jackson's work. However, it was not until 1930 when Waters, by then in Madison, Wisconsin, introduced cyclopropane, which was both expensive and explosive (49), that this CO$_2$ absorption method became widely used. However, it was difficult to maintain a gas-tight fit with the weight of the absorber attached to the mask. In addition the soda lime became quite hot, necessitating hourly cannister changes.

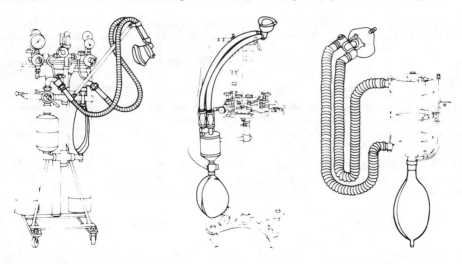

Dräger (Germany), 1925   Brian Sword, 1926   James O. Elam, 1958

Figure 15   CO$_2$ absorption breathing systems II.

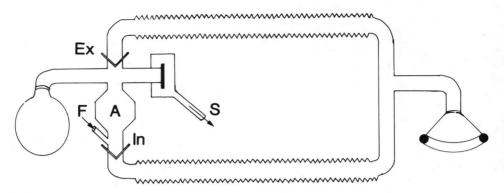

Figure 16 CO_2 circle absorption system 1958. Arrangement of components found to be efficient by Elam, Seniff and Brown (58). This diagram shows the circle system divided into its two functional halves — (1)The expiratory channel from the patient to the reservoir bag and (2) The inspiratory channel from the reservoir bag to the patient. Ex = expiratory valve; In = inspiratory valve; S = APL valve and scavenging system; A = absorber; F = fresh gas inflow.

The circle CO_2 absorption system was eagerly adopted in the US when it was introduced there by Brian C. Sword, in 1930 (Fig. 15) (50). The desire to be able to make use of cyclopropane with its benefits of speedy induction and flexibility of control of the respiration for thoracic and upper abdominal surgery, rapidly made a circle CO_2 absorption breathing system the standard equipment on most US anaesthesia apparatus.

Earlier, in 1925 in Germany, the Dräger Company used their experience with CO_2 absorption breathing systems in mine rescue apparatus to produce their Modell A, the first commercially available circle CO_2 absorption anaesthesia apparatus (Fig. 15) (51). Originally designed for use with N_2O/O_2 and ether, it was also used with O_2-acetylene anaesthesia. Unfortunately, explosions due to static buildup and the reckless use of cautery (52,53) along with the high cost of nitrous oxide inhibited enthusiasm for this system in Germany. During World War II nitrous oxide was produced on a large scale by Hoechst in Germany to provide maximum emergency power output from the Luftwaffe's aircraft engines (51). So by 1945, nitrous oxide was at last cheap and readily available for use as an anaesthetic agent.

In 1958 James O. Elam, Elwyn S. Brown and colleagues of Roswell Park, Buffalo, NY introduced the large capacity absorber (54–58) in which the void space between the granules of absorbent in each compartment was adequate to accommodate a patient's 500 ml tidal exchange (54). In their arrangement of the system's components, the overflow valve was located between the expiratory valve and the absorber (or on the Y piece). The inflow of fresh gas was between the absorber and the inspiratory valve (Fig. 16). They reported:

'While longer soda lime life was expected careful records showed an unbelievable performance. Instead of the one chamber lasting the 16 to 20 hours expected for a semi-closed system where inflow equals minute volume 60 to 90 hours per chamber was recorded in clinical use.' (58)

Thus with this arrangement of components and with a fresh gas flow (of about 5 l) equal to the patient's minute volume, the system is essentially non rebreathing, with fresh delivered to the patient and alveolar gas preferentially discarded through the overflow valve.

CO_2 removal efficiency of circle breathing systems

Although Dennis Jackson designed the carbon dioxide absorption system for economy of N_2O and O_2 consumption, modern circle systems are frequently used with 5 litre/min fresh gas flows. In many patients this would be adequate to eliminate the expired CO_2 without an absorber, provided the system's components are correctly arranged.

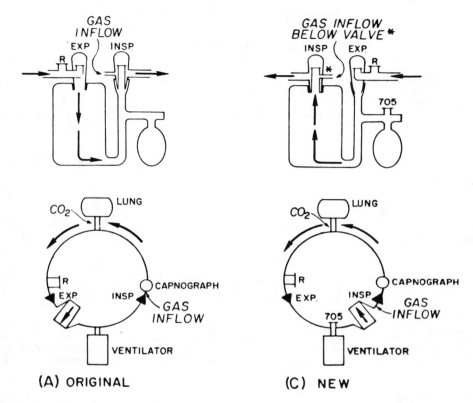

Figure 17 Foregger circle CO_2 absorption system (1976). A. The original arrangement of the system's components was inefficient for two reasons: (1) Fresh gas entered downstream of inspiratory valve (INSP), so during expiration fresh gas flowed into expiratory channel and out of the relief valve (R) without ever reaching the patient. (2) When a ventilator was used all the surplus gas passed through the absorber before being vented from the system through the ventilator's relief valve. (C) Simple transposition of the inspiratory (INSP) and expiratory (EXP) valves, relocation of the fresh gas inflow upstream of the inspiratory valve and relocation of the APL valve (705) downstream of the expiratory valve had these effects: (1) CO_2 containing surplus gas was vented before reaching the CO_2 absorbent. (2) Fresh gas accumulating in the absorber during expiration ready for next inspiration swept more expired gas out of APL valve. Thus the fresh gas was delivered to the patient and the expired gas was preferentially vented from the system. From Rendell-Baker (62).

Although the optimal arrangement of components in the circle absorption system had been defined by Brown, Seniff, and Elam (58) in 1964, Eger and Ethan (59) in 1968, Wakai and Sato in 1970 in Japan (60) and Schreiber (61) in 1972, it was clear to Soni, Malar and Rendell-Baker that this information had not been applied in the design of many then current absorption systems (62). Examination of the Foregger breathing system (see Fig. 17A) showed that the fresh gas entered downstream of the inspiratory valve and so during expiration fresh gas passed into the expiratory channel and out of the system's relief valve without ever reaching the patient. Moreover, when used with a ventilator, all expired gas passed through the absorber before the surplus gas left the system via the ventilator's relief valve. This needlessly wasted absorbent by removing CO_2 from the surplus gas before it left the system.

By a simple rearrangement of the components in accordance with these previous workers' recommendations (Fig. 17B) the lifetime of the absorbent in each half of the absorbent was lengthened from the original 7¾ hours to 19 hours (Fig. 18).

CONTROLLED VENTILATION

(5 litres fresh gas flow)

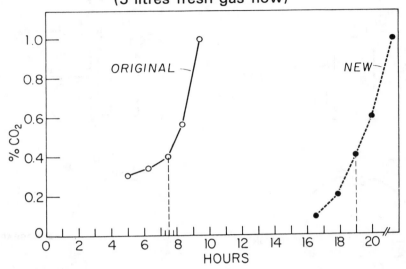

Figure 18 Effect of rearrangement of circle absorption system's components on consumption of CO_2 absorbent with a 5 litre fresh gas flow. One absorbent chamber in the original Foregger system lasted 7.75 hours before 0.4% CO_2 was detected in the gas leaving the absorber. After the rearrangement of the same components one chamber lasted 19 hours. From Rendell-Baker (62).

Humidification

Since the fresh gases delivered to the breathing system are quite dry, in an intubated patient, Chalon (63) demonstrated that damage to the bronchial mucosa from drying will occur if a condenser or heated humidifier is not used. This applies also to circle absorption systems if 4 l or more fresh gas flows are used. These fresh gas flows flush the water vapour as well as the CO_2 from the system.

In addition to the loss of humidity is the significant loss of body heat as 580 calories are lost for each millilitre of water evaporated from the bronchial mucosa. The combination of 20–25 air changes per hour provided by the air-conditioned system in the operating theatre with more prolonged surgery reinforces the need to prevent this evaporative heat loss.

Excessive breathing system compliance and wasted ventilation

If well-used rubber breathing tubes are used with a ventilator their greatly increased compliance can absorb a significant proportion of the tidal volume delivered by the ventilator. This is particularly hazardous when anaesthetizing paediatric patients with a humidifier in the system. Under these conditions Cote *et al.* (64) have demonstrated that the patient may not receive any tidal exchange. A valued feature of the Jackson Rees and other Mapleson D systems is their reduced internal volume and reduced compliance compared with all circle absorption breathing systems.

Conclusions

The various patterns of Mapleson and coaxial breathing systems which depend upon an adequate fresh gas flow for CO_2 removal were developed and are widely used in Britain and the

Commonwealth countries. They are able to eliminate rebreathing of expired CO_2 with the fresh gas flows commonly used with circle absorption systems. The circle absorption system with its large capacity CO_2 absorber, developed in the United States, is almost uniformly used there for adults. The Jackson Rees and Bain, Mapleson D breathing systems, are used mainly for smaller children. The Magill or Mapleson A system is not used at all in the USA. If the patient is intubated, most breathing systems require the use of a condenser or heated humidifier, if loss of body heat and drying of the bronchial mucosa is to be avoided. When mechanical ventilation is used, especially in babies, the compliance of the breathing system should be checked to avoid unsuspected hypoventilation. The single tube Mapleson D or F systems have the advantage here of lower compressible volume.

References

(1) Rendell-Baker L. The development, performance and safety of anesthesia breathing systems. Fifth Philip Gett Memorial Lecture. *Proc. NSW Anesthesiology Continuing Education Symposium*. Sydney, Australia: October 6th, 1984.
(2) Hewitt F. On the anaesthesia produced by the administration of mixtures of nitrous oxide and oxygen. *Lancet* 1889; **i**: 832–35.
(3) Hewitt FW. *Anaesthetics and their administration*. London: Griffiths. 1893.
(4) Hewitt FW. *The administration of nitrous oxide and oxygen for dental operations*. London, 1897.
(5) Duncum B. *The development of inhalation anaesthetics*. London: Oxford University Press, 1947, p. 484.
(6) Miller AH. Technical development of gas anesthesia. *Anesthesiology* 1941; **2**: 398–409.
(7) White SS. *Dental Cosmos* 1901; **43**: Advertisement p. 12.
(8) Teter CK. Thirteen thousand administrations of nitrous oxide with oxygen as an anesthetic. *JAMA* 1909; **53**: 448–54.
(9) Thatcher VS. *History of anaesthesia, with emphasis on the nurse specialist*. Philadelphia: Lippincott. 1953, pp. 68–76 Teter's and other early N_2O apparatus; pp. 97 Moynihan and Agatha Hodgins; pp. 128–129 Dennis Jackson's CO_2 absorption apparatus.
(10) Keyes TE. *The history of surgical anaesthesia*. New York: Schuman. 1945, pp. 69–71 Dennis Jackson and CO_2 absorption; pp. 83–86 N_2O apparatus.
(11) Crile GW. Nitrous oxide anaesthesia and a note on Anoci-Association, a new principle in operative surgery. *Surg Gynecol Obstet* 1911; **13**: 170–3.
(12) Crile GW and Lower WE. *Anoci Association*. Philadelphia: Saunders 1914 (Chapter on N_2O/O_2 anesthesia by Agatha Hodgins, CRNA).
(13) Gatch WO. Nitrous oxide–oxygen anesthesia by the method of rebreathing—with especial reference to the prevention of surgical shock. *JAMA* 1910; **54**: 775–80.
(14) McKesson EI. Nitrous oxide–oxygen anaesthesia, with a description of a new apparatus. *Surg Gynecol Obstet* 1911; **13**: 456–62.
(15) Thomas KB. *The development of anaesthetic apparatus*. Oxford: Blackwell, 1975: pp. 112–173. N_2O apparatus; p. 137 Heidbrink apparatus; p. 139 Gwathmey; p. 155 McKesson; p. 142 Marshall; p. 196 Magill apparatus for endotracheal anaesthesia.
(16) Kain ML, Nunn JF. Fresh gas economics of the Magill circuit. *Anesthesiology* 1968; **29**: 964.
(17) Gwathmey JT, Woolsey WC. The Gwathmey–Woolsey nitrous oxide-oxygen apparatus. *NY Med J* 1912; **96**: 943.
(18) Colton FJ, Boothby WM. Nitrous oxide–oxygen–ether anesthesia: Notes on administration a perfected apparatus. *Surg Gynecol Obstet* 1912; **15**: 281–9.
(19) Crile GW. Anoci Association. *17th Int Congr Med London 1913 Subsection VII (b) Part 2*. 1914. London: Hodder and Stoughton, 1914.
(20) Boyle HEG. The use of nitrous oxide and oxygen with rebreathing in military surgery. *Lancet* 1917; **ii**: 667. 'My own interest in (N_2O/O_2) is due entirely to Dr James T. Gwathmey of New York whom I met at the Congress in 1912'— 'the apparatus I use is Gwathmey's'.

(21) Boyle HEG. Experiences in the use of nitrous oxide and oxygen with rebreathing in military surgery. *Br Med J* 1917; **ii**: 653.

(22) Boyle HEG. Nitrous oxide–oxygen–ether outfit. *Proc Roy Soc Med* 1918; **11**: 30.

(23) Boyle HEG. Nitrous oxide–oxygen–ether outfit. *Br Med J* 1919; **i**: 159.

(24) Marshall G. Anaesthetics at a casualty clearing station. *Proc Roy Soc Med* 1917; **10**: 17.

(25) Marshall G. Two types of portable gas–oxygen apparatus. *Proc Roy Soc Med* 1920; **13**: 18.

(26) Boyle HEG. Nitrous oxide: History and development. *Br. Med J* 1912; **i**: 153. 'Advent of Teter and Gwathmey at conference in 1912 gave much-needed impetus to N_2O/O_2 method.' As a result he obtained a Gwathmey machine.

(27) Magill WI: Endotracheal anaesthesia. *Proc Roy Soc Med* 1928; **22**: 83.

(28) Ayre P. Anaesthesia for hare lip and cleft palate operations on babies. *Br J Surg* 1937; **20**: 131–2.

(29) Rees GJ. Anaesthesia in the newborn. *Br J Med* 1950; **ii**: 1419.

(30) Mapleson WW. The elimination of rebreathing in various semi-closed anaesthetic systems. *Br J Anaesth* 1954; **26**: 323.

(31) Willis BA, Pender JW, Mapleson WW. Rebreathing in a T piece: Volunteer and theoretical studies of the Jackson–Rees modification of Ayre's T piece during spontaneous respiration. *Br J Anaesth* 1975; **47**: 1239–46.

(32) Bain JA, Spoerel WE. A streamlined anaesthetic system. *Can Anaesth Soc J* 1972; **19**: 426.

(33) Dorsch JA, Dorsch SE. *Understanding anaesthesia equipment*, 2nd Ed. Baltimore: Williams and Wilkins, 1984: 186.

(34) Byrick RJ, Janssen EG. Respiratory wave forms and rebreathing in T piece circuits: a comparison of enflurane and halothane wave forms. *Anesthesiology* 1980; **53**: 371–8.

(35) Meaking G, Coates AL. An evaluation of rebreathing with the Bain system during anaesthesia with spontaneous ventilation. *Br J Anaesth* 1983; **55**: 487–95.

(36) Lindahl SGE, Hulse MG, Hatch DJ. Ventilation and gas exchange during anaesthesia and surgery in spontaneously breathing infants and children. *Br J Anaesth* 1984; **56**: 121–8.

(37) Lack JA. Theatre pollution control. *Anaesthesia* 1976; **31**: 259–62.

(38) Humphrey D. The Lack, Magill and Bain anaesthetic breathing systems: A direct comparison in spontaneously breathing anaesthetized adults. *J Roy Soc Med* 1982; **75**: 513–24.

(39) Miller DM, Couper JL. Comparison of the fresh gas flow requirements and resistance of the preferential flow system with those of the Magill system. *Br J Anaesth* 1983; **55**: 569–74.

(40) Humphrey D. A new anaesthetic breathing system combining Mapleson A, D and E principles. *Anaesthesia* 1983; **38**: 361–72.

(41) Dixon J, Chakrabarti MK, Morgan M. An assessment of the Humphrey ADE anaesthetic system in the Mapleson A mode during spontaneous ventilation. *Anaesthesia* 1984; **39**: 593–6.

(42) Chakrabarti MK, Whitwam JG. A new valveless all-purpose ventilator. *Br J Anaesth* 1983; **55**: 1005–15.

(43) Whitwam JG, Chakrabarti MK, Konarzewski WH, Askitopoulou H. A new valveless all-purpose ventilator. *Br J Anaesth* 1983; **55**: 1017–23.

(44) Jackson DE. New method for production of general analgesia and anesthesia with description of apparatus used. *J Lab Clin Med* 1915; **1**: 1.

(45) Jackson DE. Anesthesia equipment from 1914 to 1954 and experiments leading to its development. *Anesthesiology* 1955; **16**: 953.

(46) Jackson DE. A universal artificial respiration and closed anesthesia machine. *J Lab Clin Med* 1927; **12**: 998.

(47) Jackson DE. The use of artificial respiration in man. A report of a case. *J Med* 1930; December: 3–7, Cincinnati, Ohio.

(48) Waters RM. Clinical scope and utility of carbon dioxide filtration in inhalation anesthesia. *Anesth Analg* 1924; **3**: 20–2.

(49) Stiles JA, Neff WB, Rovenstine EA, Waters RM. Cyclopropane as an anesthetic agent: a preliminary clinical report. *Anesth Analag* 1934; **13**: 56–60.

(50) Sword BC. The closed circle method of administration of gas anaesthesia. *Anesth Analg* 1930; **9**: 198.

(51) Haupt J. *Der Drager Narkoseapparat, historisch gesehen.* Medizintechnik Sonderdruck MT 105 Dragerwerk. Lubeck, Germany.

(52) Hurler K. Eine Explosion bei Narcylenbetaubung (acetylene anesthesia). *Munch Med Wschr* 1924; **71**: 1432.

(53) Oehlecher F. Report on explosion in absorber of acetylene apparatus to Hamburg Medical Society. *Munch Med Wschr* 1925; **72**: 2170.

(54) Brown ES. Voids, pores and total air space of carbon dioxide absorbents. *Anesthesiology* 1958; **19**: 1–6. A comparison of the void space in the Roswell Park absorber and other absorbers available showing the latter's inability to accommodate the patient's 500 ml tidal volume.

(55) Nealon TF, Chase HF, Gibbon JH. Factors influencing carbon dioxide absorption during anesthesia. *Anesthesiology* 1958; **19**: 75–81. Figure 2 shows Dr JA Elam and ES Brown's 3,300 cc canister—prototype of Roswell Park Absorber.

(56) Elam JO, *et al.* Roswell Park Absorber—Anesthesia Associates advertisement. *Anesthesiology* 1958; **19**: xlii.

(57) Elam JO. The design of circle absorbers. *Anesthesiology* 1958; **19**: 99–100. Work in Progress Abstract.

(58) Brown ES, Seniff AM, Elam JO. Carbon dioxide elimination in semi-closed systems. *Anesthesiology* 1964; **25**: 31–6.

(59) Eger EI, Ethans CT. The effects of inflow, overflow and valve placement on economy of the circle system. *Anesthesiology* 1968; **29**: 93–100.

(60) Wakai I, Sato T. Experimental study on the efficiency of semi-closed circle absorption system with a pressure equalizer valve and expiratory trap. *Jap J Anesth* 1970; **19**: 1122.

(61) Schreiber P. *Anaesthesia equipment, performance classification and safety.* New York: Springer-Verlag, 1972.

(62) Soni, Malar, Rendell-Baker. In: Rendell-Baker L, ed. Problems with anesthetic and respiratory therapy equipment. *Internat Anesth Clin* 1970; **20**: 64–6.

(63) Chalon J, Ali M, Turndorf H, Fischgrund GK. *Humidification of anaesthetic gases.* Springfield: Thomas, 1981.

(64) Cote CJ, Petkau AJ, Ryan JF, Welch JP. Wasted ventilation measured in vitro with eight anesthetic circuits with and without in-line humidification. *Anesthesiology* 1983; **59**: 422–46.

15.2

The 'D-M' gas anaesthesia machine

ROD WESTHORPE
*Geoffrey Kaye Museum of Anaesthetic History,
Royal Australian College of Surgeons, Melbourne, Australia*

The first company in Australia to import anaesthetic machines was John B. Arnold Pty Ltd. In 1923 the company began manufacturing and produced an apparatus delivering gases directly from cylinders without reducing valves or flowmeters. This first Australian anaesthetic 'machine' was named the Austox machine.

In 1931 the same company, with the help of Dr Geoffrey Kaye, designed and introduced the 'D-M' Austox machine, the D-M standing for 'Dental Midwifery'. This was an intermittent flow apparatus using similar principles to that of the McKesson machine.

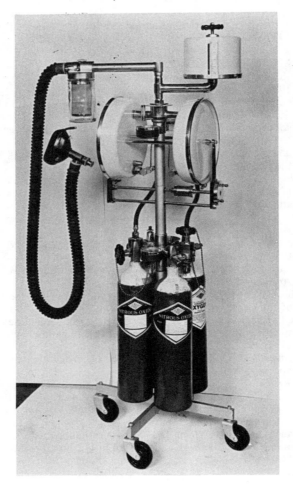

Figure 1   The 'D-M' gas anaesthesia machine.

In 1935 J. B. Arnold Pty Ltd was absorbed by another company, the Commonwealth Industrial Gases Ltd. Under the new company, the D-M machine was further modified and continued to be manufactured in one form or other until 1952 (Fig. 1).

General principles

Nitrous oxide and oxygen are piped to individual tambours, which, having a rubber diaphragm, distend. The distension is caused to operate levers which arrest the further flow of gases, leaving the tambours full. When the patient inhales, nitrous oxide or oxygen, or a mixture of the two, are caused to flow into a common mixing chamber and pass to the patient. When the tambours deflate, the levers no longer arrest the flow of gases and so refilling occurs ready for the next inhalation.

In the earliest model (1931) there were no reducing valves and each gas entered a yoke fitted with a cylinder gauge and then via a pipe with nut and tail union to its own tambour. Gas entered the tambour through a nipple occluded by a fibre faced plunger. There was also a port for the admission of air for gas–air analgesia (omitted on later models).

An additional feature allowed the pressure of gas within the tambour to be varied. An adjustable spring and pressure bar system, attached to the outer surface of the tambour diaphragms, effectively converted them into reducing valves. The spring-loading acted equally on both diaphragms and enabled a higher pressure between 0 and 40 mmHg to be sustained inside the tambours before the shut-off levers checked the flow of gases.

Later models exhibited other modifications, besides the absence of provision for gas–air analgesia, including wider bore gas channels, finer control of nitrous oxide–oxygen percentage mixtures, provision of a locking device for oxygen percentage, and oxygen flush facility. Accessories designed for use with the D-M machine included an ether vapourizer with bypass control tap, a rebreathing bag (1931) and the Austox fractional rebreather (1932).

The rebreathing bag

The fitting of a rebreathing bag to an intermittent flow machine was misguided. At atmospheric pressure, the bag was a source of uncontrolled rebreathing, while at any pressure above atmospheric, the bag became distended and non-functional.

The fractional rebreather

The object of a fractional rebreather was to reduce the consumption of gases, by rebreathing automatically any set percentage of the exhaled mixture, the machine providing the balance of the breath. The CIG fractional rebreather was rather flimsy in design compared with that of McKesson and the thin rubber bellows easily perished.

Conclusion

The D-M machine was widely used in Australian anaesthesia from 1931 until the 1960s. In 1953 C.I.G. Ltd produced the Australian version of the Boyle's machine, and the intermittent flow machines gradually disappeared from use although some remain in use in obstetric wards as demand flow devices for pain relief during labour.

16.1	A chloroform inhaler dated 1848

J. D. D. WOLFF
Bloemendaal, The Netherlands

Until recently, the Amsterdam Historical Museum had a collection of old medical instruments on view. Amongst the items was a metal object, which at first sight bore a striking resemblance to a death mask, but on closer inspection appeared to be an apparatus for giving chloroform. The adjoining leather case had the following inscription: 'Chloroforme apparaat van S. N. Dentz Jr, April 1848'.

S. N. Dentz—dentist

S. N. Dentz Jr (1817–1872) was one of a generation of dentists, living in Amsterdam. In 1857, he was elected honorary member of the Odontological Society of London. The King of Holland and the Queen of Sweden were among his patients. In 1863 he published a book in the French language: *Traité des Principales Affections de la Cavité Buccale* (1).

The Dentz apparatus

His apparatus was made of thin silverplate, in the shape of an adult face mask including the lower lip and the bridge of the nose. At the level of mouth and nostrils it was provided with many small holes, in order to make breathing possible; moreover the wall was doubled there to form two tiny boxes, also with perforated lids, opening to the inside of the mask and containing sponges to be moistened with chloroform from the outside through two funnels. The mask could be divided into a nasal part and a mouthpiece, connected by two movable hooks and a peg-and-hole fitting. The edge of the nose-piece carries the engraved words: 'Chloroform Apparaat van S. N. Dentz Jr, April 1848'. The leather case is lined with brown velvet and has a depression, containing a crystal flask, holding 5 ml of chloroform.

Discussion

We may assume that, when Dentz developed his apparatus, he was informed about the many existing inhalers of his day. Several were made simply by adopting a face-piece alone and adding wires to the inside to hold a sponge.

Chloroform was introduced by Simpson of Edinburgh in November, 1847 and, within one month, a great variety of inhalers appeared in Paris. In the advertisement page of the *Gazette Médicale de Paris* of 19 December, 1847, a '*appareil pour l'inhalation de Chloroforme*' was announced at the price of 10 Francs in pewter or 18 Francs gilded. There was even a collapsible inhaler to be carried inside a top hat. In Germany, Luer's apparatus was popular. It took the form of an inhaler of plated copper in the shape of a shell with a sponge inside.

Although Dentz's apparatus was clearly related to these inhalers, there are some original features in his design. Firstly the unique shape of the mask and the all-metal construction facilitated cleaning. Secondly, the close-fitting shape minimized dead space and obviated the—often badly functioning—breathing valves. One disadvantage of the mask was that not only inspiration, but also expiration passed through the chloroform-laden sponge thereby directing fumes towards the dentist. Thirdly, the mask has the possibility of unhooking the mouth-piece after induction and so continuing anaesthesia by the nasal route only; this was of special interest for dental work. Not until 1862 was a similar technique described by Clover. Formerly anaesthesia in dentistry was given intermittently.

The question arises why Dentz never publicized his inhaler. He must have been a man with original and scientific interests, yet anaesthesia is not maintained in his book and neither the transactions of the Odontological Society, nor the Dutch medical literature contain a paper in his name. That his apparatus was not successful and therefore unsuitable for publication is hardly likely; it fits comfortably on the face and breathing is only slightly obstructed and, besides, there are small marks on the mask which are evidence of frequent use. The impression that his inhaler was a reliable instrument for dental analgesia is fully justified.

Unnoticed and unknown this interesting apparatus went into oblivion, tucked away in a museum. The Dentz family continued in the profession of dentistry until 1916, when the last such member, named G. W. Dentz, died. The heirs presented the apparatus to the museum and it is now part of the collection of the Boerhaave Museum of Leiden.

Reference

(1) Wolff JDP. Over chloroform narcose en een Nederlandse pionier. *Ned Tijdschr Geneeskd* 1981; **125**: 1719.

16.2   Ether apparatus with an Australian flavour

CHRISTINE BALL
Alfred Hospital, Prahran, Victoria, Australia

The Geoffrey Kaye Museum contains a very large collection of ether inhalers including several original Clovers and its subsequent modifications such as Probyn Williams, Wilson Smith's and Hewitt's (1,2). Of particular interest to Australians are the Bruck inhalers which were designed and manufactured in Australia.

Bruck's inhaler

Bruck was an instrument maker in Sydney in the early 1900s. There are two Bruck inhalers in the museum, both in their original cases. The inhalers are oval shaped with the upper half made of glass to allow observation of the ether level. They consist of a central tube with controllable ports on either side. There is a cross tube leading to a face piece and bag. The measure also present in the case is important as overfilling would result in liquid ether entering the inhalation tube. The inhaler is larger than the other Clover modifications but the airways remain similar to the Clover, thereby classifying this as a small bore inhaler.

Ormsby's inhaler

Lambert Ormsby was a New Zealand surgeon who emigrated to Ireland. He described his ether inhaler in a letter to the *Lancet* in 1877 (3):

'Sir—The best and safest means of anaesthesia in surgical operations must claim the attention of every practical surgeon, and few can think of operating without considering for a moment the relative dangers of the several varieties of anaesthetics used to produce insensibility.'

The inhaler consists of an indiarubber flexible bag enclosed with a netbag designed to limit expansion. There is a soft metallic mouthpiece with indiarubber tubing around the edge. The tubing had to be purchased separately from the manufacturer. A valve can be opened to admit air if required. The body contains a wire cage into which fits a similarly shaped hollow sponge into which ether is poured. For continuous ether a recharging device was later added, not present on our specimen.

Ormsby listed the advantages of the inhaler as, simple, inexpensive, only a small quantity of ether is required to produce sleep, it prevents evaporation of ether vapour; it is portable, small and can be carried in pocket, its use results in a short time to 'complete' anaesthesia (2 mins) and it is safe.

In another letter to the Editor of the *Lancet* (4) later in 1877, Ormsby outlined his directions for use following the discovery that the inhaler had become very popular in Britain:

'1). Tell the patient before administration that the ether vapour may at first have a suffocating feel, and should not be regarded, as the sensation will only be momentary.
2). To ask an assistant to hold the hands of the patient, so as to prevent the inhaler being suddenly snatched from off the face.
3). No solicitation whatever on the part of patients should be listened to as regards giving them a breath of fresh air, as they invariably cry out for it, and the anaesthesia would only be delayed. The sliding aperture in the mouthpiece may be left open for a moment but then should be closed, so as to compel the patient to breathe and rebreathe the same ether charged air.'

He concludes by saying that none but the best anaesthetic ether should be used, SG. 0.720–0.730. The principal disadvantages of this apparatus were that it had to be removed if anaesthesia became too deep, there was considerable carbon dioxide accumulation and the potential existed for significant hypoxia.

The Ormsby inhaler was modified by Carter Braine in 1898 with aim of making it easier to clean. Essentially it is very similar except there is no net around the bag. The cap bears a small vent for admission of air but physiologically it had no advantages over the Ormsby inhaler.

Open ether masks

Open ether techniques were first introduced in the USA in 1895 but not practised in Australia until R. W. Hornaback introduced them in 1909. Of the huge collection of open ether apparatus in the Geoffrey Kaye Museum (5), only one appears to have been designed in Australia. The Coutts mask was designed in 1932. It is a large cumbersome structure, designed to allow the dome to be closed completely over the vapourizing site. This was in order to conserve ether, apparently with total disregard for oxygen lack and carbon dioxide accumulation.

Bibliography

(1) Penn HP. The Geoffrey Kaye Museum collection of portable ether inhalers. *Anaesth Intens Care* 1975; **3**.
(2) Thomas KB. The A. Charles King collection of early anaesthetic apparatus. *Anaesthesia* 1970; **25**: 4.
(3) Ormsby L. Ether inhalation. *Lancet* 1877, June 9; 863.
(4) Ormsby L. A new ether inhaler. *Lancet*, 1877, Feb. 5; 218.
(5) Catalogue of the Geoffrey Kaye Museum.

16.3   Chloroform inhalers in the Geoffrey Kaye Museum

ROD WESTHORPE
*Geoffrey Kaye Museum of Anaesthetic History,
Royal Australian College of Surgeons, Melbourne, Australia*

The Geoffrey Kaye Museum of Anaesthetic History, housed at the Royal Australasian College of Surgeons building in Melbourne, contains numerous examples of apparatus used for the administration of chloroform.

Cone masks

In 1847, Simpson placed a drachm of chloroform on to a handkerchief folded into the shape of a cup which was then placed on the face. It was not long before the cloth or handkerchief was pinned up into a cone and a marine sponge placed at the apex to absorb and act as a vaporizing surface for the chloroform. Thus was initiated the era of cone inhalers or masks with their potential for carbon dioxide accumulation and oxygen exclusion.

Rendle's cone of 1870 consisted of leather which of course was impervious to gas exchange, but it was covered with flannel for patient comfort. There was a marine sponge at the apex. In 1890, Lieutenant Colonel Lawrie devised the 'Hyderabad cone' which had a leather sheath and was lined with flannel. The liquid chloroform was introduced through the holes into the flannel. Air could also enter via these holes and the depth of depression of respiration was indicated by a feather in the expiratory cage at the top.

As the cones were being developed, the era of open anaesthesia using wire masks was also in its infancy. Their popularity remained on a par until the turn of the century when the wire masks held sway until chloroform virtually disappeared from use.

Wire masks

The wire masks were covered with cloth to absorb the chloroform and allow some gas exchange. Thomas Skinner's mask of 1862 was the first and was followed by dozens of variations.

A selection of other wire masks in the collection include Esmarch's from Germany designed in 1879 and presented in a leather compendium together with tongue forceps and a dropper which is unfortunately missing. This was probably designed for purposes of war. Esmarch's mask was extremely popular on the continent and was used up until the 1940s.

Vajna's mask of 1890 was made of glass with a lint pad stretched across the top onto which the chloroform was dropped. A flange at the base protected the patient's face from the liquid chloroform.

In 1890 Curt Schimmelbusch designed a mask consisting of a spiral wire tower. A waxed cloth cover was drawn over the tower so creating a large closed dead space. In the same year he also introduced his more familiar mask with its trough shaped rim. Impey's mask of 1908 was designed to allow surgical access during ophthalmic cases.

The best known of the wire masks is the Schimmelbusch version which survived until recent times. The reason for its survival in preference to the others appears to rest solely on the fact that it prevented liquid chloroform from running on to the face of the patient.

Tracheostomy inhaler

In 1869 Friedrich Trendelenburg of Berlin introduced his cone for use with chloroform via a tracheostomy. He later added an inflatable cuff to the tube and although never very popular, this and Hahn's similar apparatus was used successfully by both Probyn-Williams and Boyle for advanced head and neck surgery in the first decade of this century.

Controlled percentages

Clover and Snow advocated the use of controlled amounts of chloroform, Clover by the use of a 4% mixture in his widely used but rather clumsy bag, and Snow via an inhaler of his own design.

'Open' inhaler

The unmetered so-called 'open' inhalers were much more widely used. Some examples from the collection include Carter's from 1885 which was double-ended, one end for adults and the other for children with a marine sponge in the middle, and Sudeck's mask from 1900, also with a marine sponge but with the addition of primitive valves. Sir Thomas Dunhill designed an inhaler in 1911 which included early inspiratory and expiratory valves.

Vaporizers

There were two vaporizer methods used, blow-over and draw-over. The most widely used was the blow-over inhaler designed by Ferdinand Adalbert Junker in 1867. The apparatus was used for 60 years and underwent several modifications.

The original version included a graduated bottle to hold 8 drachms of chloroform. Air from a bellows passed down the long inlet tube and bubbled through the liquid then carrying the vapour via the short outlet tube to the mask. There was a hook on the top of the bottle to allow the device to be hung from the lapel or breast pocket of the anaesthetist. It was easy for either the connections to be reversed or the bottle tipped, and numerous deaths were reported from the administration of liquid chloroform, even as late as 1927.

One modification was the use of two bottles in series and another by Dudley Buxton in 1890 was to place the inlet tube within the outlet tube. He also sheathed the efferent tube in bone to prevent freezing and in 1914 added taps to the inlet and outlet tubes. Other workers added a ball valve to the inlet tube to prevent the administration of liquid chloroform through misconnection. Carter–Braine made several modifications in 1914. The bottle was intended to contain only 2 ounces of chloroform and was so designed that if it is laid on its side, chloroform would not enter the outlet tube. The flange prevented splashing and the two tubes had different fittings. The vapour could be delivered through a variety of masks preferably valved, and also through some ingenious wire masks such as Dunkley's and Gwathmey's, both dating from 1910. The vapour could also be delivered via oral or nasal tubes.

It is interesting to note that Geoffrey Kaye saw the Junker's apparatus being used during the Second World War.

The draw-over technique is epitomized by the Vernon-Harcourt inhaler. Designed in 1903 by Augustus Vernon-Harcourt, reader in Chemistry at Oxford; it was a response to the Chloroform Commission's recommendation (1901) that a maximum concentration of 2% be used.

The Vernon-Harcourt inhaler was able to deliver a fairly accurate percentage of vapour in air from 0 through to 2%. Chloroform was placed in a two-necked conical bottle and two coloured beads were dropped into the liquid. The density of these beads was such that when the temperature was within the range 16–18 degrees centigrade, one bead sank and one floated. The dimensions of the bottle were arrived at after a great deal of experimental work and were calculated to diminish the variation in the inhaled concentration of chloroform vapour caused by either abnormally shallow or deep breathing, or by variations in gas flow rate. The stopcock in the centre of the inhaler was so made that when the pointer was at the end of the arc nearest the bottle of chloroform, a maximum quantity was being delivered, namely 2%, and when the pointer was at the opposite end air only would be inhaled. The one-way valves on the two branches prevented the entrance of expired air into the apparatus.

Although ingenious and elegant the Vernon-Harcourt inhaler did not survive the Great War because of its delicate nature.

Despite reports of the adverse effects of chloroform, apparatus sold as late as 1930 included chloroform bottles as standard. The use of chloroform, mainly via Schimmelbusch masks and Junker's inhalers continued well into the 1940s.

16.4   The performance of some historic vaporizers

PETER L. JONES
University Hospital of Wales, Cardiff, Wales, UK

Abstract

The principles which govern the vaporization of volatile anaesthetics are well illustrated by the study of the performance of a number of historic vaporizers. This paper reviews those aspects of their construction which contribute to their observed performance.

Facsimile reproductions of the John Snow and Morton ether vaporizers, together with examples of the Clover inhaler, the Boyle bottle and the Schimmelbusch mask were tested under identical circumstances. Performances of these vaporizers under simulated clinical conditions provides an insight into their popularity and effectiveness. In particular, the outstanding performance of the Schimmelbusch mask during these investigations is in complete contrast to the many contemporary assertions which imply its inefficiency.

Chapter 17

THE USE OF MASKS AND TRACHEAL TUBES IN ANAESTHESIA

17.1 The design of experimental latex paediatric face masks in 1961

DONALD H. SOUCEK[1] and LESLIE RENDELL-BAKER[2]
[1]Parma, Ohio, USA and [2]Loma Linda University, California, USA

The request, in 1960, by our newly appointed paediatric surgeon that his neonatal patients with inguinal hernias be anaesthetized without intubation highlighted the dissatisfaction with paediatric face masks that had been felt for many years. Many of these had been designed merely by reducing the size of adult masks while retaining the same proportions. Infant facial contours are very different in that they lack the prominent cheek bones and nose of the adult (Fig. 1). Consequently, an infant mask designed to adult proportions often did not make a good seal resulting in poor control of anaesthetic mixtures. The dead space too, was often considerable, resulting in accumulation of carbon dioxide, which could be of serious consequence in paediatric anaesthesia. Therefore, it was decided to study the facial contours of children of a variety of ethnic and racial groups of different ages by means of direct facial moulds to determine a design which would provide optimal fit and minimal dead space.

The method will be described in three separate stages; first, making a mould of the face; second, designing a mask; third, processing a latex prototype mask.

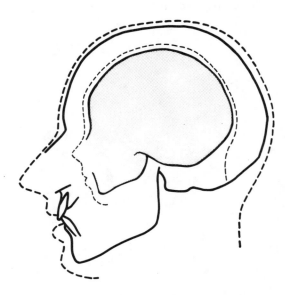

Figure 1 *Comparison of adult's and infant's facial proportions. The adult has a prominent nose and cheek bones so that an adult mask must have a deep cavity to accommodate a large nose and a pneumatic cushion to fit variable maxillary bony structures. The infant's face by contrast is much more rounded with a little nose. There are two bony points to which the paediatric mask must fit. The nasion above and the mental process below. In between these two points the baby's cheeks are like soft cushions which may be utilized to seal the mask.*

Stage 1: Making the mould

Alginate (Jeltrate), an elastic irreversible-impression material, was used exclusively as the preferred material because it can be applied directly to the skin without danger of allergic reactions. The alginate was mixed with water and the mixture was placed on the patient's face starting over the forehead and eyebrows and working down to the chin (Fig. 2) to prevent material from entering the eyes which were protected with Bacitracin ointment. Alginate was applied with the hands, being careful not to entrap air bubbles beneath the material. It was left for one of two minutes after the stickiness vanished. The patient's skin was oily enough to prevent the alginate sticking so that it was unnecessary to apply petroleum jelly.

An oral tracheal tube extending two inches out of the mouth was used to provide a secure airway. The mouth was held closed by pressure under the chin and the alginate mixture was applied around the tube. No difficulty with the mixture dropping into the nares or the oral cavity occurred.

Dental Plaster of Paris (B-hemihydrate) 100 g of powder to 60 ml of water was mixed to a creamy consistency and then placed over the alginate and around the extended endotracheal tube as a support. The normal setting time was approximately four and one-half minutes; but this could be shortened by adding sodium chloride to the powder before mixing and/or by using hot water.

The entire mask of alginate and plaster with the enclosed tracheal tube was removed from the face in one piece by gently prying it up from the edges. Thus a negative model of the face was obtained.

Dental stone (a-hemihydrate) (Castone) was mixed with water to a creamy consistency in the proportion of 100 g to 30 ml water. The negative impression was inverted and placed in a stable position on a table. If any plaster was exposed within the mould where it could come in contact with the stone, when the latter was poured into the negative impression, this plaster was coated with Vaseline to prevent chemical bonding between the two substances. No chemical

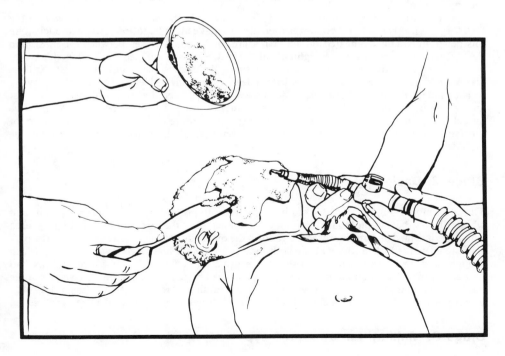

Figure 2   After induction of anaesthesia and intubation alginate impression material followed by a supporting layer of plaster of Paris is being applied to the infant's face.

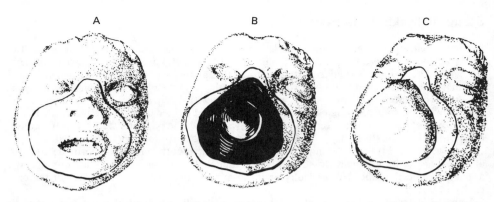

Figure 3   A. An accurate duplicate of the baby's face cast in dental stone. A line indicating the outer margin of the contact area of the future mask has been cut into the face. B. Red wax has been added over the tip of the nose and the mouth to provide an airspace from which the baby will breathe. The lateral margin between the red wax and the peirpheral line determines the airtightness of the seal between the mask and the face. C. A stone model of face with the added breathing space. This forms the inner surface onto which the mask is moulded.

bonding occurs between the alginate and stone. The stone mix was added in small increments while the mould was shaken rapidly but gently, being careful to avoid entrapping air bubbles; so that the stone penetrated every crevice of the alginate. Alginate impression material shrinks and distorts very rapidly by loss of water, therefore it was imperative to pour the stone immediately after the impression is taken. After setting for 20 to 30 minutes, the stone was separated by gently prying the substances apart. Thus a permanent positive model or cast of the face was obtained (Fig. 3).

A pencil outline was drawn on the model marking how far the mask would extend on the face (Fig. 3A). A sharp knife point was then used to make an indentation into the model along this pencil line. This delineated the outer margin of the contact area between the mask and the face which determined the airtightness of the seal. Pieces of soft red wax softened in warm water were moulded over the model from the tip of the nose to the mouth (Fig. 3B). As little wax as possible was used so as to minimize the dead space while still leaving an adequate airway.

The model with the attached dead space wax was chilled in cold water; while still very moist an alginate impression was made with dental plaster as previously described. A stone positive model was then made (Fig. 3C). In this manner, an accurate duplication of the contours of the face and inner surface of the mask's airway was made onto which the mask could be moulded.

Stage 2: Designing the mask

The latter model (Fig. 3C) was soaked in soapy water to prevent wax from adhering to it, and while still wet, heated pink base plate wax was shaped over the nose, mouth, and lateral area within the indented line previously added to form the outer edge of the future latex mask. The pink wax can be worked when soft at above body temperature but is hard at room temperature. Much thought and time was taken at this step to ensure an acceptable design. Once the wax had hardened proper symmetry and thickness was achieved by removing the surplus wax from the model with a sharp knife. After the wax mask had been shaped to the intended design (Fig. 4A), it was placed on the face model to check that no distortion had occurred in the processing.

Stage 3: Making the latex prototype

Two little-finger-sized 'sprues' of wax were attached to the upper surface of the wax mask, one over the chin and the other over the nose. The assembly was chilled in cold water for

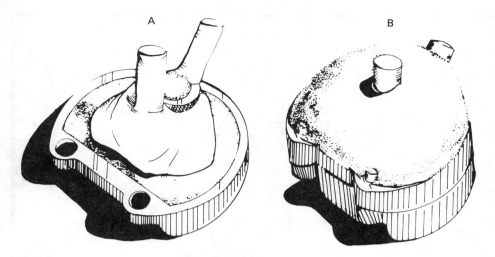

Figure 4   A. plaster-filled wax mask inverted onto plaster in base of denture flask. B. Collar has been attached to denture flask and the entire wax mask, except for sprues, has been covered in plaster.

15 minutes. Then stiff Plaster of Paris was poured into the inverted inner part of the wax mask and into the base of the denture flask, being careful to avoid trapping air bubbles between the plaster and wax. The plaster, filled mask was inverted, centred over the stone-filled base of the denture flask, and seated so the surface of the mask which rests on the face was level with the edge of the flask (Fig. 4A). The excess plaster projecting above the lower edge of the mask was removed while still moist and the surface smoothed out with the index finger.

When dry the exposed plaster was coated with petrolatum as a separating medium. The collar of the flask was placed on its base and more plaster was added covering the entire upper surface of the wax mask and part of the sprues (Fig. 4B).

When the plaster had hardened the flask was placed in boiling water for five minutes to soften the wax before being opened. Then the mould was separated and flushed with hot water and chloroform to remove residues of wax.

When the mould had cooled liquid latex was poured into it through one of the sprue holes at the top. Liquid latex shrinks during curing, therefore it was necessary to keep adding further quantities. It was allowed to set overnight as the liquid latex cures by dehydration.

The flask was gently opened and the latex face mask separated from the mould; it was allowed to cure in air for a further 12 to 24 hours. The sprues were cut off and the

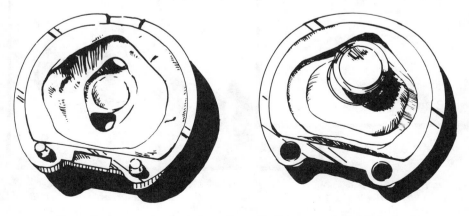

Figure 5   Inner and outer halves of mould after removal of wax by heat.

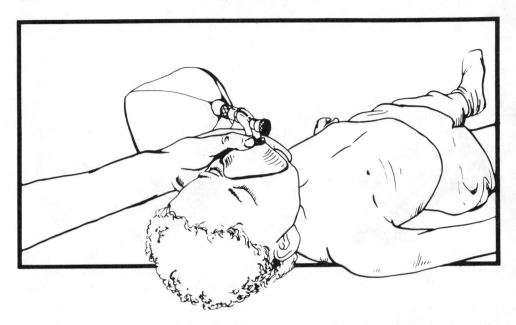

Figure 6   General anaesthesia being administered without intubation using prototype latex face mask.
These masks conformed to the child's face and required only light pressure to maintain an airtight seal.

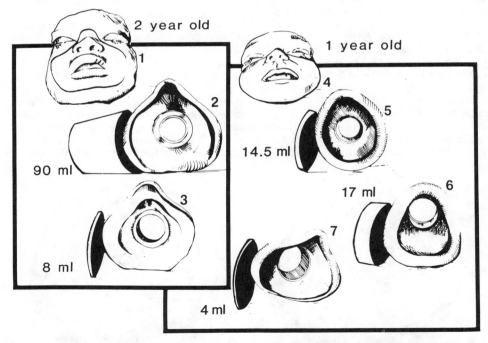

Figure 7   Comparison of dead space in masks. A. 1) Two-year-old face cast; 2) MIE Everseal mask—
dead space 90 ml; 3) RBS size 2 latex mask—dead space 8 ml. B. 4) One-year-old face cast; 5) Ohio
neonatal mask—dead space 14.5 ml; 6) MIE paediatric mask—dead space 17 ml; 7) RBS size 1 latex
mask—dead space 4 ml.

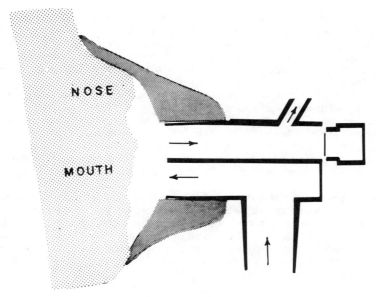

Figure 8   Mask adaptor.

mask trimmed with scissors. To produce a smooth shiny surface the mask was dipped in liquid latex.

The finished latex mask not only conformed to the child's face from which it was made, but also to the faces of children in that particular age bracket. Only enough vertical pressure to stabilize the mask was required to maintain an airtight fit (Fig. 6), permitting manually assisted respiration without leakage of anaesthetic gases.

The dead space within a variety of paediatric masks was compared to that in the latex masks (Fig. 7) as follows: the masks were matched to the correct size of stone face cast, hot wax was poured into the mask filling the dead space up to the metal connector. When chilled, the wax was removed from the mask, reheated, and poured into a gradual cylinder and measured.

Four different sizes of experimental masks from size 0 to size 3 were made to fit children from prematures to five year olds. A partitioned 15 mm–22 mm tube-mask adaptor (see Fig. 8), which separated the fresh gas from the expired gas flow, was designed to enable the masks to be used with adult or paediatric breathing systems. This paediatric 15 mm–22 mm tube-mask adaptor has since become a standard component of most adult breathing systems. Jackson Rees and other paediatric breathing systems with the new standard 15 mm size fittings were also introduced at that time.

The production versions of these masks and equipment were introduced in a scientific exhibit shown throughout 1961 and 1962.

17.2   Intubation in anaesthesia

ROD K. CALVERLEY
University of California, San Diego, USA

The ability to protect a patient's airway through endotracheal intubation ranks among the major advances in the history of anaesthesia. Before the discovery of inhalational anaesthesia, tracheotomies or endotracheal tubes were employed in experiments or during resuscitation by Galen, Avicenna, Paracelsus, Vesalius, Hook, Desault, Chaussier and others.

After 1846 tracheotomies were occasionally performed during surgery, but it was not until 1878 that an uncuffed oral endotracheal tube was used to promote unobstructed ventilation during an operation on the tongue. Years later inflatable cuffs were added to prevent pulmonary contamination and permit positive pressure ventilation.

Since 1953 double-lumen endobronchial tubes have been of great advantage in chest surgery. While the first endotracheal tubes were inserted blindly by the sense of touch, more than 100 models of direct-vision laryngoscopes have been designed since 1900. Anaesthetists may now choose from a variety of modern instruments including fibreoptic endoscopes to intubate patients with complex anatomical problems which previously might have been considered impossible for all but the most expert (or fortunate) practitioner. Every clinician who performs endotracheal intubation has access to equipment that reflects a magnificent heritage of innovation and discovery.

While new equipment continues to be introduced at an accelerating pace, most modern devices are refinement of instruments which were commonly used at the time of the centennial of ether anaesthesia in 1946. The landmark advances in intubation introduced during the first century of surgical anaesthesia which will be reviewed in this paper form a fascinating history filled with episodes of brilliant observation, forgotten or unappreciated invention, rediscovery and advance. When possible the earliest discoverer will be recognized, but in other instances the individual who successfully brought a technique into regular use will receive greater attention.

19th century contributions

Most major innovations have been introduced since 1900, but a few pioneering advances came forward in the Victorian era. Emergency tracheotomies were occasionally attempted on anaesthetized patients soon after 1846. John Snow may have been the first to administer an elective anaesthetic to a patient through a pre-existing tracheotomy. Snow also performed a tracheotomy upon an anaesthetized rabbit while studying the effects of chloroform on its heart (1).

The concern of prudent anaesthetists with the security of the airway is reflected in a report in 1877 by another British specialist, Joseph T. Clover, who corrected total respiratory obstruction in an anaesthetized patient by inserting a small curved cannula through the crico-thyroid membrane. So great had been Clover's concern over the potential for airway obstruction during anaesthesia that he was well prepared beforehand. He wrote:

'I have never used the cannula before although it has been my companion at some thousands of anaesthetic cases.' (2).

William Macewan (1848-1924)

The following year (1878) William Macewan, a distinguished surgeon of the Glasgow Royal Infirmary, was the first to employ oral endotracheal intubation electively. While this technique would be only occasionally practised for another half century, Macewan's innovation would eventually become a universally employed alternative to the mutilation of tracheotomy.

Macewan practised passing tubes by the sense of touch from the oropharynx into the trachea of cadavers before attempting the manoeuvre on an awake patient on 5 July, 1878. His first subject was a 51-year-old man with an oral tumour whom he intubated with a flexible metal tube. Immediately thereafter, his house surgeon, Dr Symington, began a historic but uncomplicated chloroform anaesthetic via the tube. After induction the surgeon inserted a sponge to protect the larynx from blood. While Macewan performed additional successful intubations for at least two cases of severe laryngeal obstruction, one due to infection and the other due to the too-rapid ingestion of a hot potato, he may have discontinued this practice following a fatality in which the patient was intubated awake, but pulled out his tube and later expired under chloroform (3).

Other early intubations for anaesthesia

A sporadic interest in peroral endotracheal anaesthesia developed in other European centres. In 1889 an Edinburgh surgeon, J. Annandale employed a gum elastic oral tube which featured a vulcanite bite block. In 1893 Victor Eisenmenger created a rigid endotracheal tube with an inflatable cuff and pilot balloon. Other cuffed tubes were fashioned by physiologists. In 1889 Henry Head made a double-lumen endobronchial tube for respiratory studies in dogs (4).

A few Americans were also interested in intubation. A physiologist, Henry Lyman, used narrow flexible tubes to insufflate air or oxygen into the airway of animals paralysed with curare. He included endotracheal insufflation among suggested remedies for respiratory failure in anaesthetized patients, but cautioned that, if any difficulty should be encountered, a tracheotomy should be performed immediately. His proposal may have been theoretical for no case reports of oral intubation are found in his anaesthesia text of 1881 (5).

Joseph O'Dwyer (1841–1898)

Four years later, however, a New York surgeon reported a successful technique of intubation. Joseph O'Dwyer contrived cunningly shaped metal laryngeal tubes which were inserted through the mouth as an alternative to the immediate and long-term risks of tracheotomy in children experiencing diphtheritic laryngeal obstruction. The first O'Dwyer tube featured an expanded superior pole which was designed to rest on the false cords. In 1888 O'Dwyer designed a second rigid tube whose conical tip covered the larynx while the end protruding from the mouth formed a T-piece. The tube was attached to George Fell's apparatus thereby permitting manual positive pressure ventilation for the successful treatment of narcotic overdose. Other modifications of the O'Dwyer tube were fabricated by Theodore Tuffier of Paris and Rudolph Matas of New Orleans for positive pressure ventilation in chest surgery.

Franz Kuhn (1866–1929)

At the beginning of the 20th century the outstanding pioneer of endotracheal anaesthesia was a German surgeon, Franz Kuhn. From 1900 until 1912 Kuhn wrote a series of fine papers and a classic monograph on intubation which, regrettably, were not widely appreciated for many years (6). In these reports Kuhn described his techniques of oral and nasal intubation which he performed with flexible metal tubes of a design similar to the coiled tubing still used for the spout of metal petrol cans. After Kuhn's death they remained in occasional use in Europe but were almost unknown to physicians of English-speaking countries before World War II when a few British military anaesthetists were captured by German forces yet continued to provide anaesthesia for their wounded comrades while incarcerated in POW camps. W. Stanley Sykes wrote a colourful appreciation of Kuhn's remarkable device:

> *'Kuhn's tube has, and I speak from personal experience, one great and solid advantage over modern methods. It does not depend upon dry batteries, which all disappear under the counter in war-time. I used it in about 40 cases in a Kriegsgefangenenlazarett, or prisoner-of-war hospital. My laryngoscope was useless, owing to the absence of batteries, my Magill tubes perished until they were unsafe to use (and the German ersatz rubber tubing was too stiff to make new ones). But Kuhn's tube, being made of flexible metal, was simple, reliable, durable, immutable, imperishable, insusceptible to damage and absolutely indestructible. There was nothing to go wrong, nothing to damage. As a war-time expedient it was excellent.' (7)*

Kuhn introduced his tubes over a curved metal stylet and directed them toward the larynx with his left index finger. He was the first anaesthetist to use topical cocaine to reduce an awake patient's discomfort during the passage of the tube. While he was aware that a cuff could be applied, he chose to seal the larynx by positioning a supralaryngeal flange near the tube's tip and packing the upper airway with an oil-soaked gauze. He recommended the nasal route for long-term intubation as he observed that a nasal tube was often well tolerated and did not require a dental guard to prevent it being 'crunched' by a restless patient.

He was the first to suggest that tracheal secretions or blood could be suctioned from the airway through a small catheter. The suction catheter could also be used to insufflate anaesthetics which would then exit the airway via the larger tube. In his routine practise of head and neck surgery Kuhn preferred an inhalation technique with bidirectional exchange of gas through a large tube instead of the continuous insufflation of gases through a narrow tube. In 1912, however, Kuhn reported an application of the insufflation technique which had been independently developed in France by Barthelemy and Dufour, as well as in America by Meltzer and Auer.

Insufflation techniques

During the next decade the continuous insufflation of gases remained popular in Europe and America despite several limitations. The shortcomings of the method included carbon dioxide accumulation, the requirement for high flow rates of inspired anaesthetics, the hazard of abdominal distention if the tube entered the oesophagus, the risk of high airway pressures and pneumothorax if the airway was sealed and the potential of aspiration if the airway was open.

Direct-vision laryngoscope

Even in experienced hands, intubation by palpation could be an uncertain and sometimes traumatic art. Prior to the introduction of the direct-vision laryngoscope, the greatest impediment to intubation had been difficulty in visualizing the cords while passing the tube. Even though indirect laryngoscopy with a mirror antedated Macewan's work, the technique could not be adapted for use during intubation. Many clinicians believed that it would be anatomically impossible to visualize the vocal cords directly. This misapprehension was overcome by the first direct-vision laryngoscope devised by Alfred Kirstein in Berlin in 1895. While Kirstein's 'autoscope' was not used by anaesthetists, it was the forerunner of modern laryngoscopes.

The impetus for Kirstein's work came in the spring of 1895 from a colleague who reported that a patient's trachea had been accidentally intubated during oesophagoscopy. Aware of the clinical potential of this observation, Kirstein promptly fabricated a hand-held instrument which consisted of a blade and a handle. The handle contained a bulb, lens and prism from Caspar's mains-powered electroscope attached at a right angle to a shortened cylindrical oesophagoscope. Kirstein soon realized that the cylindrical scope had limited application for it demanded extreme extension of the patient's neck and risked damage to teeth. Within a month he reduced these limitations by altering the cylinder to a semicircular blade which was open inferiorly. Kirstein could now examine the larynx while standing behind his seated patient whose head was placed in an attitude approximating the 'sniffing position' later recommended by Sir Ivan Magill. An examination of Alfred Kirstein's contributions appeared in a fine review by Nicholas Hirsch *et al.* (8).

A pupil of Kirstein, Gustav Killian, enthusiastically supported his concepts and came to be considered 'the father of bronchoscopy'. Endoscopic examination was further refined in Philadelphia by Chevalier Jackson who designed a 'U-shaped' laryngoscope by adding a hand grip which lay parallel to the blade. The Jackson laryngoscope became a standard instrument for laryngeal examinations and was used as an aid to the passage of insufflation tubes before surgery by Charles Elsberg, a New York surgeon, in 1912. The following year Chevalier Jackson wrote a paper directed to anaesthetists in which he advocated the direct inspection of the vocal cords with his instrument before intubation during anaesthesia (9).

The continued popularity of the 'U-shaped' Jackson scope may be somewhat perplexing to modern readers since a laryngoscope which closely approximated modern instruments was introduced in 1913. The American surgeon, Henry Janeway, produced an 'L-shaped' laryngoscope fashioned specifically for intubation. It was the first to feature an internal light source powered by batteries within the handle. The Janeway blade was straight except for a slight distal curve designed to direct the tube towards the larynx. It closely resembled a mirror image of Robert Miller's classic blade as the lateral opening was on the left side. Janeway grasped the handle with the right hand and passed an insufflation tube with the left.

Cuffed tubes

Janeway's gum elastic tracheal catheters incorporated a detachable inflatable cuff to reduce the loss of nitrous oxide (10). Three years before Janeway's paper was published another cuffed endotracheal tube had been produced in New York by G. M. Dorrance (11). Both the Dorrance and Janeway tubes seem to have been ignored by other workers of that time.

Dorrance and Janeway's clever innovations may have failed to capture wide attention because cuffed tubes and laryngoscopes lacked a sufficient market in 1913 when there were fewer than 100 anaesthetists active in the United States. Many practitioners had never attempted intubation. For many years thereafter ENT surgeons were routinely called to the operating room in some hospitals for every elective or emergency intubation while the attending anaesthetists confined their attention to the administration of anaesthetic gases and vapours. In time, however, all anaesthetists were able to learn the skills of atraumatic nasal and oral intubation by employing techniques and instruments developed by the creative genius of a few British and North American specialists in anaesthesia.

Sir Ivan Magill (1888–1986) and Stanley Rowbotham (1890–1979)

Two of the most distinguished pioneers of endotracheal intubation were self-trained British anaesthetists, Ivan (later Sir Ivan) Magill, and his friend, Stanley Rowbotham. The contributions for which each man received international recognition have been reviewed recently (12,13).

Their professional association began in 1919 when, as general medical officers without a special interest in anaesthesia, they were simultaneously seconded to the Queen's Hospital for Facial and Jaw Injuries at Sidcup near London where they accepted assignments as anaesthetists.

Rowbotham and Magill attended military casualties disfigured by severe facial injuries who underwent repeated restorative operations. There could be successful only if the surgeon, Harold Gillies, had almost unrestricted access to the face and airway. Some patients with severe abnormalities were formidable challenges, but both men were adept and appreciated the significance of fortuitous observations which they applied to extend the limitations of insufflation anaesthesia. The only alternative anaesthetic, rectal ether, left patients unresponsive for hours with an unprotected airway and was therefore rarely employed. They concentrated upon refining the insufflation of nitrous oxide/oxygen and warm ether delivered continuously by a Shipway apparatus.

While working together Rowbotham and Magill created several modifications of insufflation techniques. Before their arrival at Sidcup a single tube had been used around which the insufflated gases blew back to the surgeon's face. They learned to pass a second tube, either Silk's wide-bore pharyngeal tube or another insufflation tube, to permit the controlled escape of nitrous oxide. They then packed the pharynx to seal the airway. In this manner the lungs were protected from contamination and, as the exhaled gases were channeled from the patient, blood did not bubble back to obscure the surgeon's view. With two tubes in place the surgeon was also spared the annoyance of breathing the anaesthetic, a factor which added to Gillies's comfort and undoubtedly contributed to his endorsement of their other innovations.

Magill and Rowbotham's expertise with blind nasal intubation began after they learned to soften semirigid insufflation tubes which they passed through the nose after the nostril had been dilated with a series of lubricated tubes. Rowbotham wrote:

> *'Occasionally when the catheter is passed through the nose . . . and pushed on, the cough characteristic of its passage into the trachea occurs and on inspection the fact that it has actually passed between the cords is confirmed.'* (14)

Stimulated by this chance experience they developed the techniques of nasal tracheal intubation and, to aid in positioning the catheter, introduced Rowbotham's 'guiding rod' and Magill's 'angulated forceps'.

Although Magill recorded his first use of a wide tube in 1920, it was a few years later that he found appropriate rubber tubing of a type routinely used to carry cooking gas to a bunsen burner which he cut, bevelled and smoothed to prepare the single-lumen, wide-bore tube that anaesthetists would come to call the Magill tube. The Magill tube permitted a bidirectional respiratory pattern and soon supplanted insufflation techniques. To assist intubation Magill designed a U-shaped laryngoscope. Magill also rediscovered the advantages of cocainization of the airway, a technique which he perfected in developing his mastery of awake blind nasal intubation.

Magill's success with awake blind intubation excited the curiosity of other anaesthetists to whom Magill taught his principles at meetings of the Section of Anaesthetists of the Royal Society of Medicine. In his lectures Magill occasionally concealed, with a puckish display of humour, a few pertinent points from colleagues who might also be his competitors in seeking referrals for the limited number of private cases. As recalled by the late Dr Stephen Coffin, Magill openly described the selection of the correct tube and the advantages of the 'sniffing' position, but, in the weeks after the presentation, no member of his audience could match his success.

A few of the most determined men visited Magill to study his craft. They marvelled at his dexterity and speed, not realizing that the patient had received topical cocaine before entering the induction area. On some occasions the observer's gaze was diverted from the patient's face at the moment of intubation by an unexpected request from Dr Magill who would ask his visitor to pick up a piece of equipment from the table behind him. When the guest turned back to see the patient, the visitor was chagrined to observe the tube already in the trachea. Dr Coffin said that at least one colleague reported that the experience had taught him that blind nasal intubation could be done, but he left the hospital without knowing how Magill had passed the tube so swiftly and skilfully.

Within a short time Ivan Magill's small secrets became public knowledge, but few could ever match his mastery of the airway in the time before muscle relaxants were introduced. Throughout his professional career he continued to fabricate new devices for the advantage of all. His other innovations included endotracheal tubes for children, an L-shaped laryngoscope, a tracheoscope and wire-tipped endobronchial tubes for thoracic surgery. Sir Ivan Magill gained universal admiration for his work and was for decades recognized by his colleagues as 'The Master' until his death in his ninety-ninth year on 25 November, 1986.

Armoured tubes

One of the challenges encountered by anaesthetists was the need for wide-bore endotracheal tubes which would resist kinking when flexed, a persisting hazard of rubber tubes. In 1929 an American surgeon, Paluel Flagg, developed a metal tube whose central portion was composed of flexible metal. Dr Phillip Woodbridge improved the flexibility of the armoured tube, but the appliance found its most popular application in the form of the armoured 'Anode' tube of soft rubber reinforced with an internal wire spiral as first recommended by Ralph Hargrave of Toronto (15).

Arthur Guedel (1883–1956) and Ralph Waters (1883–1979)

Another modification that advanced anaesthetic care was the reintroduction of the cuffed endotracheal tube by two Americans, Arthur Guedel and Ralph Waters. In 1926, unaware of the prior work of Eisenmenger, Janeway and Dorrance, Arthur Guedel began a series of experiments with cuffed tubes. His goal was to combine the safety of endotracheal anaesthesia with the economy of the closed circuit soda-lime absorption technique previously introduced by Ralph Waters. Guedel subjected each step of the preparation and application of his cuffed tubes to a vigorous review. He experimented with cuffs fashioned from the rubber of dental dams, condoms and surgical gloves glued onto the outer wall of tubes. He considered three positions for the cuff—above, below or at the level of the cords—before recommending that the cuff be positioned just below the cords which would both seal the airway and prevent an inaccessible accumulation of fluid above the cuff. Ralph Waters later recommended that the cuffs be made of two layers of soft rubber cemented together at the edge. These double-layered cuffs could be slipped over the tube and replaced when a cuff malfunctioned.

While Arthur Guedel could demonstrate the safety and utility of the cuffed tube in the operating theatre by filling the nose and mouth of an anaesthesized and intubated patient with water, he felt that a more dramatic technique was required to capture the attention of a large audience unfamiliar with the advantages of intubation. He reasoned that, as the cuff would prevent water from entering the trachea of an intubated patient, a cuff should also prevent an animal from drowning even if it were totally submerged under water. He prepared the first of several public 'dunked dog' demonstrations. An anaesthetized and intubated dog, probably his own pet 'Airway', was immersed in an aquarium. After the demonstration was complete the anaesthetic was discontinued as the dog was removed from the water. 'Airway' awoke and indicated his good health by shaking water over the audience before leaving the room. With this novel display the cuffed tube gradually gained wide use (16).

At the time of the first Guedel/Waters 'dunked dog' show, a member of the audience remarked that theirs was not the first cuffed tube as he had seen one some years before but had forgotten where. This observation piqued Guedel and Waters's curiosity and led them to study a great collection of old journals to create a history of endotracheal anaesthesia which drew attention to George Dorrance and other pioneers who had anticipated their work but whose achievements had been ignored. The task must have been sometimes frustrating for the authors prefaced their report with the comment, 'The pleasure of this research has been exceeded only by the work involved' (17).

Talented observers may recognize a therapeutic opportunity when presented with what at first appears to be a misadventure. This principle was demonstrated in 1931 by an episode at Madison, Wisconsin. After a patient's tube was accidentally malpositioned in the right bronchus, Ralph Waters realized that a very long cuffed endotracheal tube could be used to ventilate one lung independently while the other was being resected (18). On learning of his friend's success with one-lung anaesthesia, Arthur Guedel proposed an important modification for chest surgery, the double-cuffed single lumen endobronchial tube which was later introduced by Emery Rovenstine. Following World War II several double-cuffed single-lumen tubes were used regularly in thoracic surgery, but were supplanted by double-lumen endobronchial tubes first reported in 1953 by Bjork, Carlens and Friberg. The double-lumen tube favoured currently is that designed by Frank Robertshaw (of Manchester, England) which is prepared in both right and left-sided versions. While these tubes were first created from rubber, Robertshaw tubes are now made of extruded plastic, a technique refined by Mr David Sheridan. Mr Sheridan was also the first to inscribe centimetre markings along the side of endotracheal tubes, a safety feature which has reduced the hazards of accidental endobronchial intubation and inadvertent extubation.

Miller and Macintosh laryngoscopes

Early practitioners of intubation were frustrated by difficulties with early laryngoscopes that were cumbersome, ill-designed to protect the patient's teeth and offered only a limited exposure of the larynx. These problems were all the more pronounced as muscle relaxants were not yet available. It was in that period, however, that Robert Miller of San Antonio, Texas and Professor Robert Macintosh of Oxford created laryngoscopes which have achieved lasting popularity. The earlier of these models was described in 1941 by Miller who created a slender, predominantly straight blade with a slight curve near the tip to ease the passage of the tube through the larynx (19).

Professor Robert (later Sir Robert) Macintosh introduced a curved laryngoscope in 1943 which is now called after him (20). Years later he wrote a note to describe the circumstances of its discovery in an appreciation of the career of Mr Richard H. Salt, the able Senior Chief Technician of the Nuffield Department of Anaesthetics. Macintosh recalled:

'. . . A Boyle-Davis gag, a size larger than intended, was inserted for tonsillectomy, and when the mouth was fully opened the cords came into view. This was a surprise since conventional laryngoscopy, at that depth of anaesthesia, would have been impossible in those pre-relaxant days. Within a matter of hours, Salt had modified the blade of the Davis gag and attached a laryngoscope handle to it; and streamlined, the end result came into widespread use.' (21)

As a result of Mr Salt's painstaking dedication to detail, the blade passed through several evolutions on its way to being formed into a shape now familiar to every anaesthetist. A fascinating display of the original and intermediate construction models of the Macintosh blade can be viewed in the Nuffield Department of Anaesthetics on Level One of the John Radcliffe Hospital, Headington, Oxford.

Since its introduction in 1943 the blade has appeared in many forms, a process which began within months of its first presentation. In 1943 the Foregger Company requested rights to copy the blade for the North American market. The inventors gave their consent freely, but, in haste caused by the pressures of other wartime activities, dispatched a prototype to New York in the expectation that Foregger's engineers would refine it. After some years Mr Salt discovered that the blade was marketed in the form they had shipped it. The variation still persists. American blades often have a deeper flange and a more pronounced curve than is seen on British models.

The Macintosh blade has since been further modified for special purposes. The curve has been reshaped in almost every conceivable way. The right angle attachment of the handle has been increased to a variety of obtuse angles. Suction tubes and manipulative arms have been added. The Macintosh blade is unique in that it is marketed with both right and left handed models. It is now available in plastic as a disposable item as well as in its familiar presentation of polished metal.

Conclusion

The many forms of the classic Macintosh blade are representative of recent advances in almost every element of anaesthetic equipment used for the control of the airway. Prisms and fibreoptic bundles now aid in difficult cases of laryngoscopy and provide anaesthetists with images beyond the expectation of the early masters of intubation. A host of special-purpose plastic endotracheal tubes have been designed to overcome the limitations of metal and rubber products which were all that were available to our predecessors. Other features designed to promote greater safety have been brought forward. Through the labours of early anaesthetists and the continuing efforts of workers still in practise, we have all gained a vital skill, the ability to perform safe intubation in anaesthesia.

Acknowledgment

I wish to recognize the generous support provided by Professor Duke B. Weeks of Wake Forest University Medical Centre, Winston-Salem, North Carolina, who brought many important points of information to my attention.

References

(1) Snow J. *On chloroform and other anaesthetics*. London: Churchill, 1858: 117.
(2) Clover JT. Laryngotomy in chloroform anaesthesia. *Br Med J* 1877; **1**: 132–3.
(3) Macewan W. Clinical observations on the introduction of tracheal tubes by the mouth instead of performing tracheotomy or laryngotomy. *Br Med J* 1880; 122–4, 163–5.
(4) Head H. On the regulation of respiration. *J Physiol* 1889; **10**: 1–70.
(5) Lyman HM. *Artificial anaesthesia and anaesthetics*. New York: William Wood, 1881: 51–61.
(6) Kuhn F. *Die perorale intubation* Berlin: S. Karger, 1911.
(7) Sykes WS. *Essays on the first hundred years of anaesthesia Vol I*. London: E & S Livingstone, 1960: 102.

(8) Hirsch NP, Smith GB, Hirsch PO. Alfred Kirstein pioneer of direct laryngoscopy. *Anaesthesia* 1986; **41**: 42–5.

(9) Jackson C. The technique of insertion of intratracheal insufflation tubes. *Surg Gynecol Obstet* 1913; **17**: 507–9.

(10) Janeway HH. Intratracheal anesthesia from the standpoint of the nose, throat and oral surgeon with a description of a new instrument for catheterizing the trachea. *Laryngoscope* 1913; **23**: 1082.

(11) Dorrance GM. On the treatment of traumatic injuries of the lungs and pleura, with the presentation of a new intratracheal tube for use in artificial respiration. *Surg Gynecol Obstet* 1910; **2**: 160–189.

(12) Thomas KB. Sir Ivan Whiteside Magill, KCVO, DSc, MB, BCh, BAO, FRCS, FFARCS (Hon), FFARCSI (Hon), DA a review of his publications and other references to his life and work. *Anaesthesia* 1978; **33**: 628–34.

(13) Condon HA, Gilchrist E. Stanley Rowbotham twentieth century pioneer anaesthetist. *Anaesthesia* 1986; **41**: 46–52.

(14) Rowbotham S. Intratracheal anaesthesia by the nasal route for operations on the mouth and lips. *Br Med J* 1920; **2**: 590–1.

(15) Hargrave R. An improved catheter for endotracheal nitrous oxide oxygen anaesthesia. *Can Med Assoc J* 1932; **26**: 218–21.

(16) Guedel AE, Waters RM. A new intratracheal catheter. *Curr Res Anesth Analg* 1928; **7**: 238–9.

(17) Waters RM, Rovenstine EA, Guedel AE. Endotracheal anesthesia and its historical development. *Curr Res Anesth Analg* 1933; **12**: 196–203.

(18) Gale JW, Waters RM. Closed endobronchial anesthesia in thoracic surgery: preliminary report. *Curr Res Anesth Analg* 1932; **11**: 283–7.

(19) Miller RA. A new laryngoscope. *Anesthesiology* 1941; **2**: 317–20.

(20) Macintosh RR. A new laryngoscope. *Lancet* 1943; **i**: 485.

(21) Macintosh RR. Richard Salt of Oxford, anaesthetic technician extraordinary. *Anaesthesia* 1976; **31**: 855–7.

Further reading

Gillespie NA. *Endotracheal anesthesia*. Madison: University of Wisconsin Press (3rd Ed), 1963.

Mushin WW, Rendell-Baker L. *The principles of thoracic anaesthesia past and present*. Springfield: Thomas, 1953.

PART V

THE HISTORY OF RESUSCITATION AND INTENSIVE CARE

Chapter 18
RESUSCITATION THROUGH THE AGES

18.1
Anaesthesia, pain relief and resuscitation in Biblical and Talmudic literature

LEON KAUFMAN
University College Hospital, London, England, UK

The period of this study extends from the Creation calculated from Biblical sources to have occurred 5747 years ago until the beginning of the 6th century AD when the Talmud reached a definitive form. The Talmud is comprised of the Mishnah which propounds the law and the Gemarrah which consists of commentaries and discussions of the interpretation of the law by various rabbinical authorities. The compilation of the Mishnah is believed to have begun at the early part of the 2nd century BC. There are two versions of the Talmud, one being assembled in Israel and the other in Babylon (Persia). The latter is more elaborate and voluminous and has become the established compendium to which reference is made on points of law and principle. The Talmud is essentially concerned with law and hence the laws of hygiene are discussed in some detail, but reference to surgical procedures are incidental and often fragmentary.

Surgery

In the Bible there is only one operation mentioned and that is that of circumcision (1,2,3). However, in the Talmud there are descriptions of the types of surgical procedures and surgical instruments and even where operations took place. Operations were performed in marble chambers (4,5) and this may refer to early operating suites. The surgeon wore a leather apron to protect himself from being soiled by blood (6). He was known to have a medicine chest and a basket for holding instruments and medicaments (7). Surgical instruments included the lancet (8) and a large ladle (9).

There are no detailed accounts of surgical operations, but amputation appears to have been performed under the influence of a 'drug' (11). There is a description of softening of the skull so that the brain could be exposed, although trephining of the skull was often performed (13). There are references to splenectomy and to suturing of the abdominal wall following rupture (15). Plastic surgery also appears to have been performed as Rabbi Elazar had an operation to remove excess fat (16).

Anaesthesia

The first reference to anaesthesia occurs in relation to the birth of Eve when 'the Lord God caused a deep sleep to fall on Adam when one of his ribs was removed' (17). The same word for deep sleep (Tardemah) also occurs later in Genesis (18) and in Isaiah (19). In the latter reference there is a suggestion of inhalation anaesthesia for 'the Lord has poured down upon you the spirit of deep sleep and closed your eyes'.

Apart from divine anaesthesia, attempts appear to have been made to carry out surgery under 'soporific drugs'. A sleeping drug appears to have been given for amputation (20) and apronectomy (21), but the nature of the drug cannot be ascertained. Other mixtures have included hyssop, juniper, aloes and myrrh which were crushed by the apothecary (22,23), but whether they were effective is doubtful.

The intoxicating effects of wine were known to Noah (24). Lot's daughters made their father insensible with wine (25), while Isaiah (26) was aware of the hangover (woe unto them) following strong drink. Wine does not appear to have been used as a major tranquillizer for surgical operations because of the unpredictability of its action, but it was administered to criminals awaiting execution (27).

There are references to powerful medicines which can either be a 'medicine of life' or a deadly poison (28). The pharmacological effects of the poppy were known to the Greeks but the earliest Biblical reference to it is on bronze coin of John Hyrkanus (135–106 BC). Poppy seeds were used as condiments (29,30).

Although the climate of Biblical lands has changed a little over the centuries the identification of plants found there is beset with difficulties (31). There are coincidental references to opion (32) which is derived from a herb, has medicinal properties and becomes deadly if given in overdose. Ladanum which was extracted as a sticky resin from an aromatic plant was applied to the skull (23). It will be interesting to speculate whether it was related to the draught of Laudanum which contains opium.

Although it had been felt that the healing of all physical ailments should be divinely inspired, Talmudic teaching permitted physicians to undertake healing (34). A volume consisting of a 'scroll of prescriptions' (35) has been lost while the 'book of cures' was deliberately hidden by King Hezekiah, possibly to avoid it falling into the hands of the unscrupulous (36).

Childbirth

Although Eve was delivered painlessly, she herself was promised pain in childbirth following the expulsion from the Garden of Eden (37). Jeremiah (38) was aware of the pains suffered during delivery in the primigravid when he exclaimed 'I have heard a voice as of a woman in travail, the anguish as of her that bringeth forth her first child'. The only means adopted of decreasing women's discomfort during childbirth was the use of the birth stool which was originally described as 'stones' (presumably put together in the form of a chair or stool) (38,39). The birth stool remained the only help that women received in labour apart from some other unidentified drugs until the advent of anaesthesia.

The mandrake referred to in Biblical sources has been identified as Mandragora, the roots of which resemble the human form and contain hyoscine. There are many superstitious rites associated with its collection and it was believed that those who plucked it out of the ground would die immediately. The apple of the mandrake which was collected by Reuben was believed to contain a love potion (40), but it has been suggested that Rachel was already pregnant and was more interested in obtaining the possible beneficial effects of the root for the impending delivery.

Post-mortem Caesarean section was encouraged to save the life of a baby of a mother dying in childbirth. In fact one was permitted to perform the operation on the Sabbath when all work was usually forbidden (41). There is however a reference to Caesarean section being performed under the influence of a drug to ease the pain of surgery. The operation was described as 'emergence (of the child) through the wall (of the abdomen)' (42). The birth of Caesar is also alluded to (43).

Resuscitation

There are two descriptions of resuscitation in Kings which might be interpreted as the modern equivalent of mouth to mouth resuscitation. Elijah who lived in the first half of the 9th century BC was called on to resuscitate a child who apparently had stopped breathing. Elijah carried him up to his bed, prayed and breathed deeply upon the child three times.

Breathing returned and the child survived (44). Elisha, who succeeded Elijah, was also involved in resuscitation of a child who appeared to have suffered from the effects of sunstroke (45). Resuscitation in this episode was less precise as Elisha had to travel a distance of some 20 miles to the scene of the dead child. But the description is impressive as Elisha put his mouth to the child's mouth, and breathed into him seven times.

Resuscitation of the newborn appears to have been attempted by blowing into the child's nostrils (46). Resuscitation of animals was also reported when 'the tube of reeds was inserted into the hole in the windpipe of a lamb which recovered' (47).

Summary

This is a brief survey of surgical procedures, pain relief and resuscitation that took place in Biblical and Talmudic times, and there is more than a suggestion that the procedures that took place were performed with high standards, and may have indeed been well ahead of their time.

References

(1) Genesis 17, 23
(2) Exodus 4, 25
(3) Joshua 5, 2
(4) Baba Mezia 83b
(5) Kethuboth 77b
(6) Kelim XXVI, 5
(7) Kelim XII, 3
(8) Kelim Xii, 4
(9) Kelim XVII, 12
(10) Shabbat 66a
(11) Baba Kamma 85a
(12) Kethuboth 77b
(13) Ohaloth II, 3
(14) Avodah Zarah 44a
(15) Chullin 56b, 57a
(16) Baba Mezia 83b
(17) Genesis 2, 21
(18) Genesis 15, 12
(19) Isaiah 29, 10
(20) Baba Kamma 85a
(21) Baba Mezia 83b
(22) Exodus 30, 25
(23) Nehemiah 3, 8
(24) Genesis 9, 21
(25) Genesis 19, 33
(26) Isaiah 5, 12
(27) Sanhedrin 43a
(28) Yoma 72b
(29) Baba Mezia 21a
(30) Baba Mezia 49a
(31) Zohary M. *Plants of the Bible* London: Cambridge University Press, 1982.
(32) Avodah Zarah II
(33) Ketuboth 77b
(34) Baba Kamma 85a
(35) Yoma 38a
(36) Berachot 10b
(37) Genesis 3, 16
(38) Exodus 1, 16

(39) Isaiah 37, 3
(40) Genesis 30, 14
(41) Arakhin 7a
(42) Niddah V, 1, 40a
(43) Avodah Zarah 10b
(44) Kings I, 17, 17
(45) Kings II, 4, 15
(46) Shabbat 128b
(47) Chullin 57b

18.2	The miracles of King Henry VI

PETER W. THOMPSON
University Hospital of Wales, Cardiff, Wales, UK

As we move from early history to modern times, we might pause on the way in the Middle Ages and, since this symposium is under Royal Patronage, look for a minute or two at one of England's more unhappy kings.

Henry VI

Henry VI was born at Windsor on 6 December, 1421, the only son of Henry V and Catherine of France. His father Henry V died in 1422 (aged 35 years) at Bois-de-Vincennes while on his way to assist Burgundy. Henry VI therefore succeeded to the throne at the age of one year, being crowned king seven years later in 1429.

Henry came under the spiritual guidance, from an early age, of the Carmelite theologian Thomas Netter who had been his father's confessor. Netter must have played a very large part in the development of Henry's undoubtedly deeply religious character. Unfortunately Henry was liable to periods of mental derangement, and he was also altogether too generous and trusting to be a successful ruler in his troubled age. He often sought refreshment in religious houses and gave much time to pious works. He was passionately devoted to the encouragement of learning and was the founder of Eton and King's College, Cambridge (1440 and 1441)— The latter is commemorated by Wordsworth who clearly regarded him as a saint:

> *'Tax not the royal Saint with vain expense,*
> *with ill-matched aims the Architect who planned—*
> *Albeit labouring for a scanty band*
> *Of white-robed Scholars only—this immense*
> *And glorious Work of fine intelligence!'*

This is not the place to rehearse details of the Wars of the Roses—sufficient to note that after the Battle of Barnet in 1471 Henry was committed to the Tower of London where he was murdered on the night that Edward IV returned—21 May, Richard of Gloucester (later Richard III) being held responsible.

The miracles

Very soon after his death accounts of miracles attributed to his intervention in response to intercession began to appear and these were particularly reported as occurring at his tomb at the Benedictine Monastery in Chertsey in Surrey which soon became a place of pilgrimage. Richard III had his body removed to St George's Chapel, Windsor, but was unable to put a stop to the rapid development of the popular devotion. The combination of miracles and devotions was the basis upon which Henry VII petitioned Popes Innocent VIII and Alexander VI for his canonization. In recent times renewed efforts have been made to this end. According to Roman Catholic Canon Law (CIC Can 2117) two to four well-authenticated miracles after death are required for the beatification of saints, though belief in any of these miracles is not demanded of the faithful as *de fide* (i.e. they can be contradicted without heresy).

The source book for information of this subject is Knox and Leslie *The Miracles of King Henry VI* (1923) Cambridge University Press. By 1500, some 174 miracles were listed in a British Library document, of which 34 were resuscitations of the dead. Among those listed were drowning (8), road traffic accidents and injury from falling tree trunks (5), hanging (4), plague (4), accidental cut throats, knife injuries, arrow wounds (3), buried in sand (2), falls from tree or roof (2), foreign body in throat (2), haemorrhage (1), lightning (1) and starvation (1). While all of these contain interest I would like to select two or three for special mention if only to show the variety of the saint's abilities.

The first in chronological order, on 31 August, 1481, was the resuscitation of a boy aged 4, after drowning in a millstream and being given up as beyond all hope. On 5 March, 1490, John Wall was run over by a wagon and spent all night apparently dead under a thicket. His body was openly exhibited for four hours and was known to have been stiff for 20 hours when he miraculously returned to life.

Thomas Fuller of Hammersmith was condemned to judicial hanging, the sentence being carried on 21 July, 1484. After suspension for one hour it was certified that there was no trace of life but, during the journey to burial, he woke up and maintained thereafter that during the whole time of his suspension the late Henry VI had kept a hand between the rope and his neck and had also supported him in the air. This was indeed a fortunate intervention since it was subsequently established that Fuller was innocent.

Cecily Featherstonehaugh was killed following the violent dashing of a horse's hooves across her forehead battering her against a stone wall into a state of unrecognizability. Her problems were no doubt added to by the forcing of spirits and treacle into her mouth. However, where this failed, intercession to the late King restored her to life and health, (her physical appearance was not specified).

Cot deaths also received attention and a six-month old boy who was 'hanging in his cradle' was effectively resuscitated on 22 August, 1491. A family which was particularly blessed were the Norths; Joan North was drowned in the Thames and was known to have been under the water for over an hour before being dragged out and recovering, while her brother was cured of a growth on his lip by Henry's intervention. And so the story goes on—of accidental cut throats, arrow injuries, carters with their brains dashed out by loaded wagons, and even death from lightning.

Conclusion

Were these miraculous interventions? Were they imagination? Was the diagnosis of death reliable? Were they mediaeval variations of the instances which are still occasionally reported even today when someone certified as dead stirs in the mortuary . . . or has Henry a genuine claim for canonization?—in which case he would make an excellent Patron Saint for Intensive Care.

18.3 The development of resuscitation in the United Kingdom

D. J. WILKINSON

St Bartholomew's Hospital, London, UK

Historical research in all aspects of anaesthesia shows time and time again how techniques are discovered, abandoned and then rediscovered.

Resuscitation is certainly no exception to this rule. Sudden death from drowning, lightning strike or even poisoning has provided a challenge for both the general public as well as for medical practitioners throughout the ages.

It has been the drowned person who has provided the majority of such hapless patients and early resuscitation techniques such as rolling the patient over the back of a horse or over a barrel was an attempt to force water out of the body and thus restore life. Hanging a patient upside down over a fire was another popular manoeuvre which was thought to promote three therapies at once. Firstly the water could drain out of the patient, secondly the patient was warmed and thirdly there was the possibility of smoke inhalation which was considered to be of fundamental importance.

Resuscitation in the 17th and 18th centuries

In 1667 Robert Hooke (1) reported a series of animal experiments in which he used a bellows to ventilate the lungs via a tracheostomy. He demonstrated how the heart would stop soon after ventilation ceased and also how it could be restarted by recommencing respiration. He even used two sets of bellows and an insufflation technique to demonstrate that the lungs did not have to move to ensure the continued function of the heart as long as they were kept expanded by a supply of fresh air. These elegant animal experiments, although often cited by historians today, had little impact on medical practice at that time.

Mouth to mouth expired air ventilation was used in 1732 to resuscitate a man who had been overcome by fumes in a mine shaft. The mine had been on fire for two days and having burnt out was being cautiously explored when one of the miners was overcome. This successful resuscitation was rereported in 1744 by John Fothergill (2) who published a small pamphlet with some ideas on how to perform resuscitation. He states that:

> *'those who to appearance are struck dead might frequently be recovered by strongly blowing into the lungs'.*

He added the belief that this inflation of the lungs in a rhythmical manner imparted motion to the heart and could be likened to restarting a pendulum which had run down.

A small pamphlet on resuscitation was published by Dr Mead in 1747 based on his original work at the turn of the century. There were at this time three main treatments to effect resuscitation, these were, warming the body, applying friction to the body and blowing tobacco smoke into the rectum. It was believed that a drowned person was only apparently dead and that their appearance reflected a loss of heat and excitation in general which could be reapplied by external means.

While adult resuscitation was slowly developing the obstetricians of that time had long been aware that the newly born infant often required some degree of resuscitation to revive them after traumatic and prolonged deliveries. A Chelmsford physician Benjamin Pugh published a book in 1753 (3) outlining his beliefs on obstetric practice and in this he described a neonatal airway, made by wrapping soft leather round a wire spring, which he introduced into the child's mouth during breech extractions thus preventing suffocation. He also described simple mouth to mouth ventilation if the child failed to breathe after delivery.

John Wilkinson (4) in 1764 devoted a section of his book, which dealt in general terms on improving the working conditions of common sailors, to methods of reviving drowned persons. Again expired air ventilation is suggested by means of a 'pipe, funnel, cane or quill introduced into the mouth'. If the victim had been immersed for a considerable period of time and was rigid and very cold, then greater stimuli had to be applied, such as the use of pointed hot irons on the skin to try and revive him. The author poses the question 'would it be amiss to try the effect of a strong electrical shock?' in these cases. This latter question reflects an upsurge in interest in electrical therapy for a whole series of problems at this time. Hawksbee had introduced an electrostatic machine in 1705 which was becoming very popular in many towns and cities for a variety of ailments.

The foundation of the Royal Humane Society 1774

In 1773 Alexander Johnson (5) published a book reporting the setting up of a society in Holland in 1767 with the aim of trying to revive drowned people. He suggested the convening of a similar body for the United Kingdom and outlined various methods of resuscitation. This work was rather overshadowed by a more accurate translation of the Dutch Society memoirs by Thomas Cogan (6) in the same year. The Dutch regime for resuscitation included warming the patient, mouth to mouth ventilation, the use of tobacco smoke enemas and vigorous rubbing of the patient.

Following the publication of these works there was a meeting at the Chapter Coffee House near St Paul's Cathedral on 18 April, 1774, when Dr Cogan and a Dr William Hawes founded a society to assist with the resuscitation of the drowned. This society was known as 'An Institution for affording immediate relief to persons apparently dead from drowning' this then evolved into 'The Society for the recovery of persons apparently drowned' and by 1776 it had changed its name yet again to 'The Humane Society'. Later George III granted Royal patronage and the Society became 'The Royal Humane Society'.

Early work of the Royal Humane Society

The Society adopted the methods of treatment found efficacious by the Dutch and encouraged the practice of life-saving by offering financial rewards for each attempted resuscitation by the general public. Various medical assistants were stationed up and down the River Thames to whom victims could be transported or who could be called out to the site of any accident.

There was a yearly report published which outlined all cases of resuscitation that had taken place and this report was augmented by the publication of a variety of essays on improved methods of treatment written by members of the Society in competition for which a variety of medals were awarded.

Within a year of its foundation the Society was considering the use of bellows for resuscitation instead of mouth to mouth breathing and in 1776 John Hunter reported the use of a double action bellows for this purpose (7). This bellows had an active expiratory phase to suck air out of the lung as well as the more obvious inspiratory phase. It is interesting that Hunter also noted how electricity could be used to restart the beating of an animal's heart.

This concept had already been tried and found effective by another member of the Humane Society. On 16 July, 1774, a three-year-old child Catherine Sophie Greenhill fell from an upstairs window onto flag stones. She was treated with electricity some twenty minutes later by an apothecary Mr Squires, having been pronounced dead earlier. After passing the electrical current through the thorax—a pulsation was noted and the child began to breathe. It was noted that the child remained in a 'kind of stupor occasioned by the depression of the cranium from the fall' but she was restored to 'full health and spirits in a week'. This is probably the first recorded successful defibrillation. The apparatus used was likely to have been that designed by Edward Nairn in 1760—a portable electrostatic generator.

The Humane Society soon adopted the use of bellows and tubes for resuscitation and they were manufactured by a variety of instrument makers throughout London initially and then countrywide. In 1785 Alexander Johnson republished his work of 1773 bringing it up to date (8). He was not an enthusiast for tracheal tubes but developed a nasal airway to which bellows could be applied for the same purpose. He expressed his alarm at the indiscriminate use of electricity which seemed to be taking place and stated that such practices should be limited to those who were medically qualified.

Royal Patronage had by now greatly enhanced its standing. In 1788 a silver medal was awarded to Charles Kite of Gravesend (9) who had developed his own resuscitation apparatus based on his belief that 'the restoring of the action of the lungs to be of the very first importance in all our attempts to recover the apparently dead'. He was not in favour of Hunter's double action bellows and showed how expiration could take place passively once the lungs had been inflated by ordinary bellows. He was, however, in accord with Hunter's repudiation of the use of tobacco as a stimulant. Kite was aware that tracheal intubation was not always easily performed by the unskilled and described a nasal airway which could be very effective when used in conjunction with cricoid pressure. This very early reference to a modern technique clearly states its use to prevent unwanted gastric distension and regurgitation. Kite also developed his own electrical machine for defibrillation very similar to the Nairn apparatus but with the added refinement of being able to store charge in a Leyden jar, a type of early capacitance.

Diagnosis of death

One of the main problems faced by those practising resuscitation at this time was knowing when to stop their attempts. Many cases were reported as being successful after several hours of continuous efforts. Kite himself believed that there was no time limit that one could apply and even putrefaction of the body should not stop the attempt as this might merely signify advance scurvy!

In 1789 a Northampton GP James Curry founded another resuscitation society to 'promote recovery from a state of apparent death'. He published a book on the subject in 1792 (10) which led to a second edition in 1815 (11). Curry tried hard to define the differences between apparent and absolute death and he disagreed with Kite in many aspects of this. He described the appearances of black swollen face, glassy or shrivelled eyes and dilated pupils as signs of permanent death and the most certain of this state was putrefaction.

He agreed with Kite on the use of cricoid pressure which he often found useful to facilitate intubation. He states that 'the use of pure air or oxygene as the French chemists now call it' was preferable to room air for resuscitation if available.

Changing attitudes to methods of resuscitation
in the 19th century

The Royal Humane Society continued to produce yearly reports which were of immense value as educational works. The practice of resuscitation was firmly established and the use of bellows and tracheal tubes was the method of choice. In 1827/28 Leroy (12,13) reported his results of a survey of resuscitation practices and a series of animal experiments. The work was presented to the French Academy of Science and showed conclusively that the application of large tidal volumes and high inflation pressures could rupture the lung alveoli. The production of a pneumothorax made resuscitation attempts hopeless and he showed how modern techniques with tubes and bellows were producing worse results than had been obtained prior to their introduction. The approval of this work by Magendie (14) and the French Academy was to doom the technique in resuscitation for decades.

By 1832 the Royal Humane Society had abandoned the use of these bellows and tubes and had reverted to rubbing and warming their drowned patients. In the same year their annual report describes a method of external thoracic compression using specially cut bandages as advocated by a surgeon called Dalrymple for artificial respiration. The Royal Humane Society continued to develop. A special receiving house was opened in Hyde Park in 1835 which was fully equipped with hot baths and all the latest in resuscitation apparatus. This house was continuously manned by trained personnel and in winter when ice skating was particularly popular, special 'ice men' patrolled the Serpentine to save those who broke through the ice.

The Dalrymple method of resuscitation was followed by a whole series of chest compression techniques of artificial respiration, all of which were taught and practised by the Royal Humane Society; these included Marshall Hall (1856), Sylvester (1861) and Howard (1871).

While these techniques were developing so was a new speciality in medicine, that of anaesthesia and within this speciality an interest in intubation was re-awakening.

Pioneering work by McEwen in Glasgow and O'Dwyer in New York in the late 1880s led to the general acceptance of the technique in anaesthesia. Artificial respiration techniques continued in parallel, Eves' rocking method of 1932 being superseded by the Holger-Neilson technique. By this time Magill and Rowbotham had described their techniques of intubation in anaesthesia and where the medical profession in the hospital environment continued with intubation—the general public were taught Holger-Neilson. It was to be 1959 before expired air, mouth to mouth, ventilation was shown to be effective for resuscitation and reintroduced.

Conclusion

It is interesting to see how the formation of the Royal Humane Society in the late 18th century led to the adoption of intubation, external chest compression, the use of cricoid pressure and oxygen therapy as well as electrical defibrillation for the apparently dead patient. Although these techniques have been adopted, then abandoned and subsequently often reintroduced decades later, the Royal Humane Society continues to have the same basic ideals as its founders had in 1774.

References

(1) Hooke R. An account of an experiment made by M Hook of preserving animals alive by blowing through their lungs with bellows. *Phil Trans Roy Soc* 2, 1667.

(2) Fothergill J. *Observations on a case published in the last volume of the Medical Essays and "of recovering a man dead in appearance by distending the lungs with air".* Edinburgh: 1744.

(3) Pugh B. *A treatise of midwifery.* London: 1754.

(4) Wilkinson J. *Tutamen nauticum or the seamans preservation.* London: 1764.

(5) Johnson A. *A short account of a society at Amsterdam instituted in the year 1767 for the recovery of drowned persons etc.* London: 1773.

(6) Cogan T. *Memoirs of the society instituted at Amsterdam in favour of drowned persons. For the years 1767, 1768, 1769, 1770 and 1771.* London: 1773.

(7) Hunter J. *Proposals for the recovery of persons apparently drowned.* London: 1776.

(8) Johnson A. *Abridged instructions for the recovery of persons apparently dead.* London: 1785.

(9) Kite C. *An essay on the recovery of the apparently dead.* London: 1788.

(10) Curry J. *Popular observations on apparent death from drowning, suffocation etc with an account of the means to be employed for recovery.* Northampton: 1792.

(11) Curry J. *Observations on apparent death from drowning, hanging, suffocation by noxious vapours, fainting-fits, intoxication, lightening, exposure to cold, etc and an account of the means to be employed for recovery.* London: 1815.

(12) Leroy J. Recherches sur l'asphyxie. *J physiologie exp pathologique* 1872; 7: 45–65.

(13) Leroy J. Second memoire sur l'asphyxie. *J physiologie exp pathologique* 1828; 8: 97–135.

(14) Magendie M. Rapport fait à l'académie des sciences sur un mémoire de M Leroy relatif à l'insuflation du poumon. *J physiologie exp pathologique* 1828; 9: 97–112.

18.4	Origins of resuscitation in the USA*

K. GARTH HUSTON, Sr
Glendale Adventist Medical Center, Glendale, California, USA

Almost all advances in medicine that occurred in early America were imported from Europe. The origins of cardiopulmonary resuscitation in the United States began in several of the larger cities on the east coast about ten years after the Royal Humane Societies were founded on the east coast of the United States—one in New York, one in Boston, and one in Philadelphia.

Massachusetts

The Merrimack Humane Society was also organized at Newburyport, Massachusetts, in 1802. It is noted mostly for the bad odes that were printed every year at the end of their sermons. It continued at least into the 1880s. In 1883, a little pamphlet was issued, *The Institution of the Merrimack Humane Society . . . with persons apparently dead from drowning or injured by accident, or in cases of accidental poisoning.* (1)

Benjamin Waterhouse, in a second edition of his lecture that he gave before the Humane Society, *Discourse on the Principal of Vitality*, (2) adds a preface in 1811. He gives a history of how, in his eyes, the Massachusetts Humane Society began. Quoting a small part of the preface he says:

> *'The Society took its origin from the following occurrences:—In the summer of 1782, a number of young persons of both sexes were drowned in the harbour of Newport Rhode-Island, by the oversetting of a pleasure boat. Four or five of these young people were taken up when they had been not more than ten minutes in the water, and yet they all perished; for there was no means used to resuscitate them. Thereupon the Author published in the Newport Mercury some account of the methods practiced by the Humane Societies of Europe, and exerted himself to form one at Rhode-Island; but nothing was effected. Three years afterwards, viz. in 1785, when sailing through the harbour of Newport with the celebrated blind philosopher, Dr. Henry Moyes of Edinburgh, he related to him the sad accident, and lamented that we had no humane society in America for resuscitating the drowned; and the ill success he experienced in attempting to establish one. "Do not be discouraged," said this extraordinary man, "but let us set about it immediately;—this very day." We accordingly did so; and by the help of his intelligent serving man, who was a good amanuensis, we committed to paper a plan of our Humane Society, and took it with us to Boston; and communicated it to a small assemblage of professional gentlemen in School-street, whence arose The Humane Society of the Commonwealth of Massachusetts, which was incorporated in 1791.'*

An independent verification of the story told by Waterhouse is in a history of the Humane Society of Massachusetts (3). In 1787, Dr Alexander Johnson sent a letter to *Gentleman's Magazine* (4) that he had received from Dr Moyes while in America:

> *'Dear Sir: Boston, November 12, 1785. In consequence of my itinerate mode of living, upon this wide and extensive continent, your acceptable letter of May 16, 1785, was put in my hands no sooner than three weeks ago. I return you my most grateful thanks for the regular communications of your productions upon the subject of recovery from apparent death. No opportunity has been permitted to escape of making them public, and explaining their principles; and I flatter myself with the pleasing hope, that by so doing, I have in some measure promoted a design which could only have originated from the purest benevolence and universal philanthropy . . . I am in hopes that a humane society will soon be established in the town of Boston; and I have reason to expect that,*

*Read by K. Garth Huston, Jr, Pasadena, California, USA

in the course of the ensuing winter, similar institutions will also be planted in New York, and Philadelphia. Some account of their success shall in due time be transmitted to you; and when I leave the Continent and return to Europe, I shall establish correspondence with some of my medical friends in, and of the principal towns in North America.'

Dr Alexander Johnson was one of the protagonists who attempted to form an organization similar to the Royal Humane Society in 1774. He entitled his organization, The General Institution. He was unsuccessful—The Royal Humane Society won out. In 1785, Dr Johnson published a small pamphlet of about 24 pages. It is called, *Relief from Accidental Death: or, Summary Instructions for the General Institution, Proposed in the Year 1773, by Alexander Johnson, M.D., to introduce and establish, in his Majesty's British Dominions, a successful practice for the recovering of persons who meet with accidents producing suddenly an appearance of death, and preventing their being buried alive (5).*

Interestingly enough, in the *Boston Magazine* for November, 1785, and continued in the December issue (6), the above pamphlet by Dr Alexander Johnson was reprinted in detail as published in the *Exchange Advertiser*, 17 November, by desire of Dr Moyes; including the woodcuts that he used for methods of resuscitation. So, Dr Moyes was indeed successful in introducing these methods of resuscitation to the general public through the newspapers in the Boston area.

Again, although Dr Alexander Johnson's ideas were the ones that were successful in proposing societies in the United States, all the societies that were formed were connected one way or another with the Royal Humane Society, and ultimately worked and operated under rules suggested by its officers.

The Massachusetts Humane Society carried on many of the traditions that were common in London at the Royal Humane Society. It has a most interesting history and there is more documentation about its founding than any other Society. They issued pamphlets, broadsides and cards and instituted an annual oration, the first one being given by John Lathrop in 1787 (7). These continued uninterrupted until 1817. Most of the orations were given by religious ministers, very few were by doctors, and they are filled with good thoughts, but very little medical information. The medical information that is in some of these, especially by the doctors, is information that comes to them from London. These occasions, like the London Society, were used as opportunities for raising money for the Humane Societies.

It gives one a great deal of confidence to realize that the man who gave the discourse in 1796, the Reverend Dr Chandler Robbins, speaks highly of a quack's virtues. Also in 1796, in a little pamphlet called, *Evidences of the Efficacy of Dr. Perkins' Metallic Tractors (8)*, in a letter dated 24 September, 1796, he speaks highly of the success he has had with Dr Perkins' metallic instruments.

An example of the impact of the Humane Societies on the lay public is a little pamphlet called, *The Wonderful Monitor or Memorable Repository, containing a curious and most astonishing account of the revivication of young Joseph Taylor (9).* It was printed in Boston, in 1788, and tells the story of a young man, of good family from Ireland, who joined the Army, fell into bad company and was caught as a highwayman. He was sentenced to death in 1788. The name he assumed so that his family would never find out about this, was young Joseph Taylor.

This is a very rare pamphlet. It is on crumbling and very unsatisfactory paper, and really cannot be handled any more, though it was reprinted in 1986 (10). The story goes into great detail about one of the local doctors in Boston who made arrangements with an Archibald Taylor for the purchase of his body for dissection and then came to talk to young Joseph Taylor the next day about burying his body for dissection also. This upset the young man so much, thinking of what was going to happen to him, that the doctor agreed to try to save his life if he would follow the methods used and suggested by the Humane Societies to see if he could be successful in saving his life. The whole pamphlet is quite interesting to read, the methods of how he was supposed to get the knot in a certain place so that it would not break his neck, etc. They got his body from the rope as soon as they could. They put him on a boat and then went through the resuscitation process and were successful.

Though this is probably fictitious, it does give evidence of what was in people's minds at that time. At the end, mention is made of the sermon given by Dr Lathrop, the year before in 1787; the methods of resuscitation that were advocated by Alexander Johnson, and some of Alexander Johnson's own comments on resuscitation.

Philadelphia

Most of the materials that had to do with the ordinary running of the societies other than the sermons are ephemeral. I have not mentioned the actual methods that were used for resuscitation. From a broadside, by the Humane Society of Philadelphia, are instructions entitled, *Directions for Preventing Sudden Death from Drowning . . . :*

> *'1. Do not hold up the body with the head downwards or roll it over a barrel.*
> *2. Strip off the wet clothes gently and wrap the body in blankets and rub at first moderately with the hand or with warm clothes for two or three hours.*
> *3. Close the mouth and one nostril completely. Blow air through the other into the lungs with ·a pair of bellows. If bellows cannot be had, air may be blown into the lungs through the open nostril from the mouth of one of the bystanders. Discharge the air which has been conveyed into the lungs by either of the above methods by gently pressing the belly upwards. This process should be repeated 20 to 30 times a minute.*
> *4. A large quantity of warm sand or ashes, mainly to keep the body warm.'* (11)

Philadelphia also seemed to be concerned about people dying suddenly from drinking cold water or cold liquors of any kind in warm weather. Perhaps this was due to the influence of Benjamin Rush (12). The directions from the New York Societies were essentially the same.

The directions given at the first Massachusetts Humane Society (13) lecture by Dr Lathrop adds the following:

> *'The smoke of tobacco thrown up the fundament should be ranked among the earliest applications. if the fumigator [and they are talking about a special machine] be used to give the tobacco smoke enema, if a fumigator should not be at hand, the common pipe will answer the purpose of applying this vapor to the bowels. So easy and important operation should be repeatedly performed as the good effects of tobacco smoke have been proven in many cases.'*

Added directions in other pamphlets consist of what we might call a reverse Sellick procedure, a common procedure used by modern anaesthetists. Cricoid pressure against the oesophagus was recommended to prevent filling the stomach with air when bellows were being used for resuscitation.

All of these directions for resuscitation; broadsides, cards, etc., are rare and not many have survived. Most of them say the same thing, from broadsides, to little pamphlets, to cards that fold that one can carry in one's pocket. Some had interesting titles. One, from the Humane Society of Philadelphia, is titled, *Do not despair* (14), and then gives directions for recovering persons who are supposed to be dead from drowning.

Most of the directions involve some means of using bellows through the nose or through a tracheal tube for resuscitation. Bellows were recommended instead of the mouth; because with bellows one gets pure air and not air that had already been partly respired with less oxygen.

Several important books were written at this time. In 1792, in New York, David Hosack wrote, *An Inquiry into the Causes of Suspended Animation from Drowning; with the means of restoring life* (15). He requested that a Humane Society be started in New York. The New York Humane Society began in 1794.

In 1799, *An Annual Oration Pronounced before the Humane Society of Philadelphia on the Objects and Benefits of said Institution; The 28th day of February, 1799* (16), by Dr Benjamin Say, President of the Society, gives an excellent review of what is being done in the way of resuscitation by Humane Societies and what their goals and objects should be in the Philadelphia area.

Edmund Goodwyn's book, *The Connexion of life with Respiration, or an Experimental Inquiry into the Effects of Submersion, Strangulation, and several kinds of noxious airs on living animals* (17), was reprinted in Philadelphia in 1805.

New York

Another English book was reprinted in New York in 1814 (18). It was originally printed in London in 1813, by Newton Bosworth entitled, *The Accidents of Human Life; with Hints for their Prevention, and the Removal of their Consequences* (19). Added to the New York addition are some of the rules of the New York Humane Society.

Student theses are generally of little medical consequences, but they do give an indication of what is currently of medical interest at a given time. Student theses by Joseph Macrery (20), Samuel Jackson (who later became a professor at Philadelphia) (21), John Oswald (22), and Daniel Legare (23) discussed resuscitation. The latter is of interest because he showed great intestinal fortitude (pun intended). His thesis had to do with the effect of tobacco fume enemas upon himself enough times until he became nauseated and quit. Other theses could be mentioned, but these give the general information that there was interest in medical schools on this subject in the United States during this time.

This is perhaps enough about the Humane Societies as a source of resuscitation and we can go on to something of greater interest.

Dr Alexander H. Stevens was for many years professor of the principles and practice of surgery at the New York Hospital. After his graduation from Yale College, he studied at the University of Pennsylvania graduating in 1811. During the War of 1812, he had gone to Europe bearing dispatches and had been captured at sea. He was taken as a prisoner of war to England and when released, he remained in that country studying under Sir Astley Cooper and Abernathy, later crossing to Paris where he worked as an intern under the famous surgeon, Boyer, whose lectures he later translated.

In a letter dated London, 29 February, 1812 (24), he mentions that around seaports, towns, and other bodies of water, there has been a problem for years about how to restore drowned people. He mentions that many texts have been written on this subject. He states that these have fallen into two groups. One has been to get the body warm and try to restore life by these methods, while others have been more interested in the actual changes that go on in the lungs and think that getting air into the lungs is the more important part of the process. He goes on:

'Others depend more on the immediate re-establishment of respiration, without which stimulants can be of no service, according to their ideas, except in a few cases, where they may get power enough to the muscles to carry it on of themselves.' . . . 'Which of these practices is most correct? It may be worthwhile to inquire.'

He also makes a point that the most proper remedies to restore the excitability of the system are sufficiently well understood and commonly practised. He says:

'It is not my intention to dwell upon them in this paper. There is little danger of not doing what is right in this respect, if we do not neglect the means which are simple and easy of application, by pursuing those which occasion a loss of time in their use.'

In addition to the use of these remedies that he is discussing, i.e., spirits, heat and warmth:

'the great desideratum is to inflate the lungs. The inventors of the numerous instruments for this purpose seem, most unfortunately, to have vied with each other in rendering them costly, complex, and difficult to manage by those who are required to use them. It often happens in New York that one of these instruments cannot be procured without a loss of much time, and even then, it cannot be applied until a physician arrives. How many cases terminate fatally in this way, which by proper means might have been successfully treated?'

He tells of a man who fell into Peckslip Dock and:

'was taken up as nearly as I could judge, in five minutes, and carried into a house. Scarcely anything was done but to tumble him about. A physician and a machine were sent for. The machine was brought, but the doctor was not at home. After much further delay a bye-stander inflated the lungs—but life had flown forever.'

Again, to quote directly for those interested in 'firsts.' This might well be considered the first example of the use of manual artificial respiration by external pressure on the rib cage.

What follows is a lengthy quotation, but it is something that I do not think is well known:

'It is well known to all who are acquainted with the structure of the human body, that air is made to enter the lungs by the removal or diminution of the pressure around them, while their internal cavities, by communicating with the atmosphere, are distended by its weight until an equilibrium takes place. This diminution of pressure arises from the contraction and consequent flattening of the diaphragm, whose convexity rises into the chest from below, and the synchronous elevation and turning out of the ribs. The first increasing the vertical dimensions of the thorax, and the latter, the anterior and lateral diameters. Persons in health may respire enough by either of these means. After a hearty dinner the diaphragm does not assist much in breathing; while on the other hand, young ladies tightly laced, respire by its means alone; the elevation of the ribs being entirely prevented. In diseases, as in inflammatory fever for example, or after exercise, the powers which move the ribs have a greater share in respiration than the diaphragm. To produce the necessary motions of the ribs in the dead subject is almost as much in the power of any person as to elevate his own, and they will as certainly determine the air to rush into the lungs. Scarcely any one has been engaged in dissection who must not have observed how easily he could move with his hands the ribs of the subject. To effect this most conveniently and completely as the patient or subject is laid on the table, and you are placed looking towards his feet, and leaning over his head, apply a hand on each side of the chest so tightly as to move only with the thorax; then bring your hands toward your body: the ribs are elevated, the chest enlarged, and inspiration has taken place. The elasticity of the cartilages now induces an expulsion of the air, which may be still more completely effected by pressing down the ribs or abdomen. This process may be repeated and respiration thus carried on to any extent as completely and effectually as by the most complicated instruments. Is it possible to devise any means to answer this most important purpose more simple, and intelligible and practicable than this? Any person may easily be made to comprehend, and taught to practise it. If it were to be substituted for the more laborious mode of inflating the lungs, I doubt not many lives would be annually saved which are now lost. It will be observed that it is equally applicable to all cases of suspended animation, whether they arise from submersion, hanging, breathing noxious airs or other causes. In the last cases, the more extended application of remedies is necessary. But these may be used by any person until a physician arrives.

'It is due to Astley Cooper, Esquire, to state that he first suggested this plan several years ago, in his public lectures in St. Thomas' Hospital. It has been pursued by one of his former pupils, and also within a few days by myself with complete success. Going down the Thames last week in a boat, I observed a crowd of people collected on the shore near the West India docks; and directed the waterman to row me to it. Soon after I landed, a man was taken up apparently drowned. He was carried to an ale house, and his clothes being stript off, he was laid upon a table in the bar room. The table was previously covered with a blanket which was pressed and rubbed against every part of his body by the people around, while I alternately elevated and depressed his ribs in the mode I have mentioned. In a little while he drew a breath by his own power. He took a little hot gin toddy, which was by this time prepared for him, and gradually recovered. The bar maid was now just returned from the apothecary, and inquiring for a pair of bellows which he had directed to be in readiness against his arrival; when I came off, leaving the man able to articulate and move his limbs.'

While people generally give credit to Marshall Hall for the first ideas of artificial respiration, Sir Astley Cooper's method pre-dated his by many years.

Again, in 1818, in a paper titled, *Reflections on the Means of Recovery After Submersion, directed by the Humane Society of New York addressed to the president and the directors* (25), Stevens states that the Humane Society has direct claim on all of its members. He says the Humane Society in general has an obligation to remedy any defects in the system for recovering the drowned. Since the older more established members had not seen any way to change their methods of resuscitation, he is going, as a younger man, to advise of his opinions on what should be done by the New York Humane Society to improve their methods. He quotes highly successful rates in Paris and in London and other major cities of Europe and states some things that he thinks would help in New York, since they have such a high incidence of failure. Stevens says:

'Your machines are unnecessarily complicated and consequently difficult to put in order and manage. They consist generally of many detached parts which must be separated that they may be placed in the boxes designed for them. These parts are very liable to be mistaken one for another. Indeed, it requires no little ingenuity to discover how the several pieces are to be fitted together; and in scenes of confusion, it is scarcely possible that less than five or even ten minutes should be consumed in adjusting them. After the unnecessary loss of so much time, even the best means will rarely succeed.'

He goes on to say that their instruments are not all alike. That the one at Beckman Slop is different from Courtland Street, and then at another area, it is different altogether; and, he says if a physician takes the time to familiarize himself with one set of instruments, and he is at another place, he has to learn another set of instruments which he may not know how to use at all.

In spite of saving on compactness, he advises that these machines be left together, ready to hand so that when they are needed, they can be put to use without spending a lot of time. He also says that it would help if all of the machines were the same. He goes on to say that the directions for restoring the dead from drowning require many alterations. He says that the directions need much help.

Alexander Stevens in the last part of his article, finally, and most devastatingly, takes each principal recommendation of the New York Humane Society and analyses it ruthlessly. He quotes the first recommendation as

'Avoid any violent agitation of the body such as rolling it on a cask or hanging it up by the heels but carefully carry it with the head a little raised to the nearest house.'

He then goes on to say that even putting the body across a trotting horse or rolling on a barrel has been proven many times to be successful, even more so than the methods recommended by the Humane Society. And, he says, it works by means of alternately compressing and expanding the chest and letting some air in and out of the lungs. He states:

'Death by drowning is induced chiefly by reason of a suspension of this process;—first for the want of air, and after the person is taken from the water, from the inability to move the chest. In these cases the primary object is to restore respiration—to do precisely that, which every animal must incessantly do, in order to live, and which the patient would do, had he not lost the power, i.e. to raise and depress alternately the chest.'

He then uses the example of a horse. If you find a horse with a rope tied around his neck tight enough that he cannot breathe, are you going to rub him and warm him and dry him and cover him with warm blankets in order to resuscitate him, or are you going to get rid of the cord around his neck? He states that every animal or human is essentially in this same condition; they are not able to breath, like an animal with a rope around its neck. He continues devastatingly through the rest of the rules using the example above.

He concludes his article with this last paragraph:

'I cannot conclude this long letter without expressing a hope that the Humane Society will lose no time in adopting such measures as are better calculated to accomplish this object of its charity . . . and I venture to express my conviction that the best means for promoting recovery after submersion will be found so simple that your society will enlarge this sphere of its humane exertions so as to include the cases of persons who are apparently dead from hanging, breathing noxious gasses, and taking poisons into the stomach.'

Conclusion

Thus, we go full circle from the early 1780s until 1818 when Alexander H. Stevens's letter was written to the New York Humane Society. The year before was the last sermon from

Massachusetts Humane Society, and 1818 was the last printed sermon from the Merrimack Humane Society.

There were probably many reasons for the lack of success and failure of the Humane Societies. Some of these have been listed by others. Lavoisier's discovery of oxygen showed that air that had already been inspired once had less oxygen. LeRoy showed bellows could cause bilateral pneumothorax and then death, which led to the decrease and disuse of the bellows and later forms of manual artificial respiration. Probably the greatest deterrent of all, was the lack of physiological knowledge that took many more years to acquire. It was not until almost 130 years later that some of the good ideas espoused by the Humane Societies were reintroduced into modern resuscitation techniques.

References

(1) Merrimack Humane Society. *The Institution of the Merrimack Humane Society, with the methods of treatment to be used with persons apparently dead from drowning or injured by accident, or in cases of accidental poisoning.* Newburyport: W. H. Huse & Co., 1883.

(2) Waterhouse B. *The Botanist. Being the botanical part of a course of lectures on natural history, delivered in the University at Cambridge, together with a discourse on the principle of vitality.* Boston: J. T. Buckingham, 1811: 233.

(3) Parkman F. *History of the Humane Society of Massachusetts: with a selected list of premiums awarded by the Trustees, from its commencement to the present time: including extracts from the correspondence, a statement of the funds, and a list of the officers and members.* Boston: S. N. Dickinson, 1845.

(4) *Gentleman's Magazine* 1787; 57 (Pt2): 1154.

(5) Johnson A. *Relief from accidental death: or, summary instructions for the general institution, proposed in the year 1773 . . .* London: T. Hodgson, 1785.

(6) Johnson A, Moyes H. Relief from accidental death: or, summary instructions for the general institution, proposed in the year 1773 . . . *The Boston Magazine* 1785: Nov–Dec: 405–08; 449–54.

(7) Lathrop J. *A discourse, before the Humane Society, in Boston: delivered on the second Tuesday of June, 1787.* Boston: E. Russell, 1787.

(8) Perkins E. *Evidences of the efficacy of Doctor Perkins's patent metallic instruments.* Philadelphia: R. Folwell, 1797: 9.

(9) Anonymous. *The wonderful monitor: or, memorable repository, containing, a curious and most astonishing account of the revivication of young Joseph Taylor.* Boston: E. Russell, 1788.

(10) Ibid. Reprinted by K. Garth Huston, M.D. (Sr and Jr) Van Nuys, California: R. Hoffman, 1986.

(11) Humane Society of Philadelphia . . . Directions for preventing sudden death . . . [Philadelphia, 1791?].

(12) Humane Society of Philadelphia. *Directions for recovering persons, who are supposed to be dead, from drowning, also for preventing & curing the disorders, produced by drinking cold liquors . . .* Philadelphia: J. James, 1788.

(13) C.f., number 7, appendix: vi.

(14) Humane Society of Philadelphia. *Do not despair.* Humane Society of Philadelphia. The managers of the Humane Society offer the following compensations, viz . . . [Philadelphia, 1806].

(15) Hosack D. *An Enquiry into the causes of suspended animation from drowning; with the means of restoring life.* New York: T. & J. Swords, 1792.

(16) Say B. *An annual oration pronounced before the Humane Society of Philadelphia, on the objects & benefits of said Institution; the 28th day of February, 1799.* Whitehall: W. Young, 1799.

(17) Goodwyn E. *The connexion of life with respiration; or, an experimental inquiry into the effects of submersion, strangulation, and several kinds of noxious airs, on living animals: . . .* Philadelphia: C. Cist, 1805.

(18) Bosworth N. *The accidents of human life; with hints for their prevention, and the removal of their consequences.* New York: S. Wood, 1814.

(19) Ibid. ——. London: Lackington, Allen, and Co., 1812.

(20) Macrery J. *An inaugural dissertation on the principle of animation:* . . . Wilmington: Bonsal and Niles, 1802. 24pp. Dissertation.

(21) Jackson S. *An essay on suspended animation.* Philadelphia: Smith & Maxwell, 1808. 81pp. Dissertation.

(22) Oswald J. *An experimental inquiry into the phenomena of suspended animal life, from drowning, hanging, and the action of noxious airs:* . . . Philadelphia: H. Maxwell, 1802. 72pp. Dissertation.

(23) Legare D. *An experimental inquiry into the effects of tobacco fumes, on the system; and their use in cases of suspended animation, from submersion.* Philadelphia: J. Oswald, 1805. 30pp. Dissertation.

(24) Mitchill SL, Miller E. *The Medical Repository . . . Third Hexade, Vol. III.* New York: Collins & Co, 1812: 325–329.

(25) Stevens, Alexander. Reflections on the Means of Recovery After Submersion, directed by the Humane Society of New York. In: Watts J Jr, Mott V, Stevens AH. *The Medical and Surgical Register: consisting chiefly of cases in the New York Hospital.* New York: Collins & Co., 1818: 105–116.

18.5

Exhortations to resuscitate in the 18th century:
civic duties in poetry and prose

T. FORCHT DAGI
United States Navy, Washington DC, USA

Europe during the 18th century was stirred by a spirit of meliorism—the conviction that human effort could make the world a better place. The resuscitation movement was one of the many undertakings that expressed this theme.

The purpose of this paper is to consider the manner in which popular support for the resuscitation movement was recruited by the resuscitation tracts of the late 18th century*. Initially, the leaders of the resuscitation movement emphasized the dangers of premature interment to induce the populace to learn resuscitation techniques. Over the next fifty years, disinterest and incredulity were overcome more effectively by demonstrating that resuscitation accurately tested and sometimes reversed apparent death. *Pari passu*, the obligation to resuscitate, which earlier had been recognized neither by physicians nor by laymen (with the possible exception of midwives, colliers and watermen, all of who apparently maintained a venerable tradition of resuscitation long before it attracted any academic or scientific interest), evolved into a civic duty. The British experience will be emphasized in this discussion.

---

*By resuscitation tracts is meant the body of didactic and almost evangelical literature of the mid-18th to early 19th centuries that conveyed the creed of the resuscitation movement and its techniques. Some were authored, but many were anonymous, published under the auspices of a national or a local humane or philanthropic organization. Resuscitation tracts ranged in style from scholarly volumes to pedantic tomes to handbooks in verse for popular use. Leaflets and mnemonic pocket cards were also issued, but these, being far more limited, are excluded.

Resuscitation prior to 1700

Records of serious attempts at resuscitation began to appear sporadically in the 16th century, although resuscitation had been practised long before. It is said that Paracelsus tried to revive a cadaver with bellows in 1530. Vesalius understood the rudiments of airway management, including tracheostomy, and in 1543, described the artificial respiration of experimental animals. In public demonstrations the hearts of decapitated roosters were shown to continue beating so long as the lungs were ventilated. Drowned dogs were restored to life (1). A resuscitation folklore unfolded, illustrated by Cerimon of Ephesus in Shakespeare's *Pericles* (Act 3, sii, 82–86):

> *'Death may usurp on nature many hours*
> *And yet the fire of life kindle again*
> *The o'erpress'd spirits. I heard of an Egyptian*
> *That had nine hours lien dead*
> *Who was by good appliance recovered.'*

Sir Francis Bacon encouraged physicians to study ways of extending life, citing several instances of successful resuscitation prior to 1638. Among the most tantalizing: '. . . a physician having hang'd a man halfe an houre, recovered him to life by rubbing and hot Baths, professing also to recover any man after halfe an houres hanging, his necke at the first falling downe beeing not broken.' (2). A gardener was revived in Tronningholm, Sweden, around 1650; he drowned in an attempt to save another person who had fallen through the ice (3). A book entitled *Helps for Soddain Accidents Endangering Life* offered simple instructions for recovering the drowned: the victim was turned '. . . upside down to let the water out . . .' (4).

Even though resuscitation texts were extant before 1700 successful resuscitations were regarded for the most part as interesting anecdotes whose further significance was ignored (5). Tozzetti, for example, alludes to a tract on resuscitation entitled *Tractutus de Morbis Subitaneis, cetra praecipites affectuum, Symptomatumque Casus, promta remedia continens*, published the previous century in Montpellier by Francesco Ranchino. Ranchino claimed to revive both the dead and the 'semi-dead.' Tozzetti compliments Ranchino for having done the best he could for his time: '*Per i suoi tempi, il Ranchino fece quanto meglio si poteva, e merita somma lode.*

The uncertainty of death

The situation started changing in 1732, after William Tossach revived a collier overcome by noxious gasses. In a case report (6), he described his life-saving method

> '. . . *he was in all appearance dead. I applied my Mouth to his and blowed my Breath as I could, but having neglected to stop his nostrils, all the Air came out at them; therefore taking hold of them with one hand, and holding my other on his breast . . . I blew again my Breath as long as I could, raising his Chest fully . . . and immediately I felt six or seven very quick Beats of the Heart . . .*'
>
> '*After about an Hour he began to yawn, as well as move his Eye-lids, Hands and Feet; . . . In an Hour more he came pretty well to his Sense, and could take Drink, but knew nothing of that had happened . . .*'

and advanced the tentative suggestion that the general public might benefit by acquaintance with this technique.

The case report did not appear until 1744, but in the interim, Tossach's success had spread by word of mouth. In 1740, Réaumur published an *Advice concerning the drowned, who appear dead* under the auspices of the Académie des Sciences in Paris (7). The same year, Jacques Benigne Winslow, another French physician, wrote *The Uncertainty of the Signs of Death and the Danger of Precipitate Interments and Dissections* (8). Because of a personal experience with premature burial in his youth, Winslow was preoccupied with this problem. Although the threat of live entombment had been recognized at least since classical times (9,10) and reiterated within recent memory (2), the appearance of Winslow's book occasioned an acute resurgence of terror, far more intense than the usual atavistic shivers of fear that periodically swept across Europe. Winslow became best known through the translations of Jacques-Jean Bruhier d'Ablaincourt (to whom authorship of was often mistakenly ascribed) (11,12), and was considered by many to be the prophet of the resuscitation movement.

An obligation to save lives

In 1745, Fothergill presented an account of Tossach's case to the Royal Society (London) (3), seeking to obtain the cachet of the Royal Society for further study of resuscitation. He emphasized the importance of the scientific method in studying how lives might be preserved:

> ' . . . *malefactors executed at the gallows, would afford opportunities of discovering how far this method might be successful in relieving such as may have unhappily become their own executioners by hanging themselves.*'

Although Fothergill was interested primarily in Tossach's method (the Royal Society was dedicated to practical knowledge) the wider implications of a reliable technique that could be utilized by the lay public did not escape him.

The interest of the Royal Society had little popular impact either in Great Britain or in the rest of Europe. The city of Florence was one of the first to attempt public involvement in this cause. An anonymous tract published in 1752 under royal decree (14) exhorted Florentines to learn resuscitation ' . . . with every confidence and with every zeal in helping their imperiled neighbour . . . .' Asserting that all episodes of sudden death should be assumed to represent an uncertain state (*Morte repentina*) during which ' . . . *men can hide an externally imperceptible languishing residual movement in the vital organs, under the appearance of a cadaver . . . ,* ' it promulgated an explicit obligation to intervene. The rational for this policy was founded on the interest of the state in preserving its population, and on practical concerns regarding the uncertainty of death. This tract was almost certainly authored by Giovanni Tozzetti, the foremost Italian resuscitationist, in response to instructions from the ducal palace (15).

A recurring problem was the difficulty in recruiting physicians who did not immediately share in this sense of urgency. Why were some physicians neither credulous nor receptive? In part they perceived resuscitation to be unproven, and in part they considered attendance at the death bed, where physicians had little to contribute, to be superfluous, and quite possibly beneath their station. In a book intended for physicians, Tozzetti wrote that he struggled to overcome:

> ' . . . *all sense of paradox and ridicule that at first glance, may appear to surround the attempt to resuscitate the dead . . .*
> . . . *observations and experiments carried out in the presence of most learned individuals*
> . . . *under the eyes of the public and authenticated by the protection and magnificence of the respective governments . . .* '

proclaim a specific professional obligation to resuscitate founded upon the:

> '*good will, charity, reason, and faith . . .* [*of physicians*] . . . *doctors, before immersing themselves in the practice of their . . . profession,* [*should become*] *fully informed of the possibility and theory . . .* [*of*] *apparent death . . . that they might keep in mind all the skills and efforts that are possible, and that must be carried out immediately . . . in order to recall the unfortunate asphyxiated* [*individual*] . . . *from the dark veil of death that oppresses him . . .* ' (15)

Tozzetti's tract, with unusual candour, indicates that physicians learned resuscitation from laymen at the water's edge. This fact alone may account for some professional defensiveness. It also states that popular opinion was swayed more by reports of success than by fears of premature burial. Physicians may thus have been reluctant to become involved in situations where laymen might compete successfully, where there was no premium on their specialized professional knowledge, and where the consequences of failure would be obvious.

An edict of obligation

In 1766, a far-reaching edict was promulgated in Zurich:

> '. . . *Experience has shown that the drowned which were considered dead and that lay for some time under water have often been restored again and kept alive by proper maneuvers. From which one rightly concludes that life has not been completely suspended in the drowned, but that there is hope to save them from death if, as soon as they are withdrawn from the water, prompt and careful help is administered. And, the love of mankind should stimulate everyone to do everything to save these unfortunates . . . '* (16)

The authority of this edict was demonstrated by its provisions regarding suicide. Suicides were traditionally regarded with revulsion: they were classified as murderers in the eyes of God and the state. These prejudices were specifically overruled in a codicil entitled, *Warnings against the Extant and Superstitious Prejudices On the Matter of Those Who Rendered themselves Lifeless by Violent Measures (namely, Suicides)* (17).

Zurich, like Florence, also recognized the importance of preserving its citizens from untimely death, but the language of this edict suggests that there was some reluctance to comply. The problem was dealt with by appealing to several higher sentiments: a more broadly defined 'Christian duty,' a sense of 'mercy,' love for mankind, and finally the promise of a handsome reward and the recognition of the state. This form of legislated altruism did not catch on. The inducement of a reward, in contrast, was widely utilized.

The establishment of humane societies in Britain*

In 1767, the first organized resuscitation society was established in Amsterdam. Dr Alexander Johnson, a contemporary, described this event in a manner intended to confront indifference towards the establishment of a similar society in Britain (18). He emphasized as the primary underlying motivation of the resuscitation movement the preservation of the human species as a whole, followed by the salvage of individual human lives, and the significance of philanthropic involvement in the national cause:

> '*it is much to be wished, that some means may be found of giving the benefit of this Valuable Institution to Great Britain and its Colonies.*
> '*If the number of accidents is proportioned to the number of persons employed on the water, this kingdom is more interested than any other nation, in the art of restoring drowned persons. The large coal-mines in Great Britain, where numbers of men are yearly destroyed by the damps, which are so commonly fatal to the miners, and the frequent instances of persons who come to an untimely end, by strangling and other casualties, render the art of restoring suffocated and strangled persons to life, of great consequence to the community.*'

Over the next several years, exhortatory tracts became increasingly utilitarian as they advocated the establishment of a British Humane Society.

> '*When any Discovery of real Utility to the World is made, it is the Duty of every Man to render it as universally known and beneficial as possible . . . The striking effects of an Institution of this kind hardly require to be illustrated . . . and the experience of success in those countries where Humanity has adopted, and where Public Beneficence has invigorated, a practice in which society is so essentially interested, opens the most pleasing prospect to the benevolent of This Kingdom, where Charity appears in its most amiable form, and is expanded in a variety that dignifies human nature . . . '* (19)

In 1774, a Society for the Recovery of Persons Apparently Drowned was finally instituted in London. Its establishment represented a victory for several related principles

---

*The general history and the chronology of the Royal Humane Society and the chronology of other humane societies in Great Britain has been discussed elsewhere and will not be considered here.

and causes, including, for example, general humanitarianism (a society-wide interest in saving lives); prudence and enlightened self-interest (the elimination of dependence on professionally trained personnel); industrial safety (insurance against fatal accidents for workers); and piety (sparing suicides the sin of murder (20).

The resuscitation movement in Great Britain went on to adopt an increasingly self-righteous tone (21). Resuscitation had clearly become a moral, as well as a practical issue. All efforts now turned to preaching the resuscitation creed, modern techniques as opposed to folk remedies, widespread popular involvement, and aggressive scepticism concerning the appearance of death. One stratagem involved the distillation of resuscitation tracts into inspirational verses such as the following:

> *'When in the stream, by accident is found*
> *A pallid body of the recent drown'd*
> *Tho' ev'ry sign of life is wholly fled*
> *And all are ready to pronounce it dead*
> *With tender care the clay-cold body lay*
> *In flannel warm, and to some house convey:*
>
> *. . . Soon, soon from slumber shall he wake;*
> *Soon, soon again of cheering health partake,*
> *And now, restor'd to partner, child or friend,*
> *Shall bless your name to life's remotest end.*
>
> *. . . When life, though latent, was not quickly seen*
> *Then thinking that the conflict all was o'er.*
> *That life was fled, and could return no more;*
> *Who much have wish'd and yet despair'd to save,*
> *Too rashly doom'd the body to the grave.*
> *More patient thou, with ardour persevere*
> *Four hours at least: the gen'rous heart will fear*
> *To quit its charge, too soon, in dark despair,*
> *Will ply each mean, and watch th'effect with care:*
> *For should the smallest spark of life remain.*
> *Life's genial heat may kindle bright again.'* (22,23)

In subsequent years, the resuscitation movement maintained an historical self-consciousness (24,25) through which it re-enforced its moral claims (26).

Soon carnivals were organized to celebrate successful resuscitations: both the rescuers and the rescued went on display. The following passage describes a parade on 22 July, 1796, by which time whole-hearted popular support had been indisputably won:

> *'Philanthropic songs, accompanied by instrumental music, excited the most sublime emotions in the minds of the hearers. What an impressive scene!—A long procession of men, women, and children, who all were indebted for their lives to this Society, proceeded in several divisions. Each of these groups followed their colours, which were adorned with an inscription. That of the first was* Thanks to the Supreme Being; *and that of the second,* Resuscitation. *The Medical Assistants were next in succession; and after these, the* Guardians of life . . . *Another division was distinguished by a flag, with the words* Divine Mercy; *and another, with that of* Humanity. *The last banner displayed the inscription,* Return to Life. *The list of restored persons was read, by which it appeared that, from 1774 to the 22nd of July, 1796, a period of twenty-two years, two thousand one hundred and seventy five persons were restored to life.'* (27)

Conclusion

The resuscitation movement elicited popular support by reiterating four major themes in the exhortatory tracts of the 18th century. The first and oldest was the dream of prolonging life. The second was an uncertainty about the signs of death. The third was a recurring fear of premature interment. The last was a passion for meliorism, and a firm belief that resuscitation provided an extraordinary opportunity for truly altruistic enterprise.

Acknowledgments

Drs Richard M. Swengel and Linda R. Dagi kindly reviewed several versions of this essay and provided valuable insights and editorial assistance.

Notes and References

(1) Baker AB. Artificial respiration: The history of an idea. *Med Hist* 1971; **15**: 336–46.

(2) Bacon F. *The historie of life and death, with observations naturall and experimentall for the prolonging of life*. London: Printed by I. Okes for Humphrey Mosley, 1638.

(3) Thomson EH. The role of physicians in the humane societies of the 18th century. *Bull Hist Med* 1963; **37**: 43–51.

(4) Keevil JJ. *Medicine and the navy, 1200–1900. Volume II: 1649–1714*. Edinburgh and London: E & S Livinstone, Ltd, 1958: 44. No year of publication is given, but it appears to date between 1550 and 1650, and refer to still older sources.

(5) Tozzetti GT. *Raccolta di teorie, osservazioni, e regole per be distinguere e prontamente dissipare le asfissie or morti apprenti, dette anche mortie repentine, or violente, prodotte da varie cause si interne, che esterne*. Firenze: per Gaet. Cambiagi Stampat. Granduc., 1773: 5–6.

(6) Tossach W. A man dead in appearance recovered by distending the lungs with air. *Med Essays and Obs Soc Edinb* 1744; **v** (part 2): 605–8.

(7) Réaumur, "Avis concernant les personnes noyées, qui paraissent mortes," cited by Baker, AB. Artificial respiration, the history of an idea. *Med Hist* 1971; **15**: 336–46. See especially note 30, p. 341.

(8) Winslow JB. *Quaestio Medico-chirurgica . . . An Mortis Incertae Signa Minus Incerta a Chirurgis, Quam ab Aliis Experimentis*, Parisiis: Quillan, 1740.

(9) '. . . *in the eighty-fourth Olympiad, Empedocles restored to life a woman who was about to be buried, and . . . this circumstance induced the Greeks, for the future protection of the supposed dead, to establish laws which enacted that no person should be interred until the sixth or seventh day. But even this extension of time did not give satisfaction, and we read that when Hephestion, at whose funeral obsequies Alexander the Great was present, was to be buried, his funeral was delayed until the tenth day.'*
     Similar legends proliferated in Rome:
               '*While returning to his country house, Asclepiades, a physician . . . saw during the time of Pompey the Great a crowd of mourners about to start a fire on a funeral pile. It is said that by his superior knowledge he perceived indications of life in the corpse and ordered the pile destroyed, subsequently restoring the supposed deceased to life. These examples and several others of a similar nature induced the Romans to delay their funeral rites and laws were enacted to prevent haste in burning as well as interment. It was not until the eighth day that the final rites were performed, the days immediately subsequent to death having their own special ceremonies.*'
     Gould GM, Pyle WL. *Anomalies and curiosities of medicine*. New York: Bell Publishing Company, 1956: 520.

(10) Death bed resuscitations were apparently quite common in Greece, for special regulations existed with respect to persons who gave the appearance of death, but recovered after their funeral rites. They were prohibited from worship or from entering the temples under any circumstances. The Romans followed Greek custom. See Ducachet, HW. On the signs of death, and the manner of distinguishing real from apparent death. *Am Medical Recorder* (Philadelphia) 1822; **v**: 39–53.

(11) Winslow JB. *Dissertation sur l'incertitude des signes de la mort et de l'abus des enterrements et embaumements précipités.* (J.-J. Bruhier d'Ablaincourt, translator) Paris: [no publisher] 1742.

(12) Winslow JB. *The Uncertainty of the Signs of Death; and the Danger of Precipitate Interments and Dissections . . . With Proper Directions, both for Preventing Such Accidents, and Repairing the Misfortunes Brought on the Constitution by Them. To the Whole is Added, a curious Account of the Funeral Solemnities of Many Ancient and Modern Nations, Exhibiting the Precautions they made use of to Ascertain the Certainty of Death.* (J.-J. Bruhier d'Ablaincourt, translator) London: M. Cooper, 1746.

(13) An abstract of the address is also to be found in: Alexander Johnson, *A short account of a society at amsterdam instituted in the year 1767 for the recovery of drowned persons; with observations shewing the utility and advantage that would accrue to Great Britain from a similar institution extended to cases of suffocation by damps in mines, choaking, strangling, stifling, and other accidents.* London: [no publisher], 1773: 117–120.

(14) Anonymous. *Istruzione al popolo circ' ai tentavi da farsi per ravvivare gli annegati ed altri apparentement morti proposta dal Collegio Medico di Firenze in essecuzione degli ordini di sua altezza reale . . . ,* Firenze: nella stamp. granducale per Gaet. Cambiagi, 1772.

(15) Tozzetti GT. *Raccolta di teorie, osservazioni, e regole per be distinguere e prontamente dissipare le asfissie or morti apprenti, dette anche morti repentine, or violente, prodotte da varie cause si interne, che esterne.* Firenze: per Gaet. Cambiagi Stampat. Granduc., 1773.

(16) Luckhardt AB. Official 'Edict' by the city of Zurich, Switzerland, 1766, A.D. *Bull Inst Hist Med*, 1938; **6**: 171–8.

(17) '. . . since . . . *there have been many people who seeing such people in the act have held back and refrained from life saving measures, not because of less love for the unfortunate fellow man, but because of an ingrained superstitious and misfounded fear that it might be held to their discredit, or should be held against them should they render this charitable help, our gracious lords and higher sovereigns suggest to the effect that everyone cease entertaining such vain and superstitious prejudices and urge him or them to help such an unfortunate individual promptly and energetically as a Christian duty and act of mercy, and, to this end, that if they perform as is wished by the state, he or they will be rewarded suitably if it can be indubitably proven . . . that they have saved the life of an unfortunate one.'* (16)

(18) Johnson A. *A short account of a society at amsterdam instituted in the year 1767 for the recovery of drowned persons; with observations shewing the utility and advantage that would accrue to Great Britain from a similar institution extended to cases of suffocation by damps in mines, choaking, strangling, stifling, and other accidents.* London: [no publisher], 1773: B2–10.

(19) Johnson A. *An account of some societies at Amsterdam and Hamburgh for the recovery of drowned persons, and of similar institutions at Venice, Milan, Padua, Vienna, and Paris, with a collection of authentic cases proving the practicability of extending the benefit of their practice to the recovery of persons visibly dead by sudden stoppages of breath, suffocation, stifling, swooning, convulsions, and other accidents,* London: [no publisher], 1774: 2–5.

(20) Anonymous. *Society for the recovery of persons apparently drowned. Instituted M.DCC.LXXIV.* Presumably London: [no author, press or locus listed], 1754: 6.

(21) '*Those who have compassionate feelings for the misfortunes of their fellow creatures, will more readily be induced to attempt the rendering of such signal good offices, when they are informed that the incontestible facts prove it to be in the power of every one to give that aid, which in the moment of distress, may tend to rescue a life, that without their assistance would be lost . . . .*

The great probability of being blessed with success, renders the attempt of such humane endeavours, a duty owing by every individual to another in particular, and to society at large.—Those therefore, who neglect or decline giving such aid, will not only be considered deficient in an essential point of humanity, but in some measure as accessary to the patient's death, by allowing the last spark of life to extinguish: a reproach which no man can, upon the least reflection, allow to be laid to his charge; even under the prejudice that none but medical men *can administer relief in such critical situations, as it is a sad apology for the loss of a life, that the* medical assistant *came too late.* Johnson A. *Relief from accidental death or, summary instructions for the general institution proposed in the Year 1773*, Maidstone: J. Blake, 1784: 5.

(22) Scherlis L. Poetical version of the rules of the humane society for recovering drowned persons. *Critical Care Med* 1981; **9**: 430–1.

(23)   *'In every instance of departed life,*
Nature, still struggling, holds a doubtful strife.
In cases the most common that we meet,
Ere death the last decisive stroke complete,
Some time elapses;—yet uncertainty
Attends that space—it long or short may be:
Therefore employ that interval to try
If yet some sparks of life may dormant lie,
And either a recov'ry safe procure,
Or from that worst of horrors thus ensure
Of quick interment. For experience shows,
That many women, from child-bearing throes,
And new-born infants, brethless long remain
In swooning's trances,—yet revive again
By means here recommended.—Then beware
None perish thro' your want of thought or care;
But try those means which every willing hand,
At any time and place, may well command.'
Specific instructions are given next:
'At first discov'ry of apparent death,
Lose not a moment for the fleeting breath
May yet be stay'd—while life's last spark remains,
Patient attend, nor spare or time or pains.
Avoid the dangerous practice now decry'd,
By ignorance and prejudice oft try'd,
Rolling with violence, nor shaking try,
Nor yet suspending—who those means apply
To force discharge of water, to the grave
Consign the wretch whom gentler means might save . . . .

' . . . With cordial drops endeavour to revive
The fleeting spirits, and life's current drive
Back to its native channels.—Try to heal,
With opiate draughts, the irritated feel,
Caus'd by reviv'd sensation.—Next attend,
With needful help, and frequent turn or bend,
Provoking motion in the languid breast,
Nor leave the body in lethargic rest.

Inject warm vapour, and blow in fresh air;
And let it likewise be your constant care
To chafe the temples, palms, on every part
Most sensible, exert that needful art.

Take a clean feather, with it, tickle, teize
The throat, and up the nose, to force a sneeze.

> *In suffocations caused by noxious air,*
> *Or bodies frost bitten,—be it your care*
> *With water icy cold, or even snow,*
> *Repeatedly apply'd, to raise a glow:*
> *Despising all absurd exploded ways,*
> *With shock electrical the dead to raise,*
> *Or seeking sheep's-blood pour'd in human veins;*
> *True judgement all those vain attempts disdains . . . .'*

Finally, there is an admonition to persist until life has been fully restored:

> *' . . . Yet stop not at the first faint glimpse of life;*
> *While struggling nature holds a doubtful strife,*
> *Continue still the means, nor spare your pain,*
> *Lest in lethargic sleep they sink again.'*

Johnson A. *Relief from Accidental Death; or Summary Directions, in verse, extracted from the instructions at large, published by Alexander Johnson, M.D. (Introducer of the Practice into the British Dominions) to divulge and generally establish a successful Treatment for recovering Persons, who meet with Accidents that produce suddenly an Appearance of Death; and to prevent them, or any others, from being buried alive:* . . . London: Logographic Press, 1789.

(24) Keith A. Three Hunterian lectures on the mechanism underlying the various methods of artificial respiration practised since the foundation of the Royal Humane Society in 1774. *Lancet* 1909; i: 745–9, 825–8, 895–9.

(25) Wilson LG. The transformation of ancient concepts of respiration in the 17th century. *Isis* 1960; **51**: 161–72.

(26) In 1792, for example, James Curry wrote:

> *'The time is within the recollection of many now living, when it was almost universally believed that* life *quitted the body in a very few minutes after the person had ceased to breath. Remarkable examples to the contrary, were indeed upon the record, but these, besides being extremely rare, were generally cases wherein the suspension, as well as the recovery of life had occurred spontaneously; . . . they were therefore beheld with astonishment, as particular instances of divine interposition, and afforded no ground to hope, that* human *means could prove at all useful under similar circumstances.—Such a view of the matter necessarily checked any rational and premeditated attempt at recovery, even in those cases where the appearance of death was evidently occasioned by the operation of external and assignable causes; and it is probably owing to the rude trials which fond attachment may have sometimes intuitively prompted, that we are indebted for the happy discovery of an essential difference between* absolute *and* apparent death. *The success which occasionally attended the artless attempts of uninformed persons, soon attracted the attention of medical men, by whom the means for recovery have been improved, and employed with such happy consequences, as to have rendered the matter an object of public concern, and highly deserving of that extensive encouragement and support which it now enjoys in this, and in several other countries of Europe . . . .'*

James Curry, *Popular Observations on Apparent Death From Drowning, Suffocation, &c, With An Account of the Means to be Employed for Recovery*, (Printed by T. Dicey and Company, for the Northamptonshire Preservative Society: Northampton, 1792) pp. v–x.

(27) Struve C. *A practical essay on the art of recovering suspended animation together with a review of the most proper and effectual means to be adopted in cases of imminent danger.* Translated from the German. London, [no publisher given] 1801: 1–16. Cited in Alexander M. 'The rigid embrace of the narrow house': Premature burial and the signs of death. *Hastings Center Report* 1980; **10** (June): 25–31, note 19.

18.6   The history of clinical thermometry

LAURIE G. ALLEN
Northwick Park Hospital, Harrow, UK

The history of clinical thermometry is rooted in the Scientific Revolution and our modern concepts are linked to two features of that era, the development of instruments to extend the five senses and the evolution of a quantitative approach to problem solving. Lord Kelvin whose statue you can see in Kelvingrove Park, Glasgow remarked that, 'When you can measure what you are speaking about and express it in numbers, you know something about it'.

The history of thermometry is an excellent example of knowing something vaguely through qualitative evaluation to knowing something concrete through quantitative scientific methods. Silas Weir Mitchell, in an address before the second congress of the Association of American Physicians and Surgeons in 1891 presented the concept that advances in medicine were due to the progressive application of quantitating devices to the care of the sick. The development of the thermometer was just such an advance and is the oldest of our quantitating devices.

The origin of the thermometer and its use in medicine

In 400 BC Hippocrates assessed temperature with his own hand. The first device used to measure temperature was the thermoscope. Four men have been attributed with its invention but Galileo, the Italian Mathematician, is usually given credit in about 1603. The heat of the hand expands the air in the glass bulb to force the fluid down the tube into the reservoir, in contrast to modern thermometers. More strictly it should be called a barothermoscope since the fluid in the reservoir is open to atmospheric pressure, it would also have been somewhat inaccurate. It was however Sanctorius, one of the other three men, who was the first to use the instrument clinically in 1611. He was also the first to apply a scale making the instrument a thermometer, the term coined by the Jesuit Father Laurechon in 1624. Throughout the 17th and 18th centuries there was much confusion over the scaling, choice of thermometric substance and site of measurement. This did little to advance its use in medicine, until in 1714 when David Gabriel Fahrenheit, a meteorological instrument maker, introduced mercury into the bore and devised the scale that bears his name. The interval of 180 degrees made it somewhat unwieldy and a centigrade scale was suggested by several workers, although it is credited to the Swedish astronomer Anders Celsius.

The clinical thermometer

The final modification, a constriction in the bore to make a maximum-reading instrument was devised by Cavendish in 1757. These accurate instruments led Bequerel and Breschet to establish the mean body temperature of a healthy adult at 98.6 °F.

Other thermometers followed—in particular the gas thermometer brought about the absolute or Kelvin Scale originally suggested by Lord Kelvin. In 1821 Seebeck had noted his effect and thermocouples were born. As early as 1871 Siemens proposed the resistance thermometer.

However, Fahrenheit's advance made accurate clinical temperature readings possible and thermometry mushroomed. A year later in 1715 Lancisi insisted that physicians should be familiar with the thermometer and microscope.

Boerhave obtained several thermometers from Fahrenheit and one of his students, Anton de Haen who later became Professor in Vienna, measured the temperature of his patients on a large scale. The work was published in 15 volumes between 1757 and 1773. However, Martine, an Edinburgh graduate, published the first accurate figures on temperature in healthy man and animals in 1738. His ideas were extended by another Scot, James Currie who was studying the effect of hydrotherapy on the temperature in typhoid fever. At this time thermometry commanded more interest in Scotland than elsewhere but, by 1840, papers on temperature in health and disease figured prominently in all the journals. By 1863 John Davy had noted the temperature variations in exercise and eating. Diurnal variation and changes with age and drugs had in fact been noted by De Haen more than a century before. By 1850 physicians and surgeons were interested. It was concluded that temperature was a better guide to health than the pulse since it was not so easily affected by the nervous system. Major works were published by Claude Bernard, Traube and Ringer and followed in 1868 by the classic work of Wunderlich, who over 15 years had made several million observations of some 25 000 cases. (Not a mean task considering his thermometer was a foot long and had to be left in the axilla for 20 minutes). Forty principles stemmed from his work and he introduced the temperature chart as used today. Harrison commented that he found fever a disease and left it a symptom.

The clinical significance of thermometry led to the need for a more portable instrument for general practice. Allbutt worked with Harvey and Reynolds of Leeds to produce just such a thermometer. Different designs were made for use in the axilla, groin, mouth, rectum, urethra and vagina. By the 1860s the axilla was the most common site until the development of germicidal agents in the late 1890s when oral thermometers became the most popular.

Electrical methods of thermometry although available by 1835 have only really been developed for clinical use on a wide scale over the last 20 years. The real concern over infection in the last 10 years has seen the development of disposable sheaths for electrical probes and single use clinical thermometers based on heat sensitive crystals. Current research is investigating continuous electrical devices for accurate measurement of skin temperature by creating a zone of zero heat flow around the probe. There is also the development of even smaller thermistors for flow studies in blood vessels and respiratory measurement.

Thermometry in anaesthesia

Tracing the origins of thermometry in anaesthesia has not been easy. However, Hippocrates used refrigeration analgesia with snow, but the first description of cooling for surgery was by an Anglo Saxon monk in about 1050.

' . . . for eruptive rash. Let him sit in cold water until it be deadened; then draw him up. Then cut 4 scarifications around the pocks and let drip as long as he will'. Although forgotten, the technique was used again in 1595 and 1807 when Larrey noticed that soldiers who had lain in snow for some time experienced painless amputation. James Arnott coined the term 'refrigeration' in 1863 and wrote a number of papers on the subject—all part of a life-long campaign against the dangers of inhalational anaesthesia. Benjamin Ward Richardson developed the 1st refrigeration spray in 1866 with rhigolene and then ether. It was so popular that the term freezing passes as a synonym for local analgesia.'

Tracing the first use of thermometers in general anaesthesia is more difficult. Nevertheless I did discover that on 15 October, 1868, there was a meeting of the New York Academy of Medicine when a Dr Neftel read a paper on 'Exact Methods of Medical Treatment in Connection with Thermometry'. In the discussion afterwards a Dr Weir reported that the thermometer had been used in surgical operations with ether and chloroform. During amputations they noted that on section of the bone the temperature fell.

In 1958 Pickering quoted that it had been said that the most effective means of cooling a man is to give an anaesthetic. The bulk of anaesthetic literature concerning thermometry has been concerned with this effect. Indeed it was noted as early as 1880 by Von Kappeler and attributed to radiation. This report stimulated others to measure temperature to contemplate the causes and devise means to prevent the cooling effect. These were so successful that by 1916 Moschowitz was able to report 12 cases of postoperative heat stroke, 2 of which had been noted by Gibson in 1900. Continued interest in the problem together with the risks of static electricity led to work on the theatre environment. Air conditioning was recommended by Huntington in 1920 and Herb concluded that an optimum temperature was 65–70 °F in theatre.

Anaesthetists have used thermometry in anaesthetic breathing circuits. During the days of open-drop cooling was a problem. Later with the development of the circle and to and fro circuits, hyperthermia commonly occurred. In 1954 Clark measured the inspired gas temperature in these circuits. It reached 102 °F in the to and fro, 97 °F in the circle and 94 °F in the non-rebreathing circuits. In 1973 Berry showed that hypothermia could result from breathing dry gases and hence there is now widespread use of humidifiers with careful temperature control in intensive care. Other areas in temperature that interest us are the mechanisms of halothane shakes described by Gozon in 1969, the reason for shivering with epidural block and the precise temperatures and length of application for thermocoagulation and cryotherapy probes.

Thermometry as a guide for resuscitation

Thermometry was also used as a clinical aid in anaesthesia. In 1947 Clutton-Brock delivered an address on the subject. He used a mercury-in-glass thermometer with no constriction reading from 80–107 °F. The bulb was ring shaped and placed on the forehead. He confirmed the vasodilation on anaesthetic induction with increased skin temperature as reported by Ipsen in 1929. He also noted that when an operation induced shock or haemorrhage, the temperature fell, and that if it fell more than 3 °F the situation was serious. Otherwise he found the temperature to be remarkably independent of the blood pressure, but that if both fell the patient was gravely ill. He concluded that the two observations enabled him to judge the need for resuscitation. The serious combination of hypothermia in shock led Boyan and Howland in 1961 to measure oesophageal temperature during massive transfusion with cold blood. Their results led them to devise a machine to warm the blood.

Ross in 1959 also found skin temperature a useful clinical guide, in particular he found that change in great toe temperature gave an early sign of hypovolaemia.

Elective hypothermia

Cooling had generated much interest and had been studied by Walter in 1862. In 1905 Simpson and Herring at Edinburgh chilled cats and noted that at 25 °C they were insensible—they coined the term 'artificial hibernation'. In 1940 Smith & Fay showed that whole body cooling halted malignant disease. This work had realized the importance of anaesthesia before cooling to stop shivering. The procedure lasted four days and temperature was monitored with a rectal resistance thermometer.

When Bigelow observed that the reduced oxygen consumption of hypothermia did not incur an oxygen debt, he suggested its role in cardiac surgery, after a successful pilot study in dogs at 20 °C. Lewis and Tauffic first reported successful surface cooling for surgery in man in 1953. Temperature measurement was critical due to the onset of ventricular fibrillation at 28 °C. Alternative means of cooling were sought and later in 1953 Gibbon reported the first successful cardiopulmonary bypass, with pervascular cooling.

The method of thermometry depended on the mode of cooling, slow surface techniques allowing rectal mercury thermometers. However, the pervascular technique required an accurate rapidly responding device such as the thermistor. Controversy followed over the best site to monitor heart and brain temperature and minimize after drop.

The finding that haemorrhagic shock was better tolerated in hypothermia was the result of a fortuitous failure in the heating arrangements in the Wilkie Surgical laboratory at Edinburgh in the winter of 1947. Combined hypothermia and hypotension under anaesthesia was used therapeutically in 1956 by McBurrows for neurosurgery. A rectal thermocouple was used to measure temperature here but hypothermia was used more commonly to treat hypotensive and shock-like states.

During the 1950s anaesthetists were pioneers in the field; they employed hypothermia for surgical cases including transplants and poor-risk cases and non-surgical conditions such as post circulatory arrest, burns and head injury. Delorme's grading of hypothermia according to depth in 1956 was helpful in management. Light hypothermia at 30–35 °C was used for hyperpyrexias such as polio, hyperthyroidism and tetanus. Intermediate at 25–28 °C allowed 5–13 minutes of surgery, with anaesthesia and muscle relaxants initially. Deep hypothermia at 15–20 °C and Drew's 'profound hypothermia' 4–6 °C were used in cardiac work.

Conclusion

Man is homeothermic, where gross changes in temperature are expected or induced the measurement of temperature is mandatory. However, since a knowledge of the patient's temperature is a proven clinical aid one is led to ask as Dr Howat did at a symposium on temperature regulation in 1973:

'Should all anaesthetised patients have not only the blood pressure, pulse rate and respiration but also the temperature of the body monitored?'.

Chapter 19
EARLY ATTEMPTS AT EXPIRED AIR RESPIRATION, INTUBATION AND MANUAL VENTILATION

19.1	The early days of expired air resuscitation

A. B. BAKER
Otago University, Dunedin, New Zealand

'Thou takest away their breath, they die, and return to their dust.' Psalm 104:29

The Bible is clear about the absence of breathing leading to death but is not at all clear about artificial breathing being useful to restore life. There are a number of oft quoted references which are mostly allegorical (1–4) or at best confusing with the distinct possibility that the best story of resuscitation by Elisha (5) in Kings II 4: 34–35 'is of resuscitation by rewarming rather than by any act of expired air respiration:

> *'And he went up and lay upon the child, and put his mouth upon his mouth, and his eyes upon his eyes, and his hands upon his hands: and he stretched himself upon the child; and flesh of the child waxed warm.*
>
> *Then he returned, and walked in the house to and fro; and went up and stretched himself upon him: and the child sneezed seven times and the child opened his eyes.'*

There are Egyptian references also quoted as early reports of expired air resuscitation but like the later Biblical references they are largely allegorical (6–8) though Jayne states that Isis resuscitated Osiris with the breath of life (9). This myth is particularly complex and on checking Jayne's references I have not been able to reach the same interpretation. The best text would appear to be:

> *'She [Isis] made light with her feathers, she made air to come into being with her wings, and she uttered cries of lamentation at the bier of her brother. She stirred up from his state of inactivity him whose heart was still.'* (6)

The Talmud also has a fleeting reference for resuscitation of babies:

> *'Hold him so that he will not fall down and breathe into his nostrils.'* (10)

The midwives' secret

Neonatal resuscitation was obviously an area of interest particularly as it is one where success will follow more often than not. The first printed medical text to be devoted entirely to Paediatrics was that in 1472 by Paolo Begellardo (or Paulus Bagellardus) (11). This text was also interestingly the first medical text to be published initially in the printed form. On page 3 of Bagellardo's *Libellus de egritudinibus infantium* is the marvellous advice:

> *'si reperiret ipsu calidu no nigru debet inflare in os eius ipso no habete respiratione'*
> (*'If she find it* [the newborn] *warm, not black, she should blow into its mouth, if it has no respiration').*

This advice no doubt was well known to the midwives of the time as Bagellardo was unlikely to be present often during delivery. Much of Bagellardo's book is based on Rhazes and Avicenna but I have not found any references to artificial respiration in either of these works.

The splendid advice by Bagellardo is unfortunately somewhat ruined by four words which end the sentence quoted above—'aut in anu eius' (or into its anus)? This brings considerable doubt to the real meaning of the usefulness of the artificial respiration. In reality both would be very good stimuli to the initiation of neonatal respiration as any stimulus tends to engender the initiation of neonatal respiration in an apnoeic newborn. Thus it can be safely assumed that this advice to expired air resuscitation would have often been used by midwives and no doubt with real effect from time to time.

The next report of expired air resuscitation is by Borelli in 1679 (12) who reported:

> 'On 24th November, 1679, a primipara was satisfactorily delivered. All seemed well when she was overcome by sudden hypothymia and appeared to die. She did not hear or feel, her pulse was scarcely noticeable . . . In this emergency I am called for; while getting the drugs . . . a most faithful servant girl—during my absence—stretches herself over the puerpera, blows her breath into her mouth which quickly calls her back to life. The lady could not remember anything of the incident. When I asked the maid how she learned of this procedure, she mentioned a similar use at Altenburg; also the midwives were using it on apparently dead babies.' (12)

Thus Borelli showed how the midwives had kept up the practise even if medical knowledge had forgotten.

The 18th century

The first undoubted therapeutic expired air resuscitation to be reported was that by Tossach (13) in 1744 who resuscitated a suffocated miner using mouth-to-mouth resuscitation. Not only was this successful but Tossach was very cautious with his claims for the technique:

> 'I must submit to better Judges to determine whether the Experiment I design to relate was the Mean of saving the Man's Life on whom it was tried; it is at least very simple and absolutely safe, and therefore can at least be no Harm, if there is not an Advantage in acquainting the Publick of it.' (13)

However, there was already published in 1740 by the Academie des Sciences (Paris) its 'Avis concerant les personnes noyées, qui paraissent mortes' (14) which advised strongly that mouth-to-mouth respiration was the best method for recovering apparently drowned persons. The Academie would no doubt have been well aware of the physiological experiments where animals could be resuscitated by doing artificial respiration from bellows. These experiments were in themselves quite an interesting history stemming from Vesalius in 1453 (15) through the frenetic activity of the early days of the Royal Society with experiments by Croune (16), Hooke (17) and Lower (18). In an earlier article I have elaborated on this and other aspects of the history of artificial respiration (19). Also around this time Jackson (20) reported secondhand a similar resuscitation.

Soon after these reports the Humane Societies of Europe came into being to promote resuscitation of the apparently drowned. The general social awareness that led to Societies in Amsterdam 1767, Milan and Hamburg 1768, Paris 1771 and London 1774 has been elegantly described by Herholdt and Rahm in 1796 (21). These Societies were soon to encourage the use of bellows and pistons instead of mouth-to-mouth expired air for resuscitation (22).

Conclusion

Expired air resuscitation was to have many further vicissitudes until modern times when two groups showed scientifically the simplicity of mouth-to-mouth respiration (23) and these visiccitudes have been described elsewhere (19). Never-the-less the formation in the 17th Century of the Humane Societies was to close the early history of expired air resuscitation.

References

(1) *Genesis* 2:7 'And the Lord God formed man of the dust of the ground, and breathed into his nostrils the breath of life, and man became a living soul.'
(2) *Ezekiel* 37:5 'Behold, I will cause breath to enter into you and ye shall live.'

(3) *Ezekiel* 37:9 'Come from the four winds, O breath, and breathe upon these slain, that they may live.'

(4) *I Kings* 17: 21–22 'And he stretched himself upon the child three times, and cried unto the Lord, and said, O Lord my God, I pray thee, let this child's soul come into him again. And the Lord heard the voice of Elijah and the soul of the child came into him again, and he survived.'

(5) *II Kings* 4: 34–35.

(6) Budge W. Translation of *The Gods of the Egyptians. Hymn to Osiris.* London: Methuen, 1904: Vol 2, 150.

(7) Budge W. Translation of *The Gods of the Egyptians*, Pyramid Text-Unas. London: Methuen, 1904: Vol 2, 204.

(8) Budge W. Translation of *Osiris and the Egyptian Resurrection.* Pyramid Text-Pepi II 868. London: Warner, 1909: Vol 1, 86.

(9) Jayne WA. *The healing Gods of Ancient Civilisation.* New Haven: Yale University Press, 1925: 65.

(10) *Gemarah Talmud Shabat* 128, 2.

(11) Bagellardus P. *Libellus de egritudinibus infantium.* Barval, 1472.

(12) Gruebel JG. *Ex halitu hominis vitae revocatio.* Ac. Nat. Cur. D2 A10 1775: 88.
    'Little can be added to the Dissertation 'de halitu humano' by Georg. Franc, a man of superlative judgement. Yet the story of Borellus may give the opportunity of describing my own observation on the effect of human breath. Borellus mentioned the case of a servant reviving his master by insufflation. On 24th November 1679 etc.'
    (I have not been able to locate this reference to Borelli's description in either of the volumes of his De motu animalium. 1680–81 Romae: Bernabo)

(13) Tossach W. 'A man, dead in appearance recovered by distending the lungs with air.' *Medical Essays and Observations*, Edinburgh, 1744: 5 (2), 605–8.

(14) Réaumur. 'Avis concerant les personnes noyées, qui paraissent mortes' 1740, quoted in full by Louis *'Letters sur la certitude des signes de le mort, ou l'on reassure les citoyens de la crainte d'etre enterres vivans, avec des observations & des experiences sun les noyés.'* Paris: Lambert, 1753. 250.

(15) Vesalius A. *De humani corporis fabrica.* Lib. VII Cap. XIX—De vivorum sectione nonnulla. Basle: Oporinus, 1543: 658 (should be 662 but error in first edition).

(16) Croune W. 1664 in T. Birch *The History of the Royal Society of London for Improving of Natural Knowledge.* London: Millar, 1756: Vol 1, 433.

(17) Hooke R. 1664 in T. Birch op. cit. Vol I p. 486, and T. Birch op. cit. Vol II p. 198, and *Phil Trans Roy Soc Lond* 1667; **2**: 539.

(18) Lower R. *Tractatus de corde, item de motu & calore sanguines et chyli in eum transitu.* Cap III Sanguines motus & calor. Amsterdam: Elzevirium, 1669: 177–8.

(19) Baker AB. Artificial respiration, the history of an idea. *Medical History* 1971; **15**: 336–51.

(20) Jackson R. A practical dissertation on drowning by a physician (attributed to Jackson). London: Robinson, 1746: 68.

(21) Herholdt JD, Rafn CG. An attempt at an historical survey of life-saving measures for drowning persons and information of the best means by which they can be brought back to life. Copenhagen: Tikiob, 1796 (trans. 1960 by DW Hannah, A. Rousing. Poulsen H ed. Aarhuus: Stiftsbogtrykkerie.)

(22) Chaussier F. of Dijon. 'Reflexions sur les moyens propres a determiner la respiration dans les enfans qui naissent sans donner aucun signe de vie, & a retablir cette fonction dans les asphyxies; & sur les effets de l'air vital ou dephlogistique employe pour produire us avantages.' *Histoire de la Société Royale de Médecine* 4, 346.

(23) Safar P, Escarraga LA, Elam JO. 'A comparison of the mouth-to-mouth and mouth-to-airway methods of artificial respiration with chest-pressure arm-lift methods.' *N Engl J Med* 1958; **258**: 671.

(24) Poulsen H, Skall-Jensen J, Staffeldt I, Lange M. 'Pulmonary ventilation and respiratory gas exchange during manual artificial respiration and expired air resuscitation on apnoeic normal adults.' *Acta Anaesth Scand* 1959; **3**: 129.

19.2   The first instruments for resuscitation

L. BRANDT, D. DUDA and M. EL GINDI
Johannes Gutenberg University, Mainz, Federal German Republic

It was during the spirit of Enlightenment in the 18th century that people began reflecting on the value of human life and its preservation in cases of misfortunes and accidents (1). In the second half of the century in nearly all European countries societies were established as having a primary responsibility for such things as, Information of the population about their rights and duties in cases of accident; Organization of lifesaving services; Improvement of resuscitation methods; Availability of instruments for resuscitation; Public promise of reward in cases of (successful or unsuccessful) resuscitation; Documentation and publication of all events concerning life-saving activities (2,3,4).

The following account will look at the first instruments and methods of resuscitation during the 18th century.

In the medicine of those times preference was given to some special forms of therapy, such as the application of cupping instruments, blood letting, insufflation of spirits, enemas and fumigation.

Blood letting

It was natural to apply some of these methods also in cases of resuscitation. Charles Kite (1768–1811) in his *Essay on the recovery of the apparently dead* (see Fig. 1) recommends blood letting as one of the first and most effective methods in resuscitation (5). He writes:

> *'Whatever objection may be urged against bleeding in the early stage of these accidents, no one will, I believe, oppose it in this* (e.g. resuscitation)*; for it is certain no remedy can answer so speedily and effectually; and it may require to be frequently repeated before the effect is produced.*
> *The part from whence the blood is to be drawn, is in these cases by no means a matter of indifference. If it is taken from the arm, the distension of the brain, for which principally this operation is performed, will scarcely be at all lessened on account of the stagnation of the blood, and the distance from the part affected; added to which, blood can seldom be procured in sufficient quality from this part. If the temporal artery is opened, no benefit will arise, because we have already shewn, that the veins only are overloaded, and that the arteries are almost destitute of blood: but the external jugular veins, although they bring the blood from the external part of the head only, yet as they immediately communicate with the superior venae cavae and internal jugulars, which receive the blood from the sinuses of the dura mater and veins of the brain, certainly ought to be preferred on these occasions.'*

If bloodletting cannot be performed, Kite recommends the application of cupping-glasses:

> *'The application of cupping-glasses to the head, neck, and breast, may be extremely serviceable, particularly if we cannot procure a sufficient quantity of blood from the jugular veins. This mode of operating, independant of the evacuation, will be attended with the additional advantage of proving a powerful stimulus.'*

As the concept of resuscitation advocated by the Societies, was made primarily for laymen and not for physicians, simple methods had priority. For example, the Amsterdam Society as well as later the London Humane Society recommended the following as resuscitation methods of first order (2): The application of warmth when the corpse had become cold; Rubbing or friction of the body; The inducement of vomiting; The oral, nasal, rectal, or cutaneous application of stimulants; The fumigation, i.e. the introduction of tobacco smoke into the rectum, and finally, the artificial respiration by mouth-to-mouth inflation with compression

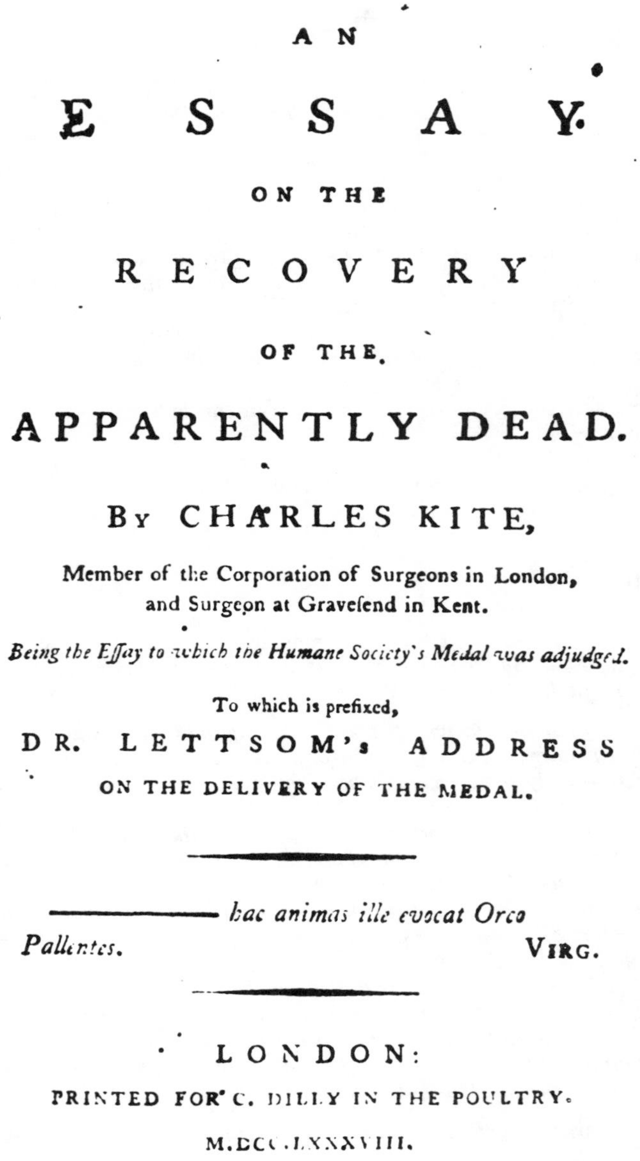

A N

E S S A Y.

ON THE

R E C O V E R Y

OF THE.

APPARENTLY DEAD.

By CHARLES KITE,

Member of the Corporation of Surgeons in London,
and Surgeon at Gravefend in Kent.

Being the Effay to which the Humane Society's Medal was adjudged.

To which is prefixed,

DR. LETTSOM's ADDRESS

ON THE DELIVERY OF THE MEDAL.

——————————

——————— *hac animas ille evocat Orco*

Pallentes.   VIRG.

——————————

L O N D O N:

PRINTED FOR C. DILLY IN THE POULTRY.

M.DCC.LXXXVIII.

Figure 1   *Title page from Charles Kite's 'Essay' (5).*

of the abdomen and the chest. Of these, fumigation and artificial respiration seem to be the most interesting ones to consider.

Fumigation

It is most probable that already at the beginning of the 17th century fumigation was a common therapy in many diseases. Special fumigation sets had been developed. The English physician John Woodall (1556–1643) in his *The Surgeon's Mate* (6) describes an apparatus for the proper

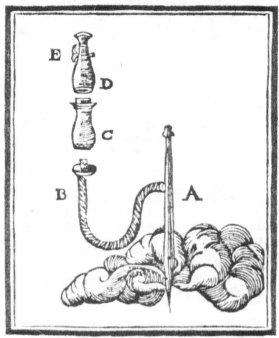

Figure 2   A 'fumigation apparatus' (3). A: The tube to be introduced into the rectum; B: The connecting tube made of leather; C: The wooden box containing the glowing tobacco; D: The mouthpiece to blow the tobacco into the rectum; E: The tap.

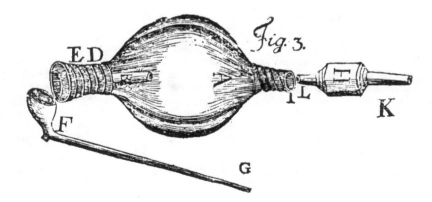

Figure 3   Alexander Johnson's 'fumigation apparatus' (7). A: The pig's bladder with two openings B and C; E: The connector to the tobacco pipe is affixed in D to the pig's bladder; F: The tobacco pipe with mouthpiece G; H: The tube for the rectum, connected with the pig's bladder in I and L; K: The cone to be stuffed into the rectum.

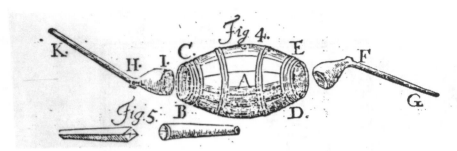

Figure 4   Another 'fumigation apparatus' by Alexander Johnson (7). A: The small barrel that is to be filled with tobacco smoke through its opening D and E with the tobacco pipe F and G; C: The barrel's second opening is connected with I to pipe H; K: The second pipe H is connected in K to the rectal tube B.

administration of tobacco smoke. This fumigation apparatus also was one of the first instruments to be used in resuscitation. A table in the resuscitation booklet of Isnard (3) shows such a fumigator (see Fig. 2). It had been developed by Thomas Bartholin (1616–1680) in the middle of the 17th century and was modified by Pieter van Muschenbroeck (1692–1761) from Leyden for it's use in resuscitation. Such a fumigation is drawn in detail on two figures in Alexander Johnson's *Collection of authentic cases proving the practicability of recovering persons visibly dead by drowning, suffocation, stifling, swooning, convulsion and other accidents* (7; see also Figs. 3 and 4).

In contrast to other methods, fumigation soon fell into disrepute. In 1788, Charles Kite wrote (5):

'Tobacco glisters, in strangulated herniae, and violent constipations of the bowels, are in universal estimation. I have sometimes, it is true, seen them succeed when every other remedy had appeared unsuccessful; but it is no less certain, that I have in many instances seen them not only fail, but produce very alarming symptoms: and in more than one case, where they were persisted in too long, death itself, unless I am much mistaken, has been the consequence.
Considering all circumstances, then, is it not a just inference, that although tobacco may at first act as a stimulus, yet it will afterwards, by its narcotic and deleterious properties, not only counteract what it has accomplished, but will abolish what before existed?'

Four years later in 1792 another physician, James Curry, in his *Popular observations on apparent death* wrote the following on the use of tobacco in resuscitation (8):

'Tobacco-smoke, injected by way of glyster, is what has been generally employed . . . and the fumigator or instrument for administering it, makes a part of the apparatus which is at present distributed by the different societies established for the recovery of drowned persons. Of late, however, the use of tobacco-smoke has been objected to, and upon very strong grounds; for when we consider that the same remedy is successfully employed with the very opposite intention, namely, that of lessening the power of contraction in the muscles, and occasioning the greatest relaxation consistent with life, it must be acknowledged to be a very doubtful, if not dangerous remedy, where the powers of life are already nearly exhausted.'

Before looking at the 'apparatus for the recovery of drowned persons' that Curry mentioned (8), another method of resuscitation, artificial respiration, has to be considered.

Artificial respiration

The importance of respiration for the maintenance of life had been accepted since ancient times (9,10). In 1714, the Danish physician Georg Detharding (1671–1747) recommended for the first time tracheotomy as a treatment in drowned persons in his *De methodo subveniendi submersis per laryngotomiam* (11). About 20 years later, 1732, the surgeon William Tossack resuscitated a coal worker by mouth-to-mouth inflation. He reported this before the Medical Society in Edinburgh in 1744 (12). John Fothergill (1712–1780) jumped at the idea and recommended it in his *Observations on a Case of Recovering a Man Dead in Appearance, by distending the Lungs with Air* (13) as the method of choice in resuscitation.

The great advances in artificial respiration by mechanical aids—bellows and endotracheal tube—have also been described (14). Artificial ventilation with bellows was proposed by John Hunter (1728–1793) who developed special two-chamber bellows for positive-negative-pressure ventilation (15). In 1782, the Royal Humane Society endorsed his opinion (2). (Hunter was also one of the first to recommend the application of electricity in resuscitation (16).)

Air was applied with the help of bellows directly into the mouth or nostrils until William Cullen (1712–1789) made the proposal to pass an orotracheal male catheter (17). He referred to Alexander Monro (1697–1767) in England and Claude-Nicolas Le Cat (1700–1768) in France, both of whom had described this method. The first to recommend it had been Avicenna (980–1037) around the year 1000 AD (9,14) for use in resuscitation (2,18) (see also Figs. 5 and 6). Charles Kite gives the following comment to endotracheal intubation (5):

> '*If any difficulty should arise in distending the lungs, it must proceed either from water in the windpipe, or a contraction or adhesion of the epiglottis. We have already pointed out the method of discovering when the first circumstance occurs; and when the latter*

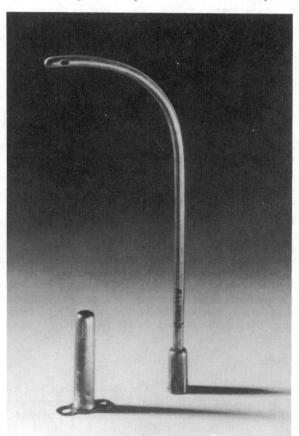

Figure 5 'A metal crooked tube, bent like a male catheter, recommended by Dr Monro' *(5)*; with kind permission of the Wellcome Museum for the History of Medicine, London.

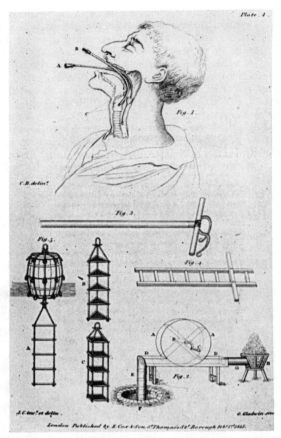

Figure 6   Depiction of an orotracheal intubation. Plate 4 of the second edition (1815) of James Curry's 'Observations on apparent death' (8).

is the case, we shall generally remedy the inconvenience by bringing the tongue forwards, which, being connected to the epiglottis by inelastic ligaments, must of course be elevated. Should any further impediment however occur, the crooked tube, bent like a male catheter, recommended by Dr Monro, and mentioned by Mr Portal, Mr le Cat, and others, should be introduced into the glottis, through the mouth or one nostril; the end should be connected to a blow-pipe, or, what will be more convenient, the pipe for the nose belonging to the elactic tube may be removed, and this instrument screwed in its place, according to the plan mentioned in the description of a pocket case of instrument for the recovery of the apparently dead, by Mr Savigny.'

Resuscitation sets

Together with his colleague John Savigny, Charles Kite developed a set of resuscitation instruments. These standardized 'Resuscitation Sets' were deposited in certain places along the Thames by the Royal Humane Society. In case of need they were available within a short time (19).

The Resuscitation Sets were evolved on the basis of the 'Fumigation Sets' of the 17th and the beginning of the 18th century. Some of these sets are still preserved and can be seen in, for example, the 'Wellcome Museum for the History of Medicine' in London (see Fig. 7).

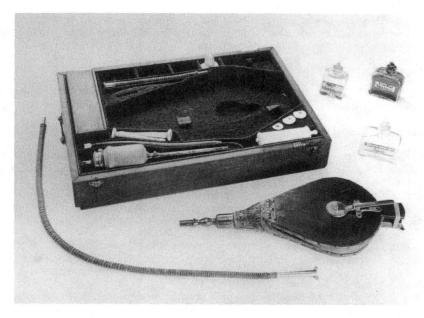

Figure 7   A 'Resuscitation Set'; with kind permission of the Wellcome Museum for the History of Medicine, London (19).

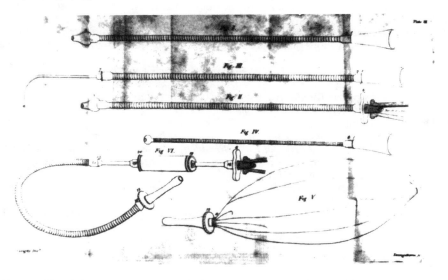

Figure 8   Plate III in Charles Kite's 'An essay on the recovery of the apparently dead' showing the contents of a 'Resuscitation Set' (5).

The contents of a 'Resuscitation Set' are described and sketched on a plate in Charles Kite's essay (see Fig. 8).

Resuscitation medicine is not an achievement of our time. Already 200 years ago outstanding physicians and scientists developed a strategy of resuscitation that, apart from the use of drugs, is still valid. This can be stressed by a sentence from the essay of Charles Kite in which he states:

*'Let it be observed, as an invariable rule, that in all attempts to recover a drowned,
our attention should be principally and primarily directed to—the administration and
proper regulation of the inflation of the lungs.'*

References

(1) Brandt L, El Gindi M, Duda D, Ellmauer S. The development of organized emergency
    medicine in the 18th century. Paper 19.3. Roy. Soc. Med Int. Congr. Symp.
    Series No. 134. London: Royal Society of Medicine, 1988.

(2) Bishop PJ. *A short history of the Royal Humane Society*. London: The Royal Humane
    Society, 1974.

(3) Isnard. *Herrn Isnards heilsamer Unterricht wie man Ertrunkenen auf die leichteste und
    sicherste Art wieder zum Leben verhelfen könne*. Straßburg: Joh. Gottfried
    Bauer, 1760.

(4) Günther JA. *Geschichte und Einrichtung der Hamburgischen Rettungs = Anstalten für im
    Wasser verunglückte Menschen*. Hamburg: Herold'sche Buchhandlung, 1828.

(5) Kite C. An *essay on the recovery of the apparently dead*. London: C. Dilly in the Poultry,
    1788.

(6) Woodall J. *The surgeon's mate or military & domestique surgery*. 2nd Ed. London, 1639.

(7) Johnson A. *A collection of authentic cases proving the practicability of recovery persons
    visibly dead by drowning, suffocation, stifling, swooning, convulsion and
    other accidents*. London, 1773.

(8) Curry J. *Popular observations on apparent death from drowning, suffocation, &c. with
    an account of the means to be employed for recovery*. London: T. Dicey
    and Co., 1792.

(9) Brandt L, Goerig M. The history of tracheotomy. Part I. *Anaesthesist* 1986; **35**: 279–83.

(10) Goerig M, Brandt L. The history of tracheotomy. Part II. *Anaesthesist* 1986; **35**: 397–402.

(11) Brandt L, Goerig M. The history of tracheotomy. Part III. *Anaesthesist* 1986; **35**: 455–64.

(12) Tossack W. *Medical essays & observations*. Vol. V, Part 2. Edinburgh, 1744: 605.

(13) Fothergill J. Observations on a case of recovering a man dead in appearance, by distending
    the lungs with air. *Phil Trans* 1744/45; **43**: 275–80.

(14) Brandt L, Pokar H, Schütte H. 100 years of endotracheal anaesthesia. *Anaesthesist* 1986;
    32: 200–5.

(15) Hunter J. Proposals for the recovery of people apparently drowned. *Phil Trans* 1776;
    66: 412–25.

(16) Duda D, Brandt L. The history of defibrillation. Paper *The Second International
    Symposium on the History of Anaesthesia*. London, 1987.

(17) Cullen W. *A letter to Lord Cathcart, President of the Board of Police in Scotland;
    concerning the recovery of persons drowned, and seemingly dead*.
    Edinburgh, 1776.

(18) Bartels I. *Die Geschichte der Mund-zu-Mund-Beatmung*. Düsseldorf: Michael Triltsch
    Verlag, 1967.

(19) Brandt L, Goerig M, Pokar H. Die ersten Notfallkoffer. *Anaesthesist* 1984; **33**: 487.

19.3   The development of organized emergency
                                              medicine in the 18th century

L. BRANDT, M. EL GINDI, D. DUDA and S. ELLMAUER
Johannes Gutenberg University, Mainz, Federal Republic of Germany

---

The dream of snatching a fellow man away from death by appropriate measures is
probably as old as mankind. In the Old Testament we already find some hints of

resuscitation efforts from sudden death (see Second Book of Kings, chapter IV; the story of Eliza).

Ancient knowledge and early inhibitions

There are very few accounts in early literature of the treatment of the so called apparently dead. Hippocrates (460–377 BC) in his *Aphorisms* describes the resuscitation of persons being hanged, and so does Galenus (129–? AD) in his work. Furthermore, he notes some other reasons for sudden death like sunstroke or death by freezing (1). Some remarks concerning the treatment of sudden death can be found in the writing *Tetrabiblon* by *Aetius of Amida* (6th century) and in the edition *De Re Medica* by *Paulus of Aegina* (7th century).

Only many centuries later were these ideas put into practice. There were several reasons. The religious people of the Middle Ages considered death, whatever its cause, as God's will. Therefore, to attempt resuscitation was considered as a protest against God's will (2). Another important reason was the existing law in the Middle Ages. If someone was found dead, the first question to be answered was not 'Is he really dead?', but was it 'Is he the victim of a murderer, is it a suicide, or did he just happen to have an accident?' It was prohibited by law to touch any corpse before a court officer had inspected it. In a declaration of the City of Amsterdam of the year 1526 no physician or pharmacist was allowed to take care of even a wound or bruise before the court officer had been informed about the accident (3). It is, therefore, not surprising that the idea of resuscitation casualties did not develop in the Middle Ages. Resuscitation at that time was an act of unchristianness and lawlessness.

The Age of Enlightenment

This attitude did not change until the 18th century. The Age of Enlightenment created new standards about the value of individual human life and its importance for the community (see also preface in Alexander Johnson's *A collection of authentic cases proving the practicability of recovering persons visibly dead by drowning, suffocation, stifling, swooning, convulsion and other accidents*; 1773). This new appreciation of life formed the basis for the development of resuscitation medicine.

In earlier centuries, men had discovered the cause of sudden death by postmortem examinations and animal experiments and these now awaited the practical applications of this knowledge (4). In those days drowning was the most frequent accident to occur, and early attempts at resuscitation were made on drowned persons. So it can easily be understood why the roots of modern emergency medicine can be traced back to countries on the seaside or with many inland waterways.

The 'Avis' of Louis XV of France and its influence

The dawn of modern emergency medicine was in the year 1740 when the French king Louis XV (1710–1774) gave his *Avis, concerant les personnes noyées, qui paraissent mortes et qui, ne l'etant pas, peuvent recevoir des secours pour étre rappelées à la vie*; a translation of which gives the general sense as follows: *A report of how to come to the help of those who are drowned* (5).

In this report the old methods of resuscitation are summed up critically and several new methods are considered, such as rewarming of the cold body, moving of the body, instillation of stimulating liquors into the mouth, irrigation of the nasal mucosa, insufflation of warm air into the mouth or into the anal orifice, and insufflation of tobacco smoke into the anal orifice. The method of anal application of tobacco smoke ('*fumigation*') was regarded as the most efficient method of all (6).

The author of the report was none other than *René Antoine Ferchault de Réaumur* (1683–1757), the inventor of one of the three classical temperature systems. Réaumur referred to experiences made in Switzerland with resuscitation of drowned persons several years before.

In fact, previously, in November, 1733, an anonymous another who wrote under the pen name 'Philantrope' had published measures and aids for the recovery from drowning in the monthly periodical *Mercure Suisse.*

The *'Avis'* of Louis XV was rapidly widely distributed. Two years after its publication the first German translation appeared with the title *Die Kunst Ertrunkene wieder zu erwecken, oder ein erneuerter und erläuterter Abdruck des im Elsaß herausgegebenen öffentlichen Berichts, wie denjenigen Personen, welche im Wasser verunglückt, und für kurze Zeit vertrunken, hülfliche Hand zu leisten sey; und auf was Art man sich bemühen müsse, solche wiederum zu ermuntern.* Again the translater used a pen name, 'Academicus curiosus'. This booklet is of greatest interest, as it advocated, in addition to the recommendations in the 'Avis', mouth-to-mouth resuscitation.

At about the same time John Fothergill (1712–1780), in London, also favoured this method with the words:

> *'It is . . . practicable by every one . . . without Loss of Time . . . without Expence, with little Trouble, and less Skill . . . perhaps, the only Expedient of which it can be justly said, that it may possibly do great Good, but cannot do Harm.'* (7)

Within a few decades the idea of resuscitation of casualties spread all over Europe. Already in 1760 a primer, translated into German and entitled *'Herrn Isnards heilsamer Unterricht wie man Ertrunkenen auf die leichteste und sicherste Art wieder zum Leben verhelfen könne'*, had been written in France (5). Nevertheless the idea of resuscitation might have fallen into oblivion in the 18th century had not a dreadful fear appeared in all social classes, namely the horror of being buried alive (5). This persisted up until the end of the 19th century and was the second compelling reason for the improvement of resuscitation and the methods of ultimately declaring a person dead.

The Amsterdam Society

The final support for bringing the idea of resuscitation to fruition in 1776, was the foundation of the *Maatschappij tot Redding van Drenkelingen* by 10 honourable citizens of Amsterdam (3). This assembly became the first Society to declare the resuscitation of apparently dead persons as their main goal. On 16 December, 1767, a proclamation was issued in all Dutch provinces. It met with a lively response. Within the first 14 months following its foundation the Society got reports of 19 successful resuscitations in Holland alone. At the end of the second year 44 cases were recorded and, on the occasion of its twenty-fifth anniversary, the Society was able to look back on no less than 990 reports of recovery from apparent death (3).

The Society became well known outside Holland. In 1768, similar associations were founded in Venice and Milan (8). In Hamburg, the first attempts to resuscitate drowned persons occurred in 1762 and the formation of a society followed in 1769 (9). Other organizations were founded in 1769 in Vienna, in 1772 in Paris, and in 1774 in St. Petersburg and London.

The Royal Humane Society

In London, in 1773, Dr Alexander Johnson (1716–1799), a practising physician, published a paper entitled *A short account of a society at Amsterdam, instituted in the year 1767, for the recovery of drowned persons; with observations shewing (!) the utility and advantage that would accrue to Great Britain by damps in mines, choaking, etc.* In the same year the Amsterdam proclamation was translated into English by Dr Thomas Cogan (1736–1818).

These two publications might have given Dr William Hawes (1736–1806) reason for inviting 32 colleagues and friends to a meeting at the *Chapter Coffee House, St Paul's Churchyard, London,* on 18 April, 1774. Dr Cogan also participated in this meeting. Together they established *The Institution for affording immediate relief to persons apparently dead from drowning.* Soon after its foundation the society was renamed in *The Society for the recovery of persons apparently drowned*, later changed to *The Humane Society* (1776), and *The Royal Humane Society* (1787) (8). Within a few years *The Royal Humane Society* became the leading international institution for resuscitation. Taking over the methods of the Amsterdam Society, it soon developed new strategies as well as new instruments for resuscitation (10) and made them acceptable all over the world (8).

Conclusion

So at the end of the 18th century resuscitation organizations were established in nearly every European country and in most colonies. A wide exchange of ideas took place between different organizations. This can be seen in the number of books that were translated into nearly all European languages. It is no exaggeration to say that the resuscitation societies in the second half of the 18th century, with their organization and their knowledge, laid the basis of modern emergency medicine.

References

(1) Eysselsteijn G van. *Die Methoden der künstlichen Atmung*. Berlin: Julius Springer, 1912.

(2) Bartels I. *Die Geschichte der Mund-zu-Mund-Beatmung*. Düsseldorf: Michael Triltsch, 1967.

(3) Mijnlieff CJ. *Die 'Maatschappij tot redding van Drenkelingen' in Amsterdam und ihre histirosche Bedeutung für die Entwicklung des Rettungswesens*. Janus 1909; **14**: 876–89.

(4) Brandt L, Goerig M. The history of tracheotomy. Part III. *Anaesthesist* 1986; **35**: 455–64.

(5) Isnard. *Herrn Isnards heilsamer Unterricht wie man Ertrunkenen auf die leichteste und sicherste Art wieder zum Leben verhelfen könne*. Straßburg: Joh. Gottfried Bauer, 1760.

(6) Brandt L, Pokar H, Schütte H. Notfallmedizin vor 200 Jahren. *Anaesthesist* 1983; **32** (suppl): 390.

(7) Fothergill J. Observations on a case of recovering a man dead in appearance, by distending the lungs with air. *Phil Trans* 1744–45; **43**: 275–80.

(8) Bishop PJ. *A short history of the Royal Humane Society*. London: The Royal Humane Society, 1974.

(9) Günther JA. *Geschichte und Einrichtung der Hamburgischen Rettungs-Anstalten für im Wasser verunglückte Menschen*. Hamburg: Herold'sche Buchhandlung, 1828.

(10) Brandt L, El Gindi M, Duda D, Ellmauer S. The first instruments for resuscitation. Paper 19.2 Roy Soc of Med Int Congr Symp Series No 134, London: Royal Society of Medicine, 1988.

Chapter 20
ARTIFICIAL VENTILATION

20.1	George Edward Fell and the development of respiratory machines

M. GOERIG, K. FILOS and K. W. AYISI
University Hospital, Hamburg, Federal German Republic

'The physician must know, what the physicians knew before him, lest he deceives himself and others.'

Hippocrates

Tracing back the history of 'modern emergency measures' and life supporting technical devices, it is clear that a history of respiratory apparatus must be reviewed (1,2).

With the beginning of the second half of the 18th-century it became more and more apparent that the success of resuscitation of human life depended on efficient artificial ventilation. The value of artificial ventilation in preserving and reviving life had been demonstrated centuries earlier. It is said, that Andreas Vesalius was the first to perform experiments with animals, which were kept alive by blowing the lungs via a tracheostome with bellows. Similar experiments were made later by well-known physicians, always demonstrating the utility of such procedures (3,4).

In 1767, concerned physicians and laymen in Amsterdam founded the Dutch Humane Society, whose aim was to study carefully different techniques of resuscitation (5). The published recommendations for these emergency situations again emphasized the importance of artificial respiration. The society gave a great impetus for further developments in the management of life-threatening situations all over Europe (5,6).

The use of bellows

The successful use of bellows for overcoming acute respiratory distress was not unusual during that epoch (3). Double bellows with a tracheotomy cannula were widely used and the advantageous effects emphasized in several publications (1,2,3,4). Widespread use was common via the laryngeal or nasotracheal route with tubes made of leather (3,4,5). If necessary and desirable, pure oxygen was administered (4). Its positive value having been discovered. This practice survived until the well-known French physiologist J. Leroy condemned the use of bellows for artificial respiration in the French Academy of Sciences in 1827 (7,8). He found that it was possible to kill animals by overvigorous ventilation producing emphysema and pneumothorax. Greatly discredited as a result of his great influence, intubations became rare and were largely abandoned. The use of bellows disappeared from the list of methods generally accepted and recommended even though Leroy, himself, had constructed and introduced a special 'safety-bellows-set' (6).

Chest compression methods

As a consequence, the various techniques of compressing and expanding the chest were introduced (8). Prone positions ensure a free airway, as the tongue and epiglottis fall forward. Intubation was therefore considered unnecessary to guarantee a free airway. The methods of Hall, Silvester and Howard became more and more accepted and were widely practised. Some of these techniques were officially recommended as the emergency measures of choice until 1958 (4–11) when expired air resuscitation was once again introduced.

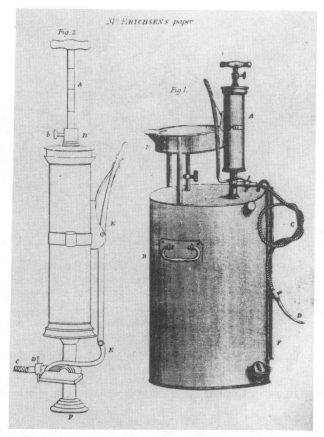

Figure 1   Erichsen's Pump for resuscitation (1845) (13).

George Edward Fell

In 1887, the Canadian-born physician George Fell published an article in the *Buffalo Medical and Surgical Journal*, entitled 'Forced Respiration In Opium Poisoning—It's Possibilities, And The Apparatus Best Adapted To Produce It' (12). Nearly half a century after Leroy's statement of discouragement, the advantageous and simple method of using bellows for performing adequate positive pressure ventilation was rediscovered.*

George Edward Fell was born in Chippova, Ontario, Canada on 12 July, 1849. In 1865, he started studying civil engineering at Buffalo, New York. For several years he was an assistant engineer. Later he took up the study of medicine and graduated at the University of Buffalo in 1882 (15,16).

Fell gave an exact description of his apparatus and described the essential conditions for its use (Fig. 2) (12). Some recommendations for its use were proposed and possible further improvements were suggested. He emphasized, that the air should pass 'through water, heated with a spirit lamp and medicated, and if desired, be treated with a suitable stimulant'.

---

*In the meantime, the only advocate of this form of ventilation had been the surgeon John E. Erichsen of London (13), who, in 1847, had designed an apparatus for this purpose. By means of his device the lungs could be inflated by a pump via a pipe in the nostril. Erichsen considered the optimum rate to be ten times a minute (Fig. 1). Unfortunately, in spite of Erichsen's excellent results in laboratory tests further research in this direction failed (8,13).

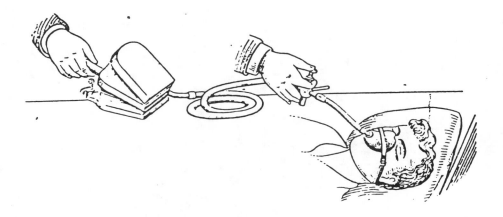

Figure 2   The original Fell-apparatus for artificial respiration (1889) (33).

To minimize negative effects to the lung tissue, he advocated the administration of 'warmed air, supplied with a thermometer to gauge the temperature of the water or air'. The administration of pure oxygen was thought to be superfluous, because:

> 'we have the reduced hemoglobin, calling for oxygen and ready to grasp it in whatever form it is offered and the supply of pure oxygen would on this account, appear superfluous, and unnecessarily complicate the apparatus.'

To facilitate the cumbersome handling by the hand or foot power of the bellows, Fell suggested an electric motor power to keep the apparatus running.

Ventilatory support in the treatment of inadequate respiration became reality. Moreover, this simple device could be kept in constant operation in some cases of respiratory failure for more

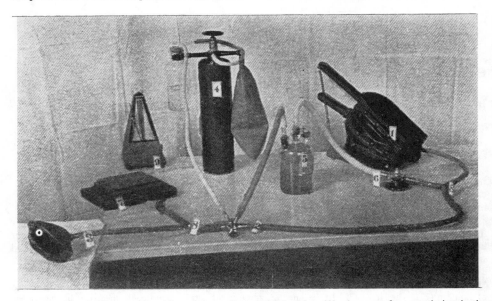

Figure 3   The Fell-apparatus with oxygen and anaesthetic tubes (1), air cup or face mask, intubation tube (3), oxygen supply apparatus (4), anaesthetic container (5), rubber manometer (7), 'Maezel' metronome (9). (ca 1900) (18).

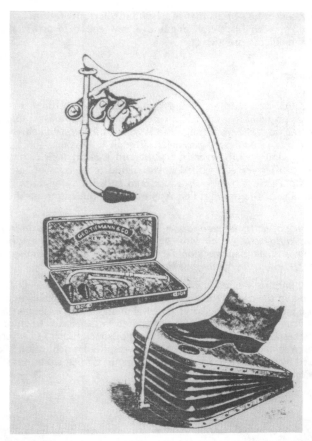

Figure 4   The Fell–O'Dwyer-apparatus for artificial respiration (1893) (20).

than sixty hours (Fig. 3). It is no exaggeration, to say that George Fell was the pioneer of long-term ventilatory assistance. In several articles dealing with problems of artificial respiration (named by him 'forced respiration' to distinguish his method from other methods of artificial respiration then in use) published some years later, he pointed out some of the difficulties he had had in gaining acceptance for his technique (16,17,18). He especially mentions 'some of Pittsburgh's ultracon-servative physicians'. During an international congress in Washington, he had great difficulties in reading his paper, in which the problems of artificial forced ventilation were discussed:

> 'The most peculiar feature of the whole circumstance was, that, even among a class of men supposed to possess the highest medical knowledge, not any of them saw the point which presented in that first case of forced respiration, in which I breathed for a man two and a half one hours with a tube in his neck. They did not grasp that point. And I now make the statement, without fear of contradiction, that there was not a paper presented at the International Congress at Washington which had a farther reaching import if to save human life is desirable than that little paper on 'Opium Poisoning', which I presented—a paper embodying in it demonstrations which would alter and advance one of the greatest medical practices of the day, a practice of wide application. It demonstrated what was before not practically accepted in medicine, that we could force air into the lungs for an almost unlimited period without danger to the delicate lung tissue . . . When I managed, however, to read my paper at Washington they did me the kindness (?) not to publish it in the proceedings . . . It was evident, that my paper either was not carefully read, or the principal point conveyed by it was not grasped by the members of the committee.' (16)

Fortunately within a few weeks of his first successful use in resuscitation, other cases followed quickly. Undisputedly, with his simple method a new epoch in artificial respiration was established in daily medicine practice (17).

Joseph O'Dwyer

In emergency cases Fell first used an air mask, until the tracheostomy was performed. The masks were made of tin or hard rubber. The inefficiency of the masks, and the well-known problem of a poor airway when the tongue falls back and the stomach is blown up by the air, were overcome by the American physician, Joseph O'Dwyer.

A few months previously, O'Dwyer had published a short article, entitled 'Intubation of the Larynx' (19). O'Dwyer was skilled in the digital techniques of insertion of tracheal tubes in cases of diphtheric airway obstruction and substituted his laryngeal tubes for the tracheostomy cannulae of the original Fell-Apparatus. Commenting on the Fell-Apparatus, O'Dwyer said:

> '*In performance of artificial respiration by any means, it is important to remember, that all we have to do, is to get air into the lungs and give it sufficient room and time to escape; the power generated and stored up in overcoming the resistance to inspiration being amply sufficient to carry an exspiration*'. (20)

The value of the apparatus was described by W. P. Northrup as Fell–O'Dwyer Apparatus (21) (Fig. 4). Success in the use of the apparatus demonstrated its efficiency for maintaining artificial respiration and the advantage over postural methods. In consequence, the indications for its use besides drug overdose were cases of respiratory arrest due to chloroform, ether or nitrous-oxide anaesthesia, cases of drowning and cases of shock. Later O'Dwyer called attention to another situation well known to every anaesthetist—respiratory depression in cases of cerebral compression, caused by cerebral haemorrhage or a tumour. Similar situations in cases of violent or sudden contusion were also mentioned by Fell:

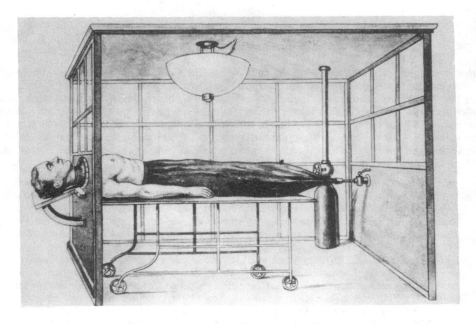

Figure 5   The negative pressure box for open chest surgery of Sauerbruch (1904) (25).

'I believe that in many cases of brain surgery all together . . . attention is given to support by artificial respiration, and now that forced respiration can be carried out in these cases another important field in which to use it is opened up. Did we not have frequent evidence of recovery from shock, I would not suggest the possibility of keeping up or saving human life in such cases by forced respiration.' (18)

Thoracic surgery

Further developments enabled the extension of surgery and the beginning of thoracic surgery. The problem of the occurrence of life-threatening pneumothorax during surgical procedures could be prevented and treated with great efficiency. These circumstances were recognized first by Rudolf Matas, who later modified the apparatus (22). By his technical device, artificial respiration and the maintenance of anaesthesia became a reality (22,23). Within a few months, the modified apparatus was used with success for thoracotomies. It became a central feature in the discussion of how the problem of pneumothorax should be best solved. The alternative to positive pressure ventilation being the cumbersome techniques of differential pressure (2,23) (Fig. 5).

The acceptance of endobronchial intubation was long delayed because the surgeons failed to learn the technique of intubation, even though the German Kirstein had advocated the use of a laryngoscope as an aid in 1895 (24). Not skilled with this method, prominent chest-surgeons at the turn of the 20th century preferred to go another, more complicated way (Fig. 5). Under the great influence of Sauerbruch and due to his forceful advocacy of the 'differential pressure technique', forced respiration was condemned (22,23,24,25,26). If necessary, artificial respiration was carried out by chest compression methods such as those of Hall or Silvester and these were still recommended in the nineteen fifties. In cases of acute poliomylitis with respiratory failure, it was not unusual to perform the method of thoracic compression for several days (14 days!) without having performed a tracheostomy (27). To facilitate this cumbersome

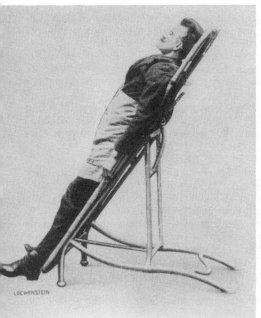
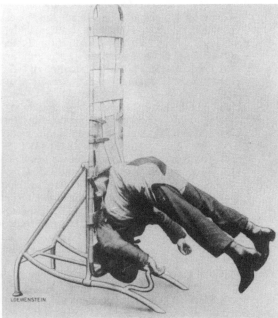

Figure 6   Artificial respiration—the apparatus of Lewin (1912) (28).

technique, the development of machines supporting the respiration by means of changing the patient's position was (Fig. 6a and b). From today's point of view, this development is hard to understand.

It seems that the evolution of respiratory machines was hampered for many years by these diametric opposing points of view. Tracing back the different efforts to develop respiratory support machines, a variety of mechanical devices were designed. Among these, highly sophisticated modern concepts have to be mentioned. One pathway led to the development of respirators closely reproducing spontaneous respiration by negative pressure created around the thorax. The first such device was described by Lewins of Leith in 1840. In 1875, a similar machine—the 'spirophore'—was produced by Woillez and used in cases of asphyxia. No changes in the principles governing breathing machines in situations of respiratory failure occurred until there was a rediscovery of positive pressure apparatus in the early 1950s (2,5,23) when the epidemics of poliomyelitis caused renewed interest of the forgotten, but well-known physiological principle, comprehensively discussed and warmly recommended years ago by George Fell. It is sad that the most important technical improvements and developments in respiratory machines became a reality long after George Fell had died on 29 July, 1918, in Chicago.

References

(1) Larcan A, Brullard Ph. Histoire des gestes et des techniques de reanimation au XVIII siecle. *Hist Sci Med* 1979; **3**: 11–20.

(2) Price JL. The evolution of breathing machines. *Med Hist* 1962; **6**: 67–72.

(3) Larcan A and Brullard Ph. Histoire des idees et development de la reanimation respiratoire au XVIII siecle. *Hist Sci Med* 1979; **3**: 1–10.

(4) Lee RV. Cardiopulmonary resuscitation in the 18th century. *Hist Med* 1972; **XXVII**: 418–33.

(5) Mijnlieff CJ. Die Maatschappij Tot Redding Van Drenkelingen In Amsterdam. *Janus* 1909; Harlem: 876–89.

(6) Bartels I. *Die Geschichte der Mund-zu-Beatmung. Düsseldorf: Universität Düsseldorf*, 1965. Dissertation.

(7) Leroy J. Second memoire sur l'asphxie. *J Physiologie Exp Pathologique* 1828; **VIII**.

(8) Keith A. Three Hunterian lectures on the mechanism underlying the various methods of artificial respiration. *Lancet* 1909; i: 745–9, 825–8, 895–9.

(9) Hall M. On a new mode of effecting artificial respiration. *Lancet* 1856; i: 229.

(10) Silvester HR. The natural method of treating asphyxia. *Med Times Gaz* 1857; **15**: 485–6.

(11) Howard B. *Plain rules for restoration of persons apparently dead from drowning*. New York, 1869.

(12) Fell GE. Forced respiration in opium poisoning—its possibilities, and the apparatus best adapted to produce it. *Buffalo Med Surg J* 1887; **XXVIII** (4): 146–57.

(13) Erichsen JE. An experimental inquiry into the pathology and treatment of asphyxia. *Edin Med Surg J* 1845; **63**: 1–59.

(14) Anonymous. Dr George Edward Fell. *Buffalo Med J* 1918; **74** (2): 73–4.

(15) Hodward JS. *Men of medicine in Erie County 1821–1971*. County of Erie, Buffalo, New York: Buffalo Medical Society, 1971: 92.

(16) Fell GE. Forced respiration. *JAMA* 1891; **16**: 325–30.

(17) Fell GE. The value of forced artificial respiration (Fell-Method) in saving human life in chloroform, ether and nitrous oxide narcosis, together with an account of a remarkable case in which it was used for four days and three nights upon a physician, resulting in saving his life. *Med Record* 1896; Philadelphia, Pa, May: 760–3.

(18) Fell GE. Artificial respiration. *Surg Gynecol Obstet* 1910; **10**: 572–82.

(19) O'Dwyer J. Intubation of the larynx. *NY Med J* 1885; **8**: 145–7.

(20) Matas R. On the management of acute traumatic pneumothorax. *Ann Surg* 1899; **29**: 409–34.

(21) Northrup WP. Apparatus for prolonged artificial forcible respiration. *Br Med J* 1894; ii: 697–8.

(22) Matas R. Intralaryngeal insufflation for the relief of acute surgical pneumothorax. Its history and methods with a description of the latest devices for this purpose. *JAMA* 1900; **34** (22): 1371–5, 1468–73.

(23) Rendell-Baker L. History of thoracic anaesthesia. In: Mushin WW, Rendell-Baker L, eds. *The principles of thoracic anaesthesia past and present*. Oxford: Blackwell Scientific Publications, 1953; 598–66. Larcan A, Brullard Ph. Histoire des idées et development de la réanimation réspiratoire au XVIIIieme siecle. *Hist Sci Med* 1979; **3**: 1–10.

(24) Hirsch NP, Smith GB, Hirsch PO. Alfred Kirstein. *Anaesthesia* 1986; **41**: 42–5.

(25) Sauerbruch F. Zur Pathologie des offenen Pneumothorax und die Grundlage meines Verfahrens zu seiner Auschaltung. *Mitt Grenzgeb Med Chir* 1904; **13**: 399–482.

(26) Sauerbruch F. Chirurgie des Brustfells. In: Angerer Ov, Bruns Pv, Freiherrn v Eisselsberg *et al.*. *Chirurgie des Halses und der Brust*. Stuttgart: Verlag von Ferdinand Enke, 1913: 766.

20.2

The development of apparatus for intermittent negative pressure ventilation

CHRISTOPHER H. M. WOOLLAM
Norfolk and Norwich Hospital, Norwich, UK

Artificial ventilation by the application of positive pressure to the airway is as old as the history of medicine. The idea of producing ventilation by the external application of positive or negative pressure has a much shorter history. It started in the early part of the last century, reached a zenith in the 1940s and '50s and was replaced by the introduction of intermittent positive pressure ventilation.

The original use of artificial ventilation was in resuscitation. It was only later that the idea was used for the treatment of chronic respiratory problems. It was not until the development of reliable electrical motors that prolonged ventilation became a possibility.

Early apparatus

Dalziel

It was a Scottish physician by the name of John Dalziel (1) of Drumlanrig who first had the idea of applying an external negative pressure to the body to produce ventilation. Dalziel's work appeared in an essay published in 1832 in the *Journal of the British Association for the Advancement of Science*. It had occurred to him that in cases of respiratory depression or failure the patient might gain relief from the application of a rhythmical subatmospheric pressure applied to the body.

He designed and constructed an air-tight box in which the patient was placed in a sitting position with the head and neck outside. The negative pressure was created by a pair of bellows inside the box. These were worked from the outside by a piston rod and one-way valve. Two convex windows were let into the side of the box so that the patient's chest movements could be observed.

There is only one account of the equipment being used. In a letter to the Editor of the *Edinburgh Medical and Surgical Journal* in 1840 (2) a Dr Lewins of Leith writes of an unsuccessful attempt to resuscitate a drowned man. The device worked so well that bystanders thought that resuscitation had been successful.

Alfred E. Jones

Where Great Britain leads the USA is never far behind. Thirty-two years after Dalziel, Alfred F. Jones of Lexington, Kentucky, patented the first American 'Iron Lung' (3). Jones made great claims for it; he stated that it had cured cases of paralysis, neuralgia, rheumatism, seminal weakness, bronchitis, dyspepsia and many other diseases including deafness! Its construction must have been very similar to Dr Dalziel's with a large syringe to create the negative pressure.

Hauke

The first cuirass was developed by the Austrian Ignez Hauke (4). He received his medical education at the Vienna Medical School where he was a pupil of Skoda and Oppolzer. He graduated Bachelor of Medicine in 1858. His first appointment was to St Anne's Hospital and he later held a post at the Crown Prince Joseph's Children's Hospital.

Hauke described and used two types of cuirass or 'Pneumatischer Panzer'. His description of the apparatus and its use in disease is rather vague. Most of the information about his work comes from the writings of Waldenburg (5). Waldenburg was Professor at The Friedrich-Wilhelms-Universitat, Berlin. Prior to the introduction of his cuirass Hauke and Waldenburg had been using positive pressure applied to the mouth via a face mask. Treatment seems to have been for periods of fifteen minutes at a time. It was used on cases of atelectasis, pneumonia and emphysema. Hauke though that negative pressure applied to the outside of the thorax might have the same effect.

The first cuirass was made of cane covered with an impermeable material. It surrounded the entire thorax and was used to apply a constant negative pressure. Hauke then realized that if he applied intermittent negative pressure in phase with inspiration he could assist ventilation in cases of respiratory failure. He constructed a second cuirass shell of sheet iron with the same air-filled rubber edge for this purpose. This shell covered the anterior part of the thorax.

He found the cuirass unsuitable for children and adults in an agitated state. To overcome this problem, he developed his tank respirator to cover the patient's whole body. The head and neck were enclosed in an elastic cap with the face left uncovered. The cap was sealed to the tank edge with adhesive tape and negative pressure was provided by a hand operated apparatus—the same apparatus that had been used to provide positive pressure by a face mask and as a spirometer.

Hauke tried the tank on nearly every type of respiratory disease, neonatal asphyxia, atelectasis, catarrhal pneumonia, tracheitis, croup and diphtheria. In diphtheria he combined treatment in his tank with the inhalation of hot dry air. He was very much against humidification and thought that it worsened the condition. Treatment seems to have been for two to three hours at a time.

Woillez

Twenty years before Hauke published his description of his tank, a young French physician Joseph Woillez working at Clermont-sur-Oise was intrigued by the sounds that Lannec described on auscultation of the chest. He sealed cadaver lungs in a metal vessel with the trachea open to the atmosphere. The vessel was attached to a bellows to evacuate the air from inside, and an endoscope was sealed into the wall to allow observation of the lungs. Despite great difficulties in obtaining an air-tight seal, Woillez managed to get the lungs to expand and contract. This led him to two fundamental conclusions. First, that, in life, air enters the lungs at a pressure not greater than atmospheric but in artificial positive pressure respiration the pressures were much higher, and, second, that the primary reason for the entry of air into the lungs is not the pressure of the air but the expansion of the thoracic cavity by the respiratory muscles.

Woillez moved to the Lariboisière Hospital in Paris in 1875 and with the aid of the famous instrument maker, M. Collin, he developed his apparatus. He called it the 'Spiroscope'. This device was followed a year later by his 'Spirophore' (6,7,8), an apparatus for ventilating the whole body. The first one was a metal cylinder surrounding the body of the patient. The cylinder was closed at one end and the other end was covered with a rubber diaphragm seal which fitted closely around the patients neck. Air was evacuated from the cylinder by means of a separate bellows with a capacity of one litre. In later models the bellows was incorporated in the cylinder. The patient's chest movements could be observed through a glass porthole and measured with a glass rod resting on the sternum and passing through the spirophore in a separate tube.

Woillez may not have known about Hauke's tank but Hauke certainly knew about Woillez. Hauke published a pamphlet in which he accused Woillez of not giving due recognition to his work (9).

The existence of the spirophore was known in this country, it is mentioned in an article in the *Lancet* published in September 1876 (10).

Bell

The problems of artificial respiration did not only concern the medical profession. Alexander Graham Bell (1847–1922), the inventor of the telephone, like all great inventors covered a wide field of subjects, including artificial respiration. This interest may have been stimulated by the death of his only son when only one-day-old on 15 August, 1851 (11).

Arthur W. McCurdy recorded conversations with Bell for the *Beinn Bhreagh Recorder* (12). In the journal of 14 August, 1910, there is an article relating one of these conversations with Bell held on 3 August, 1891.

> '*Many children, especially the premature born, die from inability to expand their lungs sufficiently when they take their first breath. There is no doubt that in many of those cases, lives could be saved by starting the respiration artificially by means of an apparatus operating in the manner described above.*'

Bell described the movement of air in normal respiration and the problems of assisted inspiration rather than expiration in artificial respiration. He goes on to describe a vacuum jacket that he invented while on a visit to England in 1882; he lent it to 'some gentleman connected with University College in London'. This man promised to experiment with the jacket, then return it to Bell—this he did not do. McCurdy recovered the jacket from Professor Yeo at King's College and it can be seen today at the 'Alexander Graham Bell Park' in Baddech, Nova Scotia. The jacket is a ridged shell in two halves with a soft lining, which is strapped around the chest. A bellows provide the negative pressure. Before Bell lent his jacket to Professor Yeo he tried it out on several drowned cats with success. He produced these results at a meeting of the 'Advancement of Science' in Montreal in the 1880s but met with very little response.

Braun

The problem of neonatal asphyxia also troubled a Dr Egon Braun of Vienna (13). He designed a wooden box with a slanting top. The box was airtight apart from an opening in the lid partially closed by a rubber diaphragm. The child was placed in the box supported by a plaster mould. The head was thrown back to bring the mouth and nose against the opening in the diaphragm. A long flexible tube was inserted into the front of the box to pump air from it. Once the child had been placed in the box, air was first blown in to it and then drawn out by sucking the tube, thus expanding the chest. Braun claimed that he had used the box successfully in more than fifty cases.

The treatment of poliomyelitis 1918–1952

Steuart

The main cause of fatal respiratory failure in children and young adults in the first part of this century was poliomyelitis. The first man to attempt to treat the respiratory failure of poliomyelitis was a South African, Dr W. Steuart (14). There was a particularly severe epidemic of poliomyelitis in South Africa in 1918 but, unfortunately, Dr Steuart had not perfected his apparatus until the outbreak was nearly over and it was ready for use only six hours after the last victim died. So, when Dr Steuart presented it at a meeting of the South African Medical Association in March 1918, no clinical trial had been done.

The principle of Steuart's apparatus was a ridged airtight box in which the child's thorax and abdomen were placed. A large bellows driven by an electric motor provided intermittent negative pressure. The child lay on a mattress in the box and the space between the child's shoulder girdle, pelvis and the box would be sealed with plaster of Paris or other suitable material, possibly plasticine or paraffin wax. The top of the box could be removed quickly in case of an emergency and was fitted with a glass panel so that the patient's chest movement could be observed. The tidal and minute volume were adjusted by moving the belt on the motor pulleys. This altered the stroke length and the rate of the bellows. The negative pressure produced could be varied by two valves in the side of the box. Unfortunately, there is no record indicating that Dr Steuart tried out his device in the next poliomyelitis epidemic but it was an important step because it was the first attempt to produce long-term artificial ventilation.

Eisenmenger

Back in Europe at the turn of the century, Dr Rudolf Eisenmenger of Piski in Hungary was developing his cuirass ventilator. A mechanical version was patented in 1927. His cuirass shell fitted from the upper part of the sternum nearly down to the pubic region. It was attached to a pair of foot-operated bellows by a flexible hose. The bellows applied alternating positive and negative pressures to the outer chest and abdomen. The device was known as 'Dr Eisenmenger's Biomotor'.

The power units of both cuirass and tank respirators were to develop into two distinct types— either a motor driven bellows or a fan vacuum-cleaner type motor. The Biomotor was powered by a half horse-power fan motor. The cuirass shell of the Biomotor had a soft sheet rubber lining. This lining was pushed into the abdomen during expiration by positive pressure. Articles on the 'Biomotor's use in various respiratory problems, particularly poliomyelitis, started to appear from 1935 onwards (15–23).

Drinker, McKhann and Shaw

Two articles (24,25) in 1928 announced the results of several years work at the Department of Ventilation, Illumination and Physiology of Harvard Medical School. An engineer, Philip Drinker, a paediatrician, Charles F. McKhann and a physiologist Louis A. Shaw had combined to develop the first really practical American Tank Respirator. The original idea had come from Drinker's ventilator for laboratory animal experiments.

The first tank was a sheet metal cylinder sealed at one end. The other end had a flat lid to which was attached a rubber collar. The patient's head and neck protruded through the collar and rested on an adjustable support attached to the outside of the tank. Inside the tank was a mattress-covered frame. This ran on rails welded into the side of the tank. An airtight seal between the cylinder and lid was achieved with commercial refrigerator locks. The sides of the cylinder had boat-type portholes for observing the patients. There were numerous other small sealed holes for manometers, blood pressure cuffs, stethoscopes etc. The original pumps were commercial products made by the Electric Blower Company in Boston. These ran continuously, and positive and negative pressures were fed to the tanks via a system of valves.

The pressure was measured by a simple water manometer and adjusted by a variable leak on the top of the tank.

The original respirator was to undergo many design changes in the next twenty-five years and many new versions were produced, e.g. Drinker Collins, Emerson Henderson and the Both. Later models were fitted with more efficient bellows-type power units.

Drinker demonstrated his respirator in the United Kingdom in 1931 (26). Siebe Gorman started manufacture of Drinker respirators in the UK in 1934. Their main use was in poliomyelitis. There were several outbreaks of the disease in this country in 1938. Ventilators were in very short supply, the only apparatus available apart from the Drinker was the Bragg–Paul Pulsator (27,28).

The Bragg-Paul Pulsator

The invention of this device was another example of a non-medical man setting his mind to and solving a medical problem. Sir William Bragg, the Nobel Prize winning physicist, had a friend with progressive muscular dystrophy. Sir William produced a pneumatic belt made from rubber football bladders which was strapped around the abdomen and lower thorax. A small air pump inflated the bladders, compressing the abdomen and thorax. Sir William enlisted the help of Robert W. Paul who improved the belt by making it of hollow rubber tubes. The belt was used successfully in many cases though unfortunately there were problems with the rubber perishing. The Admiralty bought up all available belts at the beginning of the last war for use at sea.

Both negative pressure respirators in the United Kingdom

Following the poliomyelitis epidemic of 1938 it was obvious that this country was inadequately supplied with respirators. A Medical Research Council Committee was set up to examine all respiratory assisters available, to select the best, and to decide how they should be purchased and distributed (29).

The Committee was due to meet when Lord Nuffield came to the rescue. He offered to manufacture the Both respirator at his automobile factory in Cowley, Oxford, and supply, free of charge, any hospital in the Empire who requested one. The Both had been originally designed for the South Australian Government. The brief of the Committee was changed into deciding on need and distribution of this generous offer. The conclusions were that the Both respirators were bulky and difficult to store so they should be sited at regional centres and loaned out as required. One of the first centres was the Wingfield Morris Orthopaedic Hospital, Oxford.

Cuirass respirators

Eisenmenger had patented his motor powered cuirass in 1927. No further commercially available cuirass appeared until 1930. Sahlin, working at the Physiological Institute at Lund in Sweden developed a cuirass, manufactured by Messer Stille-Werner of Stockholm. The cuirass shell was made of sheet metal with a rubber edge. It came in three sizes and bolted on to an operating table. The power unit could provide both negative and positive pressure. Flaum (30) cites a case of a 21-year-old medical student with poliomyelitis kept alive for seven months with this cuirass. Bergman (31) reported its use in 827 cases of poliomyelitis in which 127 survived.

There were several epidemics of poliomyelitis in Victoria, Australia, in 1937. At the time of the epidemic, there were only two tank respirators in the State but by the end of the year there were two hundred in operation. Aubrey Burstall, Professor of Engineering at the University of Melbourne produced the 'Burstall Jacket' (32) to provide a smaller and more easily portable respiratory aid for convalescent patients. He first demonstrated the jacket on 27 January, 1938. One week after the demonstration it went into clinical use at the Children's Hospital in Melbourne. This cuirass was made of one piece of aluminium hammered out to the shape of the thorax and abdomen as far as the waist. An inch-thick sponge rubber vest protected the patient from the shell. An airtight seal was achieved with a rubber sheet sleeve and collar. The Drinker power unit was used with the original jacket. The smaller volume required meant that several jackets could be run off one Drinker pump. This was done by drilling holes along the sides of the Drinker and attaching the Jackets by means of flexible hoses. Aubrey Burstall did not claim to have made a complete substitute for the tank but a cheaper more portable apparatus for patients in the more acute stage of the disease. He found its advantages were price, portability, ease of nursing patients in splints in ordinary hospital beds, and ease of sterilizing the unit. The disadvantages were the time needed to get the patients into the jacket (seven minutes ordinarily, and ten to twelve minutes if the patient was in splints), and the problem of getting an air tight fit.

Burstall provided a jacket for Dr Andrew Topping of London County Council (LCC). This gift led to the development of a superior cuirass jacket, the LCC cuirass (33,34). This was made in two halves bolted together with wing nuts. There were minor alterations in the arm holes and in the airtight seal. This made for easier application and more freedom for the patient. It had its own power unit: an eighth of a horse power electric motor driving a small suction bellows at a fixed rate of twenty r.p.m. with a maximum negative pressure 25 cm of water. The negative pressure was controlled by a variable leak valve on the jacket. There was a hand operated mechanism for use if the power unit failed.

Post-war development

World War II brought a halt to the development of both the tank and the cuirass ventilator and it was not until the late 1940s that further new models started to appear. All apparatus for the aid of the physically handicapped developed in the USA has to be approved by their Council of Physical Medicine. In 1947 the Council produced a list of 'standards' for all future American cuirass respirators (35). These standards covered all aspects of the cuirass from its efficiency, size, range, portability, standard of power unit, patient comfort, to the method of advertising. They pointed out that they did not consider it a replacement for the tank respirator.

1948 to 1950 saw several new American cuirasses, Blanchard's Portable Plastic Respirator (36,37), The Chestspirator (38), The Fairchild-Huxley (39), and the Monaghan (40). None of these are manufactured today. The Monaghan was available in this country until the mid-1970s.

Galloway published an article in the *American Medical Journal* in 1943, in which he recommended the use of tracheostomy in cases of bulbar poliomyelitis (41). This led to the routine use of tracheostomy in such cases in the USA. Nursing a patient in a Tank Respirator with a tracheostomy was very difficult. This problem was overcome by the introduction of the sloping front to the Tank (42).

The following year, Plum and his co-workers (43,44) at Cornell University, New York, compared the cuirass directly with the tank in 10 cases of poliomyelitis. Two of these were the acute form. They found that, compared with the cuirass, the tank could produce between 34% and 100% greater tidal volume at equivalent pressures. They also reported the findings of anterior emphysema in the lungs of polio victims dying during artificial ventilation with the cuirass.

Two papers appeared in 1953–4 comparing the cuirass with the tank respirator. In the first, Collins and Affeldt (45) took fourteen adult patients with vital capacities of 250 ml or less and tested them in the thoraco–abdominal cuirass shell and a thoracic cuirass shell. They found that if they took the tank as producing a volume of a 100%, then the thoraco–abdominal cuirass would produce 61–63% and the thoracic only 47%. They also found that with increasing negative pressure, the thoracic shell tended to dig into the upper abdomen and reduce the tidal volume. The following year, Bryce-Smith and Davis (46) compared the tidal volume achieved with the tank, a thoracic cuirass and a rocking bed in six, healthy, anaesthetized curarized patients. They found that the cuirass required much greater negative pressure to produce the same tidal volume as the tank.

Kinnear Wilson *et al.* (47,48) reviewed the availability and the use of the cuirass in Great Britain in the early fifties in two articles. They recommended its use in patients recovering from the acute phase of poliomyelitis and described the Monaghan and Kifa cuirass that had just become available in this country.

An important new power unit made its appearance in Great Britain in 1952—the Smith Clarke pump (49,50). Captain G. T. Smith Clarke was an engineer and had been director of Alvis Motors Ltd. On his retirement from Alvis he became Chairman of the No. 2 Group Hospital Management Committee. Birmingham Board approached him and asked if he would improve the 48 Both Respirators within the Region. He not only designed a vastly better power unit but went on to design a new Tank that overcame many of the disadvantages of the Both. This was called the 'Coventry' or 'Alligator' Tank.

Poliomyelitis in Denmark in 1952

The terrible poliomyelitis epidemic in Denmark in 1952 was to radically alter the treatment of respiratory paralysis. For years anaesthetists had been 'squeezing the bag' during anaesthesia to overcome respiratory depression. Now Lassen (51,52) was to prove that 'Intermitten Positive Pressure' was much the best method of artificial respiration. He described how during a period of nineteen weeks towards the end of 1952, at the Blegdam Hospital in Copenhagen there were two thousand seven hundred and twenty admissions for acute poliomyelitis. Eight hundred and sixty six had the paralytic type. Three hundred and sixteen needed some form of respiratory assistance. At the start of the epidemic the Hospital had one tank and six cuirasses. There was a time during the epidemic when seventy patients had required assistance. After the first month, Dr Lassen consulted his anaesthetic colleague, Dr B. Ibsen (53), and together they developed the technique of high tracheostomy and manual intermittent positive ventilation.

Between 1934 and 1944 the Blegdam Hospital had treated seventy six polio victims in the cuirass, with a mortality of 80%. Even the introduction of tracheostomy for the bulbar paralysis which had been so effective in reducing the mortality in the USA, had no effect on Lassen's figures. The first month of the epidemic produced exactly the same results. As soon as the technique of Intermittent Positive Pressure was started, the mortality dropped to 40%. The results were confirmed during the much smaller outbreak in Stockholm the following year.

Lassen's work really put an end to negative pressure ventilation as a treatment of acute respiratory failure. There have been isolated efforts to overcome the defects of the cuirass; particularly the problem with leaks. Mr E. J. Tunnicliffe (54) produced his Jacket in 1958. The Jacket is made of cotton and nylon mixture. Straps seal it at the arms, neck and across the buttocks. It is held off the chest by a plastic shell. The original power unit was based on a Rootes type air pump. The makers claimed that it more than doubled the tidal volume could be achieved with the same negative pressure when compared with an ordinary cuirass. This was proved by Spalding and Opie when they compared the Jacket, a cuirass and intermittent positive pressure respiration in cases of old paralytic polio and myasthenia gravis (54).

A triggered cuirass for the treatment of acute on chronic respiratory failure was introduced by Marks *et al.* (55) in 1963. The cuirass used an Emerson wrap round with a trigger operated by minute changes in pressure at the nostril or tracheostomy of the patient. They found the system unsatisfactory due to the problems of getting a good fit and the constant qualified supervision the patients required. In this country Capel (56) tried triggering but abandoned it for similar reasons.

The use of the cuirass today is limited to a few specialized units, where intermittent respiratory support can be provided by a cuirass without the necessity for a tracheostomy.

References

(1) Dalziel J. On sleep and an apparatus for promoting artificial respiration. *Br Assoc Advanc Sci* 1838; **2**: 127.

(2) Lewins R. Apparatus for promoting respiration in cases of suspended animation. *Edin Med Surg J* 1840; **53**: 255.

(3) Emerson JH. Exhibit at the Brussels World's Fair. 1958.

(4) Hauke I. Der Pneumatische Panzer. Beitrag zur 'Mechanischen Behandlung der Brustkrankheiten.' *Wiener Medizinische Presse* 1874; **15**: 785, 836.

(5) Waldenburgh L. *Die pneumatische Behandlung der Respirations und Circulationskrankheiten im Anschluss an die Pneumatometrie und Spirometrie*, Hirschwald: Berlin. 1880; 420.

(6) Leading Article. The Spirophore. *Lancet* 1876; **ii**: 68.

(7) Woillez EJ. Du Spirophore, appareil de sauvetage pour le traitment de l'asphyxie, et principalement de l'asphyxie des noyes et des nouveaunés. *Bull Acad Méd Paris, 2nd Ser* 1876; **5**: 611.

(8) Woillez M. Le Spirophore, invente en 1876. *Bull Acad Méd* 1938; **119**: 82.

(9) Hauke I. *Neue pneumatische Apparate und ihre Anwendung in der Kinderpraxis.* W. Braumüller: Vienna, 1876.

(10) Leading Article. The Spirophore. *Lancet* 1876; **ii**: 436.

(11) Bruce RV. *Alexander Graham Bell and the conquest of solitude.* London: Gollancz, 1973: 347.

(12) Special Article. Dictated notes on artificial respiration by Alexander Graham Bell. *Bein Bhreagh Recorder* 1910; **4**: 190.

(13) Doe OW. Apparatus for resuscitating asphyxiated children. *Boston Med Surg J* 1889; **120**: 9.

(14) Steuart W. Demonstration of apparatus for inducing artificial respiration for long periods. *Med J SA* 1918; **3**: 147.

(15) Hamburger F. Lebensrettung bei poliomyelitischer Atemlähmung durch den Biomotor (Eisenmenger). *Medizinische Klinik* 1935; **35**: 1132.

(16) Hellich I. Kunstliche Atmung mit dem 'Biomotor'. *Münchener Medizinische Wochenschrift* 1935; **82**: 421.

(17) Eisenmenger R. Heart failure and its treatment with the 'Biomotor'. *Wiener Medizinisch Wochenschrift* 1936; **86**: 1129.

(18) Eisenmenger R. Therapeutic application of supra-abdominal suction and compressed air in relation to respiration and circulation. *Wiener Medizinisch Wochenschrift* 1939; **89**: 1032.

(19) Fischer L, Engeser J. Pneumotachographische Untersuchungen bei Künstlicher Atmung. *Die Medizinische Welt* 1938; **47**: 1664.

(20) Eisenmenger R. American iron lung and the German biomotor. *Zeitschrift Färzlt Forbild* 1939; **36**: 654.

(21) Eisenmenger R. Soll bei Pneumonie der Biomotor Angewendet Werden? *Wiener Klinische Wochenschrift* 1940; **15**: 295.

(22) Eisenmenger R. Indications and results of artificial respiration by means of the biomotor. *Therapie der Gegenwart* 1942; **83**: 363.

(23) Fruhmann G. Circulation during biomotor respiration. *Münchener Medizinische Wochenschrift* 1951; **93**: 1849.

(24) Drinker P, Shaw LA. An apparatus for the prolonged administration of artificial respiration. *J Clin Invest* 1929; **7**: 229.

(25) Drinker P, McKhann CF. The use of a new apparatus for the prolonged administration of artificial respiration. *JAMA* 1929; **92**: 1658.

(26) Drinker P. Prolonged administration of artificial respiration. *Lancet* 1931; **i**: 1186.

(27) Paul RW. The Bragg–Paul pulsator. *Proc Roy Soc Med* 1935; **28**: 436.

(28) Bragg W. The Bragg–Paul pulsator. *Br Med J* 1938; **ii**: 254.

(29) Medical Research Council Special Report. *No. 237. Breathing machines and their uses.* London: HMSO, 1938.

(30) Flaum A. Experience in the use of the new respirator (Sahlin type) in the treatment of respiratory paralysis in poliomyelitis. *Acta Med Scand* 1936; (Suppl. 78): 849.

(31) Bergman R. Eight hundred cases of poliomyelitis treated in the Sahlin respirator. *Acta Paediatr Scand* 1948; **36**: 470.

(32) Burstall AF. New type of 'jacket' respirator for the treatment of poliomyelitis. *Br Med J* 1938; **ii**: 611.

(33) Menzies F. Mechanical respirators. *The Medical Officer* 1938; **60**: 231.

(34) Blackwell U. Mechanical respiration. *Lancet* 1949; **ii**: 99.
(35) The Council of Physical Medicine. Tentative requirements for the acceptance of respirators of the cuirass type. *JAMA* 1947; **135**: 715.
(36) The Council of Physical Medicine. Acceptability report on the Blanchard portable plastic respirator. *JAMA* 1949; **137**: 867.
(37) Huddleston OL. Use of the Blanchard mechanotherapist in treating postoperative atelactasis. *Calif Med J* 1947; **66**: 25.
(38) The Council of Physical Medicine. Acceptability report on the Chestpirator portable chest respirator. *JAMA* 1949; **141**: 658.
(39) The Council of Physical Medicine. Acceptability of the Fairchild Huxley cuirass respirator. *JAMA* 1950; **143**: 1157.
(40 The Council of Physical Medicine. The Monaghan Portable Respirator Acceptance Report. *JAMA* 1949; **139**: 1273.
(41) Galloway TC. Tracheostomy in bulbar poliomyelitis. *JAMA* 1943; **123**: 1096.
(42) Peterson RL, Ward RC. Tracheostomy in poliomyelitis simplified by a new respirator. *Arch Otolaryngology* 1948; **48**: 156.
(43) Plum F, Lukas DS. An evaluation of the cuirass respirator in acute poliomyelitis with respiratory insufficiency. *Am J Med Sci* 1951; **221**: 417.
(44) Plum F, Wolff HG. Observations on acute poliomyelitis with respiratory insufficiency. *JAMA* 1951; **146**: 442.
(45) Collier CR, Affeldt. Ventilatory efficiency of the cuirass respirator in totally paralysed chronic poliomyelitis patients. *J Appl Physiol* 1954; **6**: 531.
(46) Bryce-Smith R, Davis HS. Tidal exchange in respirators. *Anaesth Analg; Curr Res* 1954; **33**: 73.
(47) Kelleher WH, Kinnier Wilson AB, Ritchie Russell W, Stott FD. Notes on cuirass respirator. *Br Med J* 1952; **ii**: 413.
(48) Scales JT, Kinnier Wilson AB, Holmes Sellors T, Harwood Stevenson F, Stott FD. Cuirass respirators—their design and construction. *Lancet* 1953; **i**: 671.
(49) Smith RE. Modified Both respirators. *Lancet* 1953; **i**: 674.
(50) Smith-Clarke GT. Mechanical breathing machines. *Proc Inst Mech Eng* 1957; **171**: 52.
(51) Lassen HCA. A preliminary report on the 1952 epidemic of poliomyelitis in Copenhagen. *Lancet* 1953; **i**: 37.
(52) Lassen HCA. The epidemic of poliomyelitis in Copenhagen, 1952. *Proc Roy Soc Med* 1954; **47**: 67.
(53) Ibsen I. The anaesthetist view point on the treatment of respiratory complications in poliomyelitis during the epidemic in Copenhagen, 1952. *Proc Roy Soc Med* 1954; **47**: 72.
(54) Spalding JKM, Opie L. Artificial respiration with the Tunnicliffe breathing jacket. *Lancet* 1958; **i**: 614.
(55) Marks A, Bocles J, Morganti L. A new ventilatory assister for patients with respiratory acidosis. *N Engl J Med* 1963; **268**: 61.
(56) Capel LH. *Personal communication*.

Further reading

(1) Woollam CHM. The development of apparatus for intermittent negative pressure respiration. (1) 1832–1918. *Anaesthesia* 1976; **31**: 537.
(2) Woollam CHM. The development of apparatus for intermittent negative pressure respiration. (2) 1919–1976. *Anaesthesia* 1976; **31**: 666.

20.3   The development of positive pressure ventilators

LESLIE RENDELL-BAKER and JERRY L. PETTIS
Loma Linda University, California, USA

The development of ventilators has passed through many phases. The first phase which started shortly after the turn of this century was characterized by the variety of methods used to solve the problem. Queen Victoria had recently died and had been succeeded by Edward VII. The Edwardian era was a period of fashionable elegance, and optimism combined with social change. The internal combustion engine was rapidly replacing the horse as a power source and everyday inventions were making life easier. The Liberal Prime Minister Mr David Lloyd George would shortly introduce the Health Insurance scheme which for the first time enabled all working persons to enrol with the general practitioner of their choice without charge.

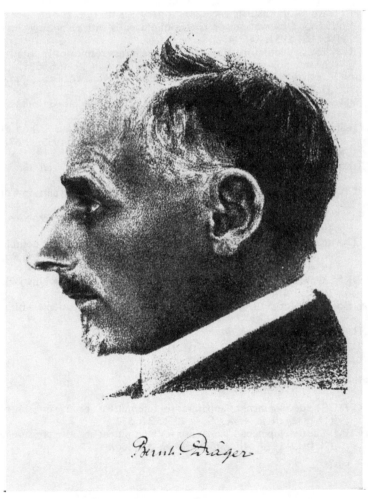

Figure 1   Bernard Dräger *(courtesy Drägerwerk AG).*

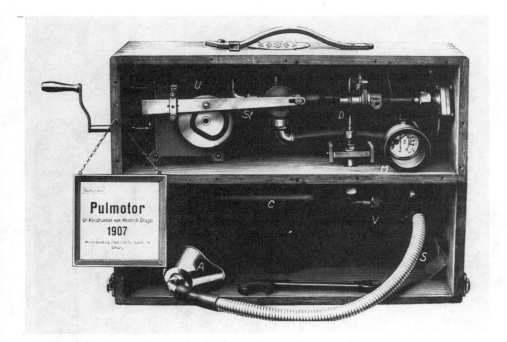

Figure 2   The Original Dräger Pulmotor 1907 *(courtesy Drägerwerk AG). This contained two venturis driven by compressed oxygen. One generated a positive pressure of around 25 cm H₂O to inflate the lungs and the other generated a slight negative pressure to assist exhalation. A cam rotated by a spring driven gramophone motor opened and closed the venturi successively, thus making the first Pulmotor a time-cycled pressure generator with a preset frequency of 15/min and an I:E ratio of approximately 1:2. Information from Dr Eric Schwanbom. Drägerwerk 1985.*

The pulmotor

It was into this environment of increased concern for personal welfare that Bernard Dräger (Fig. 1), whose company was noted for the design of mine rescue apparatus, introduced the Pulmotor in 1907 (Fig. 2). This was the first resuscitation apparatus designed to inflate the patient's lungs* since the Royal Humane Society withdrew its resuscitation bellows following Leroy's adverse reports in 1827 (1).

The original 1907 model Pulmotor had a clockwork motor that controlled the flow of oxygen from the cylinder to the positive and negative pressure venturis. The positive pressure venturi inflated the patient's lungs with the air–oxygen mixture and the other produced a slight negative pressure to assist exhalation. In 1910 the original model was replaced by an improved design which was both oxygen powered and controlled (Fig. 3). Fire and Police Rescue squads rapidly adopted this model and became proficient in its use. Unfortunately physicians rejected it, especially after the famous physiologist, Yandell Henderson, characterized the Pulmotor's use 'as a step backward towards the death of thousands'.

Thoracic surgery

At this time surgeons, who since they adopted aseptic methods in the 1880s had mastered intra-abdominal surgery, now wished to operate within the chest. However, their efforts were thwarted

*Except the 1888 Fell–O'Dwyer apparatus in the USA (1).

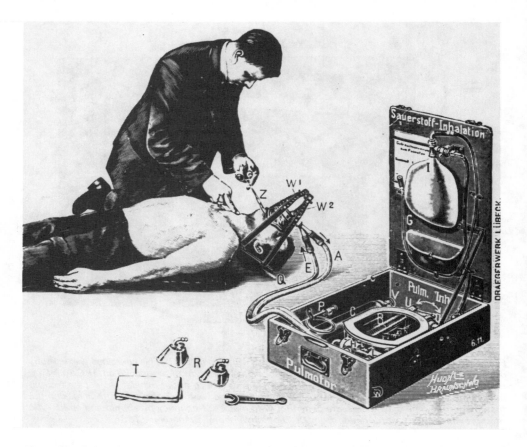

Figure 3A Dräger Pulmotor 1910 *(Drägerwerk). In this final design the gramophone motor and cam have been replaced by an oxygen pressure controlled cycling device. This type of cycling device was originally developed by the famous Swedish inventor Gustof Dalen to control the flashing lights in lighthouses. Information from Dr Eric Schwanbom Dragerwerk 1985.*

by the 'pneumothorax problem'. For no sooner would the chest be opened than the lung would collapse and patient's breathing would become disturbed. The air moved in pendulum fashion between the exposed and the unexposed lung so that hypoxia developed rapidly. Many different solutions were tried. In research labs since the time of Andreas Vesalius in 1555 (1), animals had been kept alive during experiments within the chest by inflating the lungs with bellows through a catheter inserted into the trachea. In experimental thoracic surgery, N. W. Green in New York in 1906 used a mechanical pump to inflate the animal's lungs through a cuffed tracheal tube (1,2). He noted that the animals often became apnoeic which provided a tranquil operating field.

But to intubate the human trachea was quite difficult. To avoid this difficulty the young German surgeon Ferdinand Sauerbruch in 1904 described the successful use of a negative pressure chamber to expand the exposed lung so that the patient could breathe (1,3,4,14). This seemed to prevent the pneumothorax problem from developing. Today we would call this method CPAP (continuous positive airway pressure).

Green's colleague, Henry H. Janeway (5), who had tried this differential pressure method by exposing the patient's airway to a raised pressure within a box enclosing the head, in 1909 combined a head box with rhythmic positive pressure. He also noted that the patient's spontaneous respiration ceased. In 1912 Janeway (6) described his use of an intermittent insufflation apparatus and finally in 1913 he introduced a curved bladed laryngoscope with

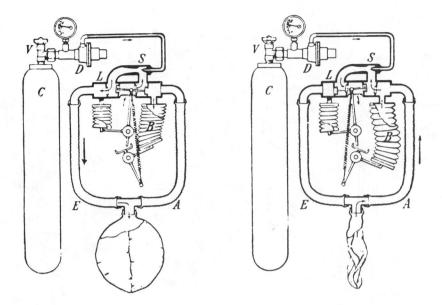

Figure 3B Dräger Pulmotor 1911 *(Drägerwerk Lubeck). During inspiration a mixture of air and oxygen at a pressure of 20 cm H₂O inflates the patient's lungs. Exhalation is assisted by a similar negative pressure of − 20 cm H₂O. The lefthand diagram shows the lung (represented by a rubber bag) being inflated. Oxygen from the cylinder passed through the venturi (S) entraining air and through the open valve (L) and the breathing tube (E) to the patient's lungs. At the same time gas mixture entered the bellows (B). When the pressure in the breathing tube reached a preset level the distension of the bellows (B) reversed the toggle mechanism thus ending inspiration (see righthand diagram).*

*   When the toggle mechanism kicked over into the expiratory position the valves were altered so that valve (L) was closed and the suction produced by the venturi assisted the outflow of gas from the lungs via tube (A).*

a battery in the handle which he used to pass his newly designed cuffed tracheal tube (7). The tube was connected to his latest apparatus which administered nitrous oxide and oxygen (N_2O/O_2) anaesthesia and also controlled or assisted the patient's spontaneous respiration.

In Leipzig, Germany, Trendelenburg's assistants Lawen and Sievers in 1910 (8) designed a piston ventilator for use in their attempts to obtain a successful outcome from Trendelenburg's heroic pulmonary embolectomy operations (9). They used a Trendelenburg cuffed tracheotomy tube and curare to control the patient's respiration during the surgery. The first successful pulmonary embolectomy was reported in 1923 by Martin Kirschner (10) to a meeting of German surgeons at which the elderly Trendelenburg was present.

World War I—1914–1918—stops development of artificial ventilation

In the First World War these surgeons left their apparatus behind in their laboratories and managed thoracic injuries as best they could without them. When nitrous oxide–oxygen apparatus became available to medical officers in the Allied Armies they found that by partially closing the expiratory valve to produce CPAP they were able to carry their patients through brief thoracic interventions. The pre-war experimental surgeons on their return from military service found there was neither time nor money for further experiments. Germany was in political and financial turmoil with extremists on all sides vying for power. There were thousands of patients with pulmonary tuberculosis for whom artificial pneumothorax and thoracoplasty

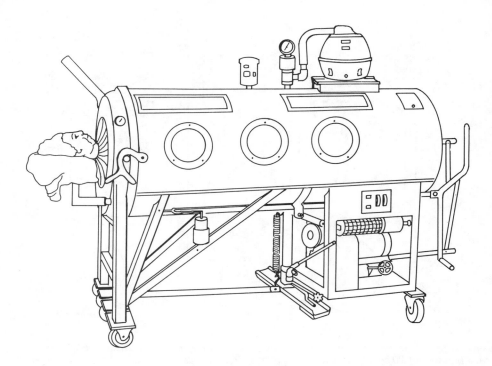

Figure 4   The 1952 Model Emerson Tank Ventilator *(J. H. Emerson Co.). John H. Emerson produced the first of his simple and robust tank ventilators during the Great Depression in 1932 in response to an acute need for affordable, reliable ventilators during an epidemic of poliomyelitis. His designs made use of readily available, economically priced plumbing, electrical and automobile components to hold down the cost. Mr Emerson made the first 'deep breath' attachment (the round device shown on top of the ventilator) for a tank ventilator in 1950 (15a) at the suggestion of Dr M. B. Visscher (16) to restore the compliance of the lungs (17). The term 'compliance' of the lungs was suggested to Jere Mead by a colleague in electronics and used for the first time in medicine in 1952 (18).*

were the treatments of choice. So no one pursued further the work of Green, Janeway, Lawen or Sievers and their promising initiatives were soon forgotten. The paintings by the pioneer German anaesthetist—Hans Killian from this period included in his autobiography (11) reflect the grim situation in his country in the 1920s. Only the Dräger Pulmotor survived from the pre-war days and physicians did not know how to use it. As a result there was a hiatus between 1913 and 1940 in the development of ventilators with the sole exception of Drinker and Shaw's 'Iron Lung'.

After unsuccessful attempts to use the Pulmotor for prolonged respiratory support in unintubated patients, Drinker in 1929 introduced his 'Iron Lung' (12,13,14). This body ventilator enclosed all of the patient except the head. It produced a good tidal exchange by raising and lowering the pressure around the patient's abdomen and thorax. Its great attraction was that it avoided the need for tracheal intubation. Iron lungs became standard equipment for artificial ventilation in hospitals from the 1930s until the 1950s in Europe and until the 1960s in the USA (Fig. 4).

The evolution of present-day ventilators

In Sweden the surgeon K. H. Giertz, formerly one of Sauerbruch's assistants who was dissatisfied with the results of the positive pressure method had been more successful with artificial respiration in his experimental thoracic surgery (19). As a result he encouraged first the ear,

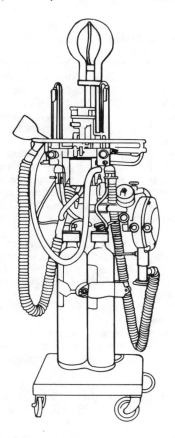

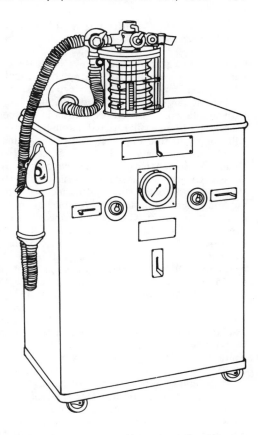

Figure 5 Frenckner, Crafoord and Anderson's AGA Spiropulsator 1940 (14,16). *This is the anaesthesia ventilator from which much of later British and US development can be traced.*

Figure 6   Blease Pulmoflator 1950 (24). *This was the first ventilator available in Britain. It was driven by an electrically powered air compressor and was pressure cycled.*

nose, and throat surgeon Frenckner and later Crafoord to work on mechanical artificial respiration as the solution of the pneumothorax problem. Frenckner developed a range of cuffed tracheal tubes to be used with an air driven ventilator he developed from the gas operated flasher mechanism used in marine automatic light buoys. This ventilator and the equipment were first described in Frenckner's monograph published in 1934 (1,20).

Clarence Crafoord who was working on his monograph *On Pneumonectomy* published in 1938 (21) developed the Spiropulsator further with Frenckner and Andersen, an engineer with the AGA company (22) (Fig. 5). Crafoord and Frenckner's routine method for thoracic surgery of intubation under topical anaesthesia with an airtight cuffed tracheal tube followed by general anaesthesia with mechanically controlled ventilation was readily accepted in Sweden. However, this was not the reception their method received in 1939 when Crafoord was invited to Los Angeles to lecture on his method and apparatus to the American Society for Thoracic Surgery (23). He demonstrated his method using mechanically controlled respiration for open chest surgery at two hospitals. Crafoord reported that, in the United States:

'Anesthesiologists argued that the most valuable signs for judging the depth of anesthesia and whether the ventilation was adequate were removed with controlled ventilation. Controlled ventilation was looked upon as dangerous and intratracheal intubation (with an airtight cuffed tube) during intrathoracic operations was considered harmful (24) as it

interfered with the outflow of secretions round the tube into the face mask as the patient was often placed 20° head down to promote this drainage.' (25)

Only the pioneer cardiac surgeons Claude Beck and Frederick Mautz of Cleveland, Ohio, who had their own ventilator (40) accepted mechanically controlled ventilation (26,27). As late as 1950 a prominent leader of American anaesthesia clearly documented, in a paper to a meeting of thoracic surgeons, the poor results, including severe carbon dioxide build-up, that occurred with spontaneous assisted respiration in open chest surgery. In spite of critical discussion of his presentation he still rejected manually or mechanically controlled respiration saying he was still hoping to find improved ways of assisting respiration (25,28,29).

In Sweden during World War II surgeons readily followed Crafoord's lead and, in occupied Denmark, Ernst Trier Morch, unable to obtain a Spiropulsator, built his own pump ventilator. British Army anaesthetists in Thoracic Surgical Units were provided with cyclopropane and Waters to and fro absorbers which they used with excellent results with the controlled respiration method described in detail by Michael Nosworthy in 1941 (31). This method was originally described by Arthur Guedel and Treweek in 1934 (32) and introduced into Britain by Ralph Waters in 1936 (33).

So by 1947 when Trier Morch spoke on the value of ventilators at the Royal Society of Medicine in London, British anaesthetists were receptive to the idea of help from a mechanical ventilator (30). This was especially so since the widespread use of large apnoeic doses of curare (34,35) with light N_2O/O_2 anaesthesia and controlled ventilation made a ventilator very desirable to busy British anaesthetists working without assistance.

Narcotic supplemented nitrous oxide/oxygen relaxant anaesthesia introduced by Neff, Mayer and Perales (36,37) in the US in 1947 and Mushin and Rendell-Baker (38,39) in the UK in 1949 only worked well when larger apnoeic doses of relaxant were used. This technique freed thoracic surgeons from the bondage of explosive anaesthetic agents and allowed them to use cautery on the lung, permitting resection of tubercular lesions under the safety of streptomycin cover.

At the end of World War II it was an engineer, J. H. Blease, who had formerly built and raced motorcycles, who introduced ventilators to Britain (40). Before the war he had made a series of anaesthesia apparatus for a Liverpool anaesthetist. When the latter died he found himself forced by the wartime shortage of skilled anaesthetists to progress from selling gas machines to using them when he was pressed into service to provide emergency anaesthesia for casualties during the heavy air raids in the Liverpool Merseyside area. Impressed by the drudgery of manually controlled ventilation during long chest operations, his inventive mind suggested a mechanical solution to the problem. His prototype (40) was demonstrated at Wallasey Cottage Hospital in 1947 and the production model Blease Pulmoflator appeared in 1950 (41) (Fig. 6).

In the USA where more modest doses of relaxant were commonly used with assisted respiration there was less urgent need for ventilators. In addition the continuing dispute about controlled respiration delayed the introduction of anaesthesia ventilators. Though the Blease Pulmoflator was introduced in Britain in 1950 the Jefferson ventilator (40) did not appear in the USA until 1956. The Engstrom ventilator appeared in Sweden in 1951; the Emerson Post-Op ventilator, its US equivalent, did not appear until 1964 (Fig. 11).

1952 Copenhagen poliomyelitis epidemic and its consequences

The city of Copenhagen, Denmark, possessed only one tank and six cuirass ventilators (42) when the epidemic of spino-bulbar poliomyelitis struck in 1952. After 27 of 31 patients treated in them had died and more patients requiring artificial ventilation continued to be admitted, the chief of the Blegdam infectious diseases hospital, Dr H. C. A. Lassen, called for help to Dr Bjorn Ibsen, Chief of Department of Anaesthesia at the Kommunes' Hospital.

On a desperately ill 12-year-old girl Dr Bjorn Ibsen demonstrated how tracheostomy with a cuffed tube permitted clearing of the airway of secretions by suction. This, followed by adequate manual ventilation with a Waters to-and-fro CO_2 absorber system, produced a prompt improvement in the patient's condition. This method of controlled respiration was

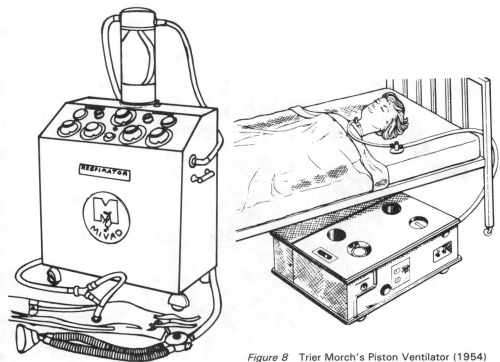

Figure 7   The Engstrom ventilator 1951 (33). *This was the first of the piston ventilators which would deliver a preset volume despite changes in compliance or airway resistance.*

Figure 8   Trier Morch's Piston Ventilator (1954) (34,35). *Designed to fit under the patient's bed this ventilator provided large tidal volumes so that uncuffed metal tracheostomy tubes could be used. The expiratory ball valve sits on the bed near the patient's head.*

by then universally used in Copenhagen for thoracic anaesthesia. By using the same method for bulbo-spinal paralysis in poliomyelitis the mortality rate was reduced from 80% to 25% (43). However, to provide manual artificial ventilation 1400 students were needed working in three eight-hour shifts so all university teaching ceased. There was an urgent need for 'mechanical students' to free the students from their life saving tasks so they could return to their studies.

In 1951 Dr Carl-Gunnar Engstrom, a Swedish infectious diseases specialist, had demonstrated his new concept—the volume ventilator (44) (Fig. 7). This was ideally suited to these patients. Engstrom and other ventilator designers rushed their apparatus into larger scale production to free the Danish students from their life-saving bondage. Engstrom's ventilator (40,45) ushered in a new era of large rugged piston ventilators designed to deliver the chosen tidal volume uninfluenced by changes in compliance or resistance. Like a steam engine their simple, robust mechanical design enabled them to run for prolonged periods with minimal attention. Ernst Trier Morch, MD, Chicago (formerly of Copenhagen), in response to their epidemic, in 1954 introduced to the USA a simple piston pump-ventilator designed to fit under the patient's bed (40,46) (Fig. 8). For the first time, using these volume ventilators, it was possible to calculate the minute volume ventilation delivered. To monitor the adequacy of the ventilation Paul Astrup, Head of the Central Laboratory of the Blegdam Hospital with Svend Schroder of the Radiometer Company designed the Astrup apparatus for the rapid assessment of the blood pH and carbon dioxide tension (47). This apparatus together with Leland Clark's oxygen electrode (48) of 1956 for the first time made readily available arterial blood gas readings from which to determine the adequacy of the patient's ventilatory exchange and oxygenation.

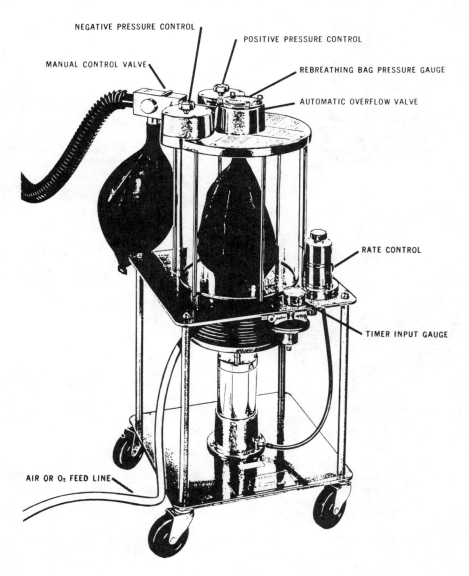

NEGATIVE PRESSURE CONTROL

POSITIVE PRESSURE CONTROL

MANUAL CONTROL VALVE

REBREATHING BAG PRESSURE GAUGE

AUTOMATIC OVERFLOW VALVE

RATE CONTROL

TIMER INPUT GAUGE

AIR OR O₂ FEED LINE

Figure 9   The Jefferson Ventilator for use during anaesthesia 1955. (Air Shields Inc.)

Developments in cardiothoracic anaesthesia

The Swedish chest surgeon Viking Bjork and Engstrom in 1955, extended the use of tracheostomy and mechanical ventilatory support for the postoperative care of segmental lung resections in patients with poor pulmonary function with excellent results (49). Bjork later devoted himself to cardiac surgery and like others found that many early open heart patients died of 'pump lung' or what we now call adult respiratory distress syndrome (ARDS). As treatment for this Bjork strongly advocated continued intubation to permit postoperative respiratory support with the Engstrom ventilator.

When John Gibbon of Philadelphia performed the first successful open heart operation in 1953 with a pump-oxygenator of his design he was already a strong advocate of mechanically controlled ventilation for open chest surgery (29). For this he used a ventilator designed by members of his cardiothoracic unit (50). In 1955 his brother's company, Air Shields, manufactured the Jefferson ventilator (Fig. 9) which was developed from this earlier prototype. This joined Morch's Surgical ventilator (51), as the first available US-made anaesthesia ventilators designed to control the patient's ventilation, rather than to assist their spontaneous efforts. In 1955 Jack Frumin, MD and Arnold St J. Lee designed and manufactured the Autoanestheton (40). This was a carbon dioxide (CO_2) servo-controlled ventilator which varied the patient's tidal volume as necessary to maintain the preset end-expiratory CO_2 level (40,52,53). Using this ventilator they could easily control the patient's arterial CO_2 level. However, in spite of an adequate inspired oxygen concentration (FIO_2), reliable oxygenation was not always achieved until they added a positive end-expiratory pressure of 7 cm H_2O. In 1957, this was the first reported demonstration of the value of a positive end expiratory pressure. Now well known as PEEP (54), it was re-discovered by McIntyre and colleagues in 1969 (55). Though a unique and intriguing design the Autoanestheton was not widely adopted and had little effect on current designs.

In 1958, Arnold St J. Lee and Jack Frumin for the first time incorporated an O_2 'fail safe' mechanism which cut off the nitrous oxide flow if the supply of oxygen failed (56,57). This was incorporated within the Frumin ventilator-anaesthesia apparatus introduced in 1958 (57). This principle was soon widely adopted on anaesthesia apparatus.

The first non-anaesthesia ventilators that could be used to control a patient's respiration post-operatively were introduced in 1957. The Bennett PRIA pressure cycled assistor-controller ventilator (42) was the first of these followed shortly by the Bird Mark 7 (42). The Bennett

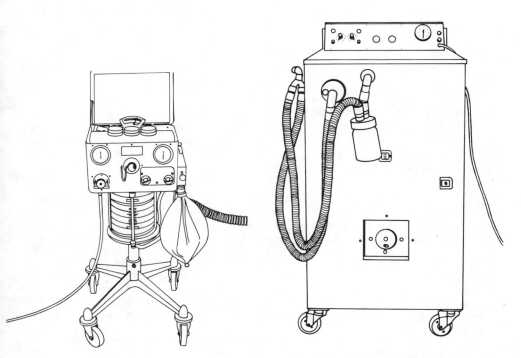

Figure 10 The Bennett B_2A anaesthesia Assistor 1957 (42). *This was one of the first ventilators which, in spite of its title of Assistor, could be adjusted to deliver a known tidal volume.*

Figure 11 The Emerson Post Op Ventilator 1964 (J. H. Emerson, Co.). *This US built volume ventilator provided features similar to the Engstrom ventilator of 1951. In addition the I:E ratio could be varied by its electronic controls.*

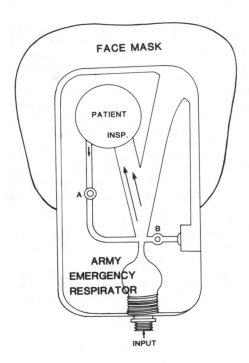

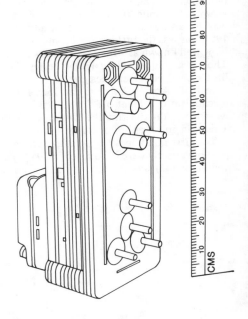

Figure 12   US Army Fluidic Emergency Respirator 1964. *Designed by Warren and Straub the gas pathways in this hand sized 'bi-stable flip-flop' were formed in a block of clear plastic. High pressure gas flowed through the lefthand channel to inflate the patient's lungs. As the pressure in the patient's airway rose a signal was transmitted back to the lefthand control port at a rate controlled by set screw A. When it was strong enough this signal switched the jet over to the righthand channel and exhalation commenced.*

Figure 13   1974 Ohio Anaesthesia Ventilator fluidic control module (55). *This 75 mm high ceramic unit formed the 'heart' of this ventilator.*

B2A anaesthesia ventilator (58) (Fig. 10) also introduced that year, was labelled an assistor. However, it could be adjusted to deliver a known tidal volume. For that reason it was used in the late 1950s by Bendixen and colleagues at the Massachusetts General Hospital. They used them to treat patients during the last poliomyelitis epidemics in Boston before Jonas Salk's vaccine eliminated this disease. By the early 1960s the Salk and Sabine vaccines had also eliminated the need for the National Foundation's Polio-Respiratory Units. Though equipped with obsolete tank ventilators and never having had the opportunity to adopt the newer Copenhagen treatment methods, their staff possessed a vast amount of skill and experience in ventilator care. This experience would have been invaluable four or five years later when hospitals' urgent needs required new Respiratory Units and ICUs to be built, equipped and staffed from scratch.

There was a similar hiatus until 1964 when Jack Emerson, responding to physicians' requests, filled the need for a US built piston pump ventilator similar to the Engstrom which had been introduced in 1951. Characteristically his Post-Op ventilator (51) (Fig. 11) was a simpler design; there was no 'bag in bottle' and the patient was ventilated directly by the piston. However, unlike the Engstrom the inspiratory:expiratory ratio could be varied at will via electronic controls. This was the first use of electronics on ventilators and foreshadowed the next generation of designs. This apparatus became the 'work horse' in many of the then newly equipped ICUs.

Fluidic ventilators

The components used in fluidic ventilators mostly have no moving parts. Flows of gas or liquid are used to carry out the sensing, logic, amplification and control functions normally performed electronically. They are thus unaffected by electronic interference. These fluidic equivalents of electronic components evolved from discussions between Raymond W. Warren, Ronald E. Bowles and Billy M. Horton at the Harry Diamond Laboratories, Washington DC in 1959 (40,59). In 1964 Barila, Meyer, Mosley and other anaesthetists from the Walter Reed Army Institute of Research, working with engineers from the Harry Diamond Laboratories, evolved prototypes for a hand-held fluidic resuscitator and a volume ventilator for anaesthesia (40,60) (Fig. 12).

The Corning Company succeeded in fabricating fluidic components by photo-etching and in 1965 produced a self-instruction 'Fluidikit' for potential industrial users to introduce them to applications of the new technology. The medical 'Fluidikit' that followed in 1972 included the design and components for a pressure/time cycled ventilator (40). The 1970 Hamilton Standard PAD fluidic ventilator prototype used a circuit similar to that given in the Fluidikit, however it never went into production. The Monaghan 225 fluidic ventilator (40) introduced in 1973 has continued in successful production. A large number of fluidically controlled (Fig. 13) anaesthesia ventilators were produced by Ohio Medical Products after 1974 (40) and by North American Drager after 1975 (40). However, in their more recent designs the fluidic components have been superseded by more versatile electronic units. Though trouble-free in use, high gas consumption, limited features and the need for more versatile alarms, more easily provided electronically, led to their demise.

High frequency ventilators

Ventilators in the past have been designed to produce normal tidal volumes at respiratory rates similar to those of spontaneous respiration, though of necessity the pressures produced within the thorax have been greater and the reverse of normal.

As patients with increasingly severe pulmonary problems required higher inflation pressures and higher levels of PEEP the number of patients on the ventilators suffering from pulmonary barotrauma or cardiovascular embarrassment has increased significantly. A method of enhancing gas exchange while at the same time not requiring such high pressures would therefore be most helpful.

It is interesting that in 1959 Emerson patented (61) just such an idea. His device was intended to vibrate the column of air to cause the gas to diffuse more rapidly within the airway and therefore aid in the breathing function by circulating the gas more thoroughly to and from the walls of the lungs. He advocated vibrations of between 500 and 1500 times per minute both during inspiration and expiration whether spontaneous or provided by a ventilator; however the apparatus was never fully tested or tried clinically.

It was the interaction between intermittent rises in intrathoracic pressure produced by the ventilator with the normal pulsation in blood pressure that interfered with the observations of two cardiovascular research groups. One in Uppsala, Sweden was studying the influence of the carotid sinus reflex on the control of the blood pressure (62) and the other in Berlin, Germany was studying the effects of pericardial pressure on cardiac performance. Sjostrand and colleagues in Uppsala, Sweden were aware that in 1908 Meltzer and Auer (63) and others (1) later had been able to reduce the anatomical dead space and ensure adequate oxygenation by insufflating oxygen through an endotracheal catheter placed with its tip just above the carina. Periodic interruption of the O_2 flow was later recognized to be necessary for adequate CO_2 removal by this method. Sjostrand and colleagues postulated that this reduction of the dead space should make it possible for a ventilator to use smaller tidal volumes at higher frequencies with lower pressure fluctuations and still provide adequate alveolar ventilation. However, to deliver such smaller tidal volumes at higher frequencies two things were necessary: (1) a high pressure supply of oxygen capable of high flows and (2) a delivery system with negligible internal compressible volume and compliance.

HFPPV

insufflation and expiratory systems

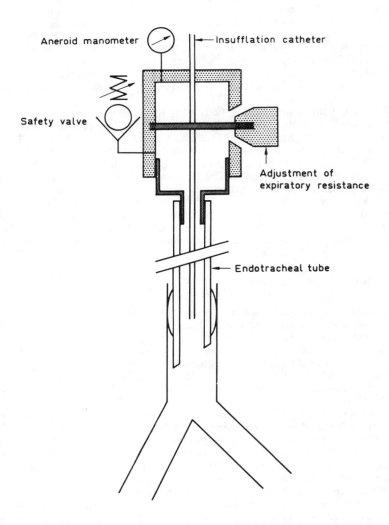

Figure 14   Sjostrand and colleagues' original arrangement (1972) for high frequency insufflation through a catheter within the tracheal tube combined with an adjustable expiratory flow resistance. From Heijman K, Sjostrand V, et al. High frequency positive pressure ventilation during anaesthesia and routine surgery in man. Acta Anaesth Scand 1972; **16**: 176.

Oberg and Sjostrand's original apparatus described in 1967 (64,65,66,67,68,69) used a catheter passed through a tracheal tube to deliver pulses of compressed air 60–80 times per minute with insufflation occupying 30% of the ventilatory cycle (Fig. 14). This combined with a positive end expiratory resistance of 2.5 cm H_2O produced a moderate and constant expansion of the lungs. This technic maintained normal blood gas levels and had no effect on the blood pressure. Within a few seconds of the start of this artificial respiration spontaneous respiration ceased without the need for hyperventilation. Spontaneous respiration returned promptly when the high frequency insufflation was discontinued.

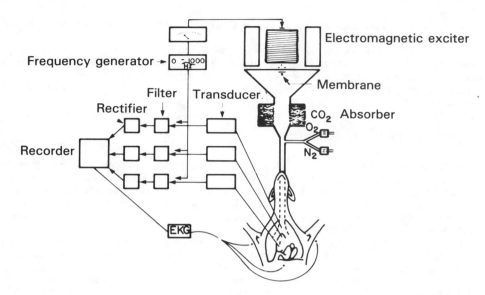

Figure 15 Lunkenheimer and colleagues high frequency oscillator 1972. Originally designed to produce high frequency cardiac excitation to measure cardiac wall stiffness by assessing transmyocardial pressure transmission during diffusion respiration. It was found that the high frequency oscillation enhanced gas exchange. Reproduced by permission of the editor from Lunkenheimer PP et al. Int Anesth Clin 1983; 21: 51–62.

A high frequency ventilator for bronchoscopy which dispensed with the insufflation catheter was introduced by Sjostrand and colleagues in 1973 (66,67). It incorporated a 'pneumatic valve' which worked on the wall attraction, or Coanda effect. This conveyed the high pressure gas impulses from the curved side connector into the lumen of the bronchoscope to ventilate the lungs even though the external (machine) end of the valve was open to atmosphere. The Siemens Bronchovent ventilator's development was based on these studies. A pneumatically controlled expiratory valve could be added to provide volume controlled ventilation using either the 'pneumatic valve' in their system H or the multi-lumen 'Hi Lo Jet Tube' in their System J. Since their pioneer publications Sjostrand and his colleagues have continued to provide leadership in this field (64,65).

High frequency oscillation

Lunkenheimer and colleagues (70,71) in Berlin, West Germany, developed a means of measuring cardiac performance based on changes in the compliance of the myocardial wall in response to pericardial pressure oscillations. Complete skeletal muscle relaxation and cessation of respiration were required so that the myocardial pressure transmission could be measured in response to intrathoracic pressure oscillations transmitted by transtracheal vibrations caused by an electro-magnetic vibrator (Fig. 15).

Lunkenheimer and colleagues were aware of Draper and Whitehead's studies on diffusion respiration in apnoeic dogs (72–75) and initially carried out their studies using diffusion respiration until by chance in 1972 they found that gas exchange was enhanced by the tracheal pressure oscillations. Though oxygenation was satisfactory irrespective of the frequency of vibration, CO_2 elimination was satisfactory only at certain frequencies between 1380 to 2400 cycles/minute (23 to 40 hertz), depending upon the size of the dog. Lunkenheimer and colleagues' later studies showed that the pressure and air flows within the various segments of the bronchial tree were not uniform; they varied with the frequencies and type of high frequency ventilator used. Their results showed the most favourable results were obtained with high frequency alternating ventilation produced by two jets, one directed down the trachea, the other directed out of the trachea (76,77,78).

Bryan, Froese and colleagues (79) in Toronto Canada used high frequency oscillation clinically with a marked reduction in pulmonary shunt in patients with chronic obstructive lung disease with no change in arterial CO_2 tension or cardiac output. They achieved excellent gas exchange during apnoea using tidal volumes of 100 to 150 ml at oscillation rates of 900 times per minute.

High frequency jet ventilation

In 1972 Smith and colleagues commenced using a high pressure oxygen jet (80) to provide artificial respiration during laryngoscopy. Later they used the same method for anaesthesia during fibreoptic bronchoscopy (81) and for respiratory support before tracheostomy (82). For this, the jet was delivered into the trachea through a 14 gauge intravenous catheter passed percutaneously through the circo-thyroid membrane (45). For both these uses traditional respiratory rates were employed.

To better manage patients receiving jet ventilation for laryngoscopy and bronchoscopy, Klain and Smith (83), in 1976, built a fluid logically controlled ventilator based on the diagrams and components in the Corning Basic Medical Fluidikit (84). This was originally designed for traditional respiratory rates up to 20 breaths per minute. However, when they became aware of Jonzon, Sjostrand and colleagues' work on high frequency ventilation published in 1970 (85) they were stimulated to try high frequency ventilation and found that their ventilator was suitable for respiratory rates up to 900 breaths per minute. For experiments with artificial respiration on dogs a 14 gauge Angiocath, with two side holes near the tip was inserted into the trachea between the first and second tracheal rings. At a frequency of 100 to 600 breaths per minute the ventilator was able to deliver oxygen at a flow rate of 17 litres per minute with a 1:2 inspiratory–expiratory (I:E) ratio producing a PaO_2 of 400–575 mm Hg and a $PaCO_2$ of 20–25 mm Hg. At a calculated minute volume of 17 litres per minute and a frequency of 400 pm the tidal volume worked out at 42 ml.

Though the PaO_2 was not much influenced by either the respiratory rate or the 1:E ratio, the $PaCO_2$ was greatly affected by both factors being lowest at a respiratory frequency of 100 and a 1:E ratio of 1:1.

Smith and Klain noted that high frequency jet ventilation could prevent aspiration of secretions from the pharynx without the use of a cuffed tracheal tube thus eliminating the need for a cuff, a common source of trachea damage.

In 1981 Smith, Klain and colleagues (86,87) introduced a multiple lumen tracheal tube for HFJV developed with the National Catheter Corporation (now called the Hi Lo Jet Tube). This also permitted suctioning of hypoxic patients without interrupting ventilatory support and facilitated fibreoptic bronchoscopy with HFJV.

Chakrabarti and Whitwam (88,89) in 1983 introduced an all-purpose jet ventilator incorporating an open Mapleson E T-piece breathing system 1.5 m in length. High pressure jet impulses delivered into the machine end of the tube did not reach the patient but inflated the patient's lungs with the humidified anaesthetic gas or air/O_2 mixture introduced into the patient end of the system. The open breathing system permitted the patient to obtain additional breaths out of phase without 'fighting' the ventilator.

Classification of high frequency ventilators

1. HFPPV—*High frequency positive pressure ventilators* (Sjostrand *et al.*) e.g. Siemens Bronchovent. Similar to a conventional ventilator but it had a minimal compressible volume delivery system and was capable of high gas flows.

2. HFO—*High frequency oscillators* (Lunkenheimer *et al.* and Bryan, Froese *et al.*) e.g. Bird VDR-4 and Mera Hummingbird. A sine wave pump or electrically oscillated diaphragm provided oscillatory movement of the same volume of gas into *and out* of the airway.

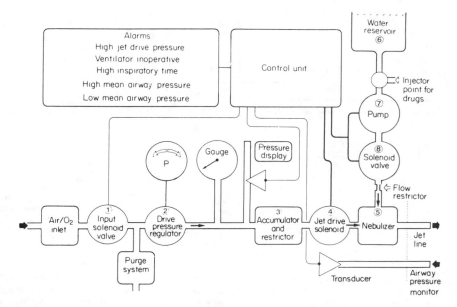

Figure 16A   Diagram of Penlon Bromsgrove High Frequency Jet Ventilator

1. *This 'fail safe' valve is normally open. It only closes if the jet drive pressure is too high, if the solenoid valve (4) fails to cycle or if the gas supply pressure exceeds the preset limit.*
2. *This is a variable pressure reducing valve that controls the driving pressure.*
3. *Accumulator and restrictor.*
4. *Jet drive solenoid. This interrupter controls the flow of gas to the patient.*
5. *Bernouilli nebulizer.*
6. *Water supply for nebulizer.*
7. *Pump to fill nebulizer with water.*
8. *Solenoid valve which opens to permit pump (7) to refill nebulizer.*

3. HFFI—*High frequency flow interruptors* Conventional ventilators able to work at the higher frequencies, fitted with low compliance breathing tubing. Unlike oscillators they provide no assistance to exhalation e.g. Siemens Servo 900C, and Infrasonics Infant Star.

4. HFJV—*High frequency jet ventilators* (Smith & Klain *et al.*) e.g. Bear Jet 150 Bromsgrove and Bunnell Life Pulse. Delivered rapid continuous pulses or jets of gas through a narrow bore tube directly into the patient's airway entraining further gas mixture from the breathing system.

High frequency ventilators can deliver gas at high flows and pressures and have very low internal compliance so a safety mechanism that detects the pressure in the patient's distal airway and stops the ventilator promptly should excessive pressure develop is essential. Mucous plugging, air trapping and inadvertent PEEP can be problems with most designs.

Indications for high frequency ventilation

There are conditions where HFJV has clear advantages such as anaesthesia for laryngoscopy, bronchoscopy, broncho-pleural fistula and with air leaks from the lungs and hyaline membrane disease in neonates; to reduce 'brain bounce' in micro-neuro surgery and to reduce respiratory movement to a minimum during destruction of kidney stones by lithotripsy. High frequency ventilation has been recommended for neonates with RDS as it permits adequate gas exchange at lower mean airway pressures. For many other conditions HFJV could probably handle the problems as well as traditional ventilators but caution dictates that each worker prove HFJV ventilation has sufficient advantages to justify the presently unknown risks of its wider usage.

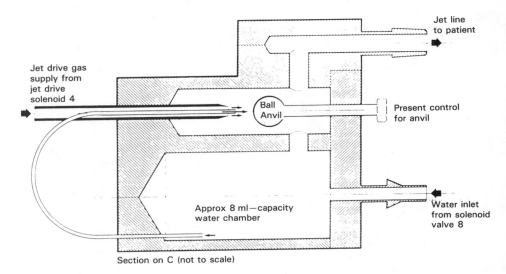

Section on C (not to scale)

Figure 16B   The Penlon Bromsgrove Jet Ventilator's Nebulizer. *Efficient humidification of the inspired gases has been a problem with high frequency ventilators. In this nebulizer the fluid in the chamber which was under the high driving pressure was actively delivered to the centre of the jet. This improved the performance over the usual pattern with a vertical aspiration tube. The compressible volume of the nebulizer was less than 15 ml with negligible internal compliance. The liquid capacity was 8 ml. At preset intervals the jet drive solenoid inhibited cutting off all gas flow to the patient. When the pressure in the nebulizer fell to atmosphere the pump recharged the nebulizer chamber with a preset volume of liquid from the intravenous infusion set.*

A simple jet ventilator using normal respiratory frequencies and based on the Bird Mark 2 control mechanism was introduced by Rendell-Baker and colleagues in 1970 (Fig. 17). It was unique in that it preserved the spontaneous respiration pattern of gas flows and the CO_2 removal efficiency of the Mapleson A breathing system while providing controlled respiration. There is little doubt that a high frequency jet ventilator with its capacity for higher gas flows would work equally well with a paediatric Jackson Rees (Mapleson D) system (Fig. 18) or a circle system (Fig. 19). The ability of a jet ventilator to deliver the tidal volume directly to the baby's airway thus eliminating unwanted compliance in the paediatric breathing system could be a considerable advantage.

Respiratory distress syndrome CPAP and IMV

In 1971 Kirby, Robinson, Shulz and deLemos (90,14) with Ed Weninger of the Bird Corporation designed the Baby Bird ventilator especially to treat neonatal respiratory distress syndrome. This was a time cycled volume ventilator with several unusual new features. It consisted of two parts, one the patient breathing system provided a continuous flow of air–oxygen mixture from which the baby could breathe spontaneously at any time. The resistance to expiration could be increased as necessary to keep the alveoli open. This was the first description of CPAP.

The other part, a Bird Mark 2 ventilator, intermittently closed the expiratory valve on the patient breathing system so that the inflowing fresh gas inflated the baby's lungs at respiratory rates up to 130 per minute. As the baby could take additional spontaneous breaths from the breathing system at any time weaning from the ventilator was accomplished by a gradual reduction in the rate and duration of inspiration so that the baby gradually resumed spontaneous respiration. This was the first use of what later became known as IMV (intermittent mandatory ventilation).

Though the original Baby Bird was entirely pneumatic, to satisfy the demand for greater sophistication in controls and alarms, the Baby Bird Mark II became entirely electronically controlled.

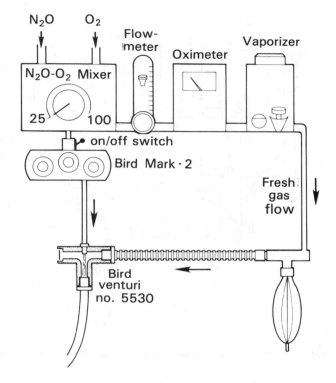

Figure 17   Rendell-Baker and colleagues' 1970 jet ventilator. *This was designed to enable the Mapleson A (Magill) breathing system to work efficiently during controlled respiration. The jet from the Bird Mark 2 control unit in passing through the venturi created a negative pressure which held the spill valve closed and entrained gases from the breathing system. The Bird N_2O/O_2 Blender delivered the same mixture of from 25% to 100% O_2 in N_2O to the Mark 2 unit and the breathing system. The Bird Mark 2 was designed for normal respiratory frequencies and delivered the desired normal tidal volumes.*

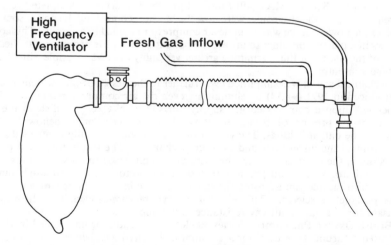

Figure 18   Use of high frequency jet ventilator with Jackson Rees System. Not shown are the N_2O/O_2 blender to power the ventilator and the provision for humidification of the gases.*

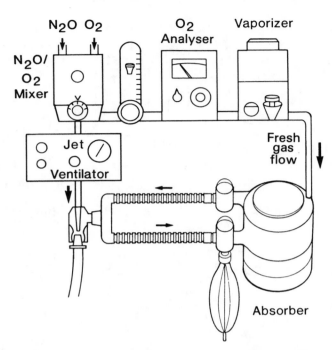

Figure 19   Use of N₂O/O₂ powered jet ventilator with circle absorption breathing system. (Rendell-Baker et al., 1970).

Electronically controlled ventilators

When Jack Emerson introduced his Post-Op ventilator (51) in 1964 (Fig. 11), his design combined a robust pump like the Engstrom ventilator but it incorporated electronic controls to vary the 1:E ratio. This design feature was not possible with a purely mechanical design like the Engstrom. These electronic controls of the Emerson ventilator foreshadowed future designs. When the Bennett MA1 (49) followed in 1967 it marked a complete break with the piston ventilators, for the electronics were now the 'master' controlling the power source 'slave'. In the MA1 the power source was a simple air compressor coupled to a venturi. This compressed the bellows in a plastic container to inflate the patient's lungs. Electronics controlled all other functions of the ventilator thus permitting greater versatility than was possible with a mechanical piston type ventilator.

The mechanical aspect was simplified even further in the design of the Siemens-Elema Servo 900, introduced in 1971 (91,14) by eliminating even the air compressor (Fig. 20). The Servo 900 depended upon a compressed gas supply (air/O2 or N₂O/O₂) to distend the reservoir bellows against the pressure of springs, and it was the force exerted on the bellows by the springs that inflated the patient's lungs. The ventilator had two electronically controlled scissor-like valves to control the inspiratory and expiratory channels. The inspiratory flow pattern, the minute volume, the respiratory rate, the inspiratory and pause times were first selected and then the ventilator's flow and pressure transducers monitored the ventilator's output. The electronic servo mechanism adjusted the opening of the inspiratory scissor valve to comply with the parameters selected. This electronic servo mechanism enabled the ventilator to compensate for changes in airway resistance and compliance.

The British Oxygen Pneumotron Series 80 electronic ventilator introduced in 1973 (92,14) incorporated a turbine-type transducer to monitor inspired gas delivery and to control by a feedback loop both flow pattern and volume delivered. A similar transducer measured exhaled volume. An alarm sounded indicating a leak if the expired volume fell below the inspired volume.

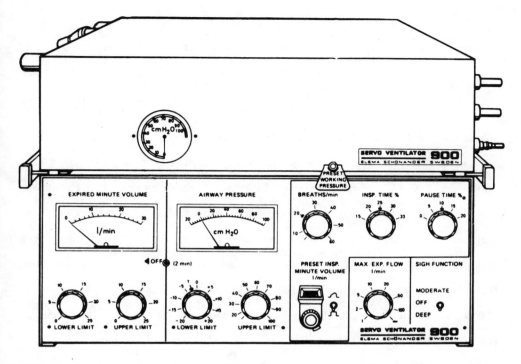

Figure 20   The Elema Schonander (Siemens) Servo 900 Ventilator 1971. *This was the first ventilator (since the Autoanestheton) that incorporated a servo mechanism able to vary the ventilator's output to compensate for variations in the airway resistance and compliance to ensure that the preset parameters were met.*

Electronic controls permitted the inspiratory wave form to be varied and an inspiratory pause to be added. This unit was compact since compressed gases provided the power to inflate the lungs and the electronic controls were conveniently arranged.

In 1974 Engstrom followed the trend away from the large piston ventilators with the introduction of the electronic Engstrom ECS 2000 ventilator (93).

Many ventilators later incorporated microprocessors such as the 1983 Puritan-Bennett 7200 to monitor the functioning of the apparatus and various patient parameters. Ventilators with microprocessors using a video screen to display the information were heralded by the Spanish MM. Pulmosystem Z800 introduced in 1980. This was followed by the Drager EV-A electronic microprocessor ventilator introduced in 1984 and the Bear 5 introduced in 1985. The shape of a curve on a video screen conveys its message to the professional observer almost instantaneously and much more readily than does a row of numbers.

In the future electronics and microprocessors with servo mechanisms will respond promptly to changes in the patient's condition and will adjust the functions of the apparatus meanwhile recording the changes and alerting the medical staff.

The change will then be complete from the simple pump to a patient treatment control centre. But there will still be need for dedicated and skilled personnel who can correctly interpret the trends so clearly displayed and who can make full use of the capabilities of these splendid machines.

References

(1) Mushin WW, Rendell-Baker L. *The principles of thoracic anaesthesia past and present* (reprints available from publisher) Springfield, IL: Charles C. Thomas, 1953.

(2) Green NW. A positive pressure method of artificial respiration with a practical device for its application in thoracic surgery. *Surg Gynec Obstet* 1906; **2**: 512.

(3) Rendell-Baker L. History of thoracic anaesthesia. In: Mushin WW, ed. *Thoracic anaesthesia*, Oxford: Blackwell, 1963: 612-7. See also: Meyer HW. The history of the development of the negative differential pressure chamber for thoracic surgery. *J Thorac Surg* 1955; **30**: 114-26.

(4) Sauerbruch F. Zur Pathologie des offenen Pneumothorax und die Grundlagen meines Verfahrens zu seiner Ausschaltung. *Mitt Grenzgeb Med Chir* 1904; **13**: 399. See also: Sauerbruch F. *Master surgeon*. New York: Crowell, 1954.

(5) Janeway HH, Green NW. Experimental intrathoracic esophageal surgery. *JAMA* 1909; **53**: 1975.

(6) Janeway HH. An apparatus for intratracheal insufflation. *Ann Surg* 1912; **56**: 328.

(7) Janeway HH. Intratracheal anesthesia. *Ann Surg* 1913; **58**: 927.

(8) Lawen, Sievers. Zar praktischen Anwendung der instrumentellen kunstlichen Respiration am Menschen. *Munch med Wchnschr* 1910; **59**; 2221.

(9) Trendelenburg F. Ueber die Operative Behandlung der Emboli der Lungenarterie. *Zentr Chir* 1907; **44**: 1402.

(10) Kirschner M. Ein durch die Trendelenburgsche Operation geheilter Fall von Embolie der Art. pulmonalis. *Verhardl Deutsch Ges Chir* 1924; **132**: 627.

(11) Killian H. *40 Jahre Narkoseforschung*. Tubingen Verlag der Deutschen Hochschlehrer-Zeitung. 1964.

(12) Drinker P, Shaw L. An apparatus for prolonged administration of artificial respiration. *J Clin Invest* 1929; **7**: 229.

(13) Drinker P, McKhann CF. The use of a new apparatus for prolonged administration of artificial respiration. *JAMA* 1929; **92**: 1658.

(14) Mushin WW, Rendell-Baker L, Thompson PW, Mapleson WW. *Automatic ventilation of the lungs* 3rd Ed. St Louis: Blackwell Mosby, 1980.

(15) Emerson JH. Respiratory problems in poliomyelitis. *Nat Found Infantile Paralysis Conf Proc*, Ann Arbor, Michigan March 1952: 11.

(16) Visscher MB. The physiology of respiration and respirators with particular reference to poliomyelitis. *Nat Found Infantile Paralysis Round Table Conf.* Minneapolis, Minnesota October 1947: 156.

(17) Whittenberger JL. Respiratory problems in poliomyelitis. *Nat Found Infantile Paralysis Conf Proc*. Ann Arbor, Michigan March 1952: 10.

(18) Ferris BG, Mead J, Whittenberger JL, Saxton GA. Pulmonary function in convalescent poliomyelitis patients. III Compliance of the lungs and thorax *N Engl J Med* 1952; **247**: 390.

(19) Giertz KH. Studier Ofver Tryckdifferensandning (rytmisk luftenblasning) via intra-thoracala operationer. *Uppsala Lakaref Forh* 22: Suppl: 1-176, 1916-17; Ommexperientella lungexstirpationer. *Uppsala Lakaref Forh* 22: 1-109, 1916-17.

(20) Frenckner P. Bronchial and tracheal catheterization and its clinical applications. *Acta Otolaryngol* 1934; Suppl 20.

(21) Crafoord C. On the technique of pneumonectomy in man. A critical survey of the experimental and clinical development and a report on the author's material and technique. *Acta Chir Scand* 1938; **81** (Suppl 54): 1.

(22) Anderson CE, Crafoord C, Frenckner P. A new and practical method of producing rhythmic ventilation during positive pressure anesthesia. *Acta Otolaryngol* 1940; **28**: 95.

(23) Crafoord C. Pulmonary ventilation and anesthesia in major chest surgery. *J Thorac Surg* 1940; **9**: 237.

(24) Crafoord C. Thirty five years experience with controlled ventilation in thoracic surgery. In: Norlander, O. P., ed. *Int Anesth Clin* 1972; **10**: 1-9.

(25) Beecher HK. Principles of anesthesia for lobectomy and total pneumonectomy. *Acta Med Scand* 1938; **90**: 146. Principles, problems, practice of anesthesia for thoracic surgery. *Arch Surg* 1951; **62**: 206-38. Reprinted as a monograph with the same title by Charles C. Thomas, Springfield, IL, 1952.

(26) Mautz FR. Mechanical respirator as adjunct to closed system anesthesia. *Proc Soc Exp Biol* (NY) 1939; **42**: 190.

(27) Mautz FR. Mechanism for artificial pulmonary ventilation in operating room. *J Thorac Surg* 1941; **10**: 544.

(28) Beecher HK. Acidosis during thoracic surgery. *J Thorac Surg* 1950; **19**: 50–70.

(29) Gibbon JH. In discussion of Beecher HK, Murphy AJ. Acidosis during thoracic surgery. *J Thorac Surg* 1950; **19**: 69.

(30) Morch ET. Controlled respiration by means of special automatic machines as used in Sweden and Denmark. *Proc Roy Soc Med* 1947; **40**: 603–5.

(31) Nosworthy MD. Anaesthesia in chest surgery with special reference to controlled respiration and cyclopropane. *Proc Roy Soc Med* 1941; **34**: 479.

(32) Guedel AF, Treweek DM. Ether Apnea. *Anesth Analg* 1934; **13**: 263.

(33) Waters RM. Carbon dioxide absorption from anaesthetic atmospheres. *Proc Roy Soc Med* 1936; **30**: 11.

(34) Gray TC, Halton J. A milestone in anaesthesia? (d-tubocurarine chloride) *Proc Roy Soc Med* 1946; **39**: 400 also *Proc Roy Soc Med* 1948; **41**: 559.

(35) Geddes IC, Gray TC. Hyperventilation for the maintenance of anesthesia. *Lancet* 1959; **ii**: 4.

(36) Neff W, Mayer EC, Perales ML. Nitrous oxide and oxygen anesthesia with curare relaxation. *Calif Med J* 1947; **66**: 67.

(37) Neff W, Mayer EC, Thompson R. Nitrous oxide anesthesia without hypoxia. *Br Med J* 1950; **1**: 1400.

(38) Mushin WW, Rendell-Baker L. Pethidine as a supplement to nitrous oxide anaesthesia. *Br Med J* 1949; **2**: 472.

(39) Mushin WW, Rendell-Baker L. Intravenous pethidine and flaxedil in anesthesia for thoracic operations. *Br J Anaesth* 1950; **22**: 235.

(40) Mushin WW, Rendell-Baker L, Thompson PW, Mapleson WW. *Automatic ventilation of the lungs*, 2nd Ed. Oxford: Blackwell, 1969.

(41) Musgrove AH. Controlled respiration in thoracic surgery. A new mechanical respirator. *Anaesthesia* 1952; **7**: 77.

(42) Lassen HCA, ed. *Management of life-threatening poliomyelitis. Copenhagen 1952–1956.* Edinburgh: Livingstone, 1956.

(43) Ibsen B. The anaesthetist's viewpoint on the treatment of respiratory complication in poliomyelitis during the epidemic in Copenhagen 1952. *Proc Roy Soc Med* 1954; **47**: 72.

(44) Sjoberg A, Engstrom CG, Svanborg N. Diagnostiska och kliniska ron vid behandling av bulbospinal polio-myelit (med film och demonstration av ny respirator) *Nordisk Medicin* 1952; **47**: 536.

(45) Engstrom CG. Treatment of severe cases of respiratory paralysis by the Engstrom Universal Respirator. *Br Med J* 1954; **ii**: 666.

(46) Avery EE, Morch ET, Benson DW. Critically crushed chests; a new method of treatment with continuous mechanical hyperventilation to produce alkalotic apnea and internal pneumatic stabilization. *J Thorac Surg* 1956; **32**: 291.

(47) Astrup P. A simple electrometric technique for the determination of carbon dioxide tension in blood and plasma. *Scand J Clin Lab Invest* 1956; **8**: 33. Read also: Astrup, Poul and Severinghaus John W. *The history of blood gases, acids, and bases.* Copenhagen: Munksgaard, 1986.

(48) Clark LC. Monitor and control of blood and tissue oxygen tensions. *Trans Am Soc Artif Intern Organs* 1956; **2**: 41.

(49) Bjork VO, Engstrom CG. The treatment of ventilatory insufficiency after pulmonary resection with tracheotomy and prolonged artificial ventilation. *J Thorac Surg* 1955; **30**: 356.

(50) Allbritten FF, Haupt GJ, Amadeo JH. The change in pulmonary alveolar ventilation achieved by aiding the deflation phase of respiration during anesthesia for surgical operations. *Ann Surg* 1954; **140**: 569.

(51) Mushin WW, Rendell-Baker L, Thompson PW, Mapleson WW. *Automatic ventilation of the lungs*, 2nd Ed. Oxford: Blackwell, 1969.

(52) Frumin MJ. Clinical use of a physiological respirator producing N_2O amnesia-analgesia. *Anesthesiology* 1957; **18**: 290–9.

(53) Frumin MJ, Lee ASJ. Physiologically oriented artificial respirator which provided N_2O/O_2 anesthesia in man. *J Lab Clin Med* 1957; **49**: 617.

(54) Frumin MJ, Bergman NA, Holaday D *et al.* Alveolar-arterial differences during artificial respiration in man. *J Appl Physiol* 1959; **14**: 694.

(55) McIntyre RW, Laws AK, Ramachandran PR. Positive expiratory pressure plateau. Improved gas exchange during mechanical ventilation. *Can Anaesth Soc J* 1969; **16**: 477.

(56) Mushin WW, Rendell-Baker L, Thompson PW, Mapleson WW. *Automatic ventilation of the lungs*, 2nd Ed. Oxford: Blackwell, 1969.

(57) Frumin MJ, Lee ASJ, Papper EM. Intermittent positive pressure respirator. *Anesthesiology* 1960; **21**: 220.

(58) Mushin WW, Rendell-Baker L, Thompson PW. *Automatic ventilation of the lungs*. 1st Ed. Oxford: Blackwell, 1959.

(59) Kirshner JM, Horton BM. A brief history of fluidics (from the viewpoint of the Harry Diamond Laboratories). *7th National Fluidics Symposium*, Tokyo, 1972.

(60) Meyer JA, Joyce JW. The fluid amplifier and its application in medical devices. *Anesth Analg* 1968; **47**: 710.

(61) Emerson JH. Apparatus for vibrating portions of a patient's airway. US Patent No. 2918917 Washington DC U.S. Patent Office, Dec. 29, 1959.

(62) Oberg PA, Sjostrand U. Studies of blood pressure regulation I. Common carotid artery clamping in studies of the carotid sinus baroreceptor control of the systemic blood pressure. *Acta Physiol Scand* 1968; **75**: 276–87.

(63) Meltzer SJ, Auer J. Continuous respiration without respiratory movements. *J Exp Med* 1909; **11**: 622.

(64) Oberg PA, Sjostrand U. Studies of blood-pressure regulation I. Common-carotid artery clamping studies of the carotid-sinus baroreceptor control of the systemic blood pressure. *Acta Physiol Scand* 1969; **75**: 276.

(65) Sjostrand U. Experimental and clinical evaluation of high-frequency positive pressure ventilation HFPPV. *Acta Anaesth Scand* 1977; Suppl 64.

(66) Eriksson I, Heijman L, Sjostrand U. High frequency positive-pressure ventilation (HFPPV) in bronchoscopy during anesthesia. *Opusc Med* (Stockh) 1974; **19**: 14.

(67) Sjostrand U. High frequency positive pressure ventilation (HFPPV): A review. *Critical Care Med* 1980; **8**: 345–64.

(68) Sjostrand UH. High frequency positive pressure ventilation. *Int Anesth Clin* 1983; **21**: 59–81.

(69) Smith RB, Sjostrand UH. High frequency ventilation. *Int Anesth Clin* 1983; **21**: 3.

(70) Lunkenheimer PP, Rafflenbeul W, Keller H, Frank I, Dickhut HH, Fuhrmann C. Application of transtracheal pressure oscillations as a modification of "diffusion respiration". *Br J Anaesth* 1972; **44**: 627.

(71) Lunkenheimer PD. Intrapulmonaler gaswechsel unter simulierter apnoe durch transtrachealen periodishen intrathoraakalen druckwechsel. *Der Anaesthetist* 1973; **22**: 232–8.

(72) Draper WB, Whitehead RW. Diffusion respiration in the dog anesthetized by penthothal sodium. *Anesthesiology* 1944; **5**: 262–73.

(73) Draper WB, Whitehead RW, Spencer JN. Studies on diffusion respiration III. Alveolar gas and venous blood pH of dogs during diffusion respiration. *Anesthesiology* 1947; **8**: 524–33.

(74) Whitehead RW, Spencer JN, Parry TM, Draper WB. Studies on diffusion respiration IV. *Anesthesiology* 1949; **10**: 54–60.

(75) Draper WB, Whitehead RW. The phenomenon of diffusion respiration. *Anesth Analg* 1949; **28**: 307–18.

(76) Lunkenheimer PP, Lunkenheimer A, Laval P, Kleisbauer JP, Ising H. Experimental studies with high frequency oscillation. In: Smith, RB, Sjostrand Ulf eds. *High frequency ventilation. Int Anesth Clin* 1983; **21**:(3) 51–62.

(77) Lunkenheimer PP, Niederer P, Whimster WF, Strohl N, van Aken H. What is really about high frequency ventilation? In: *Pulmonary problems in intensive care medicine*. Inpharzam Medical forum 1986; **10**: 43–49.

(78) Lunkenheimer PP, Bossler R, Theissen J, *et al.* Hoch frequenz beatmung: Modell einer inhomogenen Ventilation. In: Lawin P ed. *Aktuelle Aspekte und Trends der respiratoreschen Therapie*. Berlin: Springer-Verlag 1987.

(79) Butler WJ, Bohn DJ, Bryan AC, Froese AB. Ventilation by high frequency oscillation in human. *Anesth Analg* 1980; **59**: 577–84.

(80) Smith RB, Babinski M, Petruscak J. A method for ventilating patients during laryngoscopy. *Laryngoscope* (St. Louis) 1972; **54**: 553.

(81) Smith RB, Lindholm EC, Klain M. Jet ventilation for fiberoptic brochoscopy under general anesthesia. *Acta Anaesth Scand* 1976; **20**: 111–6.

(82) Smith RB. Transtracheal ventilation during anesthesia. *Anesth Analg* 1974; **53**: 225.

(83) Klain M, Smith RB. Fluidic technology. *Anaesthesia* 1976; **31**: 750.

(84) Smith RB, Klain M. Experimental high frequency jet ventilation. In Smith RB, Sjostrand U, eds. *High frequency ventilation. Int Anesth Clin* 1983; **21**: 34.

(85) Jonzon A, Oberg PA, Sedin G, Sjostrand U. High frequency low tidal volume positive pressure ventilation. *Acta Physiol Scand* 1970; **80**: 21A.

(86) Klain M, Keszler H, Kalla R. New endotracheal tube for high frequency jet ventilation. *Crit Care Med* 1981; **9**: 191.

(87) Babinski M, Bunegin L, Smith RB, Hoff BH. Application of double lumen tracheal tube for HFV. *Anesthesiology* 1981; **55**: A370.

(88) Chakrabarti MK, Whitwam JG. A new valveless all purpose ventilator. *Br J Anaesth* 1983; **55**: 1005.

(89) Whitwam JG, Chakrabarti MK *et al.* A new valveless all purpose ventilator. *Br J Anaesth* 1983; **55**: 1017–23.

(90) Kirby RR, Robison EJ, Shulz J, deLemos R. A new pediatric volume ventilator. *Anesth Analg* 1971; **50**: 533.

(91) Ingelstedt S, Jonson B, Nordstrom L, Olsson SG. A servo-controlled ventilator measuring expired minute volume, airway flow and pressure. In Nordstrom L ed. *On automatic ventilation. Acta Anaesth Scand* 1972; **Suppl 47**: 9–28.

(92) Cox LA, Chapman EDW. A comprehensive volume cycled lung ventilator embodying feedback control. *Med Biol Eng* 1974; **12**: 160.

(93) Norlander O, Holmdahl MH, Matell G, Olofsson S, Westerholm KJ. Clinical experience with a new modular Engstrom Care System (ECS 2000) ventilator. In Arias A, Llaurado R, Nalda MA, Lunn JN, eds. *Recent progress in anesthesiology and resuscitation*. Amsterdam: Exerpta Medica, 516–8.

20.4   The polio epidemic in Copenhagen 1952

OLE SECHER
University Hospital, Copenhagen, Denmark

It all started on 24 July when the first patient with poliomyelitis was admitted to the Blegdam's Hospital—the fever hospital for Copenhagen. There was nothing really unusual in this because the 'yearly epidemics' usually started at this time. Within the first four weeks the number of

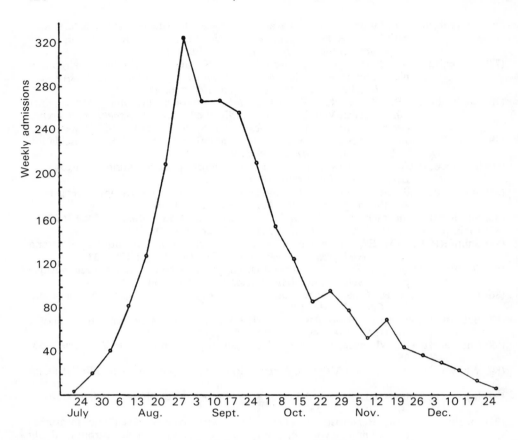

Figure 1   Weekly admissions to the Blegdam Hospital of cases of poliomyelitis.

patients admitted was steadily increasing and reached a total of about 260, which was more than previous years. The number of patients with paralysis was also unusually high as was the number of patients with affections of the respiratory function.

The first patients with this complication were treated as previously with the only available ventilators, the cuirass (six) and tank type (one) and they all died. This was not exceptional because so far only 15 patients out of 76 with respiratory affections had survived in the previous ten years (8). But gradually the number increased, and after three weeks there had been 31 patients with respiratory paralysis, out of whom 27 had died. So it became really serious, and the doctors were worried.

The 1952 Epidemic

Let me first say something about the epidemic to make it easier to understand the background for the events. The curve (Fig. 1 and Table 1) shows the weekly admissions of patients from 24 July, when the first patient arrived, until the end of December, when the number of new patients was very small. In the week from 28 August to 3 September, 335 patients came (almost 50 new cases per day). In all 2830 patients were admitted, out of whom 1235 had paralysis and 345 patients had impairment of respiration or the swallowing reflex or both. The number of patients and the severity of the disease were certainly unusual. At that time Copenhagen had a population of 1.2 million.

Table 1
Copenhagen polio epidemic 1952

Total number admitted	2830
Non-polio cases	589
Total number polio cases	2241
Non-paralytic polio cases	1006
Polio cases with paralysis	1235
Polio cases with respiratory and/or swallowing difficulties	345
Number of patients dead before new treatment	27
Number of patients treated after new principles	318
Number died during treatment	114
Number of patients survived	204
Total number of deaths	141

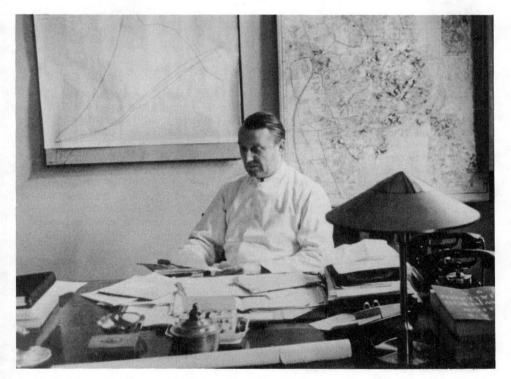

Figure 2   H. C. A. Lassen (1900–74). In the background is seen the epidemic curve and plotting on a map of Copenhagen.

Consultations

After the serious start of the epidemic the chief of the epidemic department Professor H. C. A. Lassen (1900–74) (Fig. 2) also got worried. He called in the professor of physiology, Einar Lundsgaard (1899–1968), to tell him if he thought they were doing something wrong. This was understandable, just as it was understandable that Professor Lundsgaard had no suggestions.

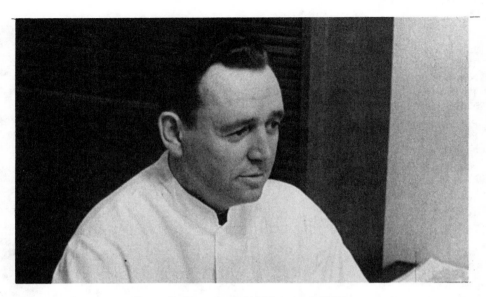

Figure 3   Bjørn Ibsen (1915–) about 1960.

In June of the same year one of the first-assistants at the hospital, Mogens Bjørneboe (1910–), had treated a child with neonatal tetanus together with Bjørn Ibsen (1915–) (Fig. 3).* The child was tracheostomized, had curare to prevent convulsions, and was ventilated. As long as this was done the child was well, but when treatment was continued in the traditional way with intravenous barbiturate, the child died from respiratory depression (2).

Bjørneboe was impressed with the results which could be obtained by such a treatment, and he suggested to Lassen that they should call in Ibsen to advise. Lassen was very much in doubt. What good could a young doctor from a discipline he hardly knew, tell old experienced epidemiologists, who had done all that was possible and even more, though they had no explanation of the cause of death? The hyperpyrexia was considered to be due to the cerebral affection *per se*. Before death the patients became warm, sweating with increased secretions and increasing levels of coma.

Next to the increasing number of patients with respiratory problems, the lack of ventilators was the most important factor for the decision to call for such a meeting with Ibsen. After it was all over Lassen expressed the situation this way:

> '*As the situation became worse we were soon faced with the intolerable dilemma of having to choose which patients to treat in the few respirators at hand, and which not to treat; we were therefore forced to seek new ways of ventilating our patients. The need for improvisation became imperative.*' (7)

A plan of action

A meeting took place on 25 August in Lassen's office. Present were Lassen, Ibsen, Bjørneboe, Fritz Neukirch (1906–) and some other doctors including Poul Astrup (1915–), who was chief of the laboratory for clinical chemistry in the hospital.

For the meeting Ibsen had brought a reprint of an article by A. G. Bower *et al.* (3) in Los Angeles, who had treated a number of polio patients with tracheostomy and an early use of

*In the spring of 1952 Ibsen had returned from a one year stay with Harry K. Beecher (1904–76) in Boston where he had trained in anaesthesia at the Massachusetts General Hospital. After his return he had worked as an anaesthetist at Rigshospitalet (University Hospital) administering anaesthesia for thoracic cases in the surgical department of Professor Erik Husfeldt (1901–84).

tank-ventilators in connection with an overpressure ventilation. By this method they had cut down the number of deaths considerably (3).

At the meeting the doctors received this information with doubts because they had tried early tracheostomy in 17 cases, and all the patients had died.

After a long discussion they went out to review the treatment of the patients. At the end they visited the pathology department where they saw four patients who had been treated with respirators. One of them, a 12-year-old boy, had lungs with almost no pathological changes, a last blood pressure of 160 mmHg and a serum bicarbonate of 44 mmol/l. This could only be interpreted as an accumulation of carbon dioxide, a clinical picture which was totally unknown to the internists. At that time most clinicians interpreted the condition as an *alkalosis* of a metabolic type.

It suddenly became obvious to Ibsen what was wrong with the treatment—the patients were underventilated due to the fact that the airways were not kept free. When the patients became cyanotic they were treated with oxygen, and the cyanosis disappeared, but the accumulation of carbon dioxide continued and it became more and more difficult for the patient to cooperate with the ventilator. The condition was identical to anaesthetized patients who were underventilated, and for this reason it should be possible to treat the patients with intubation and manual artificial ventilation with a technique used for anaesthesia for thoracic cases.

In the end it was decided that next day Ibsen should demonstrate the technique suggested by himself for future treatment.

A clinical trial

The day after, 26 August, Ibsen met Bjørneboe and Astrup at the laboratory where they planned the demonstration. For this purpose Bjørneboe had an oximeter, Astrup would make blood gas analyses and Ibsen could supply a carbon dioxide analyser and the anaesthesia equipment which was a Waters'—'to-and-fro' system (Fig. 4). This equipment was well known to anaesthetists, being used particularly for thoracic operations with open pleura due to the fact that it was easy to give positive pressure ventilation.

The plan was that Ibsen should take over the treatment of a patient who was being treated with a respirator, but who, it was thought, would probably die. For this purpose they selected a girl of 12 years (Vivi) with a pronounced respiratory insufficiency. She had atelectasis of the left lung and was fighting for breath due to secretions. Her body temperature was 40.2° and she was cyanotic.

A tracheostomy was performed under local anaesthesia and a catheter with a balloon was placed in the trachea. During this procedure she became unconscious. The airways were cleared by suction and a 'to-and-fro' system was attached, but it was impossible to ventilate her due to bronchospasm. At this time Ibsen was in a rather desperate situation, so the other doctors discreetly left the room. In order to relieve the bronchospasm and her fight for air, Ibsen gave her 100 mg thiopentone so that she stopped breathing, but could be ventilated. There was now time to clear her airways properly, and she soon regained a good colour and stopped sweating and producing secretions. When the other doctors came back they were rather astonished to see the patient in a good condition. The chest X-ray picture now showed a clear left lung.

Now that ventilation could be performed and the carbon dioxide (CO_2) level diminished, there came a drop in blood pressure and signs of hypovolaemic shock. She had a transfusion and recovered remarkably after this. With the oximeter and carbon dioxide analyser it was possible to obtain normal values. When the patient was treated again with a cuirass ventilator she went back into the former condition. The cyanosis reappeared and could be relieved by oxygen treatment, but with an increasing value of CO_2. By reapplying manual ventilation with CO_2-absorption the situation was totally reversed. To convince the epidemiologists that the theory and treatment was correct Ibsen could show that a change in ventilation was followed by changes in oxygen and carbon dioxide values.

It is interesting to note that Nielsen had written an article from Blegdam's Hospital in 1946 (8) stating that death in such case could be due to an increase in blood carbon dioxide, due to hypoventilation, increased deadspace and atelectasis caused by aspiration when the swallowing reflex is impaired. Even though it had been published six years before from the same hospital, it must have been forgotten (8).

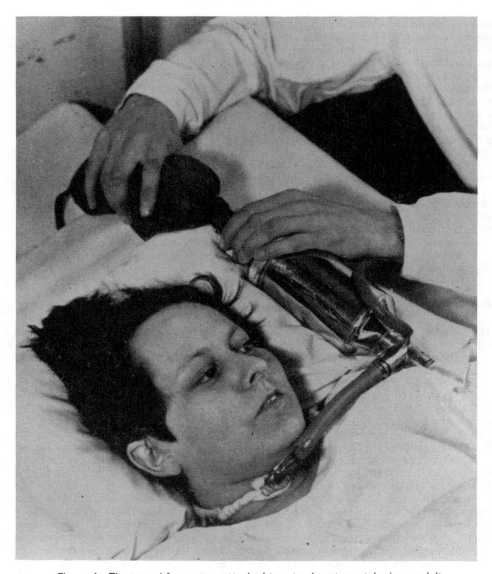

Figure 4   The to-and-fro system attached to a tracheostomy tube in an adult.

Ventilation on a large scale

After the successful demonstration it was agreed that manual ventilation was the treatment of choice. It was then decided to call in the senior anaesthesia doctors in Copenhagen. There were only six of them with, in all, about 20 others from different levels. At that time also the WHO-anaesthesia course was already established as Anaesthesiology Centre Copenhagen in 1950 (9), so in addition to the Danish anaesthetists there were ten foreign trainees who could help in the start.

Once a method of treatment had been decided, it was obvious that a group of helpers had to be organized. These were primarily medical students, but also dental students. The number of nurses had to be increased considerably (to about 250) and more physiotherapists and porters were required.

It was necessary to make up a team of four to six per patient, so each person ventilated the patient for four hours at a time. In one period there were 70 to 80 patients, who had to be ventilated, so about 450 students were involved. The anaesthesia doctors—who were entrusted with organizing all this—worked as supervisors and instructors and gave anaesthesia and intubated when the patients who were admitted had to have a tracheostomy. They also had to procure a large amount of equipment.

Later on it was possible to standardize the treatment and determine the indications for the different procedures. The standard treatment as suggested by Ibsen and followed during the epidemic was:

1. Early tracheostomy and maintenance of free airway.
2. Tracheostomy performed under general anaesthesia with intubation to avoid anoxic periods.
3. Using a rubber tracheostomy tube (a new invention) with cuff to secure manual ventilation and preventing aspiration of secretion.
4. Intermittent positive pressure ventilation with the to-and-fro system with CO_2-absorption to prevent CO_2-accumulation.
5. Removing secretion through the tracheostomy or bronchoscopy.
6. Physiotherapy.

As chief of epidemiology it was Lassen who took the responsibility for the establishing of the treatment.

Monitoring ventilation

A development of great importance in the treatment was Poul Astrup's acid-base estimation technique of arterial blood. When Ibsen had convinced the epidemiologists that it was possible to have good oxygenation together with CO_2 accumulation and a low pH in the blood, then it was logical to use these factors for a guide to when different steps in treatment should be taken (1).

The majority of patients required a great number of blood-gas estimations, and this stimulated Astrup and his coworkers to invent new and more accurate equipment and to introduce a new terminology: Standard bicarbonate and base-excess.

Results

A great number of patients had to be ventilated over a very long period. One hundred and two patients had to be ventilated for more than one month, and 40 for more than half a year. Twenty-five patients became chronic ventilator patients. Among the patients who had to be ventilated for six months or more, half were children from 1–14 years of age. It was a new group of patients, hardly seen before.

The overall death rate was 42%, and the main complications which caused death had an incidence of 8–39% and were, shock, hyperpyrexia, uraemia, kidney-stones, pulmonary oedema, ileus and hypertension.

Soon it became evident that humidification of the inspiratory air was necessary when automatic ventilators and dry gases were used. When this was done, the ventilation could take place over a very long period without respiratory problems. Also very few complications were seen from the tracheostomy tubes, when this precaution had been taken.

Subsequent developments

There was no doubt that Ibsen's suggestions regarding treatment were a success, and doctors from other countries came to study, adopt and modify that treatment. When the epidemic came to Denmark and other countries in Scandinavia and to England the following year, they were well prepared.

In 1953 Ibsen became anaesthetist, and in 1954 chief anaesthetist, at the Kommunehospital (Municipal Hospital) in Copenhagen, and here he established the first intensive care unit in a general hospital. This was probably as big a step forward as the treatment of polio. It was a natural consequence of the experience gained during the epidemic. New groups of patients could benefit from the same kind of treatment. These included cases of polyneuritis, tetanus, post-operative respiratory insufficiency chest injuries and severe poisoning; all were patients who had previously had a poor prognosis.

Conclusion

The poliomyelitis epidemic in 1952 was one of the most severe in modern times, but it certainly started some developments of great importance—intensive care units primarily for ventilatory cases, construction of mechanical ventilators, humidifiers, tubes and accessories and equipment for monitoring patients. It also showed that anaesthesia had something to offer to general medical treatment.

Sir Robert Macintosh once said to Ibsen:

'Bjørn you are the one who brought the anaesthetist out of the operating room.'

References

(1) Astrup P, Severinghaus J. *The history of blood gases, acids and bases.* Copenhagen: Munksgaard, 1985.
(2) Bjørneboe M, Ibsen B, Johnsen S. Et tilfaelde af tetanus behandlet med curarisering, tracheostomy og overtryksventilation med kvaelstofforilte og ilt. *Ugeskr Laeger* 1953; **115**: 1535-7.
(3) Bower AG, Bennett VR, Dillon JB, Axelson B. Investigation on care and treatment of poliomyelitis patients. *Ann West Med Surg* 1950; **4**: 561–82.
(4) Ibsen B. Poliomyelitis from the anaesthetist's point of view. *Proc Roy Soc Med* 1954; **47**: 72–4. *Dan Med Bull* 1954; **1**: 9–12.
(5) Ibsen B. Organisation of treatment of respiratory complications in poliomyelitis. *The Medical Press* 1954; **232**: 448–50.
(6) Ibsen B. Personal communication, 1987.
(7) Lassen HCA, ed. *Management of life-threatening poliomyelitis.* London: Livingstone, 1956.
(8) Nielsen EM. Om respiratorbehandling af respirations-pareser ved poliomyelitis anterior acuta. *Ugeskr Laeger* 1946; **108**: 1341–48.
(9) Secher O. Anaesthesiology Centre Copenhagen. In: Rupreht J, van Lieburg MJ, Lee Ja, Erdmann W, eds. *Anaesthesia—Essays on its history.* Berlin, Heidelberg: Springer-Verlag, 1985: 321–34.

21.1   The origins of today's stored blood transfusion practice:
the contribution of Albert Hustin

HENRI REINHOLD[1] and CLAIRE BERNARD-DICHSTEIN[2]
[1]Université Libre de Bruxelles and
[2]Musée, Centre Public d'Aide Sociale, Brussels, Belgium

It is not exceptional that a major discovery resulted from research initially pursuing quite a different purpose. Such was the case with the important contribution of Albert Hustin to the development of blood transfusion.

Albert Hustin

Albert Hustin (Fig. 1) was born in 1882 in Ethe, in the extreme south of Belgium. Now, 1800 people live there but, at the time, it was a village of less than a thousand inhabitants. His grandfather had been a farmer but although Albert's parents still owned the farm, they had risen in social rank; his father was the town clerk of Ethe and his mother a school teacher. Albert studied medicine at Brussels University. In May 1906, as a final year student, he had the opportunity to visit the USA. He decided to take this special opportunity and postponed his final examination until the end of the year. This was an expression of his already great intellectual curiosity, which remained a feature of his personality. He himself described it as 'angoisse scientifique' ('anguish for learning'). An account which he published of his visit to American hospitals (1), reveals an acute sense of observation and a burning enthusiasm for his medical work.

After qualification, Hustin went for further training to Paris in 1906 and to Heidelberg in 1907. In 1908, he started his hospital career at the University Hospital St Jean, under the guidance of Professor Jean Verhoogen. In 1913, he was promoted 'adjoint' (medical assistant) in the department of surgery, whose Head at that time was the famous Professor Antoine Depage. That same year he defended a thesis on the role of the duodenal hormone secretion in the triggering of the external secretion of the pancreas, timed by meal absorption (2). He thus obtained the title of 'Docteur Special de l'Université Libre de Bruxelles'.

During a ward round in 1913, Hustin was confronted with a dramatic case of a patient expiring from carbon monoxide poisoning. At the time such tragic situations were far from rare. The fuel used for lighting and cooking was mostly water gas obtained from passing steam and oxygen through red hot coke. It contained about 15% carbon monoxide and up to 40% hydrogen. It is known that a concentration of 0.5% carbon monoxide is rapidly fatal and that 0.1% causes deep coma. Pondering on this problem, Hustin wondered whether it would be possible to withdraw some of the patient's blood, maintain it for some time in its fluid state by preventing coagulation, submit it to oxygen under pressure to eliminate the toxic gas and finally to return his own purified blood to the patient (3).

Hustin's work on preventing coagulation of blood

The only method generally employed to avoid coagulation outside the body at that time was to shake it with glass beads. Hustin had used the procedure for his experiments on perfusion of the pancreas (2), but studies on intact animals had shown that the injection of defibrinated blood was not compatible with survival. Hustin therefore decided to undertake an investigation in the laboratory of physiology of the Institut Solvay in order to find a chemical method able to inhibit the coagulation of blood without altering its physiological qualities.

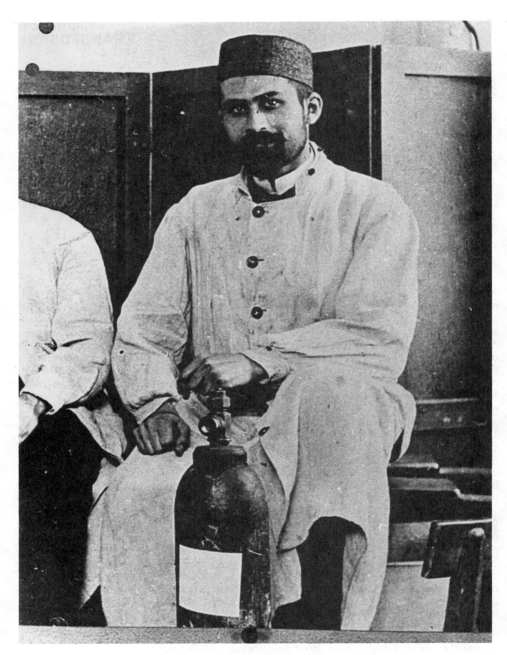

Figure 1   Albert Hustin, around the age of 30.

He started to explore the effects on blood coagulation of various solutions currently used in laboratory work. The results of these tests are summarized in Table 1. The figures show that coagulation is retarded by dilution of the blood, more so in the absence of calcium ions contained in Ringer's solution, and most by a solution in glucose without electrolytes (4). The latter diluent, nevertheless, had the inconvenience of causing a flocculation of the blood.

Table 1

The effect of various diluent solutions on the clotting time of blood

Blood (ml)	Diluent (ml)	Diluent Type	Clotting time (min)
8	12	NaCl 0.9%	5
8	12	Ringer	5
2	18	Ringer	16
2	18	NaCl 0.9%	90
2	18	Gluc. 5%	180

Adapted from A Hustin (4)

Hustin therefore set out to search for an agent possessing a dispersing effect, in order to oppose the flocculation.

In 1913, a fair amount of knowledge had been gathered in bacteriology and immunology. A colleague of Hustin in Brussels, Octave Gengou, investigating the physical chemistry of bacterial agglutination by antibodies, had made experiments with fine suspensions of solid matter such as mastic; he succeeded in slowing down precipitation of the particles by the addition of sodium citrate (5). This finding suggested to Hustin the possible effect of citrate on the flocculation of red cells induced by glucose solution. His experiments showed that adding to blood in a test tube the same volume of glucose 5% solution containing 0.2% sodium citrate, delayed the coagulation more than 30 minutes without causing flocculation, haemolysis, alteration of erythrocytes, or the production of meth-aemoglobin (4).

Hustin then proceeded to animal trials. He collected 100 ml of blood from dogs, added his glucose-citrate mixture and, half an hour to one hour and a half later, injected the fluid into other dogs. This was repeated ten times. All the animals behaved normally and none had glucosuria or albuminuria. On certain dogs he gave the injection into the carotid artery and checked that there was no thrombosis or embolism.

Having obtained these satisfying results, Hustin decided to undertake the first human trial. The details are written up in his laboratory note-book, on a page dated 27 March, 1914. The patient was a man of 20 years, severely anaemic because of bleeding from the large bowel. He received 150 ml of blood prepared by his method and was well afterwards, without any abnormal symptom.

Hustin wrote a paper on his discovery and commented on the numerous advantages of the new method. As it was the result of laboratory research, he published his first paper in the *Annales et Bulletin de la Société Royale des Sciences Médicales et Naturelles de Bruxelles* (4) (a scientific journal in publication for 72 years), in the April, 1914 issue. A nearly identical text appeared on 6 August, 1914, in the *Journal Medical de Bruxelles* (6), a periodical intended more for medical practitioners. This was important because, in 1914, the international exchange of scientific periodicals was not as wide as it is at present, although the *Journal Medical de Bruxelles* was dispatched regularly to New York.

On 4 August, 1914, the World War broke out. Two months later, on 9 October, the port of Antwerp was captured by the German army. The copies of the *Journal Medical de Bruxelles*, containing Hustin's article, reached the USA, probably with one of the last postal dispatchings leaving the harbour. Thus reference to Hustin's paper was cited in the *Index Medicus* dated 14 October, 1914 (7).

In the meantime, Belgium had become an appalling battlefield and the country was crushed by war. The Hustin family was painfully affected when on 22 August, 1914, Albert Hustin's father was executed by the German military authorities together with other citizens of Ethe.

On the other side of the Atlantic Ocean life remained normal. There was even some economic prosperity, favourable to all human activities.

The controversy about priority

As Hustin's paper shows, the importance of his discovery was clear to him and it also appeared to be so to other contemporary medical men. Soon, however, a controversy broke out, similar to that which happened in 1846, after the discovery of surgical anaesthesia, concerning the introduction of the use of sodium citrate as an anticoagulant for blood transfusion (Table 2).

On 17 December, 1914, eight months after Hustin's first publication Richard Lewisohn announced at a meeting of the New York Academy of Medicine, that he had used hirudine and sodium citrate as an anticoagulant for blood transfusion and that the latter had given good results (8). At this same session, Richard Weil also spoke of his use of citrate for blood transfusion. Neither of them mentioned Hustin, although reference to his work had appeared two months before in the *Index Medicus*. The *Annales et Bulletin de la Société Royale des Sciences Médicales et Naturelles* also arrived in America in due course and Hustin's first article (4) is referred to later by Rueck in April, 1916 (5). On 23 January, 1915, Lewisohn published his first paper on citrated blood transfusion in the *Medical Record* (10); at the end of it, he cites Hustin of Brussels, whose work he had read after he had started his own trials. A week later, Richard Weil published his first paper on the subject in the *Journal of the American Medical Association* (11). Shortly after, on 27 February, 1915, a fourth person, G. A. Rueck (5,12) claimed credit for the discovery in the *Medical Record*. Finally in Buenos Aires a fifth protagonist appeared; in January, 1915, Luis Agote described a 'new' method of blood transfusion with the use of sodium citrate, presenting it as his invention, which he may have started using in November, 1914 (13).

In fact, in the *Medical Record* of 13 March, 1915, at a time at which Hustin was not able to enter the debate, Lewisohn recognized Hustin's right of priority (14), but in later papers—one in German on 25 August, 1915 (15), and one in French on 15 October, 1919 (16)—Hustin is not mentioned.

The use of citrated blood in World War I

Notwithstanding the early dispute on priority and the enormous potential lifesaving of the new method in the theatre of war, it remained shelved for three more years. Significant experience of citrated blood transfusion only began following 2 April, 1917, when the US joined the Allies in the war, bringing over their enormous support in men, equipment and supplies.

In France, E. Hedon (17) and E. Jeanbrau (18) introduced the method in 1917. For many years, they were described in the French medical literature as the fathers of the invention. Only in 1940 did G. Jeanneney correct this (19). Even in 1951, in a popular treatise on blood transfusion, included in a collection of great discoveries and written by the highly respected authors Paul Chevalier and Jean Moulinier, Hedon is presented as inventor of the method (20).

Table 2

References to the early usage of citrated blood transfusion

Date	Author	Source
27 March, 1914	Hustin	Laboratory notes
April, 1914	Hustin	*Bull Soc Roy Sc Med Nat*
6 August, 1914	Hustin	*J Med Bruxelles*
14 October, 1914	Hustin	*Index Medicus*
17 December, 1914	Lewisohn	Meeting N.Y. Acad. Med
17 December, 1914	Weil	Id.
23 January, 1915	Lewisohn	*Med Record*
30 January, 1915	Weil	*JAMA*
January, 1915	Agote	*An del Inst Modelo de Clin Med*
27 February, 1915	Rueck	*Med Record*

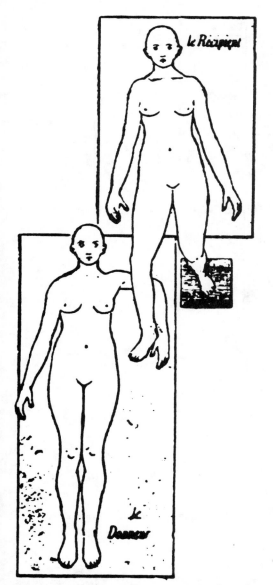

Figure 2   Transfusion by anastomosis of arteria radialis and vena saphena (23).

Discussion

Facts and dates leave no doubt on Hustin's right of priority and some striking differences exist between Hustin's publication and those of the others. Hustin describes precisely the thread of thought he followed, starting with the initial problem, progressing to experiments in test tubes and trials on animals and finally the step of clinical application. An explanation for the choice of citrate is not given in the papers of the others except by Rueck (12).

Does it mean that the other authors can be accused of plagiarism? Such a severe moral condemnation ought not to be pronounced without calling forth some palliating circumstances. Hustin's paper, cited in the *Index Medicus*, read by some, may have been brought up now and then during hospital conversations. This may have induced others to undertake personal trials. Autosuggestion may have increased misunderstanding. Several of the protagonists later contributed significantly to the development of the transfusion practice.

Hustin himself must be credited particularly for his honesty. He acknowledged that, when he searched the literature after his successful work, he found that in 1902 Sabattini (21) had described the anticoagulant properties of citrate, although he did not draw any attention to possible clinical use.

Here again there is an analogy with the history of anaesthesia. In the year 1800 Humphry Davy pointed out that breathing nitrous oxide had a soothing effect on his headaches and toothaches. He advanced the idea that use of this property could be made for surgical operations. No clinician acted on this important observation and another half century passed before the introduction of surgical anaesthesia.

The question of priority aside, the outstanding significance of the discovery of the anticoagulant properties of citrate must be stressed. Before Landsteinter (22) started in 1901 to lay down the immunological foundations of human blood groups, attempts at transfusions were bound to lead to catastrophes. The knowledge gained from the work of this brilliant scientist made blood transfusion, not only a safe, but an essential means of circulatory resuscitation, but the practice of transfusion remained highly difficult and recourse to it was exceptional. The process of coagulation, precipitated by the contact of blood with any surface other than vascular endothelium, obliged clinicians either to avoid such a contact by performing a vascular anastomosis between donor and receiver (Figs. 2, 3, 4) or to attempt to avoid the physiological process of coagulation by pumping the blood from one vessel to the other as fast as they could (Fig. 5). Coating the

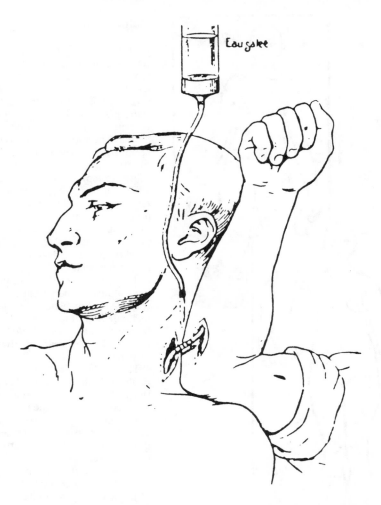

Figure 3   Transfusion by anastomosis of arteria ulnaris and vena jugularis externa (23).

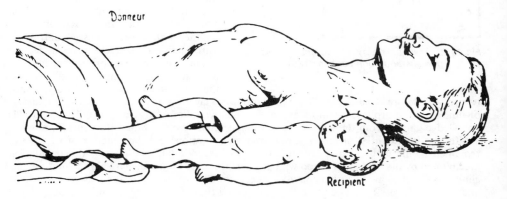

Transfusion to a child by anastomosis of arteria radialis and vena femoralis (23).

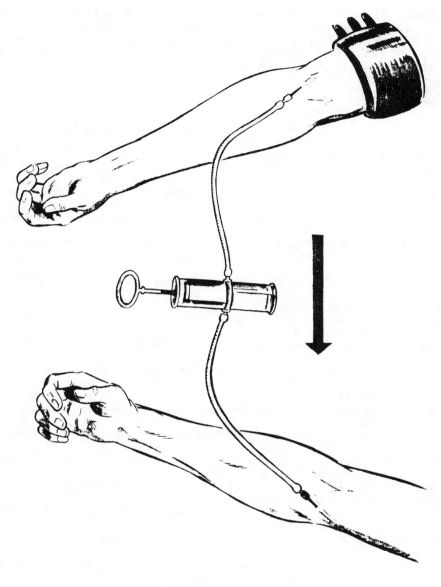

Figure 5   Transfusion from vein to vein by syringe.

instruments with liquid paraffin doubled the available time before clotting occurred. With either technique, donor and recipient had to lie next to one another, during the whole procedure and clearly, this was not compatible with the requirements of surgery and anaesthesia.

Progress in science and medicine may follow a chain to which, during the flow of years, new links are continually added. Some are small and just secure the continuity of the chain but others stand out because of greater importance. In the history of blood transfusion such notable links are Richard Lower of Oxford and Jean Baptiste Denis of Montpellier, both of whom had the audacity during the 17th century to inject lamb's blood to a patient,

James Blundell of London, who transfused blood from man to man; Karl Landsteiner, who, from the year 1900 on, defined the four main human blood groups and in 1940 identified the Rhesus factor; and finally Albert Hustin, whose discovery in 1914 made possible the use of stored blood, the creation of blood banks and the lifesaving accomplishments of today's work in the operating theatre and intensive care unit.

References

(1) Hustin A. Interne à l'Hôpital St Pierre: Quelques notes sur les hôpitaux de Philadelphie. *J Méd Bruxelles* 1906; **32**: 1–14.
(2) Hustin A. La secrétion externe du pancréas. *Arch Int Physiol* 1912–1913.
(3) Coquelet O. L'oeuvre scientifique d'Albert Hustin. In: *Livre Jubilaire au Dr Albert Hustin* Bruxelles: Imprimerie des Sciences, 1954: VII–XXXIV.
(4) Hustin A. Note sur une nouvelle méthode de transfusion. *Ann Bull Soc Roy Sci Méd Naturelles Bruxelles* 1914; **72**: 104–11.
(5) Rueck GA. The method of transfusion of blood treated with sodium citrate. *Med Record* 1916; **89**: 688–92.
(6) Gengou O. Contribution à l'étude de l'adhésion moléculaire et de son intervention dans différents phénomènes biologiques. *Arch Int Physiol* 1980; **VII**: Fascicules 1 & 2.
(7) Hustin A. Principe d'une nouvelle méthode de transfusion. *J Méd Bruxelles* 1914; **19**: 436–9.
(8) *Index Medicus* 1914 October 14, **XII**: 1115.
(9) Lewisohn R. New York Academy of Medicine. Meeting of 17 December 1914. *Med Record* 1915; **87**: 162–4.
(10) Lewisohn R. A new and greatly simplified method of blood transfusion. *Med Record* 1915; **87**: 141–2.
(11) Weil R. Sodium citrate in the transfusion of blood. *JAMA* 1915; **64**: 425–6.
(12) Rueck GA. Transfusion of blood by the gravitation method. *Med Record* 1915; **87**: 354.
(13) Agote L. Nuove procedimiento par la transfusion de sangre. *Anales Instit Modelo Clin Medicina* 1915; **1** no. 2.
(14) Lewisohn R. Priority in the use of citrated blood for infusion. Correspondence. *Med Record* 1915; **87**: 448.
(15) Lewisohn R. Eine neue, sehr einfache Methode der Bluttransfusion. *Münchener Med Wochenschr* 1915; **LXII**: 708–9.
(16) Lewisohn R. La transfusion du sang citraté. *La Presse Médicale* 1919; **27**: 593–4.
(17) Hedon E. *La Presse Médicale*, 1917 March 5.
(18) Jeanbrau E. Un procédé simple de transfusion du sang. *Bull Mémoires Soc Chirurg Paris* 1917; **XLIII**: 1571.
(19) Jeanneney G, Ringenbach G. *Traité de la transfusion sanguine*. Paris: Masson, 1940.
(20) Chevalier P, Moulinier J. *La Transfusion sanguine*. Paris: Correa, 1951 (Collection 'Les Grandes Découvertes scientifiques').
(21) Sabattini. *Bull Mémoires Soc Biologie 1902*, p. 717. (Quoted in 'Hustin A. Renouveau de la transfusion sanguine au début du XXe siècle. *Acta Chirurgica Belgica* 1960; **59**: 762–781').
(22) Landsteiner K. Über Agglutinationerscheinungen normalen menschlichen Blutes. *Wiener klinische Wochenschrift* 1901; **14**: 1132.
(23) Guillot M, Dehelly G, Morel L. *La Transfusion du sang* Paris: A. Maloine & Fils, 1917.

21.2   The history of the permanent intravenous cannula

T. GORDH
Karolinska Syukhuset, Stockholm, Sweden

Heparin was introduced in the late 1930s for prevention of thrombosis after operations. Postoperative thrombosis was then a dangerous and life threatening complication. The heparin was injected intravenously every 4 hours around the clock. Thore Olovson was a surgeon at St Görans Hospital, Stockholm, and considered these repeated injections disturbing both for the patients and the staff.

A needle for repeated injections

Olovson and an engineer (Meyer) at the instrument firm Stille-Werner in Stockholm, constructed a special needle for the purpose of repeated injections. It was simply an injection needle with a wing at the head end and provided with a rubber membrane inserted in a detachable ring (Fig. 1). This needle could be placed in a vein at the dorsal aspect of the hand, the forearm or the foot and was fixed with a tape over the wing. This needle could stay in position for several days and still be patent for injections.

The heparin injections were made through the rubber membrane without disturbing the patient. Olovson described his needle in the German periodical *'Der Chirurg'* 1940 and called it 'Heparine-needle' (1).

Use of the needle in anaesthesia

In 1940 the writer arrived back to Sweden after training with Ralph Waters in Madison, Wisconsin, USA, and started as the first anaesthetist in Sweden at the Karolinska Hospital,

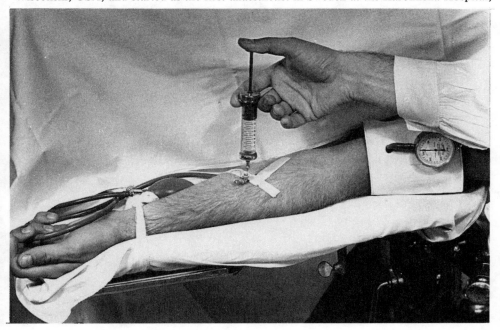

Figure 1

Stockholm. When he was shown the Olovson needle by Mr Meyer at Stille-Werner, it was like a gift from heaven. It was introduced for intravenous anaesthesia and later an inlet was added at the end for an intravenous drip and blood transfusion.

Conclusion

The Olovson needle has been modified in many ways and in many places, and has even been given other names (1). However, Olovson's simple and useful needle is the origin behind all the modifications, even the plastic disposable ones used today.

Before this needle was introduced we had to fix the syringe for intravenous anaesthesia with its needle with a tape on the forearm and even special syringeholders were devised. Intravenous fluid was seldom given and if so by the same 'cut down' method as for blood transfusions.

Olovson died this year (1987) at the age of 83 and in the obituary I wrote that anaesthetists, nurses and patients from all over the world could send him a grateful thought.

I found this needle of such important and practical value that I reported it (2) in *Anesthesiology* 1945 with Olovson as the only reference. This, and the fact that after the war many anaesthetists visited the Karolinska Hospital and saw me using the needle, maybe made them wrongly call it the Gordh needle. This paper could also have had the title 'The true story about the Gordh needle'.

References

(1) Olovson T. *Der Chirurg* 1940; **12**.
(2) Gordh T. *Anesthesiology* 1945; **6**.

Chapter 22
PULMONARY AND CARDIAC SURGERY AND RESUSCITATION

22.1	Memories of thoracic anaesthesia before the Second World War

RUTH E MANSFIELD, MBE
Brompton Hospital, London, UK

Magill (1) wrote in 1967:

> *'Many of the notable advances in chest surgery which have been made since the end of the First World War would not have been possible without concurrent advances in anaesthesia.'*

This was acknowledged by the thoracic surgeon Tudor Edwards (2) who also pointed out that methods of anaesthesia depended upon whether the pleura was opened or adherent:

> *'In the former case some method of positive pressure is essential, whereas in cases such as for chronic empyema, such a dense fibrous barrier was formed over the lung surface there was less interference with the mechanism of respiration. Hence, the use of regional analgesia with a cough reflex was feasible.'*

This paper presents personal memories of the period between 1935–1939, mainly at the Brompton Hospital. Most of the patients had pulmonary tuberculosis with a positive sputum and were in poor condition, often with an empyema or broncho-pleural fistula. Those with bronchiectasis had copious sputum which had to be controlled. There were no antibiotics, until the sulphonamides became available, and no antituberculous drugs, no relaxants, ventilators, or blood banks as we know them, (the National Blood Bank Service was not organized until after the war) and the open thorax presented the problem of paradoxical respiration and mediastinal flap (3).

Staffing

The only 'staff' anaesthetist before the War at the Brompton Hospital was the anaesthetist to the Ear, Nose and Throat Department. The thoracic departments were served by a list of visiting anaesthetists as required. These included such famous people as Ivan Magill, Langton Hewer, Frankis Evans, Rait-Smith, Machray, Rink and others.

There were no Anaesthetic Registrars, senior house officers or residents. It was only later, after the war, that part-time staff anaesthetists were appointed and a Senior Registrar was shared half-time with the Westminster Hospital. Assistance for the anaesthetist was provided by a theatre technician including the redoubtable Crowley. Crowley's job was to look after the anaesthetic machine, sterilize the endotracheal, endobronchial tubes and blockers, check the bronchoscopes, bring the patient into the theatre (as there was no anaesthetic room at that time), put up the X-rays and position the patient after induction, and postoperatively strap the chest firmly after excision of ribs, to prevent paradox. He was an invaluable help to the anaesthetist and then very badly paid (£11 a week!). Magill encouraged the upgrading of theatre technicians and the formation of the 'Association of Theatre Technicians' of which Crowley was a founder member.

Drugs

Nitrous oxide, oxygen, chloroform, and cyclopropane were used. Ether was avoided at the Brompton because of its irritating effect on the bronchial tree. Pentobarbitone, hexobarbitone

443

or thiopentone were used for induction. The local analgesic agents procaine, amethocaine, and cinchocaine, were available for regional blocks or spinal analgesia.

Monitoring and fluid replacement

Monitoring was clinical and basic, and was confined to observation of the patient's colour, pulse and blood pressure. Rectal saline was used for fluid replacement and on occasion it dripped into the surgeon's boot. Postoperatively, if necessary, a blood donor was obtained and cross-matched with the patient's blood before administration.

The surgery

The operations undertaken can be considered in two groups—those on the chest wall, and intrathoracic procedures which involved the problem of paradoxical respiration and mediastinal flap and which without controlled ventilation led to death. Earlier Sauerbruch (4) endeavoured to overcome this by having the patient and surgeon in a negative pressure chamber to keep the lung inflated while the patient's head and the anaesthetist were outside.

Operations on the chest wall

These operations were mainly thoracoplasties for pulmonary tuberculosis with cavitation to collapse the lungs, and were suitable for regional block. Premedication was with phenobarbitone 200 mg two hours preoperatively, followed by papaveretum 15–20 mg with hyosine 0.2 mg one hour preoperatively and, if not sleepy enough, a small dose of intravenous opiate was sometimes given. Procaine was used for rapid effect and amethocaine for a prolonged effect with added adrenaline for haemostasis. An intercostal block of two ribs above and below those to be resected was performed and then infiltration of the line of incision using a weaker solution. A more satisfactory method was later introduced, a brachial plexus and paravertebral block followed by infiltration.

The number of ribs resected depended on whether the underlying lung was soft and, if so, fewer ribs were resected at each stage to prevent 'mediastinal flap'.

Early cases of general anaesthesia for thoracoplasty were done under nitrous oxide and oxygen by the endotracheal route with chloroform or ethylene as adjuvant, with intermittent suction as necessary. In 1936 Waters (5) visited the United Kingdom and popularized cyclopropane in thoracic surgery. It was thought to be an advantage as it was not irritating and could be used with a high percentage of oxygen. However, although effective in low concentration, it was expensive and very explosive, so had to be given in a closed circuit with carbon dioxide absorption using a Water's (6) canister. The gas inlet was near the patient, so the bag was free for intermittent positive pressure and adequate ventilation. This was probably the 'beginning' of controlled respiration. If the pleura was opened, respiration was controlled to prevent paradoxical respiration or mediastinal flap described later by Nosworthy (3) in 1941. Because of its explosive property, cyclopropane could only be used on the chest wall and then only provided there was no leak in the apparatus. Diathermy was a prohibitive hazard.

In cases of *empyema*, rib resection and drainage was usually performed under local anaesthesia by the surgeon; if a broncho-pleural fistula was present the patient was sat up, leaning over a Mayo table or other support.

Intrathoracic operations

These presented the problems of the open pleura, paradoxical respiration and mediastinal flap, particularly if the patient was operated on in the lateral position, and also the problem of sputum control.

With general anaesthesia in the lateral position, the anaesthetist had to protect the sound lung. Endotracheal anaesthesia with intermittent suction was the only way until blockers or endobronchial tubes were introduced. Magill first used a gum elastic suction catheter with a small rubber balloon fixed to the distal end and placed in the bronchus to be resected by direct vision through a bronchoscope. On the first occasion he did not tell the surgeon what he had done and neither did the surgeon inform him when he was about to clamp and divide the bronchus. So a few words were exchanged when a foreign body was found in the specimen!

The developed Magill blocker was a long, narrow, double rubber tube with an inflatable latex cuff at the distal end, for blocking the bronchus, the small tube for inflating the cuff was moulded into the wall of the larger suction tube. A stilette through the suction tube was used for introduction through a small 8–9 mm bronchoscope and removed after a cuffed endotracheal tube was placed alongside for ventilation of the lung and lobe which remained unblocked. The lung or lobe beyond the blocker was deflated and secretions drained or sucked out.

Later Thompson designed a larger blocker which could only be introduced through an 11 mm bronchoscope and there was an increased leak between the blocker and the endotracheal tube.

When the bronchus was about to be clamped, the balloon was deflated, the blocker withdrawn, aspirating at the same time.

In 1936 Magill (7) described an armoured endobronchial tube made of latex over a wire spiral, with the lower 3 cm uncovered (Fig. 1), so that the right upper lobe, which was near the carina could be ventilated. A large cuff was inflated at carinal level and the tube was introduced under direct vision over a straight Magill bronchoscope.

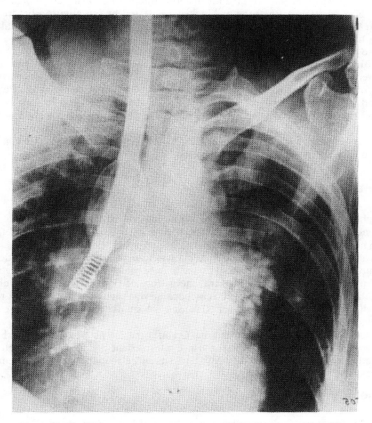

Figure 1   X-ray of the Magill armoured right endobronchial tube in position. The large balloon is at the carinal level. Ruth Mansfield, Richard Jenkins. Practical Anaesthesia for Lung Surgery, *Fig. 21.*

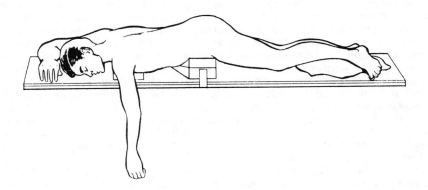

*The Parry Brown position. The diseased lung is uppermost to facilitate drainage of the secretions (after Parry Brown. Thorax 1948; **3**: 161). Ruth Mansfield, Richard Jenkins.* Practical Anaesthesia for Lung Surgery, *Fig. 17.*

Without any relaxant, the pharynx, larynx and bronchial tree were anaesthetized as for a bronchoscopy. It was then safe to give intravenous thiopentone just before bronchoscoping the patient. The position of the tube or blocker was tested by auscultation before and after positioning. To prevent coughing during the resection, the surgeon injected local analgesic around the hilum.

The prone position could be used to control secretions if the surgeon was willing to operate in this position. Overholt (8) had the affected side lower than the sound side, so that the secretions were retained. This needed an expensive Overholt table while the airway was controlled with an endotracheal tube with suction if necessary. The abdomen was left free. Parry Brown (9) described a simpler method with wooden blocks, padded with sorbo rubber. A block was placed under the shoulder girdle and another under the pelvis, leaving the abdomen free and with the affected lung uppermost and free drainage into the trachea, which was aspirated by the anaesthetist crouched under the table (Fig. 2). As blockers were unsuitable for small children with sputum, the prone position was the method of choice.

Spinal analgesia for thoracotomy

It was thought that no irritating inhalation vapours should be used on patients with lung disease, so spinal analgesia seemed a 'way out' as the patient had 'relative' control of his cough reflex but the method did not take into account paradoxical respiration with the open chest. Between 1937 and 1939 spinal analgesia was used for lobectomies but was found to be unsuitable for older patients.

Magill, having tried the Howard Jones (10) technique, changed to that of Etherington Wilson (11). After premedication he gave an intravenous dose of pentobarbitone, enough to make the patient drowsy but not asleep. 1:1500 cinchocaine was then administered with the patient sitting up with the head bent forward for 60 seconds. A small dose of 8–10 ml gave segmental thoracic anaesthesia.

We had many important visitors at that time. On one occasion I started to explain that we used the Etherington Wilson technique, when the visitor informed me that he was Etherington Wilson.

Harris and Rink (12) in 1937 used a 'unilateral spinal', also employing 1:1500 cinchocaine.

Physiotherapy

It was realized that preoperative preparation, in cases of bronchiectasis with copious sputum, helped to improve the preoperative condition of the patient. Misses McDowell, Evans and

Gaskell (13) at the Brompton, used various positions to drain each lobe affected, using percussion over the posterior aspect of the chest and vibrations in all areas daily until the day of the operation. The patient was also taught preoperatively the chest movements he had to perform postoperatively, so that the remaining portions of the lung following lobectomy or segmented resection could expand as quickly as possible and, following penumonectomy, the base of the remaining lung could be used efficiently. The patient was also encouraged to cough both pre- and postoperatively.

References

(1) Magill IW. Foreword. In Mansfield RE, Jenkins R, *Practical anaesthesia for lung surgery*, 1967.
(2) Edwards Tudor. Discussion. Anaesthesia in thoracic surgery with special reference to lobectomy. Section on Anaesthesia. *Proc Roy Soc Med* 1936; **29**.
(3) Nosworthy MD. Controlled respiration and cyclopropane. *Proc Roy Soc Med* 1941; **34**: 479.
(4) Sauerbruch F. Zur Pathologie des Offenen Pneumothorax. *Med Chir* 1904; **13**: 399.
(5) Waters Ralph. Present status of cyclopropane. *Br Med J* 1936; **2**: 1013–7.
(6) Waters Ralph. To-and-fro absorption and the Water's Canister. *Anaesth Analg* 1924; **3**: 20.
(7) Magill IW. Anaesthesia in thoracic surgery with special reference to lobectomy. Section on Anaesthetics.
(8) Overholt RH, Langer L, Szypulski, *et al*. Pulmonary resection in the treatment of tuberculosis; present day technique and results. *J Thorac Surg* 1946; **15**: 384.
(9) Brown AIP. Posture in thoracic surgery. *Thorax* 1948; **3**: 161.
(10) Jones Howard. *Proc Roy Soc Med* (Anaesth Sec) 1930; 919.
(11) Hewer C Langton. The Etherington-Wilson technique. Letter to the Editor. *Br J Anaesth* 1938; **1**: 117.
(12) Harris TAB, Rink EH. A modification of the Howard Jones technique for the use of percaine in spinal anaesthesia. *Guy's Hospital Rep* 1937; **87**: 1.
(13) Evans DF, Gaskell DV. Physiotherapy for medical and surgical conditions. *Physiol Dept, Brompton Hosp* 1960, 1962, 1964.

22.2 The first successful pulmonary embolectomy in Britain

BUDDUG OWEN
Glan Clwyd Hospital, Bodelwyddan, Clwyd, UK

It is almost eighty years since Trendelenburg (1) who was then in his sixties reported to the German Surgical Congress in 1908 his experimental research on embolectomy of the pulmonary artery and at the same time described the first two operations for pulmonary embolism in man.

After work on the cadaver he carried out animal experiments in Leipzig using long sterile strips of lung tissue which were introduced into the internal jugular veins of calves. This was carried by the blood to the heart and then blocked the pulmonary artery. Eventually he was able to operate successfully for this experimental embolism and wrote:

'The operation in the calf, on account of the form of the thorax, the situation of the pulmonary artery and the intercommunication of the pleurae presents much greater difficulty than in man. It is greatly to be hoped that, sooner or later, a successful case in the human will follow this successful case in the human will follow this successful operation in an animal.'

He and his team of assistants determined to 'try their hand at raising the dead', those patients struck down suddenly and unexpectedly when recovering from an operation, a fracture or childbirth, but this proposal was received with scepticism.

Trendelenburg's first case died in the operating theatre. The second, operated on by Sievers, his assistant, lived 15 hours and died of 'heart failure'. The third, operated on by Trendelenburg lived for 37 hours, dying of haemorrhage from the internal mammary artery. Other surgeons who tackled the problem were Schumacher, Sauerbruch, and Krüger, a pupil of Trendelenburg. Krüger's patient lived for 5¼ days, dying of infection of the left pleura.

The first successful patient was shown before the Congress of the German Surgical Society in Berlin by Kirschner (2) in 1924, but died later that year.

Five surgeons had successfully operated on eleven patients prior to Ivor Lewis's successful operation in 1938. They were Kirschner of Konisberg [1] in 1924; A. W. Meyer (3,4,5,6) of Berlin [4] 1927 [2], 1928 & 1931; Nystrom (7,8) of Uppsala [2] 1928, 1929; Crafoord (9) of Stockholm [3] 1927, 1928 & 1933 and Valdoni (10) of Rome [1] 1935.

The first successful case in the United Kingdom

The first successful operation in the United Kingdom was carried out in the North Middlesex Hospital, London by Ivor Lewis (11) on the 12th September, 1938.

The patient was a woman aged 49 years who weighed 100 kg and was admitted to the hospital on August 9th 1938 with an infected left prepatellar bursa. This was fomented for 2 days and then incised under anaesthesia.

The knee improved but eight days later the leg became tense and oedematous below the knee due to phlebitis of the internal saphenous vein.

Twelve days later she complained of pain over the left lower ribs and, after a further five days, she had developed blood stained sputum and Lewis commented 'evidently an infarct'.

A week after this on the 12th September (over a month since her admission) she suddenly told the staff nurse on the ward that she could not breathe and felt faint. The patient then grasped her throat, became blue and complained of pain in the left side of her chest. She was seen by Ivor Lewis who diagnosed pulmonary embolism and she was then taken to the operating theatre.

Forty minutes after the symptoms had started, surgery was commenced 'at leisure under local infiltration'. The 2nd and 3rd left costal cartilages were freed and removed. The triangularis sterni was cleared off the back of the 4th costal cartilage and margin of the sternum.

Lewis writes:

> 'We then waited as the patient was not yet in articulo mortis. The pulse disappeared and respiration became irregular. As soon as the patient was in articulo the pericardium was incised and split up by Meyer's manoeuvre reflecting the pleura safely with it. The heart had ceased to pulsate and only twitched irregularly. A Trendelenburg sound was passed and a rubber tourniquet tightened around the great vessels. The pulmonary artery was incised for 2 cm producing a gush of blood, a clot 40 cm long was pulled out and the lips of the incision clamped. The heart was massaged and 1 c.cm Adrenaline injected into the sinus aortae. The beat then came back at first feebly and then regularly. Respiration did not, but oxygen under positive pressure was administered all the time with a McKesson apparatus by Dr. Patrick Nagle. After Lobeline was injected into the aorta breathing started at once: it was 6 minutes since it had stopped. The circulation had probably been absent for about 3 minutes. The patient left the operating theatre 3 hours after the incision was made and was nursed in an oxygen tent for a fortnight. Postoperatively she was given 6 units of blood (12) at various times, 2 units having been taken from a son and a further 2 units from a daughter. Also her husband and brother gave one unit each.'

The patient suffered a series of complications. Clonic fits of the arms and face developed the afternoon of surgery which had not been reported in the other patients. She remained unconscious until the following day and had amnesia for a few days. There was temporary blindness and deafness and later there were psychological changes, but these had all resolved when she left hospital.

She suffered a second embolism which was treated conservatively, developed suppurative haemolytic streptococal mediastinitis and pericarditis, which was treated with sulphanilamide and drained under local infiltration with procaine, haemorrhagic pleural effusion and empyema, which was drained by rib resection under local infiltration, massive necrosis of the buttocks and scalenus articus syndrome treated by scalenotomy under local infiltration.

She was discharged from hospital on 6 April, 1939, having been in hospital for eight months and, on 26 April, 1939, she was taken to a meeting of the Royal Society of Medicine at County Hall, Westminster, prior to Ivor Lewis delivering a lecture of the operation. This was reported in the press and the *Daily Express* (12) medical correspondent wrote:

> *'It is an epoch making piece of surgery. It was a brilliant diagnosis and it required enormous courage to perform the operation.'*

Discussion

Crafoord (9) had emphasized the importance of well worked out organization and Ivor Lewis would have been aware of this for in his account he wrote that a sterile Trendelenburg tray was always kept ready indicating that he and his team were prepared to operate when the occasion arose. Lewis was later invited to contribute a chapter on 'Pulmonary embolectomy' by Rob and Smith in their textbook in 1955 (13) and another on 'Problems in Diagnosis and Management of Pulmonary Embolism' by Harley in 1960. He considered that these gave a better account of the problem than his original article in the *Lancet* (11).

Lewis pointed out that the operation is designed to save patients who succumb to the embolism from 15–60 minutes, and that the surgeon, his assistants, and the anaesthetist need regular rehearsing not only in the procedure but in speedy assembly. Oxygen and morphia are given immediately the diagnosis is made and, although he advises tracheal intubation and controlled respiration, he does not consider this practical from the beginning but that the anaesthetist should be prepared to institute it when necessary. In his view the changes of getting a patient back to the ward alive are probably about 1:10 if one sticks to the practice of not proceeding with the operation until the patient is actually dying or dead.

During the removal of the clot he advocates an assistant with a stop watch noting the time and says the circulation should not be stopped for more than 100 seconds and that 60 seconds should be aimed at. If the clot has not been removed completely in this time the tourniquet should be released after clamping the incision and cardiac massage carried out before another attempt is made.

While cardiac massage is carried out an assistant should inject 1 cc adrenaline 1:1000 and lobeline into the sinus aorta. Controlled respiration should be carried out at the same time with oxygen and carbon dioxide.

As well as adrenaline and lobeline a variety of drugs had been used to aid resuscitation by previous surgeons (3–10) which included camphor, strychnine nitrate, caffeine, and digitalis.

Lewis estimated his blood loss at 4 pints blood and had to use relatives as donors. The blood withdrawn would have been anticoagulated and transfused immediately. (Blood Banking in the United Kingdom (15) was started in Ipswich in 1938/39 by a surgeon and a pathologist, and they stored blood in a citrate medium. The National Blood transfusion Service in the United Kingdom was started in 1946 by an amalgamation of civilian and army blood transfusion services.)

Amnesia extending over the later and more distressing phase before operation, during operation and postoperatively for varying periods is a feature of all cases. Crafoord's (9) second case had some awareness as she vaguely remembered somebody had been poking about in her chest, as in a dream, and people talking.

Anaesthesia. Nystrom (8) had considered the possibility of completing the first part of the operation under local analgesia instead of waiting for the circulation to cease before starting and this is what Ivor Lewis did. In other reports, anaesthesia was deemed to be unnecessary (4,8,10) or not necessary at first. Ether (2,8) or chloroform (1) was being given when necessary either at the beginning (3) or at the end (6,8) so that the wound could be closed.

Respiration. Nystrom (8) states that in 5 of his cases which include those with unsuccessful outcomes (as also in Kirschner's (2) case) respiration was re-established as soon as the heart resumed regular action. If this should not occur he points out that artificial respiration has to be started with rhythmical insufflation of oxygen, e.g. by putting on and lifting off the mask in which a positive pressure narcosis is made, or by means of a pulmotor. Inhalation of carbon dioxide (5) is also suggested to re-establish breathing and positive pressure if the pleura is damaged. The McKesson used by the anaesthetist Dr Nagle during Lewis's case was an excellent machine for resuscitation (16). The Nargraf model had a button labelled 'Direct Oxygen' or 'Oxygen Flush' and when this was pressed and a mask held on the face, the lungs were inflated with oxygen straight from the regulating valve set at 60 lbs/square inch.

Heparin had been first isolated by McLean (17), a medical student from Baltimore, in 1916, from heart and live tissue. After carrying out two successful operations for pulmonary embolectomy, Crafoord (18) carried out the initial clinical trials of heparin in the prophylaxis of thrombosis which he reported in 1937. It was the first anticoagulant drug to be used in the treatment of peripheral venous thrombosis (19) and its value in this and in the prevention of pulmonary embolism was recognized immediately.

Cardiopulmonary bypass. The idea of a heart-lung machine came to Gibbon in 1931 while watching a case of pulmonary embolism, and embolectomy has been made much safer by the use of extracorporeal circulation.

The approach to the problem of pulmonary emboli now concentrates on prevention by early ambulation and prophylaxis by anticoagulation. The indications for surgery are massive embolism with shock which fails to respond to medical therapy with isoprenaline, oxygen and heparin. Cardiopulmonary bypass is considered a requirement for the operation of pulmonary embolectomy and carries with it a very high mortality, often exceeding 50%.

Dramatis personnae

Ivor Lewis

We can see what a challenge the operation of pulmonary embolectomy was to Ivor Lewis who was surgeon and Medical Director of North Middlesex Hospital, London, from 1933–1951. He carried out two further embolectomies at the North Middlesex (20) both of which were unsuccessful, but did not attempt the operation when he moved to Rhyl where he was Consultant Surgeon at The Royal Alexandra Hospital and Chest Hospitals at Llangwyfan and Abergele between 1951 and 1960.

In 1946 he became Hunterian Professor of the Royal College of Surgeons of England and delivered his lecture on the Surgical Treatment of Carcinoma of the Oesophagus with special reference to a new operation for growths of the middle third. This operation became known as the Ivor Lewis operation.

Lewis has two Memorial lectures named after him, one at the North Middlesex and the other at the new District General Hospital—Ysbyty Glan Clwyd—outside Rhyl. The third lecture in North Wales was delivered during a visit of the Royal College of Surgeons to Ruthin in 1986.

One of his wards in the North Middlesex was renamed the Ivor Lewis Ward in 1985. He was born in Wales in 1895 and returned to Wales (where he died in 1982) so that his children could be educated there.

Dr Patrick Nagle

What of Dr Nagle without whose efficient resuscitation the patient might well have succumbed? He graduated MBBCh BAO from the National University of Ireland, Dublin, in 1929 and became a house surgeon in the Mater Misericordiae Hospital, Dublin. From 1935–42 he was medical officer at the North Middlesex Hospital and gained his Diploma in Anaesthetics in England in 1936, being one of the first anaesthetists to do so as this examination was started in 1935.

He later returned to Dublin, becoming the first specialist anaesthetist in Ireland (21) and was Consultant at the Mater Misericordiae Hospital, Dublin, from 1946 to 1976. He died in 1980.

He became a Fellow of the Faculty of Anaesthetists of the Royal College of Surgeons of Ireland in 1960, he was a Fellow of the Royal Academy of Medicine in Ireland and was a Member of the Association of Anaesthetists of Great Britain and Ireland. He was a very humble unassuming man who never married. He was a very good teacher and a bit of a character.

It is fitting that his contribution to an historic occasion should be remembered in the International Symposium.

Postscript

In order that our brothers over the border are not left out, can I remind you that Trendelenburg (22) started his medical training in Glasgow, and qualified at Berlin. The early work on pulmonary embolectomy was carried out in Europe and this successful case was carried out in England by a Welsh surgeon and an Irish anaesthetist.

Acknowledgments

The author is grateful to Dr C. F. Bell, Mr K. J. Bladon, Librarian, Aldo Borzoni, Senior Nursing Officer, and Dr A. J. Williams for their assistance as translators. Thanks are due to those who gave their personal recollections as noted in the list of references and to Mrs Susan Hughes for her secretarial assistance.

References

(1) Trendelenburg F. Veber die operative Behandlung der Embolie der Lungenarterie. *Arch Klin Chir* 1908; **86**: 686–701.

(2) Kirschner M. Ein durch die Trendelenburgsche operation geheilter Fall von embolie der Art. pulmonalis. *Arch Klin Chir* 1924; **133**: 312–59.

(3) Meyer AW. Erfolgreiche Trendelenburgsche operation bei Embolie der Arteria pulmonalis. *Deutsche Z Chir* 1927; **205**: 1–21.

(4) Meyer AW. Eine weiterer erfolgreiche Lungembolie-operation. *Deutsche Z Chir* 1929; **211**: 352–8.

(5) Meyer AW. Trendelenburgsche Lungenembolie-operation *Med Klinik* 1928; **24**: 1380–1.

(6) Meyer AW. Eine weiterer (meine vierte) erfol greiche Lungenembolie operation (Neuer zur Technik) *Deutsche Z Chir* 1931; **231**: 586–92.

(7) Nyström G. Erfahrungen in drei nach Trendelenburg operierten Fällen von Lungenembolie. *Acta Chir Scand* 1928; **64**: 110–21.

(8) Nyström G. Experiences with the Trendelenburg Operation for pulmonary embolism. *Ann Surg* 1930; **92**: 498–532.

(9) Crafoord C. Two cases of obstructive pulmonary embolism successfully operated upon. *Acta Chir Scand* 1928; **64**: 172–86.

(10) Valdoni P. Trendelenburg's Operation for pulmonary embolism. *Policlinico (sez prat)* 1936; **43**: 913–8.

(11) Lewis I. Trendelenburg's Operation for pulmonary embolism. A successful case. *Lancet* 1939; **ii**: 1037–41.

(12) Medical Correspondent. *The Daily Express* 10 October, 1938: 13.

(13) Lewis I. Pulmonary embolectomy. In: Rob CG; Smith R, eds. *Operative surgery* Vol. III. London: Butterworths, 1955.

(14) Lewis I. Problems in diagnosis and management of pulmonary embolism. In: Harley, ed. *Modern trends in cardiac surgery*. London: Butterworths, 1960.

(15) Sheperd A. *Personal communication.*

(16) Mushin WW. *Personal communication.*

(17) McLean J. *Am J Physiol* 1916; **41**: 250.

(18) Crafoord C. Preliminary report on postoperative treatment with heparin as a preventive of thrombosis. *Acta Chir Scand* 1937; **79**: 407–26.

(19) Murray DWG, Best CH. The use of heparin in thrombosis. *Ann Surg* 1938; **108**: 163–77.

(20) Knowles G. *Personal communication.*

(21) Callaghan U. *Personal communication.*

(22) Mushin WW, Rendell-Baker L. *The principles of thoracic anaesthesia.* Blackwell: Oxford, 1953: Appx II, 160.

22.3   Origins and evolvement of cardiopulmonary resuscitation

JAMES R. JUDE

University of Miami, Florida, USA

Attempts at pulmonary resuscitation reach back to ancient times (biblical reference, Kings, 34th Verse). Andreas Vesalius (1) first carried out research in respiratory resuscitation; work repeated by Harvey, Hooke and John Hunter (1755) (2). Sudden death (cardiac arrest) was not recognized as a treatable problem or case of great interest to the medical profession until 1848 when, two months after the introduction by Simpson of chloroform as a general anaesthetic for midwifery, there occurred a sudden and unexpected death from its use in 15-year-old Hannah Greener, who underwent removal of a toenail under its influence (3). The reporters' notes at the time of the inquest are as follows:

> 'An inquest was held . . . on view of the body of Hannah Greener, a girl of 15 years of age, who died on Friday the 28th of January (1848) under the influence of chloroform, administered in order to allay sensibility while undergoing a painful surgical operation. "Mr Thomas Meggison, surgeon of Wickham, described the procedure, 'Hannah Greener died under my hands . . . while under the influence of chloroform, which I had given her for the purpose of producing insensibility during the operation of removing one of her toenails . . . She never complained of pain in the chest to me . . . I seated her in a chair and put about a teaspoonful of chloroform into a tablecloth, and held it to her nose. After she had drawn her breath twice, she pulled my hand down. I told her to draw a breath naturally, which she did, and in about half a minute, I observed the muscles in the arm become rigid, and her breathing become a little quickened, but not stertorous. I had my hand on her pulse, which was natural, until the muscles became rigid. It then appeared somewhat weaker—not altered in frequency. I then told Mr Lloyd, my assistant, to begin the operation, which he did, and took the nail off. When the semi-circular incision was made, she gave a struggle or jerk, which I thought was from the chloroform not having taken sufficient effect. I did not apply any more. Her eyes were closed, and I opened them, and they remained open. Her mouth was open and her lips and face were blanched. When I opened her eyes, they were congested. I called for water when I saw her face blanched and I dashed some of it on her face. It had no effect. I then gave her some brandy, a little of which she swallowed with difficulty (and it rattled in her throat, according to Mr Rayne). I then laid her down on the floor and attempted to bleed her in the arm and jugular vein, but only obtained about a spoonful. She was dead, I believe, at the time I attempted to bleed her' ".'

In 1858, John Snow (1813–1858) described 50 cases of death under the use of chloroform (4). Because of these iatrogenic sudden deaths, there occurred increased interest in treatment of this event. Moritz Schiff became the father of resuscitation by his work carried out in Florence, Italy, where he was Professor of Physiology (5). Experiments of 1874 (published in 1882) proved that . . .

> 'if the thorax is opened and at the same time air is insufflated into the lungs, by rhythmical compression of the heart with the hands (care being taken in so doing not to interfere with the coronary circulation) and continuous pressure of the abdominal aorta so as to bring the blood in greater quantity toward the head, it is possible to re-establish the heart beat even up to a period of eleven and one-half minutes after the stoppage of that organ.'

Closed client cardiac compression

At the Pharmacological Institute of the University of Dorpat, Louis Mickwitz (6), and subsequently Alexander Sorgerfrey (7) and Professor Dr R. Boehm (8) described the resuscitation of cats from chloroform or potassium arrest by a method of closed chest cardiac compression. Boehm described this method as follows:

> 'This is carried out in a manner of embracing with one hand the very elastic chest area of the cat, and at the same time carefully and with medium strength compression where the largest expansion area, through inblown air, has been built. At this it is without importance whether the pressure is placed more in downwards direction, where the thorax is compressed flatly, or—as I preferred—both chest walls are being directed toward each other through side-pressure. The effect of this manipulation is described in detail in the Kymograph. One can see at each compression a mercury-elevation in the manometer of 50 to 120 mm, and can artificially create desired curves in accordance to either more strongly applied, weaker, less numerous or more numerous pressure. I have also convinced myself after several unsuccessful tests about the effect the compression has on the blood circulation by incision into the carotid artery; each compression shows as a result a more or less high flow from the opened artery. It can easily be seen, that for a long time one could keep up a kind of emergency circulation; as soon as the compression is decreased, the heart refills itself from the main veins, so that again and again fresh blood will be forced out of the heart. This also is evidence to the fact, that the left heart-area still carried light-red arterial blood after one hour's unsuccessfully continued compression and artificial respiration, whilst the right heart-area and main veins show dark venous blood. This would naturally be impossible, if, through repeated compression, only one and the same blood fountain is carried back and forth through the heart.'

Dr Franz Koenig, Professor of Surgery at Gottingen, Germany, gave the first clinical description of external chest compression in *'Lehrbuch die Allgemeinen Chirurgie'* published in 1883 (9):

> 'I stand on the right side of the asphyxic patient and have somebody pull out the tongue of the patient or if this should not suffice I bring my left index finger to the floor of the tongue near the epiglottis and keep the larynx open. Then with the right hand, I conduct movements of respiration on the thorax in that manner where I stretch the thumb and the radial side of the palm over the right costal margin and the four fingers together with the ulnar portion of the hand toward the left costal margin. While I press vigorously in this manner against the costal margin, with pauses according to the rhythm of the respiration, this portion of the hand simultaneously produces a strong pressure against the heart region.
>
> Also then where apparent death has resulted from stand-still of the heart one has to revive the patient with the discussed means since neither acupuncture nor electro-puncture of the heart is to be recommended. With the methods described above we have managed to bring back to life certainly one-half dozen people in whom pulse had been absent.'

Maass (10) describes in detail the successful application of a modification of Koenig's technique in the *Berliner Klinische Wochenschrift* in 1892 in two cases. Case 1 is as follows:

> 'Heinrich, A.—9½ years old. A double hairlip had been removed from the patient in infancy . . . On 10-24-91 he returned to the hospital for repair of the split palate.
>
> On 10-26-91 he was anesthetized with chloroform and when completely relaxed the insertion of a Gutschen stomatoscope was attempted. Because of a very narrow mouth opening this was impossible and the patient awakened and screamed and resisted. Because of this he was given more chloroform, two or three applications were poured on the mask, so much that the gauze was wet. Suddenly his pupils widened, his face became cyanotic and the breathing stopped. At once his mouth was opened, the tongue drawn outward, and the epiglottis lifted with the finger. He was given artificial respiration by a surface method, however there was no radial pulse. Also no carotid pulse or heart sound could be detected. The frequency of the artificial respiration was increased to 30 to 40 per minute and the cardiac region was compressed. The airway was patent,

the cyanosis lessened quickly and the pupils narrowed, yet no pulse could be detected in neither the radial or carotid arteries. However, one could see and feel the apex pulse. If pressure in the chest was stopped, the patient would breathe at first almost normally, soon the pupils would dilate, the breathing cease, and the cyanotic color return. Pressure in the cardiac region brought always narrowing of the pupils and after long continuing also slight reddening of the cheeks and lips, only the pulse remained absent.

I continued to compress the chest in the same manner for three to four minutes, the inspirations and exhalations were becoming weaker. It appeared that a change to the Silvester method was in order. But the action of the heart weakened slightly. I applied the exhalation pressure with particular force. Despite that the respiration was very deep, the pupils remained widely dilated. As I listened the spontaneous breathing sounds that had been always present until now failed. Due to the completely dilated, reactionless pupils, the sleeping eyeballs, the corpse like appearance, the failure of the breathing and of the pulse, I must consider the patient died. I began immediately the direct compression of the cardiac region, and in the excitement very fast and powerful. The pupils rapidly contracted again, and by the continuation of fast tempo they were smaller than before and during the pauses we again had gasping breathing.

The rapid compressions were continued with only a few brief pauses for a half hour, and a change appeared, and spontaneous gasping returned in the pauses and became stronger and also more numerous.

At last, the always dilated pupils gradually narrowed, the flexion in the joints of the upper extremities gradually returned, there was the lifting of shoulder and opening of mouth wide. The pulse, however, was not felt in the carotid and in the pauses no heart sounds were heard. During the compressions the carotid pulse was not observed . . .

First after the passage of a good hour from the beginning, I believe that a vibrating motion could be felt in the carotid. I continued the resuscitation effort, the cheeks and lips which had been until now cyanotic, reddened in a short time. During a pause the patient breathed completely, quietly, and there was a rapid pulse that was clearly palpable . . . On 12-1-91 the patient entirely healthy was discharged from the hospital.'

Continued use of the closed chest methods of resuscitation did not occur, however. An attempt at open heart cardiac massage after the method of Schiff was attempted by Niehaus (11) in the late 1880s as described by Zesas (12) in 1903. The first *successful* application (13) occurred in 1901 when applied to a woman undergoing a hysterectomy in Tromso, Norway, by Dr Kristian Igelsrud. W. W. Keen (14) reported this case in the *Philadelphia Therapeutic Gazette* in 1904 together with several cases of Dr George Crile, Sr. One of these cases described the use of closed chest massage and also a pneumatic rubber suit for cardiovascular collapse.

'Sudden death during excision of exophthalmic goiter, Lakeside Hospital, February 2, 1904. Female, age 28, who had been in the hospital for nine weeks for treatment of exophthalmic goiter by medical means but had not improved. During this time the pulse varied from 90 to 150. The exophthalmia became more marked. All her nervous symptoms were greatly increased, there being delirium at times during the week past. There were attacks of syncope, though in bed and at the most perfect rest. The patient was operated upon under ether anesthesia, with every precaution against the loss of blood in the manipulation of the tumor. During the operation her condition was closely watched by her physician, Dr H. J. Lee. The heart had been beating at the rate of 144 to 150 per minute during the entire operation. After the completion of the dissection, and after almost all the ligatures had been tied, the patient went into a sudden collapse. The heart's action entirely ceased; the respiration continued for less than a minute later. A pneumatic rubber suit as a precautionary measure, had been put on but not inflated, before the operation was begun. Rhythmic pressure upon the thorax over the heart was at once made, and the rubber suit inflated as rapidly as possible. After an interval of between five or six minutes the heart slowly began to recover its beat and circulation was

re-established. It was intended to use the infusion of adrenalin, which was ready to be given just as the heart began beating. Spontaneous respiration was resumed. The operation was completed and the patient was sent to bed with circulation supported by the rubber suit, which was gradually decompressed during the period of one and a half hours. Following this the patient did well.'

Dr Crile (15,16) also introduced the use of adrenaline to cardiac resuscitation. The clinical application of closed chest cardiac resuscitation was thereafter lost as open chest became the applied clinical method.

Tournade, Rocchisani and Mely (17) conducted animal research at The Faculty of Medicine in Paris in 1934 on closed chest resuscitation as did Gurvich and Yuniev (18) in Moscow at The Institute of Resuscitation.

Closed chest cardiac defibrillation

The year 1926 brought developments in the electrical industry in the United States which gave impetus to research that ultimately led to the development of the external cardiac defibrillation and clinical application of external cardiac massage (ECM). There had occurred with increasing frequency fatal electrical accidents by employees in the electric power industry. On advice of The Rockefeller Institute, a research study was begun on the effects of electricity on the human body at the Johns Hopkins University. Dr R. Hooker (19) began experimental studies in the treatment of ventricular fibrillation with drugs in 1927 and in 1928 together with W. B. Kouwenhoven and O. R. Langworthy (20) began studies of the effects of electric shock on nerves and the heart. Prevost and Battelli (21) in 1899 had been the first to describe death in ventricular fibrillation from electric shocks. Dr Kouwenhoven (Fig. 1) described the development of the open chest cardiac defibrillator in 1964 (22):

'In 1930, the effects of electric currents on the heart were studied. It was found that small electric shocks were particularly hazardous and often would throw the heart into ventricular fibrillation, whereas a more powerful shock would completely depolarize the myocardium and arrest the arrhythmia. This later fact confirmed the findings of Prevost and Battelli.

Experiments in closed chest defibrillation, using the dog as the experimental animal, were conducted, with electrodes strapped on opposite sides of the shaved chest and with concomitant artificial respiration. It was found possible to arrest the arrhythmia, but unless the countershock was applied while fibrillation was still vigorous, the heart would be too hypoxic to resume effective contractions. The time limitation caused by hypoxia was a severe handicap to the closed chest method of defibrillation. Consequently thoracotomy and direct massage of the exposed heart was performed, since it was well known then that it was possible to maintain adequate circulation by rhythmically squeezing the heart with the hand.

The open chest cardiac defibrillator, using A.C. countershocks with a duration of 0.1 second, and delivering about 1 amp at 130 to 150 volts, evolved.

This later became a standard effective technique for treating clinical ventricular fibrillation.'

Dr Claude Beck in 1947 first applied Dr Kouwenhoven's internal defibrillation successfully in a human (23). David Leighninger (24) described this great contribution of Dr Beck at the first Wolf Creek Conference on Cardiopulmonary Resuscitation as follows:

'In 1947, Beck was operating on a 14-year-old boy for a severe funnel chest. The preoperative ECG showed T-wave inversion in leads II and III. Anesthesia was nitrous oxide and ether. The pulse rose to 160, so the patient was given lanatoside-C, 1.6 mg. The pulse returned to 80, where it remained for the duration of a 2-hour operation. During closure of the skin, the pulse suddenly became imperceptible. The chest was quickly opened and Beck noted the heart was feebly fibrillating. The heart was pumped by hand and defibrillation attempts were made. After 70 minutes of hand-pumping, the heart

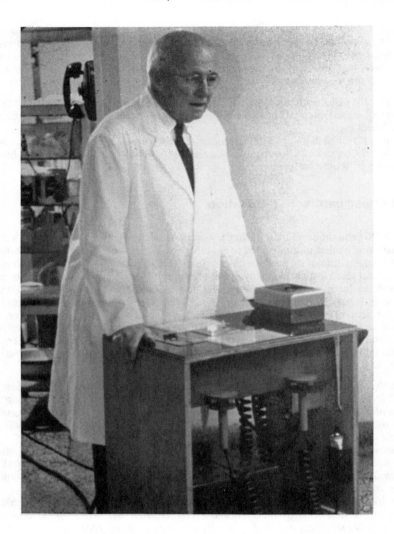

Figure 1   William Kouwenhoven with A.C. External Defibrillator, 1957.

was successfully defibrillated. Three hours later, the patient was awake and rational.
This was the first successful defibrillation of the human heart with recovery of the patient.
He lived a normal life of about 20 years, and died while still a relatively young man
of causes unknown to me.'

Open chest cardiac defibrillation

Open chest defibrillation had the obvious drawback of requiring major surgery to get to the
heart. Because of this, Dr Kouwenhoven was requested by the Edison Electric Institute in 1951
to attempt to develop a defibrillating device that could be used with the chest closed. At the
time, Dr Kouwenhoven was Dean of the School of Electrical Engineering of Johns Hopkins
University. His research was carried out at the old Hunterian Research Laboratory at the medical
school in association with Dr W. R. Milnor (25). Dr Kouwenhoven described the A.C. external
defibrillator development as follows (22):

'With the exposed hearts, monophasic capacitor shocks of 5 watt seconds at 500 or more volts defibrillated the ventricles in a high percentage of cases, provided fibrillation had not continued more than ½ minute. In the closed chest tests, the energy of the countershock needed to be of the order of 400 watt seconds at several thousand volts. If the heart was allowed to remain in fibrillation for more than a minute the chances of successful recovery decreased greatly in both the open and closed chest experiments. Therefore, attention was turned to alternating currents. A closed chest defibrillator was developed. This defibrillator delivered a countershock of 5 amp for 0.25 second at a potential of 440 volts. The energy of the countershock was sufficient to defibrillate a normal heart even if it had been in fibrillation for several minutes without circulation of oxygenated blood. The device weighed about 280 pounds and was mounted on a movable table. It was first used in 1957.'

Dr Paul Zoll in Boston was working also on an external defibrillator that was first used successfully in 1955 (26). Subsequently, the research work of Gurvich and Yuniev in Moscow in 1940 on capacitor discharge shocks directly to the fibrillating heart led to the development of the portable external compact defibrillator by Dr Kouwenhoven in 1957 (27).

Dr W. Kouwenhoven

Dr W. Kouwenhoven is the founder of modern resuscitation beginning with his work on the effects of electricity on the heart and extending to the development of the internal and external defibrillator and the discovery of external cardiac compression in his laboratory. He was born on 13 June, 1886, in Brooklyn, NY, and received his Bachelors and Masters degree at Brooklyn Polytechnic Institute in 1906 and 1907 and his PhD under Professor Arnold at the Karlsruhe Technische Hochschule in 1914. He became Dean of the School of Engineering at Johns Hopkins University in 1939, a position from which he retired in 1953. His work continued in the Hunterian Laboratory at the Johns Hopkins Medical School until his death at the age of 89 (10 November, 1975).

External defibrillation and external cardiac compression combined in animal experiments

The lifetime work of Dr Kouwenhoven culminated with the discovery of external cardiac massage (compression) in the spring of 1958. A typical experiment became applied serendipity: an anaesthetized dog was strapped to the research table in the supine position with an ECG attached as well as a femoral artery cannula which was attached to a recording transducer. The chest was shaved in preparation for fibrillation/defibrillation paddle application. The trachea was intubated and artificial positive pressure ventilation maintained: The animal's heart was put into ventricular fibrillation with a low voltage alternating current across the thorax and after a period of time (30 seconds), the defibrillator paddles applied. The animal had a highly angled chest wall (breast) and the heavy paddles applied on each side and pressed together caused an increase in the recorded femoral artery pressure. Noticing this, Dr Kouwenhoven and Guy Knickerbocker (Fig. 2) repeated the electrode pressure and the femoral arterial pressure again increased. The animal's heart was readily defibrillated when the shock was applied. Review of the records revealed that the possibility existed that artifically some circulation might have occurred by the pressure of the electrodes. Further studies revealed this to be the case and that the heart could remain in an oxygenated fibrillation state for periods of many minutes and yet be successfully defibrillated, something not before possible. Thus was reborn external cardiac massage (ECM) which was originally described eighty years earlier. Guy Knickerbocker informed the author (who was then in his final two years at the National Institute of Health) of their findings during one of his weekend visits to the Hopkins Laboratory. The author shortly returned to residency training at Hopkins and further experiments were made with the hand replacing the electrodes for the 'external cardiac massage'. The length of time the animal heart could be kept in ventricular fibrillation was extended incrementally to 15 minutes

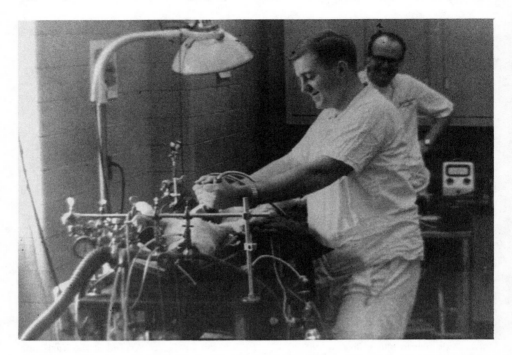

Figure 2   Johns Hopkins University School of Medicine, Hunterian Laboratory: Guy Knickerbocker applying defibrillation shock to experimental animal, 1956.

and ultimately over one hour and yet defibrillation occur with external countershock and the animal survived with an intact central nervous system. The effects of various pharmacological agents (adrenaline, calcium chloride, sodium bicarbonate and others) on pressure, circulation and defibrillation were also studied under the situation of prolonged external cardiac massage of the fibrillating heart.

Clinical application in man

The first clinical application was in an obese 35-year-old female who had been admitted from the Emergency Room for surgery for acute cholecystitis. The author was the operating resident in this case and when the woman had sudden loss of respiration and pulse during halothane anaesthesia induction, we applied ECM together with ventilatory support. In the past under such circumstances the left chest would have been opened and open chest cardiac massage applied. In this case, the ECM was successful and in a few minutes resumption of spontaneous cardiac activity resulted. An ECG showed no cardiac damage and the operation was completed without incident with normal recovery. While this case had no recorded documentation, in the next several months, multiple well documented cases (ECG and aterial pressure) of arrest and resuscitation with ECM occurred.

While traditionally cardiac resuscitation by the open chest method had been restricted to the operating theatre, Dr Claude Beck had resuscitated a dentist who had 'dropped dead' in the hospital lobby on 22 June, 1955, by application of open chest cardiac massage (28). External cardiac massage was especially applicable to other than operating theatre cases. Typical of such early cases are the following:

(1) B.B., 67, (Fig. 3) had recently been discharged from the hospital after recovery from a myocardial infarction. Shortly after sitting down for dinner in his home in East Baltimore, he suddenly developed chest pain and shortness of breath. The Emergency Fire Rescue were called and shortly before they arrived, he became pulseless and apnoeic. His son, a coal miner

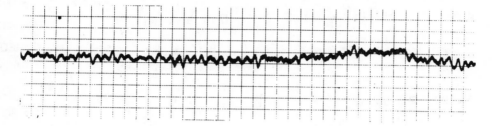

BB 67 WM I   JHH 844231   MYOCARDIAL INFARCTION

VENTRICULAR FIBRILLATION - 20 Min.

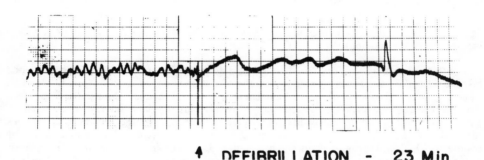

↑ DEFIBRILLATION - 23 Min

Figure 3   B.B., age 67, ECG on arrival at Johns Hopkins Emergency Room and after defibrillation shock.

trained in artificial respiration by the Silvester arm-lift and chest pressure method, applied this rigorously. The Fire Rescue squad found the patient without spontaneous respiration or palpable pulse. They began external cardiopulmonary resuscitation. He was transferred to the nearby Hopkins Emergency Room when he was found to be in ventricular fibrillation. Twenty-three minutes after the patient had become pulseless at home, he was given a 440 capacitor discharge 50 watt-second biphasic shock and went into idioventricular and then sinus rhythm. He was given also sodium bicarbonate and quinidine for treatment of a myocardial infarction. After a relatively benign course, he was discharged twenty-three days later. This was the first case of resuscitation from sudden death from myocardial infarction where a rescue squad had applied life saving CPR.

(2) M.F., (Fig. 4), a 29-year-old man was admitted for further diagnostic studies of cyanotic congenital heart disease previously diagnosed as pulmonary stenosis with a single ventricle and an atrial septal defect. Thirteen years earlier a right subclavian-to-pulmonary artery shunt had been successfully performed. An ectopia cordis and bifid sternum had been surgically corrected nine years before. On admission his general condition was quite good but he had marked exercise intolerance and mild congestive failure. The heart was enlarged and there appeared to be dextrocardia. The subclavian-to-pulmonary artery shunt was functioning well. Cardiac catheterization was carried out by percutaneous right femoral vein catheterization. The catheter entered the left atrium through an interatrial communication. The catheter then entered a ventricle and went out the aorta. Cardiac irritability developed but responded to Pronestyl and waiting. Suddenly ventricular tachycardia followed by ventricular fibrillation ensued. The patient became comatose immediately.

EXTERNAL CARDIAC MASSAGE

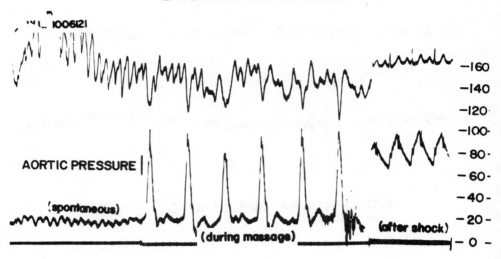

Figure 4   M.F., age 29, ECG above and arterial pressure below showing effect of ECM and resuscitation after 15 minutes.

Mouth-to-mouth respirations and external cardiac massage were immediately begun. Good systolic arterial pressures were obtained with the cardiac massage of 80 to 100 mm of Hg. Two externally delivered 440-volt alternating current shocks of 0.25 second's duration had no effect. An endotracheal tube was now inserted and positive pressure oxygen administered. Adrenaline, 1 mg, was injected percutaneously directly into the heart blood. Another electric countershock restored a transitory nodal rhythm followed again by ventricular fibrillation. A fourth countershock after 250 mg of Pronestyl and 44.6 mEq. of sodium bicarbonate intravenously restored a supraventricular rhythm with good pulse and blood pressure. After about 30 minutes a sinus rhythm appeared. He awakened and had no evidence of central nervous system deficit from the 15 minutes of cardiac arrest and massage. He was discharged unchanged from his admission status of 12 days. This early patient, because he was so closely monitored in the cardiac catheterization laboratory, gave very firm evidence of the effectiveness of CPR.

(3)   J.H. a 66-year-old-woman with a history of Adams-Stokes syncopal attacks of two years' duration was admitted for studies of the possibility of implanting a permanent pacemaker. Her case was especially well documented by the Marburg (Private Service) Hopkins House staff who had been trained in CPR in Dr Kouwenhoven's laboratory. Her admission electrocardiogram showed nodal bradycardia of 48 to 50, ST changes compatible with digitalis effect, and prominent U waves suggestive of hypokalemia. Her serum potassium was found to be 2.8 mg per 10 ml. She was treated with potassium chloride and isoprenaline. Digitalis was withheld as she also had occasional bigeminy. Thirty hours after admission, at 11.34 p.m., the patient's pulse which had been 50 per minute, was recorded at 40 by the nurse. Immediately thereafter the patient began to take gasping breaths which soon stopped and the nurse could obtain no pulse. Within one minute a house officer present on the ward began mouth-to-nose expired air ventilation and external cardiac massage. The anaesthesiologist was called and an electrocardiograph and defibrillator were obtained. The standby pacemaker was temporarily tried but had no effect. At 11.45 p.m. an electrocardiogram revealed ventricular fibrillation. Respirations were now spontaneous and the anaesthesiologist administered oxygen.

The patient became completely conscious shortly after the onset of cardiac massage and inquired of the staff as to what they were doing to her chest, complaining by yelling and fighting. A cut-down was placed in the greater saphenous vein at the ankle for administration of drugs and fluids. At 12.00 midnight, 25 minutes after the onset of the cardiac arrest, a single 440-volt

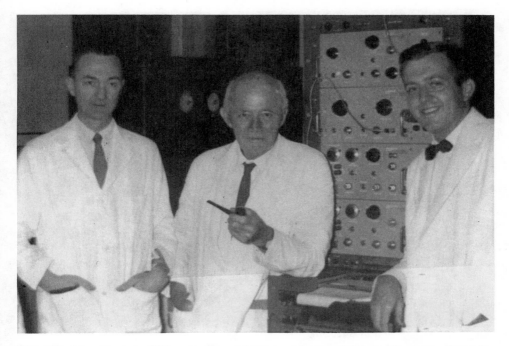

Figure 5 James R. Jude, William B. Kouwenhoven and G. Guy Knickerbocker in The Hunterian Laboratory, (1960).

alternating current countershock of 0.25 second's duration was administered externally to the thorax between the apex and base of the heart. No drugs had been administered to this time. Spontaneous coordinated cardiac action resumed, together with a palpable pulse and blood pressure of 110/60 mmHg. Sodium bicarbonate, 44.6 mEq, was given by the venous cut-down as was 1 g of calcium chloride. The pulse rate returned to 50 to 60 per minute. The bradycardia was subsequently initially controlled with drugs and then by venous catheter pacemaker. There was no sign of central nervous system deficit. Chest X-rays revealed no evidence of thoracic trauma and the patient complaining of only slight sternal soreness. Eight days after the cardiac arrest a permanent pacemaker was implanted without incident. She was discharged three and a half weeks after the arrest.

Such cases gave impetus to wide training of hospital and of hospital rescue personnel in CPR. In the laboratory, Dr Kouwenhoven established a regular training program utilizing dogs for practice by medical student and other medical groups (Fig. 5). His training of the Baltimore Fire Rescue under Captain Maroc McMahon led ultimately to the out-of-hospital CPR applied by Emergency Medical Technicians and more recently the lay public.

Publication and international developments in cardiopulmonary resuscitation

The first journal communication was in the issue of *The Journal of the American Medical Association*, 9 July, 1960 (29). This caused such interest in the medical profession that a marathon poster board type presentation was made at the American Heart Association meeting in October, 1960 at St Louis, MO. Thereafter the three investigators, Dr Kouwenhoven, Guy Knickerbocker and myself (Fig. 6) made extensive trips throughout the United States and Puerto Rico for the American Heart Association giving teaching programmes, frequently with the use of laboratory resuscitation demonstration on animals. The Maryland Heart Association, which was a financial contributor to the original research, as were the Edison Electrical Institute and the National Institute of Health, formed a committee chaired by Dr Leonard Sherlis on

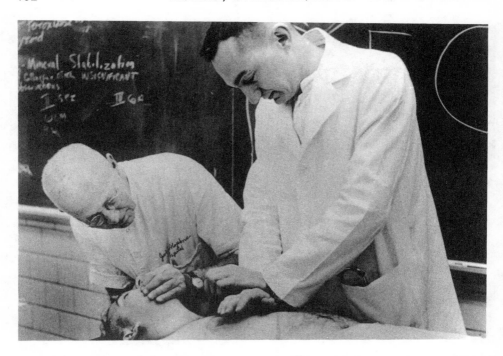

Figure 6   Dr James Jude applies ECM, Dr W. B. Kouwenhoven gives mouth-to-mouth ventilation and G. Guy Knickerbocker is the patient in a demonstration of ECM, (1961).

cardiac resuscitation whose purpose was to foster training and application of CPR. This was followed by a similar committee of the National American Heart Association which evolved into the American Heart Association Committee on CPR and Emergency Cardiac Care. Standards and guidelines for Cardiopulmonary Resuscitation and Emergency Cardiac Care were formed in the United States through national conferences in 1966, 1973, 1979 and 1985. Internationally, there was an International Symposia on Emergency Resuscitation in Stavanger, Norway, in August of 1961 under the sponsorship of Asmund Laerdal, whose training manikin, Resusci Anne, has provided the basic CPR training manikin for most of the world. A second International Symposium on CPR also sponsored by Laerdal was held in Oslo, Norway in 1967.

Circulatory resuscitation did not evolve in a void by itself. Changes in pulmonary resuscitation allowed its simple application to be effective. Jim Elam first applied mouth-to-mouth resuscitation in 1946. He described its renewed use at the First Wolf Creek Conference on Cardiopulmonary Resuscitation in October of 1975 in Blainsville, Georgia (30):

> *'During the poliomyelitis epidemic in Minnesota in 1946, I did mouth-to-mouth breathing as an instinctive reflex many times on patients with combined spinal-bulbar paralysis at times of equipment failure. The tank respirators and medical personnel were in short supply.*
>
> *I don't recall ever getting tired doing mouth-to-mouth; on one night I was stuck with this chore for three hours. There was absolutely no physiologic theory applied. The method was natural improvisation on the spot.'*

Elam continued to apply mouth-to-mouth and mouth-to-mouth endotracheal tube resuscitation in his anaesthesia practice. Later he proved with Peter Safar at Baltimore City Hospital the oxygenation proficiency of the technique with volunteer medical students (31). Archer Gordon, who had been a proponent of the Holger-Nielson method of artificial pulmonary resuscitation quickly was converted to a powerful disciple and provided multiple training movie films on mouth-to-mouth and then combined with external cardiac massage in complete CPR. Archer Gordon also was instrumental in advising Asmund Laerdal in the modification of his Resusci-Anne to the teaching of both mouth-to-mouth ventilation and external cardiac massage.

CPR had emerged quite quickly from the laboratory to clinical application but not without thorough evaluation as to its credibility and safety. This was demanded by our professor, Dr Alfred Blalock, at Johns Hopkins. Only when he was sure of the physiological soundness and lack of risk to benefit was it reported, at the Surgical Forum of The American College of Surgeons in 1960 and The American Surgical Association in 1961, and the free communication to the JAMA in 1960.

The development of a simple and widely applicable method of cardiopulmonary resuscitation had widespread implications to the care of acute myocardial infarction. One of the most important of these was the establishment of the first coronary care unit by Dr Hughes Day in Bethany Hospital in Kansas City, Kansas, in 1962. His idea was to keep the high risk patients under monitoring so that when they had cardiac arrest, resuscitation could be immediately applied (32). Most of all, however, there were innumerable scientists and clinicians who verified the research, made beneficial changes, and taught the technique to all who would listen. The First Wolf Creek Conference on Cardiopulmonary Resuscitation brought all those investigators together in 1975 (33). The second in 1980 and especially the third in 1985 showed an attrition in the 'old guard' and emergence of a new generation of resuscitators. The practice of medicine was changing and resuscitation once initiated could be carried on by application of new scientific, mechanical and pharmacological techniques almost indefinitely. The ethics and legal implications and questions of use, non-use or abuse were increasing dramatically. In a manner of speaking, we had created a quandary over making the decision as to resuscitate, not resuscitate or to discontinue resuscitation.

The future direction of resuscitation, at least in the United States, is in good hands with the National Conferences on standards and guidelines for Cardiopulmonary Resuscitation and Emergency Cardiac Care last held in 1985 (34). Sponsorship by the American College of Cardiology, The American Heart Association, The American Red Cross and the National Heart, Lung, and Blood Institute has assured adequately cross fertilization and, hopefully, a consensus.

References

(1) Vesalius A. *De Humani Corporis Fabrica*. Basel, 1555.

(2) Harvey W. *Movement of the heart and blood in animals* (translation by K. J. Franklin). Oxford, 1957.

(3) Beecher HK. The first anesthesia death, with some remarks suggested by it on the fields of the laboratory and the clinic in the appraisal of new anesthetic agents. *Anesthesiology*, 1941; **2**: 443.

(4) Snow J. *Chloroform and other anaesthetics*, London: Churchill, 1858.

(5) Schiff M. Über direkte Reizung der Herzoberflache. *Arch Ges Physiol* 1882; **28**: 200.

(6) Mickwitz L. *Vergleichende Untersuchungen über die physiologische Wirkung der Salze der Alcalien und alcalischen Erden* (dissertation), Dorpat, 1874.

(7) Sorgenfrey A. *Ueber die Wiederbelebung und Nachkrankheitenu nach Scheintod* (dissertation), Dorpat, 1876.

(8) Boehm RV. Arbeiten aus dem pharmakologischen Institut der Universitat Dorpat. XIII. Über Weiderbelebung nach Vergiftungen und Asphyxie. *Arch Exp Path* 1878; **8**: 68.

(9) Koenig F. *Lehrbuch Allgemeinen Chirurgie*, Gottingen, 1883: 60–1.

(10) Maass Dr. Die Methode der Wiederbelebung bei Herztod nach chloroformeinathmung. *Ber Klin Wschr* 1892; **12**: 265.

(11) Niehaus: *Reported by Zesas* (12).

(12) Zesas DG. Über Massage des freigelegten Herzens beim Chloroformkollaps. *Zbl Chir* 1903; **30**: 588.

(13) Igelsrud K. Tromso, Norway, 1901; first successful case. *Reported by Keen* (14).

(14) Keen WW. Case of total laryngectomy (unsuccessful) and a case of abdominal hysterectomy (successful) in both of which massage of the heart for chloroform collapse was employed, with notes of 25 other cases of cardiac massage. *Ther Gaz* 1904; **28**: 217.

(15) Crile GW. The resuscitation of the apparently dead and a demonstration of the pneumatic rubber suit as a means of controlling the blood pressure. *Trans South Surg Gynec Assn* 1904; **16**: 362.

(16) Crile G, Dolley DH. An experimental research into the resuscitation of dogs killed by anesthetics and asphyxia. *J Exp Med* 1906; **8**: 713.

(17) Tournade AL, Rocchisani L, Mely L. Etude experientale des effets circulatoires qu entrainent la respiration artificielle et le compression saccade du thorax chez le chien en état de syncope cardiaque. *C R Soc Biol (Par)* 1934; **117**: 1123.

(18) Gurvich NL, Yuniev SG. Restoration of a regular rhythm in the mammalian fibrillating heart. *Am Rev Soviet Med* 1946; **3**: 236.

(19) Hooker DR. Clinical factors in ventricular fibrillation. *Am J Physiol* 1930; **92**: 639.

(20) Hooker DR, Kouwenhoven WB, Langworthy OR. The effect of alternating electric currents on the heart. *Am J Physiol* 1933; **103**: 444.

(21) Prevost JL, Battelli F. La mort les courants electriques-courants alternatifs a haute tension. *J Physiol Path Gen* 1899; **1**: 427.

(22) Jude JR, Kouwenhoven WB, Knickerbocker GG. External cardiac resuscitation. *Monographs in the Surgical Sciences* 1964; **1**: 66.

(23) Beck CS, *et al*. Ventricular fibrillation of long duration abolished by electric shock (Herzflimmern von langer Dauer, welches durch Elektroschock unterbrochen wurde), *JAMA* 1947; **135**: 985.

(24) Leighninger DS. Contributions of Claude Beck. In: Safar P, ed. *Advances in cardiopulmonary resuscitation*. New York: Springer-Verlag, 1977: 259–62.

(25) Kouwenhoven WB, Milnor WR. Treatment of ventricular fibrillation using a capacitor discharge. *J Appl Physiol* 1954; **7**: 283.

(26) Zoll PM, Linenthal AJ, Gibson W, *et al*. Termination of ventricular fibrillation in man by externally applied electric countershock. *N Engl J Med* 1956; **254**: 727.

(27) Kouwenhoven WB, Milnor WR, Knickerbocker GG, Chestnut WR. Closed chest defibrillation of the heart. *Surgery* 1957; **42**: 550.

(28) Beck CS, Weckesser EC, Barry FM. Fatal heart attack and successful defibrillation. New concepts in coronary artery disease. *JAMA* 1956; **161**: 434.

(29) Kouwenhoven WB, Jude JR, Knickerbocker GG. Closed chest cardiac massage. *JAMA* 1960; **173**: 1064.

(30) Elam J. Rediscovery of expired air methods for emergency ventilation. In: Safar P, ed. *Advances in cardiopulmonary resuscitation*. New York: Springer-Verlag, 1977: 263–5.

(31) Elam JO, Greene DG, Brown ES, *et al*. Oxygen and carbon dioxide exchange and energy cost of expired air resuscitation. *JAMA* 1958; **167**: 328.

(32) Day HW. An intensive coronary care area. *Dis Chest* 1963; **44**: 423–7.

(33) Safar P, ed. *Advances in cardiopulmonary resuscitation*. New York: Springer-Verlag, 1977.

(34) Montgomery WH, Donegan J, McIntyre KM. Proceedings of the 1985 National Conference on standards and guidelines for cardiopulmonary resuscitation and emergency cardiac care. *Circulation* 1986; **74**: Monograph No. 126.

22.4   The history of defibrillation

D. DUDA, L. BRANDT and M. EL GINDI
Johannes Gutenberg University, Mainz, Federal German Republic

The history of defibrillation is closely related to the observation, understanding and production of electrical power and its effects on animals and human beings. Several ways for the generation of electricity have been found throughout the centuries.

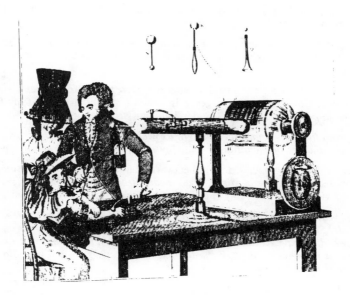

Figure 1   Stimulation of a girl's paralysed arm with electrical shocks from a Leyden jar (George Adams'
An essay on electricity, 1799).

Like so many other things the phenomenon of electricity, was already known to the ancient Greeks. The philosopher and scientist *Thales of Miles* (624–574 BC) described the phenomenon of static electricity which was produced by the friction of amber (1). So from the word 'elektron' which is the direct translation of 'amber' our term 'electricity' was derived.

More than 1000 years passed until the static electricity was rediscovered by the German Otto von Guericke (1602–1686), the mayor of Magdeburg. He produced static electricity by means of a sulphur globe which rotated while he rubbed it with his hand (2,3).

In the 18th century, the so called Age of Rationalism, very important discoveries concerning the different ways of producing and using electricity were made.

The Italian Luigi Galvani (1737–1798) observed, among others, the contraction of frog muscles at the moment they came into direct contact with two different metals (1,2). Allessandro Volta's (1745–1827) correct interpretation of this observation led at least to the production of *Galvanic Electricity* by means of the *Voltaic Pile* (1,2).

Early use of electricity in medicine

The 'Leyden' or 'Kleist-jar' was invented almost at the same time, but independently, by the German Ewald von Kleist and the Leyden physician Pieter van Musschenbroek (1692–1761) (3). This device is the oldest form of electrical condenser, (4) constructed of a glass jar which has tin foil covering on its inner and outer wall. With this bottle electrical shocks were applied to the human body for medical reasons including the treatment of paralysed limbs (Fig. 1). Other sorts of condensers which were also used for medical reasons were the electrostatic disc generator and, from the 19th century onwards the magneto-electric generator (4).

Resuscitation of the apparently dead

One of the first to be convinced of the beneficial effects of electricity for '*the revivification of the human body*' was Benjamin Franklin (1706–1790), the famous American philosopher, scientist and politician. In his '*Experiments and Observations on electricity*' (5) he wrote to Peter Collinson in London in the year 1749:

> '*If any should doubt whether the electrical matter passes Thro'the substance of bodys . . . a shock from the electrified large glass-jar taken thro'his own body will probably convince him.*'

Apparently Franklin's experiments and observations were known to Charles Kite (1768–1811) (6), member of the Corporation of Surgeons in London. In the preface of his *Essay on the recovery of the apparently dead* in 1788, Dr Lettsom wrote:

> '*Franklin from the New Hemisphere taught us wield the artillery of the skies and direct its fire to aid and restore debilitated man, by its penetrating and nervous energy.*'

In this essay, which was associated with the award of a silver medal of the Humane Society, Kite recommended: '*The general stimulus are heat, electricity and friction*'.
Kite also reported about probably the first case of electrical defibrillation:

> '*. . . a three year old child, which fell out of a window . . . was taken up to all appearance dead . . . Mr. Squires . . . very humanly tried the effects of electricity. He could apply the shock which he gave to various parts of the body without any happy success; . . . on transmitting a few shocks through the thorax, he perceived a small pulsation; . . . at least the child was restored to perfect health.*'

Kite concluded:

> '*Electricity is the most powerful stimulus we can apply . . . are we not justified in presuming . . . that it will be capable of reproducing the motion of the heart . . . that means accomplish our great desiration, the renewal of the circulation? . . . [We should] apply shocks of not more than one third or half an inch, from a vial containing about twenty-four inches of coated surface. These should be transmitted particularly through the diaphragm and the intercostal muscles, the heart, the brain and spinal marrow.*'

The Leyden jar was thus the first instrument to be used for defibrillation and detailed instructions for use were provided.
In the year 1792 James Curry (7), a member of the Royal Medical Society of Edinburgh, published his *Popular observations on apparent death*. He realized that:

> '*. . . In the suspension of life by falls, blows or lightening . . . both cavities of the heart ceased to act at the same instant [so that it seems to be possible . . .] . . . to renew their contractions whenever their sensibility is restored . . . Stimulants of every kind have this tendency, but none so much as electricity. . . .*'

Curry gave concrete instructions in the reports of the Royal Humane Society for the years 1787, 1788 and 1789:

> '*The shocks employed should at first be moderate and gradually be increased in strength as may be found necessary. The brain, spinal marrow and heart are the parts to which they ought chiefly to be applied.*'

In the second edition of his book in the year 1815 (8) Curry concluded in note 29:

> '*M. Abildgard affirms . . . that fowls struck down by an electric shock through the head . . . were completely recovered again by a similar shock through the breast and back. A second shock given through the head had no effect in bringing them to life. . . .*'

Joseph Berut's (9) instruction where to apply electricity to the heart (Vienna, 1819) appears very modern:

> '*It must be taken care that the heart is exposed to the influence of electricity and . . . the positive chain has to be positioned between the 4th and 5th left rib while the negative must be positioned between the 2nd and the 3rd right rib. The Galvanism promises to be effective even if other sorts of electricity were useless. Among the saving instruments a Voltaic pile with at least 100 pairs of discs should be available. . . .*'

At the end of the 19th century, Prevost and Battelli (10) resumed the work of Joseph Priestley who in 1766 had made extensive studies on the lethal effect of battery discharges in animals. At the beginning of the 20th century, the same Prevost and Batelli prepared the ground for the clinical use of defibrillation. In systematic studies on condenser and alternating current (AC) discharges in animals, they found out that ventricular fibrillation is not induced when large current flows through the body and, if present, it can be stopped by a high voltage countershock.

Modern developments

Stimulated by these findings, Hooker, Kouwenhoven and Langworthy from the Johns Hopkins University (11) experimented with alternating and direct currents in dogs and sheep in the year 1932. Their results were that:

> *'alternating 60 cycle currents up to 0.4 amperes and 1100 volts applied for 5 sec will cause fibrillation . . . and currents of 0.8 to 1.0 amperes with electrodes directly on the heart is sufficient to arrest fibrillation. In the intact animal it was found necessary with the electrodes on either side of the thorax to use a current strength of approximately 6–7 amperes to arrest fibrillation.'*

In 1937, Beck and Mautz (12) published their experimental success, a successful AC countershock in the dog. Their clinical observations were reported '. . . with special reference to ventricular fibrillation occuring during cardiac operations', and in 1947 Beck (13) reported the first successful defibrillation of the human heart:

> *'The heart is then placed between two large electrodes and ordinary 110 volts A.C. with 1.5 amperes is momentarily impressed through the heart between the electrodes. . . . We are reporting the first case of complete recovering after prolonged ventricular fibrillation. We present it with the hope, that following Beck's suggestion, operating rooms will be equipped to handle cases of sudden ventricular fibrillation and that personnel will be trained in the method. Speed and precision in Technique are important.'*

From this first successful case report to the commercial production of defibrillators many technical problems had to be overcome. So the experiments of Mackay, Mosslin and Leeds in 1951 (14) were undertaken, 'that the design of a more useful and effective defibrillation apparatus could be obtained'. DC apparatus for external defrillation was also considered.

'The termination of ventricular fibrillation in man by externally applied countershock' was introduced into clinical practice in 1956 by Zoll and Linenthal (15). One year before one of the first commercially available DC defibrillators was produced by Edmark.

Conclusion

With this important step in the development of defibrillation this account is concluded, but not without reminding one of the considerable consequences of this invention. Without it modern invasive cardiology, advances in cardiac surgery and especially emergency medicine as we now know them would not have been possible.

References

(1) Der neue Grimsehl. *Physik für höhere Lehranstalten I*. 5th Ed. Stuttgart: Ernst Klett, 1966.
(2) Diepgen P. *Geschichte der Medizin I und II*. Berlin: Walter de Gruyter, 1949.
(3) *Meyers Enzyklopädisches Lexikon in 25 Bänden*. 9th Ed. Mannheim: Bibliographisches Institut, 1982.
(4) *Brockhaus Enzyklopädie in 20 Bänden*. Bd. 10, Wiesbaden: F. A. Brockhaus, 1970.
(5) Franklin B. *Experiments and observations on electricity made at Philadelphia in America and communicated in several letters to Mr. P. Collinson of London F.R.S.* London: E. Cave, 1751.

(6) Kite C. *An essay on the recovery of the apparently dead*. London: C. Dilly in the poultry, 1788.

(7) Curry J. *Popular observations on apparent death from drowning, suffocation, &c. with an account of the means to be employed for recovery*. London: T. Dicey and Co., 1792.

(8) Curry J. *Observations on apparent death from drowning, hanging, suffocation by noxious vapours, fainting-fits, intoxication, lightning, exposure to cold, &c., &c. and an account of the means to be employed for recovery, to which are added, the treatment proper in cases of poison; with cautions and suggestions respecting various circumstances of sudden danger*. London: E. Cox and Son, 1815.

(9) Berut J. *Vorlesungen über die Rettungsmittel beym Scheintodt und in plötzlichen Lebensgefahren*. Wien: Carl Gerold, 1819.

(10) Prevost JL, Batelli F. La mort par les décharges électriques. *J Physiol Pathol Gen* 1899; **1**: 1086–129.

(11) Hooker DR, Kouwenhoven WB, Longworthy OR. The effect of alternating electrical currents on the heart. *Am J Physiol* 1933; **103**: 444–54.

(12) Beck LS, Mautz FR. The control of the heart beat by the surgeon. *Ann Surg* 1937; **106**: 525–37.

(13) Beck CS, Pritchard WH, Feil HS. Ventricular Fibrillation of long duration abolished by electrical shock. *JAMA* 1947; **135**: 985–6.

(14) Mackay RS, Mooslin KE, Leeds SE. The effects of electric currents on the canine heart with particular reference to ventricular fibrillation. *Ann Surg* 1951; **134**: 173–85.

(15) Zoll PM, Linenthal AJ, Gibson W, Paul MH, Norman LR. Termination of ventricular fibrillation in man by externally applied electric countershock. *N Engl J Med* 1956; **254**: 727–32.

22.5

An essay on the history of extracorporeal circulation in Germany

M. EL GINDI, L. BRANDT, D. DUDA and W. DICK
Johannes Gutenberg University, Mainz, Federal German Republic

---

The history of extracorporeal circulation (ECC) is mainly the history of the development of its fundamental components—the oxygenator, the roller pump and the anticoagulants. Other factors such as hypothermia, extracardiac suction and the great advances in anaesthetic techniques are also very important but cannot be discussed here. This paper is limited to the development of the fundamental components of ECC in German speaking countries up until 1939 when World War II started. These discoveries have had an important influence on the development of modern extracorporeal perfusion apparatus.

The oxygenators

The film oxygenator

When Dennis *et al.* (1) 1951 performed the first total bypass in man they used oxygenators with rotating screens, and when Gibbon (2) 1954 performed the first successful total bypass in man he used oxygenators with vertical stationary screens. Developments of the rotating disc oxygenators by Melrose (3) 1953 and by Cross *et al.* (4) 1956 dominated the 1960s as cardiac surgery spread widely around the world.

The forerunner of these 'film-oxygenators' was the one described 1885 by von Frey and Gruber in *Ein Respirationsapparat für isolierte Organe* (5). This was developed in order to be able to supply isolated organs with oxygen.

The oxygenator consisted of a glass cylinder 70 cm long and 14 cm in diameter, diagonally mounted and capable of longitudinal rotation. The blood was introduced at the upper end, distributed itself in a thin film over the inner surface of the rotating cylinder, and was collected at the lower end of the vessel. Covered by 210 ml of blood in a film 0.55 mm thick, the inner surface of the glass cylinder extended over 0.42 m² and rotated at 30 rpm. The oxygenator was located in the middle of the system. Blood circulation was maintained by a motor driven syringe and conducted through two valves. The isolated organ was placed into a tank. Venous blood flowed into the oxygenator, and arterialized blood was collected at its lower end and pumped back into the organ. Air circulation was provided by two pressure and suction pumps. Oxygen was delivered from a reservoir. Carbon dioxide was eliminated by four bottles containing 'barita solution'. The closed air circulation system allowed volumetric measurements of oxygen uptake. Carbon dioxide output was determined by means of titration. Air and blood samples could be taken. This apparatus is generally regarded as the original forerunner of ECC (6).

The bubble oxygenator

In its modern form this derived from the work of Clark *et al.* (7) 1950, and the disposable helical reservoir bubble oxygenator, which pointed the way to the future and was described by De Wall *et al.* (8) 1956.

In 1882, von Schröder (9) criticized the method of arterialization of blood described by Bunge and Schmiedeberg, in which the venous blood was shaken in a balloon in order to be arterialized. This method did not allow the continuous flow of blood, and large quantities were needed. Von Schröder described a bubble oxygenator in which venous blood was passed through a 'Wulff's bottle' from above while air was supplied from below. He also tried to solve the problem of the foam which built up due to mixing of blood with air by connecting the Wulff's bottle with another one from above in series so that the foam could pass out, if only partially, to the second bottle and did not pass to the organ. Oxygenated blood was drawn off from below. In his experiment, Von Schröder could arterialize 52 litres of blood in 5½ hours (i.e. 150 ml blood per minute).

The lung as an oxygenator

Between 1952 and 1956 the autologous or the heterologous lung as an oxygenator was clinically used by Dodrill *et al.* (10), Mustard *et al.* (11), Cohen *et al.* (12) and Campbell *et al.* (13).

In 1890 Jacobi (14) described the perfusion apparatus of von Frey and Gruber as a complicated construction, which was difficult to handle and expensive. He then described a method using a kind of bubble oxygenator and, in 1895, he developed a new perfusion apparatus employing dogs' lungs or lobes of pigs' and calves' lungs as oxygenators (Fig. 1). The apparatus consisted of two circular systems. The first circuit was concerned with the perfusion of an isolated organ. The second circuit was dedicated to the oxygenation of the blood by passing it through the lungs. Both circuits were connected together by a tap. Two rubber balloons representing the left and right heart were alternately compressed by a motor driven rocker thereby providing flows through both circuits. Venous blood was arterialized by passing it through the animal lungs (see Fig. 1). The priming volume of this system amounted to about 800 ml. When used with whole blood it permitted oxygenation for about 4–6 hours.

It can therefore be said that, about a century ago, three systems of oxygenators were already in use in the German speaking countries, namely the bubble oxygenator, the film oxygenator and the lung as an oxygenator.

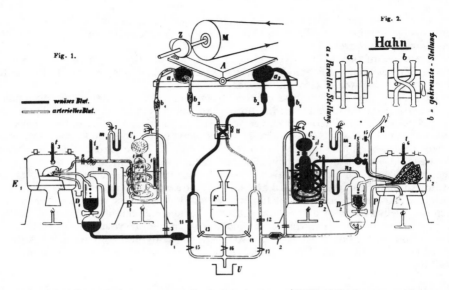

Figure 1   *Jakobi's perfusion apparatus for isolated organs, 1895 (15): A: motor driven rocker; a^1, a^2: rubber balloons; $b^1 - b^4$: four valves; E^1: the isolated organ; E^2: the lung; H: tap.*

The pump

The Dale and Schuster pump dating from 1926 (16) was the best known at that time. It was the one used by Gibbon at the beginning. From 1939 onwards Gibbon used De Bakey's roller pump (17) constructed by him in 1935. It was a pump with a continuous flow in contrast to the other pump of Dale and Schuster. The roller pump, which now usually bears De Bakey's name was first invented by the German surgeon Beck in 1925 (18) for use in blood transfusion,

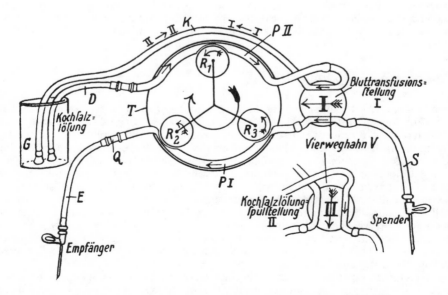

Figure 2   *A sketch of Beck's blood transfusion pump 1925 (18).*

and was known in Germany as the *Beck'sche Mühle*. It consisted of three rollers and two tubes (Fig. 2). Via the first tube the donor's blood was pumped to the recipient. Intermittent flushing was provided with sodium chloride solution in the opposite direction by the second tube and was directed by stopcock.

The anticoagulants

Anticoagulants are also an important component so that without their development ECC would not have been possible. When Dennis *et al.* (1) performed their first total bypass in man the anticoagulant heparin was used. This anticoagulant was extracted from the liver of the dog in 1916 by MacLean and was later named 'Heparin' by Howell (19).

The first known anticoagulants were the leeches. They were first used in Bavaria, Mecklenburg and Böhmen in Germany. At that time the leeches were also sent in the 17th century from Germany to France in order to do bloodletting. From 1803 leeches were also exported to Russia and from 1840 to destinations all over the world. In 1895 Jakobi, while describing his new perfusion apparatus and the different parts of it for the different uses, mentioned that this apparatus in combination with anticoagulants (leeches extract) could be applied to living animals, in order to undergo haemodynamic measurements. In 1903 'Hirudin' was extracted from the leeches. In 1921 the anticoagulant properties of the drug 'Germanin' (Bayer 205) were described by Brukohnenko (20) and in 1927 he described successful blood transfusions in rabbits while using this drug instead of sodium citrate which was usually used at that time. He spoke of 'Germanised Blood'.

Conclusion

It is clear that the fundamental components of ECC were originally developed to a great extent in the German speaking countries. Other factors also important to ECC, such as endotracheal anaesthesia, described in 1870 by Trendelenburg and in 1911 by Kuhn (21,22), and cardiac catheterization described by Forssmann in 1929 (23) were developed in Germany. In spite of this, and most probably because of both the political situation in Germany at that time and the outbreak of World War II, the first successful ECC in man was done by Gibbon in 1954 in the Mayo-Clinic in Rochester, USA.

References

(1) Dennis C, Spreng DW, Nelson GE, *et al*. Development of a pump oxygenator to replace the heart and lungs: An apparatus applicable to human patients and application to one case. *Ann Surg* 1951; **134**: 709.

(2) Gibbon JH, jr. Application of a mechanical heart and lung apparatus to cardiac surgery. *Minn Med* 1954; **37**: 171.

(3) Melrose DG. A mechanical heart–lung for use in man. *Br Med J* 1953; **ii**: 57.

(4) Cross ES, Berne RM, Hirose J, *et al*. Evaluation of a rotating disc type reservoir oxygenator. *Proc Soc Exp Biol Med* 1956; **93**: 210.

(5) Frey M von, Gruber M. Untersuchung über den Stoffwechsel isolierter Organe. Ein Respirationsapparat für isolierte Organe. *Arch Anat Physiol* 1885; **9**: 519.

(6) Rodewald G. History of Extracorporeal circulation. In: Hagl S, Klövekorn WP, Mayr N, Sebening F, eds. *Thirty years of extracorporeal circulation*. München: Deutsches Herzzentrum, 1984: 25.

(7) Clark LC, Gollan F, Gupta VB. The oxygenation of blood by gas dispersion. *Science* 1950; **3**: 85.

(8) De Wall RA, Warden HE, Read RC, *et al*. A simple expandable artificial oxygenator for open heart surgery. *Surg Clin North Am* 1956; **36**: 1025.

(9) Schröder W von. Über die Bildungsstätte des Harnstoffs. *Arch Exp Path Pharm* 1882; **15**: 364.

(10) Dodrill FW, Hill E, Gerich RA, *et al.* Pulmonary valvuloplasty under direct vision using the mechanical heart for a complete bypass of the right heart in a patient with congenital pulmonary stenosis. *J Thorac Surg* 1953; **26**: 584.

(11) Mustard WT, Chute AL, Keith JD, *et al.* A surgical approach to transposition of the great vessels with extracorporeal circuit. *Surgery* 1954; **36**: 39.

(12) Cohen M, Warden HE, Lillehei CW. Physiologic and metabolic changes during autogenous lobe oxygenation with total cardiac bypass employing the azygos flow principle. *Surg Gynec Obstet* 1954; **98**: 523.

(13) Campbell GS, Crisp NW, Brown EB. Total cardiac bypass in humans utilizing a pump and heterologous lung oxygenator (dog lungs). *Surgery* 1956; **40**: 364.

(14) Jakobi C. Apparat zur Durchblutung isolierter überlebender Organe. *Arch Exp Path Pharm* 1890; **26**: 386.

(15) Jakobi C. Ein Beitrag zur Technik der künstlichen Durchblutung überlebender Organe. *Arch Exp Path u Pharm* 1895; **36**: 331.

(16) Dale HH, Schuster EHJ. A double perfusion pump. *J Physiol* 1928; **64**: 356.

(17) De Bakey M. A simple continuous flow blood transfusion instrument. *New Orleans Med Circ J* 1934; **87**: 386.

(18) Beck A. Über Bluttransfusion. *Münch Med Wschr* 1925; **72**: 1232.

(19) Howell WH, Holt E. Two new factors in blood coagulation: Heparin and Antithrombin. *Am J Physiol* 1918; **47**: 328.

(20) Brukhonenko S, Steppuhn O. Experimentelles zur Anwendung von Germanin (Bayer 205) bei Bluttransfusionen. *Münch Med Wschr* 1927; **74**: 1316.

(21) Brandt L. Endotrachealtuben zur Intubationsnarkose im 19. Jahrhundert. *Anaesthesist* 1983; **32** (Suppl.): 389.

(22) Brandt L. Die Geschichte der Intubationsnarkose unter besonderer Berücksichtigung der Entwicklung des Endotrachealtubus. *Anaesthesist* 1986; **35**: 523.

(23) Forssmann W. Die Sondierung des rechten Herzens. *Klin Wschr* 1929; **8**: 2085.

22.6   The introduction of cardiac anaesthesia
                                   to an Australian children's hospital

RICHARD J. BAILEY
Royal Alexandra Hospital for Children, Camperdown, New South Wales, Australia.

The Royal Alexandra Hospital for Children, Sydney, was founded in 1880. It occupied a site in Glebe until 1907, when it moved into larger premises at Camperdown, a site it still occupies.

Ligation of patent ductus

Although small numbers of lung resections were performed in the early 1940s, using endotracheal ether anaesthesia and assisted spontaneous ventilation, the first cardiac operation, a ligation of patent ductus, was not carried out until May, 1947. Details are missing, the method of anaesthesia is unknown, but the anaesthetist was A. D. Morgan.

Two similar operations were performed in 1948, and five in 1949. One of these latter patients received, after morphine and atropine premedication, and a blood transfusion started in the ward, a thiopentone, curare induction, followed by endotracheal cyclopropane, changing to nitrous oxide–oxygen prior to incision. The anaesthetist for most of these patients was C. A. Sara.

Although ligation of patent ductus was performed in greater numbers during the next few years the procedure was not always uneventful. One of the patients, after induction with thiopentone and tubocurarine, was intubated and ventilated with cyclopropane. At this stage, the patient collapsed. Despite successful resuscitation, the operation was deferred until six months later, when the child was given nitrous oxide, oxygen and ether, changing to oxygen, ether after endotracheal intubation. The ductus was tied successfully.

Blalock's procedure

The first Blalock anastomosis was carried out about August, 1949. Again details are unavailable, but the history of a four-year-old, operated upon a year later, gives us an indication of the technique used. As the dangers of high haematocrits were well appreciated, a normal saline infusion was started some two days prior to anaesthesia. Premedication was with nembutal (pentobarbitone), morphine and atropine, followed by a nitrous oxide, oxygen induction. Ventilation was controlled initially using cyclopropane, following on with nitrous oxide, oxygen and ether.

Early valvotomy operations

In 1952, we see the first instances of valvotomy, one of which is specified pulmonary valvotomy. Both patients were anaesthetized by A. D. Morgan. The operative technique involved inflow occlusion, that is, clamping both venae cavae to prevent blood entering the right heart. The resultant low cardiac output could be generally tolerated for a few minutes, while a small knife was inserted through a ventriculotomy, splitting the valve. The second of these patients unfortunately died on the operating table.

Coarctation of the aorta

The first resection of coarctation of the aorta that I find recorded, was performed in 1954. A. D. Morgan was the anaesthetist again, ordering for premedication quinidine, nembutal and atropine. Induction was with his favourite nitrous oxide, oxygen, ether, followed by intubation and controlled respiration with circle absorption. A year later, we note that gallamine was used for a similar operation.

Hypothermia

With the return to Australia of Surgeon Douglas Cohen in January 1956, after specialized cardiac surgical training, and the appointment of Victor Hercus as honorary anaesthetist, the numbers of cardiac operations jumped markedly. At this stage also, the use of ether was superseded, being replaced with nitrous oxide, relaxant techniques.

As the time allowed for valvotomy or atrial septal defect (ASD) closure was short, it was realized that the use of hypothermia to reduce the body's metabolism would allow more time for surgery, while protecting the heart and brain from injury (1). Hercus was closely involved in this development, assisted by a refrigeration engineer, Mr Viv Ebsary. Ebsary not only constructed the necessary machine, but also supervised its running during the surgery. He also manufactured various elements of the bypass machine, which was being developed at this same time.

The anaesthetic record of a seven-year-old girl, for closure of an ASD on 14 November, 1957, managed by Hercus and Verlie Lines, notes that she received pentobarbitone, morphine and atropine premedication. Induction was with thiopentone, then tubocurarine, nitrous oxide, oxygen, and pethidine. After intubation with a number 4 cuffed Magill orotracheal tube, her ventilation was controlled using a Waters' to and fro canister. Other than problems with recurrent ventricular fibrillation during rewarming, she did very well.

Other records available from about this time, show similar anaesthetic techniques for closure of an ASD, this time using coronary perfusion to assist myocardial protection, and for resection of coarctation of the aorta, utilizing trimetaphan for control of blood pressure.

It was well appreciated by Hercus that increased muscle tone and shivering can generate much body heat, so that high doses of relaxant were necessary. A detailed description of the management of the hypothermic technique was published in 1959 (1).

The introduction of cardiopulmonary bypass techniques

In 1957, Bahnson and Spencer from Johns Hopkins Hospital, Baltimore, visited Sydney, operating at Royal Prince Alfred Hospital on 10 patients using cardiopulmonary bypass. These patients, mainly children, all recovered after successful surgery. Also in 1957, Sir Russell Brock visited St Vincent's Hospital, demonstrating surgery, using his venovenous technique of hypothermia.

Spurred on by these exciting demonstrations, the team at the Children's Hospital began experiments, using a simple machine constructed by an engineer, John McDonald. The patients were sheep at the McMaster Institute at the University of Sydney Veterinary School, with Hercus anaesthetizing. Vivid descriptions remain of one of his duties, that of visiting the abattoirs in the early morning to collect sheep's blood to prime the bypass machine.

In early 1959, Ebsary, after seeing a heart–lung machine ordered from overseas, felt that he could build one as good or better, at less cost and with a much more reliable maintenance program. This machine was built in a little over six months, coupled with the Kay-Cross disc oxygenator (2). Its success was reflected in its being marketed throughout Australia, New Zealand and South-East Asia.

The first cardiac procedure on cardiopulmonary bypass at the Children's Hospital was undertaken on 10 December 1959, for the closure of a ventricular septal defect (VSD). Hercus and Lines were the anaesthetists for this seven-year-old boy. Premedication with paraperetum and hyosaine gave a satisfactory result. Induction with intravenous thiopentone and gallamine allowed intubation with a number 4 cuffed Magill tube. Ventilation was controlled using an adult Waters' canister for carbon dioxide absorption, and nitrous oxide, oxygen and halothane for anaesthesia. The bypass record shows that the time on total bypass was 24 minutes. The child recovered well, indicating the prowess and dedication of the team involved—anaesthetists, surgeons and pump specialists. Although this patient required subsequent surgery on bypass two years later, for closure of a residual VSD. He was discharged from the cardiac clinic in 1965, aged 13 years, with normal effort tolerance, and able to play sports.

From this point, the number of procedures on cardiopulmonary bypass increases markedly, 29 being the total for 1960.

Table 1

Cardiac operations RAHC Camperdown 1947–1960

	1947	1948	1949	1950ᵃ	1951	1952	1953	1954	1955	1956	1957	1958	1959	1960
PDA	3	2	5	5	12	7	16	15	16	33	40	35	28	42
Tetralogy			1	1	3	2	2	1	—	12	14	8	13ᶜ	19
Pulm. valvotomy						2	—	—	—	6	6	8ᵇ	5	5
Coarctation								1	1	1	4	6	5	3
Vasc. Ring											1	—	—	—
ASD											2	7	7	8
VSD													1	16
C Cath						2	—	9	50	49	73	98	95	100
LV Punct												3	2	3

ᵃ Figures incomplete
ᵇ Includes 2 aortic valvotomies
ᶜ Includes 2 revisions

Summary

The development of cardiac anaesthesia in a children's hospital developed over a twelve-year period from endotracheal ether for an occasional ductus ligation, through relaxant plus hypothermia techniques to allow longer time for valvotomies and ASD. Closure to the introduction of cardiopulmonary bypass, for more leisurely and accurate intracardiac surgery.

References

(1) Cohen D, Hercus V. Controlled hypothermia in infants and children. *Br Med J* 1959; **1**: 1435–9.
(2) Cohen D, Hercus V, Ebsary VR. The Royal Alexandra Hospital for Children Heart–Lung Machine, *Med J Aust* 1960; **2**: 734–6.

22.7   The history of oximetry*

J. SEVERINGHAUS
University of California, San Francisco, USA

Abstract

In 1860 the relation of blood colour to oxygen-transport by haemoglobin was demonstrated by Stokes and Hoppe-Seyler. In 1876, von Vierordt recorded the reduced Hb spectrum of light passing through his hand when he stopped the circulation. In 1932, Millikan and Roughton in Cambridge constructed a photoelectric colorimeter to measure blood oxygen saturation, during rapid O_2-Hb reactions *in vitro*, the first to introduce the idea of compensating for light and density changes by using a second O_2 insensitive wavelength. In Germany beginning in 1932 Nicolai, Kramer and Matthes constructed *in vivo* saturation meters, first for exposed arteries, then for the ear. Millikan's ear 'oximeter' in 1940, developed for military aviation, used red and (accidentally) infra-red light. Squire, Goldie and Wood built oximeters with pneumatic cuffs to obtain a bloodless zero, conceptually anticipating pulse oximetry. Reflection oximetry, developed about 1950 in Groningen, Netherlands led to the application of fibre optics to oximetry in 1962 by Polanyi. Using multiple wavelengths, carboxy haemoglobin and methaemoglobin were also measured in cuvette oximeters, from which Shaw developed the first pre-calibrated ear oximeter (Hewlett Packard).

In 1971 Takuo Aoyagi in Tokyo at Nihon Kohden Corporation attempted to eliminate arterial pulsatile 'noise' in his earpiece dye dilution curves by subtracting infra-red signals. He observed that the compensated noise varied with oxygen saturation and realized that

---

* The substance of this paper was published in historical reviews in a series on the history of blood gases and acids and bases. Full references will be found in:
1. Severinghaus JW, Astrup PB. The history of blood gas analysis VI: Oximetry. *J Clin Monitoring* 1986; **2**: 780.
2. Severinghaus JW and Honda Y. The history of blood gas analysis VII: Pulse oximetry. *J Clin Monitoring* 1987; **3**: 135.
3. Astrup PB, Severinghaus JW. *History of blood gases, acids and bases*. Copenhagen, Munksgaard, 1986.

it might be used to compute the arterial oxygen saturation. In his first pulse oximeter Aoyagi used 900 nM IR (rather than the isobestic 805 nM), hoping to also record dye dilution curves with the same device. It was commissioned and tested by surgeon Nakajima. A similar pulse oximeter was developed by Minolta, but early models were not successful. Shimada *et al*. showed that multiple internal scattering invalidated the theoretic (Beer's Law) equations. Pulse oximeters became practical and accurate when bright small light emitting diodes and sophisticated microchip computer programmes were introduced about 1980. New and Lloyd demonstrated the potential importance and enormous market for oximetry in anaesthesia and neonatology.

PART VI

BIOGRAPHY

Chapter 23
BEFORE 1846: THE PATHFINDERS

23.1

Thomas Beddoes (1760–1808),
tuberculosis and the medical pneumatic institutor

NORMAN A BERGMAN
Oregon Health Sciences University, Portland, Oregon, U.S.A.

Many individuals from the era of 'anaesthesia prehistory' helped to set the stage for the ultimate introduction of clinical anaesthesia in 1846 (1). A most important and pivotal role was played by Thomas Beddoes (1760–1808). Beddoes began operation of a Medical Pneumatic Institution at Bristol in 1798. His expectation was to obtain cures of diseases previously considered incurable by using therapeutic inhalation of gases and he engaged Humphry Davy as Medical Superintendent.

Davy had already developed an interest in nitrous oxide gas and, at the Pneumatic Institution he conductd extensive chemical investigations on this gas and proved its respirability. He also identified its effect on consciousness and its analgesic properties. Beddoes, too, experimented with nitrous oxide and the many celebrities from the fields of literature, industry, and science who inhaled nitrous oxide under the supervision of the Institution staff acknowledged publicly their predominantly pleasant experiences with the gas (2). The consequent frivolous use of nitrous oxide, and subsequently of diethyl ether, over the next half-century for demonstration and entertainment purposes, led directly to the introduction of clinical anaesthesia into medical practice (3). Thus, because of the essential role of Beddoes's Medical Pneumatic Institution in the discovery and dissemination of knowledge concerning properties of nitrous oxide, the circumstances surrounding the founding and operation of this facility are highly relevant to the history and development of anaesthesia.

By 1793 Beddoes had come to believe that several diseases which were of major concern to the 18th century physician were caused by excess or deficiency of oxygen in the body. Of these, pulmonary tuberculosis, the dreaded consumption or phthisis, was of greatest concern to him. In a series of publications from 1793 to 1798 he presented his theories on the aetiology of tuberculosis and proposed a cure based on the resulting conclusions. These ideas were eagerly accepted by his medical associations as well as members of the wealthy business, literary and landed classes with which he was associated. These individuals provided generous financial support and other types of aid which permitted founding of the Pneumatic Institution in 1798. It is not difficult to imagine why Beddoes's writings received such enthusiastic reception. Tuberculosis was rampant in England at the time of the industrial revolution. The peak was reached shortly after the turn of the 19th century and the mortality was appalling (4). There was no cure. There was scarcely one family with which Beddoes was aquainted which did not have one or more members afflicted with consumption. Hope of relief from this anguishing illness offered by a distinguished scientist and physician could not have failed to attract tangible expressions of support and encouragement which enabled the speculations to be tested. It is therefore of interest to examine Beddoes's career as well as his theories and ideas which led him to conclude that the primary inciting cause of pulmonary tuberculosis was an excess of oxygen in the body and that it could be cured by pneumatic means.

The career of Thomas Beddoes

Beddoes seemed to be particularly well qualified to tackle the problem of consumption because of his wide-ranging education and associations with distinguished contemporaries in medicine and chemistry. He received his BA degree from Oxford in 1781 and then studied medicine in both London and Edinburgh. At the latter institution he became a disciple of John Brown and retained his Brunonian beliefs and practices for the remainder of his career. Beddoes was awarded the MD degree by Oxford University in 1786 and, during this same year, he travelled on the continent and enjoyed a prolonged visit with Antoine Lavoisier and his brilliant wife. Beddoes was appointed Reader in Chemistry at Oxford in 1787 and remained in that post until his political beliefs (primarily support of French revolutionary republicanism) forced his resignation in 1792. He was a popular and inspired teacher and attracted large numbers of students to his chemical lectures (5). His previous scientific publications had included an annotated description of the work of John Mayow as well as English translations of selections from the works of Scheele, Spalanzzini, and Girtanner and, on the basis of these solid academic credentials, it seems probable that Beddoes' subsequent medical writings were likely to have been regarded as authoritative and worthy of careful attention.

Beddoes and Tuberculosis

The initial exposition of his ideas on tuberculosis appeared in his pamphlet 'Observations on the Nature and Cure of Calculus, Sea Scurvy. Consumption, Catarrh and Fever. etc.' dated Oxford, 30 July, 1792 (6). In the section of the manuscript on consumption, after a brief philosophical introduction, he immediately proposed without further explanation that the only possible starting point from which to approach tuberculosis was the observation that the onset of pregnancy may slow and ameliorate the course of tuberculosis—a proposition which is now known to be untrue (7). He wrote:

'The only circumstance in phthisis, from which, in our present state of ignorance, we can hope to reason to any purpose, has always appeared to me to be the occasional effect at least of pregnancy in suspending the progress of phthisis; for if we could once discover how pregnancy produces this singular effect, we might be led to discover also a method of superinducing and prolonging the same change of the system at pleasure.' (6)

Beddoes next identified the particular physiological alteration which he considered improved consumption during pregnancy as systemic oxygen lack caused by increased body oxygen demand in association with diminished ventilatory capacity:

'The fetus has its blood oxygenated by the blood of the mother through the placenta. During pregnancy there seems to be no provision for the reception of an unusual quantity of oxygen. On the contrary, in consequence of the impeded action of the diaphragm, less and less should be continually taken in by the lungs. If therefore a somewhat diminished proportion of oxygen be the effect of pregnancy may not this be the way in which it arrests the progress of phthisis; and if so, is there not an excess of oxygen in the system of consumptive persons? and may we not, by pursuing this idea, discover a cure for this fatal disorder?' (6)

The conceptual leap from physiological changes of pregnancy to consumption is enormous. This type of reasoning, however, was not peculiar to Beddoes. It is characteristic of the 18th century intellectual milieu in which he was educated and worked. To paraphrase an applicable quotation: 'To find fault with . . (the) . . theory, therefore, is to make a criticism rather of the age than of the man.' (9)

Beddoes next described physical signs and symptoms which he believed confirmed the state of oxygen lack in the pregnant subject. These included the thickened and darkened state of the blood and the so-called stigmata of pregnancy: (hyperpigmented spots and blotches covering the legs and thighs of pregnant women, pigmented striae on the abdomen and thighs and darkening and pigmentation of the face—the mask of pregnancy). These changes were thought to be related to scorbutic spots (subcutaneous haemorrhages in scurvy). Scurvy was another disease which Beddoes proposed was caused by oxygen deficiency. Beddoes appears to have regarded all darkness or pigmentation of the skin as attributable to oxygen lack and suggested a possible relationship between these stigmata of pregnancy and scurvy, arguing that pregnant women have an instinctive dislike for foods of animal origin and prefer vegetables and fruits. The latter types of foods were believed to contain oxygen in a form available to the body.

He then asked whether the inference from the supposed deficiency of oxygen in pregnant women was confirmed by appearances of phthisical patients indicating any redundancy of oxygen. He answered affirmatively:

> '. . the clear, bright and florid hue of the flushed hectic countanance, so diametrically opposite to the scorbutic complexion affords some presumption of a state of the blood, equally receding, but in an opposite direction from the standard of health.' (6)

Next placed in evidence were experiences and anecdotes relating inhalation to different gases and the course of tuberculosis. Beddoes' personal practice indicated that inhalation of oxygen, although possibly transiently beneficial in consumption, quickly aggravated cough, haempotysis, chest pain and fever. Joseph Priestley and Dr William Withering had treated consumption with fixed air (carbon dioxide gas) with considerable benefit but no cure. Other factors to be considered were a possible mutual exemption from tuberculosis conferred by scurvy and *vice versa* as well as an apparent remarkably low death rate from consumption among sailors continually exposed to wet and cold (believed to be aggravating circumstances in consumption) but also particularly vulnerable to scurvy.

Experimental evidence for the relationship between hyperoxia and tuberculosis included the observations by both Priestley and Lavoisier that small animals confined in oxygen lived longer than animals confined under similar circumstances in ordinary air but died long before the atmosphere of oxygen was exhausted. Other animals subsequently placed in the container seemed to do well. At autopsy of the original animals, the tissues, particularly the lungs, appeared extremely florid and turgid with blood. Could not consumption originate from a similar effect occurring more slowly? Other arguments along similar lines were presented.

Proposals for treatment of tuberculosis based on the above considerations were then presented. Beddoes suggested that the diet of the consumptive patient should be that known to promote scurvy. Eating of salty meats and oily foods was advocated while avoidance of vegetables and stimulants was advised. A second important therapeutic measure was inhalation of a gas mixture containing a lower concentration of oxygen than that of atmospheric air; The oxygen concentration of the atmosphere could be lowered by the addition of either azotic air (nitrogen) or hydrogene air (hydrogen). Patients should be removed from airy spacious apartments and should sleep in small, confined rooms with a cool temperature.

During the course of tuberculosis, if a marked loss of pulmonary tissue occurred the rate of progress of the disease might slow. Presage of the value of pulmonary collapse therapy was evident in Beddoes' presentation of cases in which tuberculosis was improved when the patients sustained either spontaneous or traumatic collapse of one side of the thoracic cage. He differentiated between the dyspnoea of asthma (dark skin) and of phthisis (red, flushed skin)—even in conditions of dyspnoea hyperoxygenation is evident in phthisis!

Beddoes enthusiastically emphasized his newly proposed method of therapy:

> 'the more you reflect the more you will be convinced that nothing would so much contribute to rescue the art of medicine from its present helpless condition as the discovery of the means of regulating the constitution of the atmosphere. It would be no less desirable to have a method of reducing the oxygen to 18 or 20 in a hundred than of increasing it in any proportion.' (6)*

On 17 January, 1793, Erasmus Darwin of Derby, one of the most renowned English physicians of the day, sent a letter to Thomas Beddoes. He inquired concerning any possible new ideas relating to the causes and treatment of tuberculosis which might have surfaced since publication of 'Calculus, Sea Scurvy, Consumption etc.'. He also asked about the nature of the apparatus which had been constructed to carry out the pneumatic treatments. Darwin generally concurred in the theories previously set forth by Beddoes. He praised his work and encouraged him to

---

* Beddoes, on the basis of Lavoisier's analysis, believed that the atmosphere contained 28% oxygen.

advance and continue in pneumatic medicine. This inquiry initiated the next publication of Beddoes: 'A Letter to Erasmus Darwin, M.D. on a New Method of Treating Pulmonary Consumption and Some other Diseases hitherto found Incurable'. This communication is dated: 'Hope-square, Bristol Hotwells, 30 June, 1793.' (10)

Beddoes offered several additional observations supporting his theories on the relationship between oxygen excess and tuberculosis in this publication. He concluded that the phthisical patient would take longer to drown or to suffocate in unfit airs than normal persons because of their preexisting condition of hyperoxygenation. An anecdotal case supporting this contention was presented. He then stated that consumption is less common in the southern than in the northern districts of France and that the overall incidence of consumption was higher in England than in France. This difference was attributed to the French mode of cookery which tended to divest foods of oxygen or to combine the oxygen more tightly than English cooking. French chefs permitted bread to rise longer, cooked food longer, and used oils and sauces generously, which were believed to be deficient in oxygen and to promote scurvy. The incidence of consumption was also lower in warm than in cool climates.

Beddoes maintained that the incidence of consumption was much more frequent in his time than in previous eras in England. The inhabitants were believed to breath a freer and purer air than their ancestors:

> *'You see then that subjects of our Edwards, and our Henrys, and good Queen Bess may have found, in being more free from so formidable a disease than their delicate and airy posterity, some compensation for the confined air and filth in which they passed their existence.'* (10)

Pertinent details of other cases of consumption were presented by Beddoes. He reported results of pneumatic therapy which had been performed. The most detailed was that of a physician's son who was treated by both pneumatic and dietary means. Although Beddoes was plagued by technical difficulties and the patient ultimately succumbed, the symptomatic relief and improvement following individual treatments was remarkable. A typical prescription for inhalation might have been about one part of hydrogen mixed with eight parts of atmospheric air. Darwin's inquiries about the apparatus used for preparation and handling of gases were answered. Beddoes was extremely optimistic about the future of medical practice wrought by new discoveries in pneumatic chemistry.

Further thoughts on tuberculosis and pneumatic means of therapy were advanced in 1795 in the book *Considerations on the Medicinal Use of Factitious Airs and on the Manner of Obtaining Them in Large Quantities*. James Watt was a co-author of this work with Beddoes (11). Watt had devised the apparatus used to collect, store and administer the therapeutic gases. During his discussion of properties and physiological effects of breathing different gases, Beddoes again emphasized the propensity of oxygen to cause pulmonary inflammation and the value of the atmosphere of 'low standard' for the treatment of consumption. Watt, despite the lack of medical qualification, also gave advice on the therapeutic value of several gases. Many different diseases amenable to treatment by pneumatic means were enumerated and numerous reports of cases treated by inhalation of factitious airs were presented.

The Medical Pneumatic Institution

The idea of founding a hospital to provide a greater volume of clinical material to evaluate pneumatic medicine occurred to Beddoes in 1793. Several appeals for financial support for this undertaking occurred over the next few years. The Medical Pneumatic Institution opened its doors in 1798 in Bristol with a long list of distinguished backers but the interest in pneumatic medicine had already peaked about 1795 and was waning when the activities at the hospital began. Expectations of pneumatic cures for various ills failed to materialize and tuberculosis continued to ravage society for many years. The principle importance of the Medical Pneumatic Institution was its role as a monumental milestone on the path towards the introduction of clinical anaesthesia as related previously. After the departure of Davy in

1801 the hospital became a Preventive Institution. Beddoes' later ideas on prevention of tuberculosis based upon concepts such as cleanliness and proper balanced diet make greater sense to the modern practitioner than his early speculations on hyperoxia and consumption (12). Nevertheless, it was probably these early conjectures on tuberculosis which attracted the interest and support of the public by offering some glimmer of hope in an otherwise dismal situation.

References

(1) Bergman NA. Forerunners of modern anesthesiology. *Pharos* 1985; **48**: 8–12.
(2) *Davy, Humphry. Researches, chemical and philosophical; chiefly concerning nitrous oxide.* London: J. Johnson, 1800: 373–559.
(3) Smith WDA. *Under the influence.* Park Ridge, III: The Wood Library-Museum of Anesthesiology, 1982: 19–41.
(4) Cartwright FF. *A social history of medicine.* London: Longman, 1977: 120–6.
(5) Stock JE. *Memoirs of the life of Thomas Beddoes, M.D. London:* John Murray, 1811: 42.
(6) Beddoes T. *Observations on the nature and cure of calculus, sea scurvy, consumption, catarrh, and fever etc.* Philadephia: T. Dobson, 1777. (First printed: London: J. Murray, 1793.)
(7) Rich AR. *The pathogenesis of tuberculosis.* Springfield, III: Charles C. Thomas, 1951.
(9) Hall CR. *A scientist in the Early Republic: Samuel Latham Mitchill, 1764–1831.* New York: Columbia University Press, 1934: 36.
(10) Beddoes T. *A Letter to Erasmus Darwin, M.D. on a new method of treating pulmonary consumption and some other diseases hitherto found incurable.* Bristol: Bulgin and Rosser, 1793.
(11) Beddoes T. Watt J. *Considerations on the medicinal use of factitious airs and on the manner of obtaining them in large quantities.* Bristol: Bulgin and Rosser, 1794–1796.
(12) Jacobs MS. Thomas Beddoes and his contribution to tuberculosis. *Bull Hist Med* 1943; 13: 300–12.

23.2   William Allen (1770–1843) the Spitalfields genius

PETER COE
Guy's Hospital, London, UK

William Allen was born at home in Spitalfields, City of London on Wednesday, 29 August, 1770. His father was a silk manufacturer in the city and both his parents belonged to the Society of Friends (Quakers). His father was keen that he should succeed him in his silk company, while his mother wanted him to become a Quaker religious leader. In fact William's interests were to lie elsewhere. At the age of fifteen he entered his father's business where he worked for three years. By this time he was pursuing an interest in the Sciences, (by the age of fourteen he had already constructed a home-made telescope, having an interest in astronomy, and had performed simple chemical experiments).

The Plough Court pharmacy

The Allen family were friendly with a fellow Quaker, Joseph Gurney Bevan, who owned a chemical establishment at Plough Court in the City of London, and in 1792 William Allen finally abandoned the silk trade and settled in Plough Court as Bevan's apprentice (1–5).

Plough Court as Allen knew it was a cul-de-sac off Lombard Street, entered via an archway, [2]. Three houses faced into the yard, having been built in 1668 following the Great Fire of London, on land owned by the Haberdashers Company. Number 2 Plough Court was the birthplace in 1688 of the poet Alexander Pope and in the modern thoroughfare a plaque commemorates this. Silvanus Bevan acquired number 2 Plough Court in 1715 when he opened the first apothecary's shop there. As the business grew he took the lease of number 3 Plough Court, to provide space for chemical manufacture.

The Plough Court pharmacy was handed down through the Bevan family to his grandson Joseph Bevan, who is said to have been born in the same room as Pope. As he had no heir, he was succeeded by Samuel Mildred in 1794, when he retired because of ill health at the early age of 40 years.

William Allen had been apprenticed to Bevan and lived at the Plough Court pharmacy from 1792.

In 1795 he entered into partnership with Mildred and by 1797 had encouraged Mildred to take early retirement with a golden handshake of £500, enabling him to set up partnership with his friend and fellow Quaker Luke Howard.

This was a happy partnership, but Howard became more interested in the manufacture of heavy chemicals, and in 1806 the partnership was amicably terminated and Howard left to set up a factory in Ilford, leaving Allen the owner of the Plough Court pharmacy. Meanwhile he attended the classes of Mr Bryan Higgins, a London chemist and physician, who lectured on the Sciences. By 1795 he had been elected a member of the Physical Society at Guy's Hospital and had become a physician's pupil at St Thomas's Hospital. The success of his business prevented him from completing these studies. His main interest was chemistry and in April 1799 he assisted in the formation of the British Mineralogical Society. In 1800 he began the study of Botany, becoming a fellow of the Linnean Society only two years later.

Allen and chemical philosophy

Allen attended lectures at the Royal Institution in Albemarle Street, London, and his circle of friends included scientists and physicians and in 1796 they formed the Askesian Society at Plough Court. The object of the Society was to elucidate, by experiment, either facts generally understood, or to examine and repeat any novel discoveries, and to improve themselves by philosophical exercises. The meetings were held twice a month in the winter season, and each member in turn had to produce a paper for reading and discussion upon some subject of scientific inquiry. Many of the papers were afterwards published in *Tilloch's Philosophical Magazine*. The society lasted twenty years, the founder members included William Allen, Luke Howard and William Hasledine Pepys. Later on they were joined by Astley Cooper, surgeon at Guy's Hospital, William Babington, physician and mineralogist at Guy's Hospital and Humphry Davy, who was to become a close friend to Allen.

William Allen had attended meetings of the Guy's chemical society in early 1795 and was elected into the Society in April 1795. In October 1795 he became a member of the Physical Society at Guy's Hospital, and formed the Askesian Society one year later.

Allen's lectureships

Dr Babington called at Plough Court in January 1802 and offered Allen a partnership in his lectures on Chemistry at Guy's Hospital. Allen was initially unsure whether to accept but, after advice from Astley Cooper and Joseph Bevan, he agreed and one month later gave his first lecture. He was nervous about giving the lecture, and awoke feeling distressed and low, his anxiety was heightened by the presence of Dr Babington in the lecture theatre and by the arrival of Astley Cooper after the lecture had started, but the students received him well (1). By May his lectures had become very popular and up to 180 students crowded into a theatre to hear him give the last lectures of that term. Allen appears to have been both a good and popular lecturer although always nervous beforehand, and would often sit up all night preparing notes for his lecture the next day. The lecture course was based on Chemistry in the morning and Physics in the evenings. He continued to lecture twice a week at Guy's until 1826, when the demands of his business, family, and public work forced him to give up the lectureship.

In 1803 Allen was elected as one of the Presidents of the Guy's Physical Society and in November the same year was asked by Davy to undertake a lecture course at the Royal Institution along the lines of the lecture course at Guy's; after a little hesitation Allen accepted, giving his first lecture on 24 January, 1804. The first lecture course he gave was on natural philosophy and he was very popular, continuing to lecture at the Royal Institution until 1811. He lectured mainly on natural philosophy, mechanical inventions and their history, but also would stand in for his friend Davy if he was absent, lecturing on Pneumatics on one occasion (1).

Allen and chemical research

Nitrous oxide

Humphry Davy had been experimenting with nitrous oxide around this time and had shown that the gas could be respired. The members of the Askesian Society had expressed an interest in this and on 27 February, 1800, (Allen's diary), they repeated Davy's experiment of breathing nitrous oxide. Present at Plough Court were Astley Cooper, William Allen and other members of the Society. Allen's own description of the experiment follows:

> 'We all breathed the gaseous oxide of azote, it took a surprising effect on me, abolishing completely at first all sensation. Then I had the idea of being carried violently upward in a dark cavern, with only a few glimmering lights. The company said my eyes were very fixed, face purple, veins in the forehead very large, apoplectic stertor etc. They were all much alarmed, but I suffered no pain and in a short time came to myself'.

This account is published in many books, (1–6), but Allen's own diary also records a previous experiment with nitrous oxide. W. H. Pepys provided Allen with much practical help for his experiments, and is recorded as making the new gas from nitrate of ammonia for an Askesian meeting on 28 January, 1800, when Allen and a certain Mr Tupper breathed nitrous oxide and noted it's effects as being remarkably inebriating. William Allen included nitrous oxide in his lecture course at Guy's and in 1806 his lecture 'of nitrous oxyd gas' (6,7) stated that it was:

> 'procured from the decomposition of nitrate of ammonia, with a gentle heat. Soluble in double its volume of water, to which it communicates a sweet taste. Remarkable for the intoxicating effects which it produces in respiration'.

Additional handwritten notes by George Hickman, a Guy's medical student attending the course that year include:

> 'this gas had been thought to be irrespirable but Davy has proved that it may, when respired it produces a most curious sensation. It should not be exhibited to hysterical persons, it has been known to produce ill effects—tho in the common number of persons it produces only temporary effects'.

It is interesting to note that despite the presence of one of the great surgeons of the time during the experiments, the possibility of using the gas in a clinical capacity to reduce the pain of surgery was never considered. Astley Cooper was one of the most innovative surgeons of the time, but in these pre-antiseptic days, spent more time in the dissecting room than the operating theatre. The incidence of wound infection was high and surgery was only undertaken in life or death situations, so the role of a drug in rendering the patient insensible to pain may not have been foremost in their minds.

Oxygen, carbon dioxide and respiration

William Allen was elected Fellow of the Royal Society in 1807. Along with William Hasledine Pepys (another Quaker chemist), he undertook chemical experiments using the Eudiometer a simple device designed by Pepys (8) which could measure gas absorption during a chemical reaction.

They delivered a paper on respiration to the Royal Society in 1808 describing the changes produced in atmospheric air and oxygen by respiration. They used a spirometric method of delivering the air and collecting it after respiration for chemical analysis. They were able to calculate the amount of carbon dioxide in the expired gases by using absorption into lime water in the eudiometer, and oxygen content by absorbing the oxygen over ferrous sulphate. The conclusion of the experiment was that the only change that occurs to air when it is breathed is the substitution of carbon dioxide for a proportion of the oxygen and that water was not produced by union of oxygen and hydrogen in the lungs. One variation of the experiment was to allow one subject to totally rebreath into the spirometer—they describe the result as follows:

'in less than a minute the subject found himself obliged to take deeper and deeper inspirations and at last the efforts of the lungs to take in air became so strong and sudden, that the glass was in some danger of being broken against the side of the gasometer. A great sense of oppression and suffocation was not felt in the chest, vision became indistinct, and after the second minute his whole attention seemed to be withdrawn from surrounding objects, and fixed on the experiment. He now experienced that buzz in the ears that is noticed in breathing nitrous oxide, and after the third minute had only sufficient recollection to close the cock after expiration. This secured the result of the experiment, but he had become so perfectly insensible that on recovering, he was much surprised to find his friend and the assistant on the table in the act of supporting him'.

The air from the gasometer was analysed and found to contain 10% carbon dioxide, 86% nitrogen and 4% oxygen, this experiment led them to state that as oxygen diminishes in quantity perception gradually ceases and they surmised that life would be completely extinguished on the total abstraction of oxygen (9). The sensation of breathing a hypoxic mixture also sounded not surprisingly like the sensations described by Allen when breathing pure nitrous oxide earlier on.

Allen and Pepys presented a paper in 1809 describing an experiment to prove that the lungs did not collapse fully on expiration as had been thought previously. From a cadaver experiment they concluded that an adult's lungs had a residual volume of more than 100 cubic inches of air (10).

Allen and social reform

Allen was one of the philanthropic Quakers of the time who were concerned with social reform. His friends included slavery abolitionists William Wilberforce and Elizabeth Fry. They met frequently at Plough Court and their campaigning eventually led to the Abolition of Slavery Bill passed in 1807. As a Christian he could not accept capital punishment, and in 1808 he formed the Society for the Abolition of Capital Punishment.

At home he and Joseph Lancaster collaborated in establishing a school in Borough Road, London, this opened in 1808 aiming to educate the children of the local poor by the monitorial system. His co-operation with Robert Owen, now credited as being the founder of Infant Schools in Great Britain was less successful. The aim was to run a cotton mill at New Lanark near Glasgow as a worker's co-operative, but the Christian Allen could not reconcile himself with the agnostic Owen, and the partnership was dissolved by Allen.

After this disappointment he established a school of industry at Lindfield in Sussex which opened in 1825. The principles of this school were embodied in the Education acts of the 1950s some 125 years later. A small boarding school for boys was also set up and Allen taught at the school himself, treating the boys as if his own family.

Abroad Allen travelled Europe widely as an evangelist for the Society of Friends. During a visit to Russia he was introduced to Czar Alexander Ist, and they developed a close friendship that lasted until the Czar's death in 1825.

Allen also counted amongst his friends the Duke of Kent. When the Duke ran into financial difficulties, Allen and some of his friends acted as trustees. The Duke's daughter, Victoria, became Queen in 1837 and would have known Allen as one of her father's closest friends.

Allen's family life

William Allen, married three times. His first wife died 5 days after giving birth to their daughter Mary in 1795; they had only been married a year. His second wife was Charlotte Hanbury whom he married in 1806, thereafter taking up residence at the Hanbury family home in Stoke Newington, North London. Charlotte's nephews also lived in this home and became as sons to Allen. One of them, Daniel Bell Hanbury, joined the Plough Court pharmacy which he took over after Allen's death. The other, Cornelius Hanbury, also worked at Plough Court and in 1822 married Allen's daughter Mary, thus the families of Allen and Hanbury became linked both by marriage and business, and this union eventually led to the expansion of the Plough Court pharmacy into the modern pharmaceutical company of Allen and Hanburys. Charlotte died whilst they were abroad in 1816.

In May 1823 his grandson William Allen Hanbury was born, but his daughter died following childbirth. Allen received much support from a widow, Grizell Birkbeck, a lifelong Quaker friend of Allen and she became his third wife in 1826, until her death in 1835.

William Allen's health and mental faculties which had been so good, eventually deteriorated and he died on 30 December, 1843, at the age of 73 years, just before the clinical use of nitrous oxide and ether to relieve the pain of surgery was reported (6). The Spitalfields genius was buried in the Quaker burial ground, Yoakley Road, Stoke Newington, where today a small worn stone, marks the spot.

References

(1) *The life of William Allen* (in three volumes). London: Charles Gilpin,1846.
(2) Chapman-Huston D, Cripps EC. *Through a city archway, the story of Allen and Hanburys 1715-1954*. London: Murray, 1954.
(3) Wilks S and Bettany GT. *A biographical history of Guy's Hospital*. London: Ward, Lock, Bowden and Co, 1892.
(4) Fayle J. *The Spitalfields genius, the story of William Allen FRS*. London: Hodder and Stoughton, 1884.
(5) Cripps EC. *Plough Court, the story of a notable pharmacy, 1715-1927*. London: Allen and Hanburys, 1927.
(6) Smith WDA. *Under the influence. The history of nitrous oxide and oxygen anaesthesia*. London: MacMillan, 1982.
(7) Babington W, Allen W. *A syllabus of a course of chemical lectures read at Guy's Hospital*. London: W. Phillips, 1802.
(8) Pepys WH. A new eudiometer. *Phil Trans Roy Soc Lond* 1807; **97**: 247–59.
(9) Allen W, Pepys WH. On the changes produced in atmospheric air and oxygen gas, produced by respiration. *Phil Trans Roy Soc Lond* 1808; **98**: 249–81.
(10) Allen W, Pepys WH. On respiration. *Phil Trans Roy Soc Lond* 1809; **99** 404–29.

23.3	Davy's contribution to inhalational anaesthesia

DAVID P. COATES
Sir Humphry Davy Department of Anaesthetics, Bristol University, UK

Humphry Davy was not an anaesthetist: 'Philosophy, Chemistry, and Medicine are my profession' he said. However, his contribution to the understanding of the chemical and physiological properties of nitrous oxide opened the door for its subsequent medical use in a way that was barely conceivable at the time of his fundamental but precise initial investigations. It is tempting to conclude that he had the foresight to predict the revolution that the introduction of anaesthesia was to come that was not to occur for nearly 50 years, when he wrote:

> *'As nitrous oxide in its extensive operation appears capable of destroying physical pain, it may probably be used with advantage during surgical operations in which no great effusion of blood takes place.'*

To fully comprehend his contribution, one has to consider the scientific knowledge and principles pertaining at the time. Born in rural Cornwall, 300 miles from London, in 1778, Davy was educated at local schools. He was apparently not an exceptional pupil but displayed an aptitude for languages and especially enjoyed poetry. Indeed, the latter remained a life-long interest and, in the midst of his hectic scientific work in Bristol at the turn of the century, he contributed to Southey's *Annual Anthology* and criticized and revised several works by Coleridge, Southey and Wordsworth.

From the biography by Paris it appears that the time Davy spent between leaving school, at the age of 16, and becoming an apprentice to an appothecary and surgeon in Penzance allowed him the opportunity to develop his inquisitive personality and formulate his ambitions. At that stage he intended to go to Edinburgh to qualify as a physician. During his apprenticeship, he studied widely. His voracious interest in chemistry was initiated by reading Lavoisier's *Traite Elementaire* in the original French just before his 19th birthday in December 1797. This work introduced a new theory of chemistry and contradicted the still widely held phlogiston theory. Stahl had ascribed the ability of a substance to burn to the presence of phlogiston; the residue was said to be dephlogisticated. It must be borne in mind that, in these days, interest in scientific matters was displayed as much for the philosophical benefit of thought provocation and debate as for the intrinsic value of an exact conclusion. For example, Coleridge and Wordsworth began to study chemistry for the intellectual relief it provided and to rest their minds from the passions of poetry. Prompted by his readings, Davy undertook a series of experiments designed to investigate various properties of light, heat and gases. Gregory Watt, whose father, James, had developed the concept of steam power, was staying with Davy at this time. He suffered from poor health, probably as a result of tuberculosis, and was hoping to gain benefit from the country air. It was Watt who put Davy in contact with Beddoes in Bristol in April 1798. They corresponded about Davy's experiments, Beddoes was favourably impressed and the post of superintendent to the recently commissioned Pneumatic Institution was offered. Davy left for Bristol in October 1798 and his rapidly written experimental conclusions were published early in 1799 in *Contributions to Physical and Medical Knowledge, Principally from the West of England, Collected by Thomas Beddoes, MD*. The time from the dawning of Davy's interest in chemistry to his arrival at the Pneumatic Institution was two years; he was just 20 years old.

Work at the Pneumatic Institution

The Pneumatic Institution was established to enable the assessment of the prevailing concept, that various gases could have therapeutic properties when inhaled. In 1794, Beddoes and James Watt had published the pamphlet *Consideration on the Medicinal Use of Factitious Airs and on the Manner of Obtaining them in Large Quantities*. A supplement was added two years later that included a reprint of a book on nitrous oxide by an American, Samuel Mitchill. Davy had read the original in 1798 and this had directed his attention to the dephlogisticated nitrous gas (nitrous oxide) described by Joseph Priestley. Mitchill had postulated a theory of Contagion, by which he had attempted to prove that nitrous oxide, which he called oxide of septon, was the principal factor responsible for contagious diseases, and capable of producing disease when respired or applied to skin or muscle. Priestley had thought nitrous oxide '. . . was in the highest degree noxious to animals' and the Society of Dutch Chemists later came to a similar conclusion.

It was with this background that Davy started his research. He immediately proved that nitrous oxide could be breathed safely. Having carefully manufactured the gas personally, he inhaled it and recorded the effects. Great importance was placed on the purity of the gas. He described in great detail the decomposition of ammonium nitrate with increasing temperature to produce respirable nitrous oxide and he developed a technique for obtaining and storing the gas in sufficient quantities for experimental and medicinal use. Similar methods and apparatus were used at least half a century later by the early anaesthetists who had to manufacture their own gas. Nitrous oxide is still manufactured commercially from ammonium nitrate with stringently controlled purification of the resultant gas.

The results of his exhaustive endeavours, which included chemical analysis and physiological investigation of amphibians and mammals, were published in *Researches, Chemical and Philosophical chiefly concerning Nitrous Oxide or Dephlogisticated Nitrous Air, and its Respiration* in 1800. He makes several references to the analgesic properties of nitrous oxide in relieving head and tooth ache and describes how he gained relief from the chest pain and oppressive sensation associated with breathing a gas mixture containing a significant concentration of carbon monoxide.

The reason that he did not pursue his celebrated contention regarding the use of nitrous oxide to relieve the suffering associated with surgery has long been debated. He, unlike Beddoes, was not medically qualified and the Pneumatic Institution did not aspire to surgical remedies. He could, however, have extended the scope of his animal experiments to include investigations of the analgesic property of the gas during surgical operations. It is surprising, in view of his thorough attitude to scientific research, that apparently he chose not to investigate personally these possibilities further. It was the excitatory properties of the gas that were considered to be most important and it was only used for medicinal, as opposed to pleasurable purposes, in patients being treated for '. . extreme debility produced by deficiency of common exciting powers'. Even though Davy benefited personally from the analgesic properties of the gas and believed 'it may *probably* be used with advantage', it may have proved very difficult to convince a sceptical audience, to whom the concept of pain-free surgery was an impossible dream, that such a possibility even existed. There was undoubtedly a variation in the physiological response of healthy patients to inhalations of the gas due in part to its purity and oxygen content and the amount of rebreathing that could have occurred during its administration. Pallor, cyanosis and weakening or quickening of the pulse were assiduously recorded signs. They were most frequently demonstrated after the prolonged inhalation of the gas which would have been necessary to provide surgical anaesthesia. Beddoes may not have wished to pursue the concept in case it brought disrepute to his establishment.

If it is surprising that Davy chose not to investigate the possibility further, it is perhaps even more remarkable that no one else did following the publication of his well received *Researches*.

Davy proved, at an early stage of his research, that nitrous oxide was absorbed by the blood. He conducted a number of experiments to investigate this phenomenon quantitatively. This necessitated the measurement of lung volumes. He used Clayfield's mercurial air holder which is not dissimilar in design to a modern spirometer and has a volume of 3.25 litre. With practice, he found that he could repeatedly exhale to a residual volume that varied by only about 25 ml. (*Inter alia* he recognized that posture could significantly influence lung volumes.) He then breathed pure nitrous oxide from the air holder. He commented that, due to the inevitable intoxication that took place, he could not reliably breath the gas for more than 45 seconds without breaking the gastight seal with his mouth. He measured the amount of nitrous oxide remaining in the air holder, taking into account the carbon dioxide and nitrogen that it now also contained. The difference between this and the original volume had been taken up by his body. From the description of two experiments in *Researches*, he showed the rate of uptake to be about 1.3 litres/min. He realized also that some of this would be in the airways and not actually in the blood and so he endeavoured to establish his own residual volume including the dead space. This involved some alarming experiments with pure hydrogen which he had previously shown not to be absorbed. His results indicated a total lung volume of only about 2 litres but he was a small man and he commented that:

'This capacity is probably below the medium, my chest is narrow, measuring in circumference, but 29 inches, and my neck is rather long and slender'.

Conclusion

Davy spent just over two years at the Pneumatic Institution before departing to take up the post of Assistant Lecturer in Chemistry, Director of the Laboratory and Assistant Editor of the

Journals at the Royal Institution in London in March 1801. He was appointed Professor of Chemistry there 14 months later and, in November 1803, he was elected a Fellow of the Royal Society shortly before his 25th birthday. His interests, although remaining catholic, moved away from medicine and he did not complete a formal medical education. He never again had sufficient time to devote to a single subject in the way that he had been able to do in Bristol. Although he died, in 1829, before the advent of anaesthesia, his researches in chemistry and physiology made a definite, if inadvertent, contribution to scientific anaesthesia. He was the first to establish a safe and reliable method of manufacturing uncontaminated nitrous oxide and he investigated and described the physiological effects of inhaling the gas. He also determined its rate of uptake by the blood, a factor that had to wait another 150 years to be investigated further by Severinghaus and he made determined efforts to measure his own lung volumes even to the extent of developing hypoxaemia when breathing pure hydrogen. There is no doubt that he recognized the analgesic properties of nitrous oxide and almost certainly anticipated the possibility of anaesthesia.

23.4   A nitrous anaesthetic declined:
                                    Sir Humphry Davy, PRS, (1778–1829)
                          portrayed by Sir Thomas Lawrence, PRA (1769–1830)

GEORGE S. BAUSE
Yale University School of Medicine, New Haven, Connecticut, USA

Most anaesthetists have encountered patients who were reluctant to receive anaesthesia. In 1821 the President of the Royal Academy (PRA), Sir Thomas Lawrence, declined to breathe the nitrous oxide offered to him by the President of the Royal Society (PRS), Sir Humphry Davy (1). The factors leading to Lawrence's refusal of laughing gas are a compelling addendum to anaesthetic history.

The Richards family connection

On 15 March, 1975, near the coal mining region of Reading, Pennsylvania, in the United States, the author accompanied Mrs Margretta Lena Richards Drumheller to see her paternal uncle, Robert J. Richards. At 95 years of age, Mr Richards was finally succumbing to the 'black lung' disease induced by his years of inhaling coal dust in the mines. Bedridden and receiving home oxygen, Mr. Richards nonetheless seemed determined to share some of the Richards family history with his niece. He proudly revealed that his great-uncle had invented a miner's lamp which prevented gas explosions in the mines. Mrs Drumheller revealed subsequently that Mr Richards's brother, her father, was named John Davy Richards (2). This fact was confirmed by a thorough inspection of the German Protestant Cemetery of Mahonoy City, Pennsylvania.

Mrs Drumheller's second husband, Guy Benjamin Drumheller, volunteered that his wife actually had a Davy lamp passed down through the family to her in their basement at home (3). He pressed Mr Richards as to whether this was the miner's safety lamp. Mr Richards had not seen the lamp, but he did recall that in his youth he had seen a portrait of his great-uncle next to an early model of the lamp. Family members had related to Mr Richards that the inventor of the safety lamp had offered to 'gas' the painter of the portrait, but that the artist had refused. Mr Richards could not fathom 'why anyone would willingly expose himself to firedamp outside of a coal mine.' (1)

Robert J. Richards succumbed a short time later to his black lung disease. It is perhaps ironic that the invention of the miner's safety lamp by Sir Humphry Davy had indirectly facilitated the choice of mining as a vocation for many of Davy's American relatives. Robert J. Richards, John Davy Richards, and a host of men in the Richards family were afflicted with black lung disease (2).

On 18 December, 1982, near the artists' haven of New Hope, in Lahaska, Pennsylvania, the author located an oil portrait of Sir Humphry Davy from a Richards family estate (3). This portrait appeared to be the one that Robert J. Richards had seen in his youth. The portrait, *Sir Humphry Davy, Bart., from Lady Davy*, had been painted in 1821 as a unique 'one quarter' of life-size oil of Sir Humphrey standing next to his safety lamp. The artist was Sir Thomas Lawrence, PRA. By this time I had deduced that Davy's great-nephew, Robert J. Richards, had been describing Davy's efforts at administering nitrous oxide, not 'firedamp' or methane as we now call it, to an unwilling Lawrence. Remember that Coleridge, Southey, Wordsworth, and Roget had all inhaled nitrous oxide and had all reported its benefits. Understanding why Lawrence declined inhalation of nitrous oxide requires an in-depth look at this careful man.

Sir Thomas Lawrence, PRA

Son of an English solicitor turned innkeeper, Sir Thomas Lawrence was born on Redcross Street, Bristol, in 1769. By four years of age, Lawrence was entertaining his father's guests, pencilling their portraits with astonishing skill. By 1782 Lawrence's reputation as a child prodigy had preceded him to Bath, where he undertook chalk pastel. As both pugilist and portrait artist, Lawrence began sparring there with Britain's boxing champion, John 'Gentleman Jackson,' years before Lord Byron was to do so.

Besides boxing, Lawrence had a lifelong passion for collecting the old masters' works of art. This avocation brought him to near-bankruptcy several times. The President of the Royal Academy, Sir Joshua Reynolds, admonished Lawrence in London that:

> *'it is very clear that you have been looking at the old masters, but my advice to you is to study nature, apply your talents to nature.'* (4)

Inspired by the President's advice, Lawrence exhibited seven crayon portraits in 1787 at the Royal Academy and enrolled there as a student. Lawrence's single 1788 oil portrait of Mr Darsey was eclipsed by the brilliant group of thirteen oils he displayed the following year. One of these, *Lady Cremorne*, led to Lawrence's first royal commission, when he was:

> *'commanded by Her Majesty to . . . come down to Windsor and bring . . . painting apparatus . . .'* (5)

Lawrence soon caught the public's eye with his 1790 portraits of Queen Charlotte, Princess Amelia, and the romantic *Miss Farren*. Under the pseudonym 'Anthony Pasquin,' John Williams satirized Sir Joshua Reynolds years later as having said, 'This young man has begun at a point of excellence where I left off.' (6)

Peter Pindar recorded vividly the King's dismay in 1791 when the Royal Academy initially refused Lawrence early election as an Associate:

> *'Refuse a Monarch's mighty orders!—It smells of treason—on rebellion borders! 'Sdeath, Sirs! it was the Queen's fond wish as well, that Master Lawrence should come in!'* (7)

The King corrected this injustice the following year when, on Sir Joshua's death, Lawrence succeeded Reynolds as Painter-in-Ordinary to His Majesty George III. In an 'attempt to correct the National Taste,' Anthony Pasquin lampooned that:

> *'Mr. Lawrence began his professional career upon a false and delusive principle. His portraits were delicate but not true, and attractive but not admirable—and because he met the approbation of a few fashionable spinsters (which, it must be admitted, is a sort of inticement very intoxicating to a young mind) vainly imagined that his labors were perfect—his fertile mind is overrun with weeds . . .'* (8)

In 1794 as a newly admitted Royal Academician, Lawrence unveiled *A Gypsy Girl*. Popularly juxtaposed with Gainsborough's 'Blue Boy,' Lawrence's 'Pinkie' portrait the following year immortalized Miss Mary Moulton Barrett, the aunt of Elizabeth Barrett Browning. Lawrence was greeted as a Regency portrait painter who specialized in portraying beautiful ladies and

490 *The History of Anaesthesia, eds. R. S. Atkinson & T. B. Boulton*

pretty children. Nonetheless the public was fascinated by Lawrence's self-described masterwork, the enormous *Satan Calling His Legions*. An anonymous poet mused:

> *'Lawrence beware how you impart*
> *Unto the world a second evil,*
> *For once, 'tis said, your magic art*
> *Made all mankind adore the Devil.'*(9)

The Demon was modelled, in fact, in a narrative rather than portrait style after Lawrence's boxing mentor 'Gentleman Jackson.' Anthony Pasquin lampooned hapless Lawrence's Satan as:

> *'a mad German sugar-baker dancing naked in a conflagration of his own treacle; but the liberties taken with his infernal Majesty are so numerous, so various, and so insulting, that we are amazed that the ecclesiastic orders do not interfere in behalf of an old friend.'* (6)

The disappointing reception for his *Satan* had a sobering effect on Lawrence's later work.

Sir Thomas Lawrence presented the Royal Academy with nine to ten portraits a year over a span of thirty-three years. His prolific painting showed an astonishing variability in quality, perhaps reflecting his recurring financial difficulties. Prince Metternich and the Duke of Wellington were portrayed brilliantly in 1815, and the Prince-Regent, soon to be George IV, after seeing his own portrait, knighted Lawrence. As Sir Thomas, then, Lawrence sojourned to the Continent, where he painted the likenesses of the Austrian, Prussian, and Russian victors of the Napoleonic Wars. He travelled onward to Rome and captured both Pope Pius VII and Cardinal Gonsalvi on canvas. On his return to England in 1820, Sir Thomas Lawrence was elected President of the Royal Academy.

Lawrence's portraits and subjects

For a fee of 150 guineas (5), Lawrence had been commissioned soon after his return to Britain to celebrate in three-quarter of life-size the baronetcy of Sir Humphry Davy. Now as President of the Royal Academy, Lawrence was commissioned by Lady Davy in December of 1820 to commemorate Sir Humphry Davy's election as President of the Royal Society with a smaller one-quarter life-sized oil of the same pose of her husband.

When he sat for Lawrence, Davy made a point of recounting his experiences with the gas, including his 26 December, 1798, inhalation of twenty quarts of unmingled nitrous oxide:

> *'A thrilling extending from the chest to the extremities, was almost immediately produced. I felt a sense of tangible extension highly pleasurable in every limb; my visible impressions were dazzling and apparently magnified, I heard distinctly every sound in the room and was perfectly aware of my situation. By degrees as the pleasurable sensations increased, I lost all connection with external things; trains of vivid visible images rapidly passed through my mind and were connected with words in such a manner, as to produce perceptions perfectly novel. I existed in a world of newly connected and newly modified ideas: I theorised; I imagined that I made discoveries.'* (10)

In the sixth stanza of his poem 'Spinosism,' Davy seemed to set to verse his sensations of inhaling nitrous oxide:

> *'To breathe the ether; and to feel the form*
> *Of orbid beauty through its organs thrill;*
> *To press the limbs of life with rapture warm,*
> *And drink of transport from a living rill!'* (11)

Lawrence, Davy and the poets

Lawrence was well aware of the poet as well as natural philosopher hidden within Sir Humphry Davy. It was common knowledge that Sir Humphry relished conversations he had with the Lake Poets. Mr Cottle of the Cottle and Biggs publishing firm introduced Samuel T. Coleridge to Sir Humphry Davy. When Cottle pressed Coleridge to compare Davy to 'the cleverest men,' Coleridge responded:

> *'Why Davy could eat them all! There is an energy, an elasticity in the mind which enables him to seize on, and analyze all questions, pushing them to their legitimate consequences.*

> *Every subject in Davy's mind has the principle of* vitality. *Living thoughts spring up like turf under his feet.'* (11)

Holding Davy in such high esteem, Coleridge convinced Wordsworth to ask Davy 'to look over the proof sheets' of the second volume of Wordsworth's *Lyrical Ballads* (12). Rather fond of Davy's nitrous oxide, Coleridge was surprised by the effects of his third exposure to the gas:

> *'The third time I was more violently acted on than in the other two. Towards the last, I could not avoid, nor indeed felt any wish to avoid, beating the ground with my feet; and after the mouth-piece was removed, I remained for a few seconds motionless, in great extacy.'* (10)

Of the Lake Poets, Robert Southey had the most intense relationship with Davy's nitrous oxide. After inhaling nitrous oxide, Southey was reported to have exclaimed:

> *'the atmosphere of the highest of all heavens to be composed of this gas.'* (13)

His initial enthusiasm was short-lived:

> *'Now after an interval of some months, during which my health has been materially impaired, the nitrous oxide produces an effect upon me totally different. Half the quantity affects me, and its operation is more violent; a slight laughter is first induced, and a desire to continue the inhalation, which is counteracted by fear from the rapidity of respiration; indeed my breath becomes so short and quick, that I have no doubt but the quantity which I formerly breathed would now destroy me. The sensation is not painful, neither is it in the slightest degree pleasurable.'* (10)

Coleridge, Southey, and countless other prominent figures presented their tales of nitrous oxide adventure to Lawrence. Upon revealing his curiosity about the gas to Sir Humphry, Lawrence found Davy increasingly fascinated with the idea of administering the gas to Lawrence. Lawrence declined Davy's offer, because, unlike the visionary Romantics, Coleridge and Southey, Lawrence felt he could neither spare the time from his busy schedule nor risk distracting his concentration from portraiture. Lawrence reasoned the way he rhymed:

> *'While to retrieve the past neglected time,*
> *My days I give to unremitting toil,*
> *And shake the rust from off my better mind,*
> *Which too distracting thoughts have left to soil.'* (4)

One distraction which piqued Lawrence was the possibility that he as PRA would be overlooked when the time came for formally celebrating the coronation ceremony of George IV. Lawrence would later write to the Clarenceux King of Arms, Sir George Nayler, that the President of the Royal Academy had 'strong claims, altho' not by Right or Precedent . . .' to participate in the procession. (14) Heartily concurring with Lawrence, Davy expressed his interest in having both the PRA and the PRS take part in the coronation. After all, both Lawrence and Davy had been knighted by the Prince-Regent, soon to be King George IV. When Lawrence realized Davy's support for the PRA's participating, Lawrence felt some obligation to return the favour. However, the PRA remained uncomfortable about what to expect from the PRS's gas.

For that matter, not everyone Lawrence had encountered had experienced salutary effects from inhaling nitrous oxide. In particular, two of Lawrence's sitters, Sir James Mackintosh and James Watt, had related to Lawrence the disturbing nitrous oxide experiences of Gregory Watt and Josiah Wedgwood. Somewhat disenchanted, the Scottish engineer James Watt confessed his disappointment in nitrous oxide as he sat for his regency portrait, which was exhibited by Lawrence at the Royal Academy in 1813. (15) Though a staunch supporter of Davy, Watt had complained to Lawrence that Davy's gas, as pneumatic therapy, had done nothing to improve the health of Watt's stricken son, Gregory. Earlier the younger Watt's tuberculosis had been severe enough to force his retreat from Scotland to the south. James Watt had been instrumental in providing Dr Thomas Beddoes with apparatus for his Pneumatic Institute in Bristol. As Kenneth Bryn Thomas noted:

> *'Watt had a consumptive son, Gregory, who had been under treatment by Beddoes, and James Watt, impressed by the physician's knowledge of pneumatic medicine, was willing to come to his aid in designing apparatus which was made at the Birmingham factory of Boulton and Watt.'* (16)

Along with his associate William Clayfield, the elder Watt had successfully designed inhalational apparatus including oiled silk bags, the tubing and the containing gasometer. (17) On administering nitrous oxide to Boulton and the younger Watt, Davy was bitterly disappointed to report that 'Mr R. Boulton and Mr G. Watt have been much less affected than any individuals.' (10) As James Watt recounted to Lawrence, Gregory Watt had succumbed to tuberculosis by 1804. Upon learning of the younger Watt's death, Davy had lamented, 'Oh! there was no reason for his dying—he ought not to have died.' (19)

That same year, in 1804, Lawrence had exhibited his portrait of Sir James Mackintosh at the Royal Academy. (15) Perhaps anticipating James Watt's complaints by some nine years, Sir James Mackintosh likewise delivered to Lawrence a harsh review of the effects of Davy's gas. The portrait Lawrence was painting of Mackintosh had been commissioned by Josiah Wedgwood, one of Davy's first recipients of nitrous oxide. As both Mackintosh and subsequently Wedgwood underscored in their conversations with Lawrence, Mr Wedgwood had not been pleased with his personal experience of the gas. In fact, Davy's supervisor and the founder of Bristol's Pneumatic Institute, Dr Thomas Beddoes, was the first person to publish the rather unpleasant sensations that Mr Josiah Wedgwood had experienced from the gas (13). In a letter addressed to Davy, Wedgwood recorded his dismay on 23 July, 1798, after inhaling six quarts of nitrous oxide:

> *'I then had 6 quarts of the oxide given me in a bag undiluted, and as soon as I had breathed three or four respirations, I felt myself affected and my respiration hurried, which effect increased rapidly until I became as it were entranced, when I threw the bag from me and kept breathing on furiously with an open mouth and holding my nose with my left hand, having no power to take it away though aware of the ridiculousness of my situation. Though apparently deprived of all voluntary motion, I was sensible of all that passed, and heard every thing that was said; but the most singular sensation I had, I feel it impossible to accurately describe. It was as if all the muscles of the body were put into a violent vibratory motion; I had a very strong inclination to make odd antic motions with my hands and feet. When the first strong sensations went off, I felt as if I were lighter than the atmosphere, and as if I was going to mount to the top of the room. I had a metallic taste left in my mouth, which soon went off'* (10)

Wedgwood had donated a thousand pounds to Beddoes in support of the Pneumatic Institute. Thus, with some chagrin, Davy observed that:

> *'Mr. Josiah Wedgwood has since repeated the trial, the effects were powerful, but not in the slightest degree pleasant.'* (10)

Lawrence's attitude

Both the general uncertainty of the nitrous oxide experience and the ambivalence of those who inhaled the gas dissuaded Lawrence from accepting Davy's offer.

> *'It is remarkable that, in the latter part of his life, when his great practice might have been expected to make him more rapid in the completion of his works, the increased pains he took, arising no doubt from his improved perceptions, acquired for him the character of slowness . . .'* (4)

Lawrence prided himself on the precision of his draftsmanship. He feared any feelings of becoming powerless before an unexpected end and, frankly, dreaded the apoplectic fate experienced three years earlier by his brother, Major William Read Lawrence (4). In summary, Sir Thomas Lawrence feared loss of control, disruption of his work schedule, and distraction of his thought processes—fears not unlike those expressed by patients facing modern general anaesthesia.

Davy's portrait

Undaunted by fear, Lawrence's brush portrayed Sir Humphry Davy with a romantic dignity. Sir Thomas's brilliance in crayon and pencil portraiture formed a foundation for his efforts in oil (4). In all media, Lawrence demonstrated his precision in drafting faces and hands. From potboiling youth to Academician, Lawrence remained entertaining and ingratiating. His efforts as courtier were mirrored in the superficial elegance of his portraiture. Lawrence's flattering portrait of Davy bears out this observation. The simplicity of the painting's background belies Lawrence's thought in executing it. The swirl of clouds and sky represents Davy's early investigations into therapeutic gases at Bristol's Pneumatic Institute. By twenty-one years of age, Sir Humphry Davy had described the anaesthetic properties of laughing gas, observing:

> *'As nitrous oxide in its extensive operation appears capable of destroying physical pain, it may probably be used with advantage during surgical operations in which no great effusion of blood takes place.'* (10)

Below the painted horizon one sees the expanse of earthly elements, six of which were discovered by Davy. Through electrolysis of salt solutions. Davy isolated more chemical elements than any man before or since—sodium, potassium, calcium, barium, boron, and strontium. In the portrait's foreground and, to his contemporaries, in the forefront, the lifesaving miner's safety lamp invented so recently by Davy. As painted by the admiring Lawrence, this later prototype of the Davy lamp was credited with saving thousands of lives from methane gas explosions in the coal mines. Lawrence demonstrated that:

> *'a vast deal more of his time than is commonly supposed, was spent in gratuitous drawings or paintings, of which he made presents to his friends.'* (19)

In the end, Lawrence donated the smaller portrait to the Davy household. Lady Davy then presented the smaller portrait to John, her brother-in-law (1), who had distinguished himself as Medical Inspector-General of the Army by popularizing clinical use of thermometry and hydrometry and by demonstrating the etiology of spontaneous pneumothorax (20). As editor of Sir Humphry's works, Dr John Davy prized the one-quarter size portrait of his older brother, especially after Lady Davy presented the larger portrait to the Royal Society (21).

Conclusion

The mutual respect shared by Sir Thomas Lawrence and Sir Humphry Davy mirrored the striking parallels in their lives. Each man sprang from the lower classes and moved, at some point, from Bristol to London. Both men were almost entirely self-taught, and both rose at an early age to the presidency of their respective Royal organizations. Both men were knighted by the Prince-Regent, soon-to-be George IV. While pressing his claims that he, as President of the Royal Academy, had a right to participate in the ceremony marking the coronation of George IV, Lawrence reminded the Clarenceux King of Arms, Sir George Nayler, that:

> *'You do me privately, infinite kindness, if in the civilization of past Ages, Art has had distinction, press my claims, and publickly, do me Justice.'* (14)

Royalty indeed acknowledged Lawrence's claims and on 19 July, 1821, Sir Thomas Lawrence, President of the Royal Academy, walked ceremonially at Westminster Abbey. Abreast of him, just six months after sitting for his regency portrait, marched Lawrence's alter ego, the President of the Royal Society, Sir Humphry Davy (22). Both men were to die childless, yet Davy with his discoveries and Lawrence with his portraits each left a vast legacy to mankind.

References

(1) Richards RJ. Personal communication. 15 March, 1975.
(2) Drumheller MLR. Personal communication. 15 March, 1975.
(3) Darby P. Personal communication. 18 December, 1982.
(4) Williams DE. *The life and correspondence of Sir Thomas Lawrence, Kt*. London: Henry Colburn and Richard Bentley, 1831; vol. 1.
(5) Compton H. Correspondence to Thomas Lawrence. September 1789.

(6) Pasquin A. *Critical guide to the present exhibition at the Royal Academy*. London: Symonds & McQueen, 1797.

(7) Pindar P. *The works of Peter Pindar, Esq*. London: John Walker, 1794; vol. 3: 11.

(8) Pasquin A. *A liberal critique on the present exhibition of the Royal Academy*. London: Symonds & McQueen, 1794: 28.

(9) Layard GS, ed. *Sir Thomas Lawrence's letter-bag*. London: George Allen, 1906: 226.

(10) Davy H. *Researches, chemical and philosophical; chiefly concerning nitrous oxide, or dephlogisticated nitrous air, and its respiration*. Bristol: Biggs and Cottle, 1800:

(11) Carlyon C. *Early years and late reflections*. London: Whittaker and Co., 1856; vol. 1.

(12) Wordsworth W. Correspondence to Humphry Davy. 28 July, 1800.

(13) Beddoes T. *Notice of some observations made at the Medical Pneumatic Institution*. Bristol: Biggs and Cottle, 1799.

(14) Lawrence T. Correspondence to Sir George Nayler, Clarenceux King-of-Arms. 8 May, 1821.

(15) Armstrong W. *Lawrence*. London: Methuen & Co., 1913.

(16) Thomas KB. *The development of anaesthetic apparatus*. Oxford: Blackwell Scientific Publications, 975: 108-9.

(17) Beddoes T, Watt J. *Considerations on the medicinal use and the production of factitious airs*. London: Johnson, 1794-96.

(18) Kendall J. *Humphry Davy: 'Pilot' of Penzance*. London: Faber & Faber, 1954: 71.

(19) Campbell T. Correspondence to D. E. Williams, Esq. 10 November, 1830.

(20) Ross RS. John Davy: physician, scientist, author, brother of Sir Humphry. *Bull His Med* 1953: **27**: 101-11.

(21) Robinson NH. *The Royal Society catalogue of portraits*. London: The Royal Society, 1980: 82.

(22) Goldring D. *Regency portrait painter*. London: MacDonald, 1951: 290-1.

24.1   Finding the real Crawford Long (1815-1878): The discovery of an historical photograph

M. S. ALBIN, J. RAY and S. SMITH
University of Texas Health Science Center, San Antonio, Texas, USA

Dr Crawford Williamson Long (1815-1878) has been called the father of modern surgical anaesthesia because of his use of ether on 30 March, 1842, during a procedure for removal of a neck tumour performed on James Venable in the town of Jefferson Georgia. The second case (1) reported by Crawford Long using ether occurred on 6 June, 1842, again on James Venable, and again the removal of another small tumour. In these cases, ether was used 2 years prior to the use of nitrous oxide by Horace Wells (2) and four years before ether by Morton (3).

The photograph

In January, 1986, one of the co-authors on the paper, Scott E. Smith, MD, discovered a small photograph print (2 by 3 inches) at a book fair in Austin, Texas, which he purchased and donated to the Dolph Briscoe Library of the University of Texas Health Science Center, San Antonio, Texas, USA. The photograph can be classified as a ferrotype or tintype since it consisted of a photographic emulsion coated on a thin plate fabricated of a metallic iron compound. The ferrotype process was developed in 1854 and was preceded by the daguerreotype, in which the image was taken on a silver or silver emulsion copper plate. The ferrotype image shows a staged demonstration of an amputation under ether anaesthesia (Fig. 1) and was probably taken between 1854 and 1861, the year of the outbreak of the Civil War in the United States.

The photograph features a barefoot black man posing as a patient lying in the supine position on a packing box, and one tourniquet can be noted directly above the knee with the second placed at mid-calf. Three individuals can be seen standing along the left side of the patient's body. At the head is the 'anaesthetist', a cleanshaven individual wearing a waistcoat over a shirt and tie, and applying a cloth to the face of the patient with the right hand, while apparently taking the pulse with his left hand. The head of the patient rests on a sheet or small pillow and a bottle lies on the box to the right of the patient's head, ostensibly containing the ether. The surgeon is holding up the left leg with his left hand at the ankle, and his right hand is holding an amputation knife pointed down towards the packing box. The surgeon has a full beard and moustache and is dressed with a waistcoat and jacket over a shirt. Standing slightly back between the surgeon and anaesthetist is an 'assistant' holding a pair of scissors in his right hand and either a probe or a silver nitrate stick-cautery in his left hand. This individual has a moustache and appears to be wearing a smock over his undershirt.

Who is who and what is what?

The discovery of this unusual piece of history raises several interesting questions concerning the participants in this photograph. First, which individual is the surgeon Crawford Long, since other known likenesses of Long bear resemblance to both the surgeon and anaesthetist in the picture? Secondly, what is the significance of the wording on the packing box used to perform the 'surgery'? Our research has provided some tantalizing clues, though not conclusive evidence.

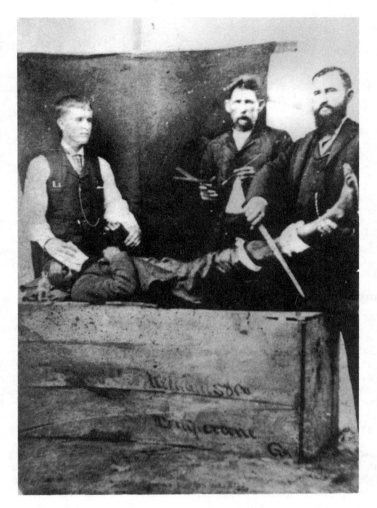

Figure 1   A ferrotype photo of a staged demonstration of a leg amputation under ether (circa 1854?).

We know that Crawford Long was 26 years of age when he carried out his first operation on James Venable in Jefferson, Georgia, less than a year after he had bought his practice from Dr Grant in 1841. Long remained in Jefferson for a period of eight years leaving there in 1850 to spend a year in Atlanta, Georgia. In 1851, Crawford Long and his family moved to Athens, Georgia where he practised medicine for the remainder of his life. In Athens, Long operated a drugstore and shared a practice with his younger brother, Robert, also a physician. The two brothers had their offices located in the back rooms of the pharmacy.

What about the identity of the anaesthetist in the photograph? A portrait of Crawford Long painted from a crayon drawing of him, at the age of 26 (Fig. 2) reveals a striking resemblance to the individual in the photograph giving the ether anaesthetic. A portrait of Dr Long (Fig. 3) at about the age of 60, also appears to resemble the surgeon in the ferrotype. Since Crawford Long's approximate age at the time was between 39 and 45, it is most likely that he was the surgeon in the photograph and that his brother Robert, bearing a real familial likeness, was the anaesthetist. We have not as yet been able to identify the 'assistant' holding the scissors and probe.

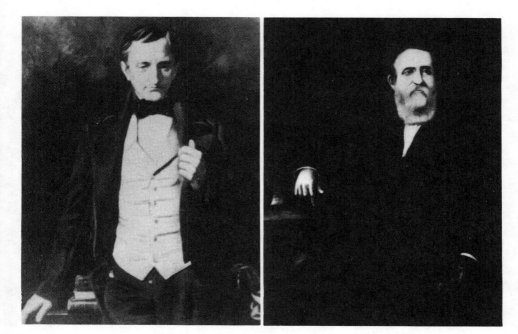

Figure 2   Portrait of Crawford Williamson Long.   Figure 3   Portrait of Crawford Williamson Long.

The wording on the packing box in the foreground is also intriguing and one can note 'Williamson' on the first line, 'TEMPERANE' on the second and 'Ga' on the third. The box is evidently a shipping crate and the words on the side an address. Williamson was, of course, Long's middle name, but it is unclear why it appears alone here. Magnification of the space preceding 'Williamson' offers us a possible clue since it appears that a word may have been smudged off. Could this word have been 'Long'? We are currently trying to see whether some new analytical techniques will help us to identify the existence of this word or words. Speculating that 'Temperane' was a misspelling of 'Temperance', we found that there were in fact 3 towns called Temperance in Georgia, one of them relatively close to Athens. Furthermore, the Temperance in question was located in Greene County near Union Point, a rail terminal, and also near Crawfordville (a possible family connection?). The letters 'Ga' obviously refer to the State of Georgia.

The photograph shown here (Fig. 1) is the only one known to have been taken while Long was actively engaged in practising medicine in Athens, Georgia. A crayon drawing was made of him while Long was 26 years of age (Fig. 2) and a full length portrait (Fig. 3) was painted by F. B. Carpenter (4) when Long was 60, the age of his death. Dr Marion Sims (5) was also responsible for persuading Long to have full length photographs made before he died which were used after his death as a guide in the carving of busts and sculptures (6) of his likeness.

References

(1) Long CW. An account of the first use of sulfuric ether by inhalation as an anaesthetic in surgical operations. *South Med Surg J* 1849; **5**: 705–13.

(2) Wells H. *A history of the discovery of the application of nitrous oxide gas, ether, and other vapors, to surgical operations*. Hartford, Connecticut: J. Gaylord Wells, 1847: 25.

(3) Bigelow HJ. Insensibility during surgical operations produced by inhalation. *Boston Med Surg J* 1846; **35**: 309–17.

(4) O'Donovan WR. The discoverer of anaesthesia. *Harper's Weekly*, September 15, 1979; 725.

(5) Sims MJ. Discovery of anaesthesia. *Virginia Med Monthly* 1877; **4**: 81–100.

(6) Sykes WS. *Essays on the first hundred years of anaesthesia*, Ellis, Richard H. ed. Edinburgh: Churchill Livingstone. 1982; **3**: 10.

24.2   John Snow (1813–1858) and his book
'On the inhalation of the vapour of ether in surgical operations'*

AKITOMO MATSUKI
University of Hirosaki, Hirosaki, Japan

In September, 1980, the 7th World Congress of Anaesthesiologists was held in Hamburg under the presidency of Professor E. Rugheimer, University of Erlangen. In this congress, a panel discussion entitled 'Anesthesiology: Past and Future' was held and the chairman was Professor

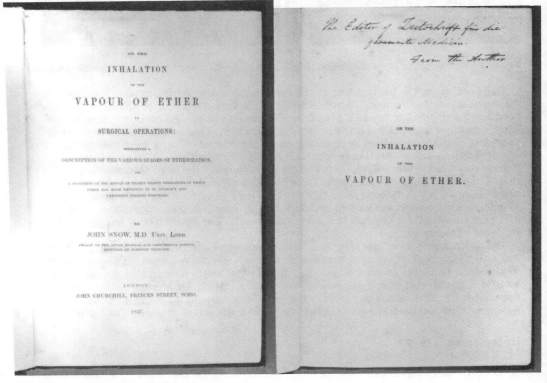

Figure 1   Front page of John Snow's book on
ether anaesthesia.

Figure 2   Autograph by John Snow.

*The Organising Committee of the Second International Symposium on the History of Anaesthesia wish to convey their thanks to Professor Akitomo Matsuki who so kindly presented a copy of his reproduction of John Snow's book to every registrant at the Congress.

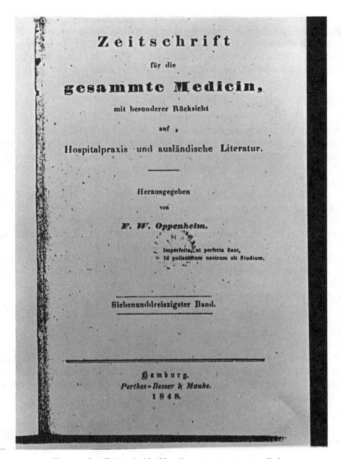

Figure 3   Zeitschrift für die gesammte medicin.

R. Frey, University of Mainz. The thirteen panellists, pioneers in this field from all over the world, presented interesting stories of anaesthesiology and related sciences in their own countries. These painstaking presentations were enthusiastically received by the audience.

Among the panellists, Professor Sir Robert Macintosh, Emeritus Professor of Oxford University, was most impressive. He carried his eighty-three years easily and explained lucidly the British story of anaesthesiology. He emphasized the important role of the United Kingdom in the evolution of anaesthesiology and attributed its beginning to the life-long endeavours of the two pioneers, John Snow and Thomas Clover. He emphasized the importance of John Snow's achievements and his place in history. This is firmly established by his first monograph entitled 'On the inhalation of the vapour of ether in surgical operations' published in 1847. The book is based entirely on his scientific observations and reflects the careful nature of his work. Sir Robert concluded his presentation by stating that this classic work should be read at least once by every anaesthesiologist because it is the best classic in this field.

A strange coincidence

At the time of this congress the writer was studying the history of anaesthesiology in the United Kingdom with particular reference to the transfer of information about ether anaesthesia from the United States and it was a fortunate coincidence that he came across a medical book shop in the congress hall. There was an old book out of reach the title of which could not be seen. On closer examination, to the astonishment of the writer, it proved to be the very book by John Snow of which Professor Macintosh had spoken (Fig. 1). In addition John Snow's autograph could be clearly seen on the front page (Fig. 2). This particular volume had been dedicated to Dr Oppenheim, the editor of *Zeitschrift für die Gesammte Medicin* (Fig. 3).

The book and its reproduction

The historical and contemporary significance of Snow's book *On the inhalation of the vapour of ether in surgical operations* has been widely recognized. The Wood Library Museum published a reprint edition of the book under the auspices of American Society of Anesthesiologists and Professor Ole Secher of Denmark, made private reprints to distribute among his friends as a Christmas gift in 1986.

Although Snow's book has been reproduced in the United States and in Europe, it is still an uncommon volume, especially in Asia and Oceania, and so the writer determined that the present time was opportune for further reproductions to be made.

The author's edition of Snow's original book is slightly different in binding from those reproduced by The Wood Library Museum and Professor Secher.

Firstly Dr Robinson's article, which appeared in 2 January issue of *The Medical Times* in 1847 is included, and indicates when Snow began to be interested in anaesthesia. Secondly it contains the death certificate of Snow, a review of Snow's book written by Dr Oppenheim for *Zeitschrift für die Gesammte Medicin* in 1847.

Conclusion

It is the writer's hope that the present reproduction of John Snow's book and its distribution to various countries, including the United Kingdom, may contribute not only to the progress of the historical study of surgical anaesthesia but also to the establishment of close relationships between those foreign countries and Japan.

24.3   Some interesting patients of John Snow (1813–1858)

R. S. ATKINSON
General Hospital, Southend on Sea, Essex, UK

John Snow lived from 1813 to 1858 and kept a diary of his clinical cases for the last 10 years of his life. These diaries (1) consist of three closely written volumes and give details of the name, age, occupation and site of anaesthesia as well, as a description of the administration of the anaesthetic itself in varying detail. All the chloroform anaesthetics except for the first 46 are recorded here as well as a number of administrations of ether and amylene.

John Snow became the leading anaesthetist in London and among his patients there are a number of important or otherwise interesting personages.

Her Majesty Queen Victoria

Snow's most famous patient was undoubtedly Queen Victoria who had been on the throne of England since 1837 and who had married Prince Albert of Saxe-Coburg and Gotha in 1840.

They were to have 9 children and, in the case of the last two, John Snow administered chloroform during the labour.

The entry for Thursday, 7 April, 1853, concerns the Queen. Snow received a note from Sir James Clark a little after 10 a.m. asking him to go to the palace. He remained for some time in an adjoining room, but at twenty minutes past twelve commenced to give a little chloroform with each pain, pouring about 15 minims of the drug on to a folded handkerchief. Chloroform was given only during the second stage, and never to the extent of quite removing consciousness. Dr Locock, the obstetrician, thought that the chloroform might have prolonged the interval between pains, but the infant, Prince Leopold, was born at 13 minutes past one o'clock (the clock in the room being 3 minutes before the right time). The Queen, Snow says, expressed herself much gratified with the effect of the chloroform.

Snow was called to the palace again on Tuesday, 14 April, 1857, when the Queen's ninth and last child was born. Labour commenced about 2 a.m. and Snow commenced the administration of chloroform at 11 o'clock. Prince Albert had already administered a very little chloroform at 9 or 10 o'clock. This time Snow poured about 10 minims of chloroform on to a handkerchief folded in a conical shape when each pain occurred and the Queen expressed great relief from the vapour. There is a note, however, that later the Queen kept asking for more chloroform, complaining that it did not remove the pain, though she did sleep between pains. Princess Beatrice was the last child born to Queen Victoria.

Mrs Thomas—daughter of His Grace, The Archbishop of Canterbury

There is no doubt that the administration of chloroform to Queen Victoria did much to silence criticism that relief of pain during childbirth was wrong on moral and religious grounds. Indeed on 20 October, 1853, Snow was called to administer chloroform to the daughter of the Archbishop of Canterbury at Lambeth Palace. The patient, a Mrs Thomas, was in fact under the care of her physician because she had extensive cavities in the lungs and thus had a tendency to cough during the inhalation of chloroform. The seal of approval was thus given by the highest personages of both Church and State.

Snow's practice

Snow administered chloroform at a variety of addresses in London and for a number of surgeons, though most commonly for Sir William Ferguson of King's College Hospital, who served on the Council of this Royal College from 1861 to 1877 and became President in 1870. The operations were normally short, though sometimes hazardous as when the surgery was concerned with the maxilla and thus anaesthetist and surgeon got in each other's way.

Snow was also interested in the possible value of chloroform inhalations in non-surgical conditions. He tried it out to control such a diversity of conditions as lockjaw, convulsions, and even acute mania. He also administered the drug to a child with whooping cough. However, any relief obtained could only be temporary.

The Most Honourable the Marquess of Anglesey KG

One of his famous patients was the Marquess of Anglesey (2). In his prime, then the Earl of Uxbridge, he had been the commander of the cavalry under Wellington at the Battle of Waterloo. In the closing minutes of the battle, on 18 June, 1815, Uxbridge was struck by a grapeshot on the right knee. In the popular version, Uxbridge exclaimed, 'By God, Sir, I've lost my leg!' Wellington takes the telescope from his eye for a moment before resuming his scouting of the battlefield and said, 'By God, Sir, so you have!' The leg was amputated and buried in the village of Waterloo where the tomb can still be seen today. Uxbridge recovered, and with a series of artificial legs lived to a ripe old age, holding many great offices of state. At the coronation of Queen Victoria in 1838 he was one of the four Knights of the Garter who held the golden canopy over the Queen at her anointing. At the opening ceremony of the Great

International Exhibition held in Hyde Park, he was seen arm in arm with the Duke of Wellington, both now grand old men.

In later years he was troubled considerably by trigeminal neuralgia or 'tic douloureux' for which he sought many cures without permanent relief. His amputation stump also pained him and, on Thursday, 25 April, 1850, when the Marquess was almost 83 years of age, Snow applied chloroform to the stump without much effect, so that he proceeded to inhalation which was repeated several times, occasionally to the point of unconsciousness, both before and after his dinner at 8.30 p.m. Following a good night's sleep he was much better. During the treatment, Anglesey, in his capacity as Master of the Ordnance, received a despatch containing an account of the death of an artilleryman while receiving chloroform, but Snow records that this did not deter his distinguished patient.

Mrs Baker

Finally I would like to draw your attention to a patient called Mrs Baker. Last year the Faculty was offered for purchase a silver card case. This had originally been presented by Mrs Baker to Mr Pettigrew FRCS, who removed a fatty lump from her side. It is interesting to read in Snow's casebook that on the same day, 14 February, 1850, he administered the short chloroform inhalation referred to in the inscription on the case.

References

(1) Atkinson RS. The 'lost' diaries of John Snow. In: Boulton TB, Bryce-Smith R, Sykes MK, Gillett GB, Revell AL eds. *Progress in Anaesthesiology*, Amsterdam: Excerpta Medica Foundation, 1970.
(2) The Marquess of Anglesey. *One-leg. The life and letters of Henry William Paget, First Marquess of Anglesey, K.G.* London: Cape, 1961.

24.4   J. F. Heyfelder (1798–1869).
                                        A pioneer of German anaesthesia

ULRICH VON HINTZENSTERN
University of Erlangen, Erlangen, Federal Republic of Germany

---

Johann Ferdinand Heyfelder was born on 19 January, 1798, in Küstrin. He studied medicine at various places in Germany. After a one-year stay in Paris he settled as a general practitioner in Treves, 1822. At that time he wrote scientific articles, too, and because of his perfect knowledge of French he was able to publish translations of the newest medical and original French papers.

He gave up working as a general practitioner in 1831 and undertook a research on cholera in several cities under the royal government of Treves. One year later he did the same in France.

In 1833 he received a command to be appointed as Physician in Ordinary of the Prince of Hohenzollern and to be public health officer of the princely government in Sigmaringen. There he reformed the local medical affairs in the Prussian manner. He also practised as a physician at a watering place called Imnau.

The Prince of Hohenzollern wished to get rid of him in 1841 without awarding him a lifelong pension. The Prince therefore arranged for Heyfelder's appointment as Professor in Ordinary of

Surgery and Ophthalmology of the University of Erlangen against the wishes of the local faculty. There Heyfelder made himself respected as an excellent surgeon and scientist and developed what was for his time, a modern way of teaching students. However, because of his pig-headed and discontented nature he had numerous quarrels with many colleagues of his faculty and, consequently in 1854 he was superannuated after further vigorous disagreements.

He entered a Russian service in 1855 and became Chief Surgeon of the Finnish army and later Professor in Ordinary at Petersburg. He came back to Germany, shortly before his death on 21 June, 1869, at Wiesbaden (1).

The first ether anaesthetics in Germany

The age of modern anaesthesia began on 16 October, 1846. W. T. G. Morton successfully publicly demonstrated the use of ether for surgery at Boston, Massachusetts. The Professor of Ordinary of Internal Medicine at Erlangen—Karl Cannstatt—is said to have referred Heyfelder to publications concerning this development. Heyfelder is said to have expressed contempt that this should be tried out by English dentists. It is said that only when Cannstatt had tested the narcotic action of ether on himself and volunteers did Heyfelder pay attention to the revolutionary importance of the discovery for operative surgery (2). After having tested the action of ether on himself he had an inhaler made. This apparatus was constructed from a pig's bladder and a glass tube.

On 24 January, 1847, Heyfelder was the first to anaesthetize a patient with sulphuric ether in Germany (3). The patient was the 26-year-old shoemaker's journeyman, Michael Gegner. Heyfelder described him as 'pale, shrunken and not strong, suffering for a long time from a voluminous cold abscess on his left buttock.' First he inhaled the ether via his mouth with closed nostrils. After 3 minutes Heyfelder interrupted the administration because of a fit of coughing. Then the glass tube of the inhaler was put in the right nostril and the inhalations continued. After three and a half minutes mydriasis was observed, one and a half minutes later bradycardia occurred. After two further minutes, the heart rate rose again. Five minutes later the patient collapsed, after two further minutes sensation was very much decreased but the patient remained conscious. Because of another coughing-fit inhalation had to be interrupted for two minutes and then continued via the left nostril. In the following three minutes the pulse was palpable only with difficulty, whereupon inhalation was tried via the mouth again. A new violent coughing-fit necessitated cessation of the narcosis without achieving the incision of the cold abscess. The following day Heyfelder succeeded in carrying out surgery on the same patient under ether despite repeated interruptions due to coughing-fits. The patient did not feel any pain and said that he had dreamt during the operation. Therefore, the new drug was recognized to be effective (4).

On 6 February, Jakob Herz, one of Heyfelder's assistants, reported in a newspaper article about the first results of 24 administrations of sulphuric ether (5). By 17 March, 1847, Heyfelder had undertaken 121 surgical procedures under ether. The majority of the operations were teeth-extractions, the minority, more complex operations such as the treatment of a harelip or of lip cancer, the resection of the shoulder joint, etc.

Heyfelders monograph

Heyfelder described in detail 108 of these inhalations in a little book entitled *Die Versuche mit dem Schwefeläther* (The experiments with sulphuric ether) (4). This monograph published in March, 1847, represents one of the first complete dissertations on sulphuric ether in the German literature. In a special chapter he analysed the development of various physiological and psychological parameters during etherizations. His accurate observations led him to the conclusion that individual differences are so important that no generally accepted standards can be stated about the manifestations subsequent to etherization. In particular, Heyfelder defined 4 stages of consciousness under etherization:
1. Complete insensibility and unconsciousness, often combined with complete collapse.

2. A strongly pronounced reduction of sensibility occurring with partial or total loss of consciousness.
3. Exaltation without consciousness.
4. Exaltation with consciousness combined with normal or increased sensation.

Concerning the duration of the inhalation, Heyfelder believed that the patient should inhale as long as he still appeared to be sensible and conscious. The inhalation should be resumed only when the action of narcosis recognizably decreased.

Heyfelder also examined the blood and urine of some etherized patients and reported that he did not find any important or specific alteration. He concluded his dissertation with the demand that only physicians should be allowed to administer sulphuric ether for anaesthesia. Heyfelder also considered the presence of an experienced assistant to be necessary, particularly for long-lasting operations during which the inhalations were given repeatedly. In the last chapter Heyfelder precisely depicts the construction and application of two inhalers with which he had had very good results.

Further investigations by Heyfelder and his colleagues at Erlangen

Stimulated by Heyfelder's clinical activities with sulphuric ether his colleagues on the faculty, the analytical chemist Ernst von Bibra and the physiologist Emil Harless intensively studied the biochemical and physiological action of sulphuric ether. Their results were published in April, 1847 (6). Together with Heyfelder's dissertation these articles made the Faculty of Medicine of the University of Erlangen respected because of its important scientific contribution to the application of sulphuric ether (7,8).

In 1847, Heyfelder was probably the first to apply 'salt-ether' in man. After 4 administrations he concluded that: salt ether worked more quickly but for a shorter time than sulphuric ether (9). The advantages of salt ether were its application without problems and ease of induction. He was, however, convinced that salt-ether would not be used generally though it had some advantages in comparison with sulphuric ether. Its disadvantages were its high volatility, its price and the difficulty of getting it in a pure form (10).

From December, 1847, Heyfelder started to use chloroform. He was now able to perform more major operations, for example the total resection of the hip-joint.

He published his book on *Die Versuche mit dem Schwefeläther, Salzäther und Chloroform* (The experiments with sulphuric ether, salt ether and chloroform) (10). In this he describes a great number of anaesthetic administrations using these 3 agents. In the chapter dealing with chloroform he writes on unexpected problems occurring at first. The use of the sulphuric ether-inhalers turned out to be the reason. After having recognized that chloroform could be dropped on a cloth, which was lightly pressed on the patient's mouth and nose, Heyfelder found out that the physiological and psychological actions were very similar to those of sulphuric ether. However, Heyfelder believed that chloroform was better tolerated by the patients and caused less side effects. The most important disadvantage he described was the disagreeable awakening after chloroform. In contrast to ether anaesthesia chloroform administration was smooth—at first excitation occurred in some cases but then general muscular relaxation always followed with complete insensibility and unconsciousness. In his summary Heyfelder arrives at the conclusion, that chloroform is undoubtedly superior to sulphuric ether mainly because it is a quicker acting and longer lasting agent and leads to a deeper narcosis. Moreover its application was much easier for it needed no special apparatus. However, because of its great anaesthetic potency, Heyfelder particularly demanded great caution in the application of chloroform. Explicitly he expected an assistant for chloroformizations, whose only duty was to supervise the inhalations and the patient—a forerunner of the modern specialized anaesthesiologist.

References

(1) Heidacher A. *Geschichte der Chirurgischen Universitätsklinik Erlangen*. Bonn: Semmel, 1960: 69–84.

(2) Pfaff E. *Aus Pauline Braters Mädchenjahren.* München: Beck, 1931: 151–68.

(3) Walser H. *Zur Einführung der Äthernarkose im deutschen Sprachgebiet im Jahre 1847.* Zürich: Universität Zürich, 1957. 10. Dissertation.

(4) Heyfelder JF. *Die Versuche mit dem Schwefeläther und die daraus gewonnenen Resultate in der chirurgischen Klinik zu Erlangen.* Erlangen: Heyder, 1847.

(5) Herz J. Schwefeläther. *Allgemeine Zeitung* 6 February 1847: 290 (col 2).

(6) v. Bibra E, Harless E. *Die Wirkung des Schwefeläthers in chemischer und physiologischer Beziehung.* Erlangen: Heyder, 1847.

(7) *Zeitschr ges Medicin* 1848; **37**: 117–29.

(8) Vierodt K. Recension zu E. v. Bibra und E. Harless. *Arch physiol Heilkunde* 1848; **7**: 249–53.

(9) Heyfelder JF. Versuche mit dem Salzäther. *Arch physiol Heilkunde* 1847; **6**: 441–6.

(10) Heyfelder JF. *Die Versuche mit dem Schwefeläther, Salzäther und Chloroform und die daraus gewonnenen Resultate in der chirurgischen Klinik zu Erlangen.* Erlangen: Heyder, 1848.

24.5   John Tomes (1815–1895)—Anaesthetist 1847

O. P. DINNICK

The Middlesex Hospital, London, UK

In 1847, John Tomes was surgeon-dentist at the Middlesex Hospital in London, but he later became Sir John Tomes and the doyen of his profession. His career has been reviewed at length elsewhere (1) and can only be summarized here.

He was born in 1815 near Stratford on Avon where he went to school. He was apprenticed to an apothecary at Evesham for five years before completing his studies at the new Medical School at the Middlesex Hospital, where he served as house surgeon. He then decided to specialize in dentistry and, in 1840, was appointed surgeon-dentist to Kings College Hospital but after three years he resigned and returned to his old hospital. In 1858 he was also appointed to the Dental Hospital of London of which he was a founder and where he inaugurated regular clinical demonstrations.

His major and enduring scientific contributions concerned the microscopical structure of teeth; indeed, while still a student, he delivered an important paper on this subject to the Royal Society—of which he later became a Fellow. Equally enduring were his designs for dental extraction forceps which have remained substantially unchanged ever since. He also invented an ingenious machine for carving artificial teeth—which earned him a gold medal from the Society of Arts.

In 1845 he delivered a celebrated series of lectures on Dental Physiology and Surgery which were described as having 'marked a new era in dentistry.' (2) An expanded version of these lectures was published in 1848 (3) and became the basis of his later 'System of Dental Surgery'. (4).

Tomes's public and ultimately successful energies (he had a large private practice) were long devoted to establishing dentistry as a profession. Unlike some of his contemporaries with a similar aim, he felt that dentistry could not be divorced from surgery and he was largely instrumental in persuading the Royal College of Surgeons to institute, in 1860, the Licentiate in Dental Surgery (LDS) diploma for which he was one of the original examiners. Tomes had previously been a founder and a secretary of the Odontological Society of which he was later twice President but it was not until 1878 that Parliament established the Dental Register, though by that time he had retired from active practice. He then became the first President of the British Dental Association and an Honorary Fellow of the Royal College of Surgeons and was knighted for his services to his profession nine years before his death in 1895.

Tomes the anaesthetist

Tomes was also described as 'being much occupied with the question of general anaesthesia' (2) and on 25 January, 1847, he gave the anaesthetic for the first 'Operation without Pain' reported from the Middlesex Hospital—a lithotomy by J. M. Arnott (5).

Tomes's first use of ether

The patient was a man of 68—the oldest up to that time recorded in Robinson's* book (6) and the operation was unusually long—12 minutes—and difficult, as the stone crumbled and required several insertions of the forceps and of a spoon to scrape out 'matter like mortar'. The bladder was also washed out and it was noted that, unlike the voluntary muscles, those of the bladder were not relaxed by the anaesthetic: this discrepant effect was commented on by a French contemporary (7) and may sometimes cause problems today! The operation was justifiably described at the time as one 'where the efficacy of the ether was put to as severe a test as it had yet been subjected to' (8).

The anaesthetic was remarkable in another way, for Tomes used the ether inhaler 'invented by Mr Bell, chemist, of Oxford Street, who was present and assisted Mr Tomes in its application' (8). Mr Bell was, of course, Jacob Bell, the founder of the Pharmaceutical Society and editor of its Journal: he had described his inhaler on 13 January (9) and, as will be recounted, was concerned with another of Tomes's anaesthetics.

However, the relationship between these two great men remains unknown: though both aimed to advance their respective professions by petitioning Parliament for appropriate legislation, no correspondence between them has been discovered and Bell left no diary (10,11). That Bell's firm supplied the rectified ether (and probably other drugs) used at the Middlesex is a possible, but seemingly inadequate, explanation for the association. No other connection between Bell and the Middlesex has been identified, except that he later attended its weekly Board meeting on behalf of the St Marylebone Vestry, over problems in the streets outside the hospital (12).

For Tomes to have chosen such a difficult case as that lithotomy for his first anaesthetic seems out of keeping with his scientific outlook and the description of him as a 'man imbued with the seriousness of life', (1) and suggests that he may have had some previous anaesthetic experience with dental patients. Indeed, that he should have had such experience is to be expected, as Robinson, Tracey and many others, had given anaesthetics for dental extraction before 13 January (13).

This expectation is confirmed by Tomes's diary—or more correctly by his obituarists' interpretations of that document, which cannot now be traced and which was described by one of them as 'somewhat fragmentary' (14). The same author summarized the relevant entries as:

> *'after sundry experiments with it [ether] for tooth extractions at the Middlesex Hospital, some successful, some not, we then read: "Gave ether to Arnott's case of lithotomy, eight minutes and insensibility came, the operation commenced and lasted twelve minutes. (Jan. 14th)"'.*

The date is incorrect if it was intended to refer to Arnott's case as this was on 25th. The same error was made by another obituarist (15) who interpreted the diary as:

> *'after using sulphuric and sometimes chloric ether in the out-patients room for dental operations, we find "Jan. 14th. Gave ether to Arnott's case . . . [as above]"'.*

---

*James Robinson was also a scientific dentist and administered the first anaesthetic in England in Gower Street on 19 December, 1846.

A third author (16) said that a mixture of the two ethers was tried during the initial experiments.

Chloric ether

One such experiment was described by Tomes in his book of 1848 (3):

> 'Previous to the discovery of the anaesthetic effects of chloroform Mr J Bell brought to the hospital a little chloric ether or terchloride of carbon as it was then called, that its effects might be tested. A female patient from the venereal ward . . . was speedily rendered apparently insensible . . . and a first permanent molar was removed. She did not seem to feel the operation—there was no expression of pain. In a few minutes . . . [she] . . . regained her consciousness. She then said that the operation gave her great pain and described it so accurately that no doubt remained that she felt the usual amount of pain; but the power to move, she said, was suspended; . . . The ether was given in the morning; during the day she fainted several times, had headache, and felt generally unwell, and was very angry at us for giving her the ether. She said that she had never fainted before, and that the ether made her ill. As the disposition to faint was doubtless due to the ether, I did not again use this drug. Chloric ether consists of chloroform with 80% alcohol.'

Unfortunately Tomes gave no date for this unhappy incident but it seems probable, as suggested by his obituarists, that it took place before 25 January, 1847. That date is also compatible with Bell's statement published on 1 February (17), that:

> 'Chloric ether had been tried . . . [and though it continued . . .] in some cases with success, . . .'

the latter cases could have been those mentioned by Tracey on the same date (18). From the above account, unlike those written thirty-eight years later (15,16,19), it would seem that Tomes used that drug only once: he did not mention how it was given and one can only speculate that Bell's inhaler was used.

No other reports about Tomes's earliest dental anaesthetics have been discovered. A search of the Middlesex Hospital archives—which contain clinical records dating back to 1745—frustratingly revealed that all those for 1847 are missing (12). Nevertheless, in spite of the minor inconsistencies in the interpretations of his diary, and of the lack of any independent confirmation, it would seem reasonable to accept them as evidence that he did indeed give some anaesthetics for dental extractions before he undertook Arnott's case on Monday, 25 January, 1847.

Further early 'Operations without pain' at the Middlesex Hospital

In the weeks that followed the successful lithotomy, a further twenty-two 'Operations without Pain' were reported from the Middlesex (20)—fifteen of them at length (21,22,23) although anaesthesia could not be induced for two patients and was incomplete for two others. Unfortunately, the authors of these reports did not name the anaesthetist and, though in many instances it was almost certainly Tomes, that assumption is not confirmed by his diary though the entries therein are compatible with it. As one obituarist's interpretation records:

> 'In the ensuing weeks he gave ether many times with varying success and on "February 23rd, gave ether to eight patients with great success; Earl of Cadogan (a governor of the hospital) and many others present."' (15)

However, the house surgeon's report (20) lists but three surgical patients on that day so presumably the other five were dental extractions.

It is of course possible that all the anaesthetics mentioned in the diary were for dental patients but there are four factors which taken together strongly suggest the contrary. Firstly, it is very difficult to believe that, after his triumphant lithotomy anaesthetic, he did not then give others for his surgical colleagues, secondly, eight of the operations, including the last in the report on 26 March, were by his friend Arnott, thirdly, Bell's inhaler was again used in twenty of the twenty-two cases and finally his biographer (2) clearly refers to '. . . ether . . . for operations for general surgery.' It is therefore reasonable to conclude that Tomes did anaesthetize some of these surgical patients—though the exact number remains unknown.

There are no further relevant extracts from his diary and no other records have been found to show if he continued to anaesthetize general surgical cases after the end of March, 1847. He certainly would have ceased to do so by November when chloroform largely replaced ether, as his biographers mention only 'ether in 1847 at the Middlesex Hospital' (1,2).*

Tomes's book *Dental Physiology and Surgery* 1848 and later publications

Nevertheless, Tomes's interest in anaesthetics for dental operations was maintained. He not only administered chloroform in his practice—as Snow recorded (24)—but he also devoted eighteen pages to anaesthesia in dental extractions in his influential book *Dental Physiology and Surgery* published in July, 1848. Contemporary book reviews and the publishers' circular (25) showed that five other surgical textbooks had been published in England between January 1847 and July 1848, but only three mentioned anaesthesia—all in 1847. South (26) in February was far from enthusiastic, Druitt (27) in April wrote the longest contribution—two and a half pages, while Lizars (28), six months later, offered virtually no advice but described and illustrated an inhaler. None of these authors unequivocally claimed to have given any anaesthetics themselves. Thus Tomes's was the first surgical book to be published in this country in which anaesthesia was discussed authoritatively and at length.

In *Dental Physiology and Surgery* Tomes paid tribute to Morton, quoted verbatim from Warren, Snow ('a great authority') and Simpson, and added some observations of his own on the changes in the circulation and respiration caused by anaesthesia. After a description of a satisfactory administration of chloroform, he noted that 'ether is but now rarely used' and concluded that 'its use should be discontinued in ordinary cases of extraction of teeth.'

There followed six pages on the possible adverse effects of chloroform but the first example concerned the girl who received the chloric ether, as already recounted. Induction difficulties with struggling, as well as postoperative nausea and vomiting were discussed but Tomes was particularly concerned about prolonged recovery with long-lasting mental changes, of which he recounted four examples—though none were from his own practice. He pointed out that dentists did not usually become aware of such problems 'but unfortunately there are many examples where the medical attendant does.'

He then referred to the first two reported deaths from chloroform, only briefly to the one 'You will remember . . . near Newcastle-upon-Tyne', but in some detail to the second one in Cincinatti which concerned a patient for dental extractions. He continued:

> *' I have brought before you the untoward results that occasionally follow the inhalation of chloroform, not with a view to prejudicing you against its use in proper cases but to guard you against using it needlessly.'*

He admitted that the incidence of death from chloroform was not known,

> *'But supposing even one in ten thousand were killed and we cannot tell which one that will be, it is, surely unwise to take even that risk merely to avoid pain that is very bearable and will not last more than three or four seconds.'*

He added that the possibility of nausea for a day or of disturbance of the mind for a week or two afterwards should also be considered when assessing the need for anaesthesia. However, he made it clear that this cautious attitude was applicable mainly to the straightforward extraction of one tooth. When the operation promised to be difficult or when several teeth were to be removed, then the risk of an anaesthetic was 'perhaps warranted.' These restricted indications for chloroform anaesthesia were still advocated in 1860 (29,30). Tomes's caveats

---

*In 1853, the duty of giving chloroform to surgical patients at the hospital was assigned to Tomes's brother-in-law, Septimus Sibley, the registrar.

on the dangers of chloroform were also commended at the time (31) and, as is well known, were later shown to have been well founded.

Tomes also discussed anaesthetic techniques for dental extractions and stressed that only the minimum amount of chloroform should be used, partly because he considered that only analgesia was required and partly to achieve the rapid recovery which was so important for an outpatient. He rejected Simpson's rapid induction technique in favour of Snow's more gradual method but preferred the former's simple funnel shaped sponge to any of the 'almost endless variety of instruments for exhibiting chloroform.'

He also stressed three points that are still valid today; that the patient should have an empty stomach, that strict silence should be kept during the procedure and that the patient should lie down until fully recovered. However, he was less specific about treating the complication which so concerned him for 'when permanent depression follows narcotism, stimulants and generous living would seem to be the answer.' (This advice would seem equally appropriate for the unfortunate anaesthetist!). So ended Tomes's chapter of 1848.

He did not again write about anaesthesia in any depth. In his 'System of Dental Surgery' of 1859 (4) he said only that:

'The subject of general anaesthesia by inhalation of the vapour of chloroform or ether, need not be specially discussed in connection with dental operations. The agents capable of producing anaesthetic effects have taken their place among the many subjects used by the surgeon; and in works devoted to materia medica and therapeutics their respective merits are fully discussed.'

He was equally brief about the newly advocated techniques of local analagesia by cold or electricity, which he correctly foretold would cease to be used when their novelty had worn off.

There were three further editions of Tomes's *System of Dental Surgery'* (32,33,34), successively revised and enlarged by his son, Charles, but with one exception, the expanded discussions on anaesthesia were not relevant to the elder man's earlier anaesthetic practice—indeed the last edition was published two years after his death.

That exception is a long sentence in the second (1873) edition (27) as its content and style strongly suggest the hand of the senior author—the more so the unambiguous imperative in its final clause was attenuated in the later editions:

'The subject of general anaesthesia, as induced by the inhalation of the vapour of chloroform, or of ether, or of nitrous oxide gas, does not call for a lengthy discussion in these pages, inasmuch as, since a patient under the influence of any anaesthetic agent demands the undivided care and undistracted attention of the administrator, the operator should never administer such agent single handed; so that the exhibition of anaesthetics forms no part of the duties of the practitioner in his capacity of dental surgeon.'

That last forthright injunction forms a suitable conclusion to this account.

Conclusion

John Tomes's close involvement with anaesthesia was relatively brief and he made no lasting technical innovations, nevertheless his contributions were not without contemporary influence. He should still be remembered for his pioneering anaesthetics in January, 1847, for his association with Jacob Bell and with chloric ether, and for writing the first authoritative discussion of anaesthesia in an English surgical textbook.

Acknowledgments

The writer is indebted to Miss K. Arnold-Forster, Museum Officer of the Pharmaceutical Society of Great Britain, Mr J. A. Donaldson, Honorary Curator of the British Dental Association Museum, and Mr W. R. Winterton, Archivist of The Middlesex Hospital, for kindly searching their respective records on my behalf.

References

(1) Cope Z, *Sir John Tomes. A pioneer of British Dentistry*. London: Dawsons, 1961.
(2) D'Arcy Power. *Dictionary of national biography*. London: Smith Elder & Co. 1899, **57**: 6.
(3) Tomes J. *Dental physiology and surgery*. London: John W Parker, 1848.
(4) Tomes J. *A system of dental surgery*. London: John Churchill, 1858.
(5) Rogers JH. Operations without pain. *Lancet* 1947; **i**: 132.
(6) Robinson J. *A treatise on the inhalation of the vapour of ether*. London: Webster & Co, 1847.
(7) Lach FJ. *de L'éther Sulphurique*. Paris: Labé, 1847; 250.
(8) Anonymous. Painless operations at the Middlesex Hospital. *London Med Gaz* 1847; **4** (New Series): 218.
(9) Bell J. *Pharmaceutical J* (Meeting Report), 1847; **6**: 355.
(10) Donaldson JA. *Personal communication*.
(11) Arnold-Forster K. *Personal communication*.
(12) Winterton WR. *Personal communication*.
(13) Clendon JC, Tracey SJ, Waite. *Pharmaceutical J* (Meeting Report) 1847; **6**: 354–7.
(14) Anonymous. Sir John Tomes (Obituary). *Nature* 1895; **52**: 396.
(15) Anonymous. Sir John Tomes (Obituary). *Br Dent J* 1895; **16**: 462.
(16) Anonymous. Sir John Tomes (Obituary). *Br Med J* 1895; **2**: 396.
(17) Bell J. [Editor's footnote]. *Pharmaceutical J* 1847; **6**: 357.
(18) Tracey SJ. [Correspondence]. *London Med Gaz* 1847; **4** (New Series): 258.
(19) Anonymous. Sir John Tomes (Obituary). *Lancet* 1895; **ii**: 352.
(20) Rogers JH. Operations without pain. *Lancet* 1847; **i**: 367.
(21) Rogers JH. Operations without pain. *Lancet* 1847; **i**: 184–5 & 237–8.
(22) Anonymous. Operations without pain. *Lancet* 1847; **i**: 210–2.
(23) Tuson EW. Clinical Notes. *Medical Times* 1847; **16**: 231–2.
(24) Snow J. *On chloroform and other anaesthetics*. London: John Churchill, 1858; 314.
(25) *Publishers circular*. London: Sampson Low, 1847 and 1848.
(26) South J in Chelius JM. *System of surgery*. (Translator's postscript). London: Renshaw; 1847 Vol. 2, pt. XVI and Philadelphia: Lea and Blanchard, 1847; Vol. 3. 768.
(27) Druitt J. *The surgeon's Vade Mecum*, 4th Ed. London: Henry Renshaw. 1847; 547–50.
(28) Lizars J. *The system of practical surgery*, 2nd Ed. Edinburgh: WH Lizars and London: S Highley, 1847; 184–5.
(29) Anonymous. *Dental Review* 1860; **2**: 359.
(30) Richardson BW. *Dental Review* 1860; **2**: 591.
(31) Anonymous. Dental physiology and surgery, by J Tomes. (Book Review). *London Med Gaz* 1848; **7** (New Series): 540.
(32) Tomes J, Tomes CS. *A system of dental surgery*, 2nd Ed. London: J and A Churchill, 1873.
(33) Tomes J, Tomes CS. *A system of dental surgery*, 3rd Ed. London: J and A Churchill, 1887.
(34) Tomes J, Tomes CS. *A system of dental surgery*, 4th Ed. London: J and A Churchill, 1897.

24.6   Dr E. D. Worthington (1820–1895)
                                                          pioneer Quebec anaesthetist

A. J. C. HOLLAND
McGill University, Montreal, Quebec, Canada

In Quebec, as in the rest of the world, the first few years of anaesthesia saw no full-time specialists but there were many doctors who gave anaesthetics as part and parcel of their medical duties.

Early practitioners of the art of anaesthesia needed to possess both courage and ingenuity—courage to perform a procedure which by no means had universal approval, and ingenuity to devise ways and means of administering relatively unknown anaesthetic agents in as safe a way as possible.

A doctor who had these qualities in full measure was Dr E. D. Worthington, MD, FACS. He was in practice for fifty years in the town of Sherbrooke about 50 miles from Montreal, and was one of the first, if not the first, to administer ether and later on chloroform in the Province of Quebec.

Biography

Like so many who practised medicine in Quebec, Dr Worthington was born in Ireland—in Ballinakill, Queen's County on 1 December, 1820, and came to Canada with his parents at the age of two. They settled in Quebec City which was then part of Lower Canada (not Quebec Province) and it was here that Dr Worthington began his medical studies (1).

There were no medical schools in Canada at the time so that in 1834 Dr Worthington was indentured for seven years as a medical student with Dr James Douglass of Quebec City. This was reduced to five years in order that he could accept an appointment as assistant surgeon to HM 56th Foot and subsequently to HM 68th Light Infantry.

He resigned his commission to proceed to Edinburgh where he won the silver medal in his year for medical jurisprudence. He was in 'Auld Reekie' (as Edinburgh was known), during the Snowball Riots which saw three days of fighting between 'town' and 'gown' in the winter of 1842, and his student days were eventful to say the least. Nonetheless he received a Doctorate in Medicine from St Andrews and a licentiate of The Faculty of Physicians and Surgeons of Glasgow, and of the College of Surgeons of Edinburgh (2).

He returned to Canada sometime in 1845 and received the license of the Montreal Medical Board. Almost immediately he located in Sherbrooke east of Montreal and practised there for nearly half a century.

He received the MA from University of Bishop's College and, in 1868 the CMMD from McGill University. For some years he was one of the Governors of the College of Physicians and Surgeons of Lower Canada and helped instigate the organization of the Canadian Medical Association.

This outline of Dr Worthington's medico-political career gives no idea of Dr Worthington the all round surgeon, general practitioner, and anaesthetist, who was the doyen of the medical profession in his area for many years.

He was a prolific writer both on medical and non-medical topics, and some of his writings were collected into book form and give a fascinating picture of the life of a truly general practitioner, who had to be prepared to go everywhere and do anything, at a time when transport was primitive in the extreme, and medical facilities virtually nonexistent (2).

Dr Worthington and anaesthesia

The writings which deal with anaesthesia showed that he himself used it, or supervised its use, for most of his surgery from 1847 on. He thought that he had performed the first capital operations under ether (14 March, 1847) (3) and chloroform (24 January, 1848) (4) in Canada and it seems from his descriptions that he was both surgeon and anaesthetist.

The descriptions of his anaesthetics are clear and succinct. They are remarkable for his appreciation of the need of a valve system to prevent rebreathing, and for his awareness of the side effects of the drugs he was using:

> *'A large ox-bladder, with a stop-cock attached, a mouth-piece, made of thick leather, covered with black silk and well padded round the edges, with a connecting long brass tube that had done service as an umbrella handle in many a shower, formed an apparatus that, though rude looking, and bearing marks of having been got up in haste, presented withal a very business-like, and, for the country, tolerably professional appearance.*

A couple of ounces of ether were poured into the bladder, which was then filled with air from a bellows. Not having time or ingenuity sufficient to construct a double valve, the objection to inhaling carbonic acid gas again into the lungs was done away with, by simply allowing the patient, after a full inspiration from the bag, to expire through the nose, for three or four times, when the nostrils were kept closed, and the breathing confined to the bladder.' (4)

It is interesting that Dr Worthington, like others, did not produce full unconsciousness in his patients, at least initially, but rather a 'twilight' state with insensibility to pain combined with a retained ability to respond to commands.

'About six full inspirations sufficed to produce a complete effect; the eyes turned up under the upper lid and became fixed; his wrist was pinched, and he was asked if he felt pain; he laughed, and said, "Oh no, I just feel—no pain at all!" The operation was then commenced, and terminated without his evincing, in any way, that he was at all conscious of the least feeling of pain. He retained his consciousness, talked rationally, and made some very witty remarks in answer to questions put to him, converting the scene from one of a most painful to one of an excessively ludicrous character. Both during the operation, and afterwards, he expressed himself as knowing perfectly well what was doing, and the different stages of the proceeding, but at no time did he feel pain.' (3)

Dr Worthington may not have been the first to use ether in Quebec—Dr Douglas, his old mentor in Quebec City, and Dr Nelson of Montreal probably preceded him (5,6)—but he was almost certainly the first to use chloroform on 24 January, 1848, when he anaesthetized a lady for reduction of a dislocated hip. This anaesthetic was only partially successful, but on the following day he anaesthetized a child, with complete success for removal of a tumour from the head. A little later (we do not know exactly when) he was also successful with an anaesthetic for a woman in premature labour.

As with the descriptions of this ether anaesthesia, Dr Worthington discussed in some detail the technique that he used and offered very sensible ideas on the type of apparatus that he thought was best suited to the giving of chloroform (5).

Conclusion

A list of Dr Worthington's academic achievements, although considerable, gives very little idea of the man himself and the universal esteem in which he was held by the people of Sherbrooke. At his death, *The Medical Age* wrote

'His whole life was intimately interwoven with the medical history of Canada, and was an integral part of the history of the Province of Quebec. It is the lot of few men to be so noble, so distinguished, so loved, and so missed.'

From the outset, Dr Worthington appreciated the value of anaesthesia as few did. It is a highly reasonable conjecture to think that his popularity and reputation for humaneness were due not only to his personal qualities but also to his use of anaesthesia for surgical procedures. Although a surgeon by training and inclination, he could also truly be called a pioneer anaesthetist.

References

(1) Editorial. The late Doctor Worthington. *The Medical Age* (Detroit, Michigan) 1895; **13:** 177-9.
(2) Worthington ED. *Reminiscences of student life and practice.* Sherbrooke: Walton and Co, 1897.
(3) Worthington ED. Case of amputation of leg—the patient under the influence of sulphuric ether vapour. *Br Am J* 1847; **3:** 10.

(4) Worthington ED. Cases of chloroform. *Br Am J* 1848; **3**: 326–7.

(5) Editorial Note: Employment of sulphuric ether vapour in Montreal, Quebec and Sherbrooke. *Br Am J* 1847; **2**: 238.

(6) Nelson H. Experiments with the sulphuric ether vapour. *Br Am J* 1847; **3**: 34–6.

24.7   T. W. Evans (1823–1897) and
J. T. Clover (1825–1882) and their common patient

OLE SECHER
University of Copenhagen, Denmark

Thomas Wiltberger Evans (1823–97) (Fig. 1) was born in Philadelphia, where he got his education as a dentist. Samuel Stockton White (1822–79) was a fellow student and friend. He later became the manufacturer of gas machines for dental use establishing the well-known firm of S. S. White in Philadelphia (2). Most likely they produced some of the equipment used by Colton (15) (see later) and Evans.

Evans in Paris

In 1847 when Evans was 24 years old he went to Paris, where he joined the first American dentist there, Cyrus Starr Brewster from Charleston, who had a successful practice (2,5). In 1848 Evans treated for the first time Charles Louis Napoleon Bonaparte (1808–73), a nephew of the great Emperor. That was the year of the revolution and Louis Napoleon became President in December that year. He was President 1848–51, when he by a *coup d'état* became Emperor until 1870. He married the 27-year-old beautiful Spanish Countess Eugenie-Marie de Montijo (1826–1920) in 1853 (2,6,8).

In 1850 Evans was able to establish his own *'practice elegance'* at Rue de la Paix, where people of importance and royalty from Europe were treated including Edward Prince of Wales who later became Edward VII of England (1841–1910) (2).

Evans also became friendly with the Imperial Family and in 1869 he was in the Empress's party when she opened the Suez Canal (the builder of the Canal—Vicomte Ferdinand de Lesseps (1805–94)—was of her mother's family—a sort of honorary uncle) Evans also undertook diplomatic missions for the Emperor (2,4).

Evans was a very imaginative person who wrote books, not only on dental treatment, but also on the equipment for field ambulances for the army.

In 1867 the World Exhibition took place in Paris and he was active in exhibiting medical equipment for ambulances. He also bought with his own money an ambulance, which was exhibited by the Americans, and donated it to the French army (2,4).

Gardner Quincy Colton (1814–98) of New York, who had reestablished nitrous oxide as an anaesthetic for dental cases also came to the Exhibition and exhibited some nitrous oxide equipment. Evans got very interested in this and soon Colton taught him how to use it in his practice even for bigger operations.

Evans in London

In March 1868 Evans went to London to demonstrate the use of nitrous oxide at the Dental Hospital, Soho Square, at Moorfields Eye Hospital and, privately, in Dr Robert Hepburn's

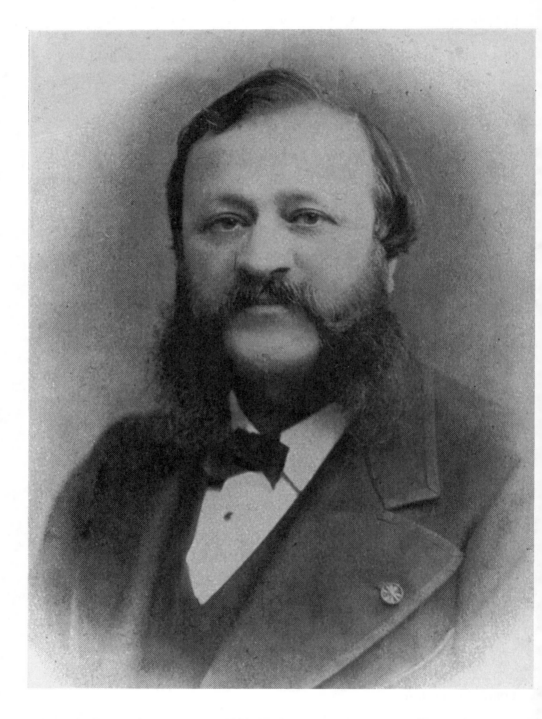

Figure 1   Thomas Wiltberger Evans, 1823–97. The picture is from around 1875, published in his Memoirs.

(1810–1901) home. The nitrous oxide was produced by a generator manufactured by *A. W. Sprague* of Boston, USA (15) in a room in the Langham Hotel, where here Evans filled the bags (7,12).

Later in 1868 Evans donated £100 to the Dental Hospital 'to be used for the purchase of apparatus and materials to manufacture the gas' (12).

The demonstrations went well and during these Evans met Dr Joseph Thomas Clover (1825–82) for the first, but not last time. Clover had at that time taken over John Snow's (1813–58) position as the accepted expert in anaesthesia in London and the man to call for (10). After the demonstration Clover made his own apparatus for administering nitrous oxide later in 1868 (12). Among those who were critical was Benjamin Ward Richardson (1828–96) (7). Evans went back to Paris and continued his lucrative practice.

The Franco-Prussian war

When the Franco-Prussian war broke out on 19 July, 1870, Evans was very active in establishing the American ambulance together with his friend, another American dentist, Edward A. Crane (2).

The war was a catastrophe for the French. On 1 September, at the battle of Sedan, the Emperor became a prisoner of war. When the news came to Paris a revolution started, and 4 September, the people went to the Tuileries, where the Empress Eugenie was staying. She wished to stay, but her staff were able to persuade her to leave.

The escape of the Empress Eugenie

Two friends of the family, Richard Metternich (1829–95) the Austrian ambassador, and Castantino Nigra (b. 1827), the Italian ambassador, came to her help. The Empress and a trusted lady-in-waiting (Madame Lebreton-Bourbaki) came out through one of the sidegates and got into a cab. They first visited trusted persons from the court staff, but they were not home, and then they tried Dr Evans, who was living at the corner of Avenue de l'Imperatrice and Avenue Malakoff in his big house 'Bella Rosa'. Dr Evans was not at home, but his servant let them in—it was then five o'clock. An hour later Dr Evans returned with his friend Edward A. Crane. It was decided that the ladies should stay overnight and that the next day they should try to get out of town in Dr Evans's carriage with his trusted coachman Célestin and make for the Channel and England (2,4,8).

The next day (5 September, 1870), they left early in the morning and got out of the city without difficulty. After two days and staying in an inn on the way they came to Deauville where Mrs Agnes Evans was on a month's holiday in the Hotel de Casino. In the harbour Dr Evans found a British gentleman, Sir John Montagu Burgoyne (b. 1832), who had picked up his wife in his yacht 'Gaselle'. After some time they were persuaded to take the French party across the Channel with Dr Evans and the French party. Dr Crane returned to Paris (2,4).

The crossing was rough and when they came ashore at Rye on the south coast of England the Empress had to consult a doctor. It turned out to be the same doctor who had seen the 75-year-old King Louis-Philippe (1773–50) when he escaped in 1848 (2).

Dr Evans was now busy finding a place to live and, in the end, he bought Camden Place, Chislehurst, where the ladies moved in. He and his wife had to stay in England until after the collapse of the Commune at the end of March, 1871. During this time he visited the Emperor Louis Napoleon at Wilhelmshöhe, near Kassel, where he had been made a Prisoner of War after the battle at Sedan.

The illness of the Emperor Louis Napoleon

Years before the war the Emperor had suffered from a bladder stone, which had been treated by his French doctors. His personal doctors, Dr Henry Conneau (b. 1803) and François Remy Lucien Corvisart (1824–82) (a nephew of Napoleon's famous physician, Jean

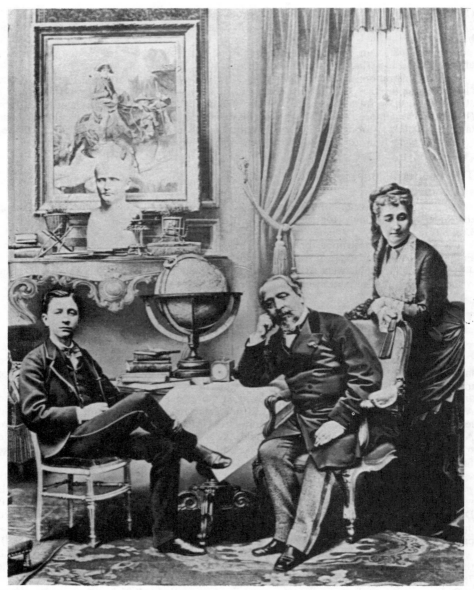

Figure 2   The Imperial family at Camden Place. Prince Eugén Louis, the Prince Imperial (1856–79), was killed by the Zulus in a guerilla war in South Africa when he was serving the British army in the artillery.

Nicholas Corvisart (1775–1821)) regarded the condition as a catarrh of the bladder. The leading surgeon, Auguste Nélaton (1807–73) of the Hôpital St Louis,* took the same view but two other doctors, Philippe Ricard (1800–89), an expert of venereal diseases, and Professor Germain Sée (1818–96), a specialist in heart and nervous diseases, were of the definite opinion that the Emperor had a bladder stone (13).

*Nelaton had become famous when, in 1862 he had removed a bullet from the foot of Guiseppe Garibaldi (1807–82) the Italian liberator (9).

At the battle of Sedan and in the period before it, Louis Napoleon had such severe bladder trouble and pain, that he, who was an excellent horseback rider, could not sit on his horse, and had difficulty taking decisions. His condition was bad, he was anaemic due to bleeding from haemorrhoids; he was probably at that time uraemic and he was passing very bloody urine. When he was sent to Wilhelmshöhe, his two trusted doctors went with him. Here Louis Napoleon spent six months until he was released in March, 1871, and could travel to England and be united with Empress Eugénie at Camden Place (2) (Fig. 2).

The half year had improved the Emperor's health and he remained well for the next 18 months, but in the autumn of 1872, he deteriorated and could neither ride nor walk. Sir William Gull (1816–90), Guy's Hospital, who had attended him for some time called in the surgeon Sir James Paget (1814–99) of St Bartholomew's Hospital (13). He recommended that Sir Henry Thompson* (1820–1904), University College Hospital, who was considered the leading specialist in diseases of the bladder, was consulted, and he examined the Emperor on 24 December, 1872. He decided that a further examination must be carried out under anaesthesia, so he repeated the examination on 26th with Clover,† who gave most of the anaesthetics for Thompson in his private practice, administering chloroform. Thompson diagnosed a bladder stone the size of the seed of a date and it was decided to crush the stone and have it removed. This took place on 2 January, 1873, in the afternoon. A number of the doctors were present. Sir Henry Thompson operated, assisted by Dr Foster and Dr Clover who administered chloroform. The crushing with a lithotrist went well, but not all the debris were removed so it was decided to repeat the operation on 6 January. The emperor was at that time uraemic and had attacks of rigor. Again under the influence of chloroform by Dr Clover the stone pieces which obstructed the urethra were removed. The following day further pieces passed, but it became evident that the urethra was obstructed once more, but some passage was obtained by introducing an instrument (13).

On Thursday morning the 9th all his doctors including Thompson and Clover were again present, but the patient was very much changed for the worse and died at 10.45 a.m.

Thus Clover anaesthetized the Emperor three times and every time he used the chloroform apparatus with the big bag. In this way he could give a very constant concentration.

Postscript

The Emperor Napoleon III was buried on 12 January, 1873. Evans came over from Paris, as a friend of the family, when the Emperor became ill. He gave medical advice and consoled the Empress and most likely attended the operations, when Clover gave the anaesthetics. He was also present at the funeral (2).

Evans and Clover in this way met a couple of times professionally.

Acknowledgments

Professor I. C. Christoffersen, MD and Chief Dentist Leif Marvitz have kindly helped me with literature, and Dr R. K. Calverley, San Diego, and librarian Lee Perry, Seattle, with information on the Clover/Snow collection.

References

(1) Calverley RK. Personal communication 1986.

*Thompson had been asked to go to Brussels in 1863 where King Leopold I (1790–1865), the uncle of Queen Victoria (1819–1901), was suffering from a bladder stone. He was treated for this at the castle of Laken, but Thompson crushed the stone without anaesthesia. Clover was not present, but it had been agreed that he could go if it was considered necessary (3,13).

†Clover gave anaesthetics to many members of the Royal Family during his career. They included Alexandra Princess of Wales in 1867 and Princess Beatrice in 1872—the youngest daughter of Queen Victoria for whom the latter had received chloroform at her birth in 1857 (1,11,14).

(2) Carson G. *The dentist and the Empress. The adventures of Dr Tom Evans in gas-lit Paris.* Boston: Houghton Mifflin Co, 1983.

(3) Cope Z. *The versatile Victorian. Being the life of Sir Henry Thompson Bt. 1820–1904.* London: Harvey & Blythe Ltd, 1951.

(4) Crane EA, ed. *The memoirs of Thomas W. Evans. Recollections of the second French Empire.* Vol. 1 & 2. London: Fisher Unwin, 1905.

(5) Davenport WS. The pioneer American dentists in France and their successors. *Revue d'histoire de l'art dentaire* 1965; **3**: 99–116.

(6) Duff D. *Eugenie & Napoleon III.* London: Collins, 1978.

(7) Duncum BM. *The development of inhalation anaesthesia.* Oxford University Press, 1947.

(8) *Empress Eugenie's memoires.* Danish edition: Gyldendalske Boghandel 1920.

(9) Guthrie D. *A history of medicine.* London: Thomas Nelson & Son Ltd, 1945.

(10) Marston AD. The life and achievements of Joseph Thomas Clover. *Ann Roy Coll Surg Engl* 1949; **4**: 267–80.

(11) Secher O. *Chloroform-anaesthesia to a Royal family (Danish).* Med-hist Årbog Copenhagen 1987: 107–125.

(12) Smith WDA. *Under the influence. A history of nitrous oxide and oxygen anaesthesia.* London: Macmillan Publishers Ltd, 1982.

(13) Stevenson RS. *Famous illnesses in history.* London: Eyre & Spottiswoode, 1962.

(14) Thomas KB. The Clover/Snow collection. *Anaesthesia* 1972; **27**: 436–49.

(15) Thomas KB. *The development of anaesthetic apparatus.* Oxford: Blackwell, 1975.

24.8   Little known Liverpool contributions (1761–1862)

T. CECIL GRAY
University of Liverpool, Liverpool, UK

In the 18th and 19th centuries there was a remarkable group of Liverpool practitioners who made small but interesting contributions to the story of anaesthesia and resuscitation. Sometimes these were near misses, at others they were prophetic.

David Waldie

The story of how David Waldie suggested to Simpson that he should try chloroform as an anaesthetic is well documented and need not be repeated; however, I wish to make three points. First, Waldie is usually described as a chemist; he was in fact a doctor—a contemporary of Simpson at Edinburgh Medical School. Second, when his laboratory was burnt down after his discussion with Simpson, it not only meant that he could not send his pure chloroform to Simpson, but also that he was deprived of any chance of forestalling him in the use of chloroform as an anaesthetic. He was able to give an anaesthetic, but, delayed by the fire, his first demonstration of chloroform was sixteen days after that of Simpson. Third, one of the preparations tried by Simpson before chloroform was 'chloric ether'. He had been introduced to this so-called 'diffusible stimulant' in 1845 by another Liverpool physician, Richard Formby, who had learnt of the prescription from some visitors from the USA. Dr Brett, the Director of the laboratory at the Liverpool Apothecaries' Hall, made it for him by distilling chloride of lime with spirit. When Waldie took over the laboratory in 1839, he improved the product by making first chloroform and then adding alcohol to it: hence his offer when he met Simpson in October, 1847, to send him some pure chloroform.

Hugh Neill

Who was the first to describe the analgesic effect of ether? An audacious claim was made by a colourful Liverpool Eye surgeon, Hugh Neill (1). He was of distinction in his field but an inveterate publicist. In 1840, he published a pamphlet on the treatment of deafness and the relief of pain in the inner ear by the insufflation of ether into the Eustachian tubes. This was not an original procedure; a French and a German surgeon had described it some twenty years before. In 1847, Neill published another book, this time on cataract in which he writes of his previous pamphlet:

> *'It is strange if a thousand copies of my little work . . . regularly shipped and entered through the Customs and extensively circulated [in the USA], it is strange that such a pamphlet declaring the efficiency of Aether-vapour in relieving pain should have been five years in Boston, and yet that its suggestions, apparently, should not have been seen— at any rate acknowledged—by the new discoverer.'*

Neill claims himself 'As an humble pioneer—towards its complete discovery'. A contemporary reviewer of his book dismissed this as 'An utterly absurd and ridiculous claim'.

Mathew Turner

One who did not make any claim but was probably the first to note the pain-relieving potential of ether, was Mathew Turner who published a paper in 1761 entitled 'An Account of the Extraordinary Medicinal Fluid called Aether' (2). He practised in Liverpool where one of his patients was Josiah Wedgwood, the founder of the factory which has been making beautiful china and porcelain ever since. In an 1863 biography of Josiah, Turner is described as:

> *'A good surgeon, a skilful anatomist, a practised chemist, a draughtsman, a classical scholar and a ready wit [who] did much to foster a literary and artistic taste among the more educated classes of Liverpool.'*

He is known to have introduced to chemistry no less a man than Joseph Priestley, the discoverer of oxygen (3). In his pamphlet, he describes ether as a:

> *'Highly penetrating vapour—vaporised at less than body temperature [and] perceptible by its smell as it passes through the pores of the skin several hours after taking.'*

He recommended it for many conditions including fits, headaches, 'hooping' cough, asthma, pleuritic pains and deafness. His methods of administration were topical and oral. But, significantly, he also describes its administration by sniffing it mixed with oil of lavender or on pledglets of cotton wool or rag stuffed up the nose; there can be no doubt that the relief of pain, when given thus, was due to its inhalation. I wonder if anyone else knows of an earlier account of this action of ether?

James Currie

Another 18th century physician of Liverpool was James Currie MD, FRCP (Edin), FRS. Like Mathew Turner he was of radical mind and humanitarian, being involved in the anti-slavery movement to such a degree that, at one time, his life was under threat. An enthusiastic supporter of Paine's *Rights of Man*, he persuaded fellow humanitarians, who formed an influential group, to have regard of the suffering of the insane, and was largely responsible for founding the first asylum in the town. Outraged by the conditions under which French prisoners from the Napoleonic war were kept in the Borough gaol which housed not less than 4000 of them, his correspondence with the Prime Minister, Pitt, resulted in considerable improvement in the conditions of their captivity.

He qualified in Glasgow but had studied medicine in Edinburgh where, as a student, he gave two papers on the effect of cold on the body. This was to be an interest throughout his career and, apart from drawing your attention to so remarkable a man, is the reason why he is of interest to anaesthetists. He pioneered the taking and recording of the temperature in febrile patients and with another Liverpool physician, Dr Brandreth, enthusiastically advocated the treatment of fevers by douching with cold water and by cold drinks. But his special interest for us today lies in his experiments on the effects of immersion in cold water which were stimulated by observations on sailors rescued from drowning in the River Mersey (4). To elucidate why cold killed some and not others, he carried out a series of pretty drastic experiments. Two young men were immersed in a bath of water at 44° F in the open air on raw, cold days for periods up to 30 minutes while their pulse and oral temperature was recorded. The unfortunate subject was taken out of the cold bath and plunged into one warmed to 97° F and, on one occasion to 109° F. These drastic exercises were certainly not very humanitarian but they and the discussion of the results make for fascinating reading. One of his observations must surely be of interest to anaesthetists. He records it as follows:

> *'That after a person is long chilled in cold water, the first effect of passing through the external air into the warm bath is first a fall of [temperature] whilst in the air and after this a still greater fall [when put] in the warm bath followed later by a speedy rise.'*

Those who have been involved in hypothermic techniques, particularly in the early days of surface cooling, will recognize this as surely the first recording of the 'after drop' of temperature which is seen when active cooling is stopped.

Alfred Higginson and others

Other Liverpool men of interest who might be mentioned are Thomas Skinner, who is well recognized for having designed the first wire frame mask for the administration of ether and chloroform in 1862, thus preceding Shimmelbusch, Bellamy Gardner, who also designed a mask and others. There is no space to consider their contributions in detail here, however, and this chauvinistic survey will be concluded by mentioning Alfred Higginson. He was a Liverpool surgeon with a remarkably inventive brain and is remembered in this country for his invention in 1840 of the enema syringe named after him and which is still in use. After attending the first demonstration of ether anaesthesia in Liverpool on 10 January, 1847, he constructed an ether inhaler from an ear trumpet and pig's bladder. He was greatly interested in respirology and, when Hutchinson defined the 'Vital Capacity', he designed a spirometer for its measurement. To us perhaps his most interesting invention was what he called a 'Pneumatic Chest'—an apparatus for maintaining artificial respiration. He showed this device to a meeting of the Liverpool Medical Institution in 1843 and in the Minutes it is described as 'An air tight box upon which a pair of bellows is placed for the alternated introduction and withdrawal of air. The effect is to force air into abstraction of air from the box' (Fig. 1). The patient's head was, of course, outside the box. His manuscript 'An Essay on the subject of Suspended Animation and the best means of restoring life as well as the most approved apparatus to be used for that purpose, communicated to the Liverpool Literary and Philosophical Society, Feb. 19th 1844. Addressed to the Royal Humane Society on Nov. 29th 1842' is in the possession of the Liverpool Medical Institution. What a pity his invention was not taken up and perfected.

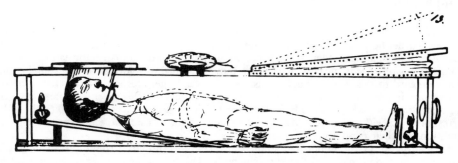

Figure 1   The 'Pneumatic Chest'.

References

(1) Neill H. *A report upon deafness when resulting from diseases of the eustachian tubes with the modern methods of care*. Liverpool: John Walmsley, 1839: 197–205. (Available in the Library of the Liverpool Medical Institution.)
(2) Turner M. *An account of the extraordinary medicinal fluid called aether*. 1761. (Pamphlet available in the library of the Royal Society of Medicine.)
(3) Turner Mathew (1718–1789). *Dictionary of national biography*, 1899: 350–1.
(4) Currie James *Medical reports effects of water cold and warm as a remedy in fever and other diseases*. 2nd Ed. Liverpool, 1798. (Available in the Library of Liverpool Medical Institution.)

25.1	The contribution of the pioneers in neurosurgery to the development of neuroanaesthesia

Macewen (1847–1924), Horsley (1857–1916),
Krause (1857–1937) and Cushing (1869–1939)

ELIZABETH A. M. FROST
Albert Einstein College of Medicine, New York, USA

When neurosurgery was identified as a specialty within surgery just under 100 years ago, anaesthetic services, although generally available were poorly organized. Administration, techniques and drug effects were ill defined. Certainly, no attempts had been made to adapt anaesthesia to surgical requirements.

From the researches of the pioneers of neurological surgery came not only a better understanding of the specific anaesthetic needs of the patient with cranial disease, but advances of lasting importance to the whole field of anaesthesiology.

Significant contributions were made by four surgeons.

Sir William Macewen

William Macewen, a Scot, born on the Port Bannantyne side of Skeoch Wood on the Island of Bute in 1848 and acknowledged as the chief pioneer of neurological surgery (1), made significant advances in the devlopment of anaesthesia in general and emphasized the importance of specialty training.

Shortly after William Macewen's graduation in 1869, he worked as medical superintendent of the Glasgow Fever Hospital at Belvedere. There, prompted by his involvement in the care of many patients with diphtheria, he began his investigations of the possibilities of peroral intubation of the larynx. In this, he was influenced by Pierre Desault, the French surgeon, who in the late 18th century demonstrated that foreign bodies such as tubes could be tolerated by the larynx in the conscious individual (2). After extensive cadaveric work, Macewen applied his knowledge clinically.

On 5 July, 1878, he passed a tube into the trachea of a patient prior to the induction of chloroform anaesthesia. The upper laryngeal opening was packed with gauze which encircled the tube to prevent entrance of blood.

> '*The assured patency of the air passage was a source of comfort to everyone concerned and the respiratory currents were both felt and heard as they traversed the tube. The after result of the operation was admirable.*' (2)

In a second case of epithelioma of the fauces, tubes were passed prior to surgery and the patient responded well to their presence. At a meeting of the Glasgow Medico Chirurgical Society in 1879 he read a paper 'On the Introduction of Tubes through the Mouth instead of Tracheotomy or Laryngotomy.' (3). These case reports were published the following year in what was considered perhaps a more prestigious journal (4).

Macewen's tubes were made of flexible brass and were about nine inches long and three eighths of an inch in diameter although he also described the use of graded sizes of gum elastic catheters, especially in acute situations (5). The tube was guided into the larynx by a finger which depressed the tongue and epiglottis. Macewen also noted that a metal tube could be placed through the nose and a catheter then passed through the tube which could be guided by a finger into the larynx (4). To secure a tight fit, he recommended that a tight bag or gauze or muslin pack encircle the tube although Macewen clearly described endotracheal anaesthesia the idea was not to be developed for 40 years (6).

This neurosurgeon made even more significant contributions in his dedication to training in anaesthetics. His predecessor, in the Chair of Surgery at Glasgow University, Joseph Lister had published a paper in 1861 on the benefits and safety of chloroform (7). Macewen, who had been a student of Lister and dresser on his wards for one year prior to the latter's departure for Edinburgh, was undoubtedly influenced by his stern admonition on the inherent dangers of chloroform in unskilled hands. Although students of medicine were required to have a certificate of proficiency in vaccination prior to graduation, no formal training in anaesthetics was required (2). On 9 October, 1882, Mr McEwan, Chairman of the Glasgow Royal Infirmary Board of Governors proposed at the quarterly meeting that the pathologist should deliver a course of lectures on anaesthetics at the beginning of each winter session, and that all assistants should hold a certificate attesting to knowledge of this subject. The resolutions were amended by the omission of 'pathologist' in November 1882 (8).

In 1883, an elderly patient died during surgery under chloroform anaesthesia. McEwan published the case and insisted that residents should not be permitted to administer chloroform. A bitter debate, published during March, 1883, in the *Glasgow Herald*, followed between McEwan, firmly supported by Macewen, Mr James Morton and Dr Leishman, staff members of the Royal Infirmary. As a consequence, a special committee of the Managers of the Glasgow Royal Infirmary was formed on 1 March, 1883. Under the leadership of Professors W. T. Gardner and John Cleland a letter was sent on 16 March, 1883, to medical superintendents of 40 hospitals and medical schools in the United Kingdom enquiring as to their practice in the administration of chloroform. A questionnaire attached sought information as to formal regulations with respect to the use and administration of anaesthetics, availability of special instruction, qualifications of persons administering anaesthetics and the presence of specialist anaesthetists. The response rate was a remarkable 50%. The report submitted by the committee under the convener, John Ure recommended that all assistants in surgery, in additional to prior formal certification, be trained practically in the administration of anaesthetics. All anaesthetics and untoward effects were to be recorded in the Operations Book. The resolutions were accepted in May, 1883 (8).

William Macewen immediately adopted these policies. In 1884 at the beginning of each session, a week was devoted to systematic lectures on anaesthetics including a review of Macewen's experimental work. He insisted that each student should administer at least 12 chloroform anaesthetics under his own direct supervision (9). In this he certainly refuted Silk's statement in 1892 that there was 'no systematic instruction in anaesthesia in Scotland, Ireland and the provinces' (10).

By 1890, the question of anaesthetic administration was still very important in the public mind. The demand had been made that two physicians should be present at all cases in which the administration of an anaesthetic was necessary. Macewen opposed this practice, noting the difficulties imposed on remote areas where a second doctor might be many miles away, but again emphasized that formal training for all students in anaesthetics was essential (2).

Macewen was particularly noted for his clinical acumen and tenacity in reporting physical signs. After a long series of observations, he mapped out pupillary changes in response to anaesthetics, cerebral injuries and intoxication. In his choice of anaesthetics, Macewen preferred chloroform. His dislike of ether was based on its stimulant action on the heart and salivary glands (11). He felt that the cardiac depressant effect of chloroform was of no importance and even advantageous and could be reversed by ether if necessary. He noted especially that in acute inflammatory cerebral disease, anaesthetics had to be used cautiously as prolonged or deep anaesthesia could increase oedema in an already oedematous brain. Chloroform was to be given gradually and could be supplemented by morphine, 1/8th grain (7.5 mg) by suppository. However as the effects of even small doses of morphine could be very long lasting this drug could be omitted.

An interesting speculation has been raised—had William Macewen accepted the offer of the new Chair of Surgery at Johns Hopkins Hospital in Baltimore in 1889, a post subsequently filled by William Halsted, how might the course of neurosurgery and anaesthesia in both countries have been affected? (12).

Sir Victor Horsley

Quite different from the poor seafaring family of William Macewen, the family of Victor Horsley was well established in London. He was given his first two names, Victor Alexander, by Queen Victoria (13). Thwarted in his childhood ambition of becoming a cavalry officer, he opted for the profession of physician and surgeon (14).

As a house surgeon to John Marshall at University College Hospital, London, in 1880, he began a long series of experiments on his own brain. He was himself anaesthetized some 50 times and he devised ways of recording and signalling his experiences. It is reported that the hospital authorities noted an increased consumption of gas (15). Undoubtedly today such behaviour would demand instant suspension and drug rehabilitation!

Of special interest are his observations on nitrous oxide anaesthesia, published in *Brain* in October, 1883:

> . . . *'experimenting on myself . . . the anaesthesia was complete and pushed until rigidity and sometimes cyanosis resulted. The recovery of consciousness was very frequently attended with considerable muscular spasm and semi-coordinated convulsive struggles and excitement.'* (16)

It was to be many years before these detrimental effects of nitrous oxide on the central system were realized and emphasized (17).

Between 1883–1885 Horsley investigated the different intracranial effects during surgery of chloroform, ether and morphine sulphate. He concluded that ether caused a rise in blood pressure, increased blood viscosity and prompted excessive bleeding, dangerous postoperative vomiting and excitement and thus should not be used in neurosurgery. He felt that morphine was of value because of the apparent decrease in cerebral blood flow and the more readily controlled haemorrhage in the surgical field (18). His preference was for chloroform. He advised the 'judicious use of chloroform to control haemorrhage'.

His first operation at Queen's Square Hospital was on 25 May, 1886. The patient, identified as James B, 22 years old, suffered from intermittent status epilepticus due to head trauma sustained as a child (19). Under chloroform anaesthesia, Horsley removed the scar in the brain and the surrounding brain substance to a depth of 2 cm (19). The outcome was most successful except for one factor noted by the physician Dr Hughlings Jackson:

> *'Here's the first operation of this kind that we ever had at the Hospital; the patient is a Scotsman. We had the chance of getting a joke into his head and we failed to take advantage of it.'* (20)

Horsley felt that major intracranial surgery should be undertaken in two stages to minimize shock and recognized the value of hypotension which he achieved by increasing the depth of anaesthesia (20). In his earlier operations he combined morphine with chloroform but later he used only chloroform because of the respiratory depressant effects of the former (21). However, death under chloroform was not uncommon and between 1864 and 1912, eight committee and commissions were convened to study this drug.

In 1901, the British Medical Association appointed a Special Chloroform Committee including Waller, Sherrington, Harcourt, Buxton and Horsley among others. It had been shown that rather less than 2% chloroform vapour in air was sufficient to induce anaesthesia and much less was required for maintenance. The debate centred around the need for an apparatus to exactly determine the percentage of vapour as opposed to simply sprinkling the drug on a fold of lint. The issue was that of science dictating to practice. Horsley was insistent that the percentage should be controlled and used a vaporizer designed by Vernon Harcourt, a physical chemist, that delivered 2% as a maximum. During craniotomy, Horsley ruled that chloroform administration should be reduced to 0.5% or less after removal of the bone (22). He felt that exact determination of the percentage delivered was of particular importance in patients with raised intracranial pressure that might make fatal a concentration that would be safe under normal circumstances. A cylinder of oxygen was adjusted to the inhaler, in the belief that capillary bleeding might be reduced by giving oxygen instead of chloroform. His anaesthetist, from 1904 to 1914, Dr Mennell noted that Horsley's demand for reduced concentrations often made it necessary for assistants to restrain patients intraoperatively (23).

Horsley was also involved politically, again with anaesthetic implications. The National Antivivisection Society had organized the British Union for the Abolition of Vivisection in 1884 (20). An ardent spokeswoman, Miss Frances Cobbe, published a book '*The Nine Circles from Dante's Inferno*' in 1892 in which she attacked the English scientists for inhumane treatment of animals. At a church congress on Folkestone in October, 1892, Horsley responded that in reviewing the 26 experiments cited, all had been performed under ether or chloroform anaesthesia (20). Even in his early works, he had always recorded the administration and affects of anaesthetics on his animals (20). He concluded that the brain surgery he subsequently performed could not have been undertaken had it not first been performed on animals under anaesthetics. The verbal conflicts were reported in *The Times* on 8 October, 1892 (20).

In 1907, he gave evidence before the Royal Commission on experiments on animals. He argued effectively for vivisection under three headings: 1) the need to teach students how to operate; 2) the need to teach students how to give anaesthetics and; 3) the working out of new methods in surgery (20). His evidence covered 31 pages and was incorporated in the final Act.

Professor Fedor Krause

Fedor Krause, born in Friedland in 1857, has been acclaimed the founder of German neurological surgery. He worked as assistant to Richard Volkman at the Surgical University Hospital at Halle from 1883 to 1892 before going to Altona (Germany) and then to Berlin (24,25). During his time with Volkman, he saw the use of a morphine-chloroform combination but he was not convinced that it was advantageous for neurosurgical procedures. From 1889 he preferred chloroform alone (26). However, he recognized the value of morphine in small doses for postoperative pain in adults. Although he appreciated the greater overall safety in use of ether, he advised against its use because of venous bleeding. Rarely, he conceded, ether might have a place in the care of patients with non-compensated heart lesions being operated for removal of the Gasserian ganglion.

Like Horsley, he suggested increasing the concentration of chloroform to cause hypotension and decrease bleeding. He noted that in cases of intracranial tumours, sudden death might occur if respiration ceased. He preferred to use a Roth-Dräger oxygen/chloroform apparatus which allowed administration of 100% oxygen which he considered especially important for patients with cardiorespiratory problems.

Like Horsley and Macewen, Krause emphasized that the brain was not sensitive to pain and only very light narcosis was necessary. However, anaesthetic concentrations had to be increased during surgery of the scalp, periosteum and dura (26). In questioning the use of local anaesthesia, a technique advocated by some surgeons, he considered that pain was not the only problem. Preparation for surgery, a positive attitude and psychological status must all be carefully controlled. In particular, he noted that death might be caused by severe mental disturbance prior to anaesthesia. He concluded that a rapid, aseptic surgical technique, minimal blood loss, maintenance of normothermia (especially avoidance of hypothermia) and general narcosis were essential to a good outcome).

However, in some circumstances, local anaesthesia particularly procaine ½% with 1% adrenaline (15 drops per 100 cc) could be used for spinal surgery. The method had been recommended by H. Braun (27). Krause injected the solution above and below the spinous processes in 4 aliquots of 5 ml. The anaesthesia produced was satisfactory until it was necessary to detach the dura from the inner surface of the vertebral arch. Use of the laminectome caused less pain, however, the technique:

'*is only effective in patients who can exercise a certain degree of self control.*' (28)

The use of spinal anaesthesia as described by Augustus Bier (29) was rarely necessary, especially not if compression of the cord existed.

Harvey Cushing

As a second year medical student at Harvard Medical School, Harvey Cushing was asked to substitute for Frank Lynam at the Massachusetts General Hospital for two weeks. Dr Lynam noted that Cushing:

. . . '*was not as anxious for the position as I had expected, said that he had anaesthetized only a couple of times but consented to try it.*' (30)

The first case on 10 January, 1893, a woman with a strangulated hernia, stopped breathing and died on the table shortly after administration of ether. Lynam assured Cushing that death was the usual outcome in such cases. Cushing was unconvinced as was a fellow student, Amory Codman. In 1894 at the suggestion of their chief, Dr F. B. Harrington, Cushing and Codman devised charts for recording pulse, respiration and temperature during anaesthesia (31,32). Codman later noted that Cushing's fatal case was the one that first interested him in brain surgery (33).

During his residency at the Johns Hopkins Hospital, Cushing remained interested in neurosurgery and in 1900 went on an extended educational tour of Europe. While in Berne visiting Theodore Kocher, he realized that increased intracranial pressure resulted in a higher systemic arterial pressure (34). He visited the Ospidale di St Matteo in Padua and was impressed by a 'home-made' adaptation of Scipione Riva-Rocci's blood pressure device which had evolved from those described by Vierordt, Marey and Basch. He sketched the instrument and on his return to Baltimore in September, 1901, almost immediately developed a new anaesthesia chart that incorporated the recording of blood pressure (35,36).

At that time, in the United States, the Gaertner tonometer was in use at Cleveland, mainly because of George Crile. Possibly the first programme on blood pressure, 'Considerations of blood pressure,' was held in the Boston Medical Library on 19 January, 1903 (36). As a result of the papers presented by Crile and Cushing advocating the routine use of blood pressure recording, a committee was formed by Harvard Medical School to investigate the suggestion. The committee decided after long deliberation that the skilled finger was of much greater value clinically for determination of the state of the circulation than any pneumatic instrument, and the work should be put aside as of no significance (37). Cushing later commented on this decision by quoting from Oliver Wendell Holmes' Stethoscope Song:

> *'Now such as hate new fangled toys*
> *Began to look extremely glum;*
> *They said that rattles were made for boys*
> *And vowed that his buzzing was all a hum.'*

Fortunately the rest of the world did not concur with the Harvard decision. In 1930, in a letter to Ralph Major in Kansas City, Cushing whimsically remarked:

> *'I am sure that the general use of a blood pressure apparatus in clinical work has done more than harm. Just as Floyer's pulse watch led to two previously unknown diseases, tachychardia and bradycardia, so the sphygmomanometer has led to the uncovering of the diseases, (God save the mark) of hypertension and hypotension, which have vastly added to the number of neurasthenics in the world.'* (38)

Dr Cushing attached great importance to continuous auscultation of the heart and lungs—a technique which he learned from his anesthesiologist, Dr S. Griffith Davis (39).

With regards to his choice of anaesthesia for neurosurgical cases, he remained sceptical about the safety of ether mainly because of continued intraoperative mortality. Students of the Medical School at Johns Hopkins were permitted to administer ether just as had been the case at Harvard and Cushing, as assistant resident, under William Halsted could not change the practice. Thus he experimented with block anaesthesia by cocaine infiltration of nerve trunks, a technique based on work by Halsted (40). He popularized various local anaesthetic techniques and coined the term 'regional anaesthesia.' In 1929, a patient from whom he had removed a large intracranial cyst, as a demonstration for Pavlov, reported:

> *'One of the secrets of Dr Cushing's success is that he uses nothing except a local anaesthetic which permits the normal functioning of the heart and other organs during the operation'* (41).

Conclusion

The evolution of neuroanaesthesia is closely linked to the development of neurosurgery itself. The contributions of these four neurosurgeons, namely an understanding of monitoring, recording, airway control, the effects of anaesthetic agents on intracranial contents, and appropriate training, have formed the basis for the recognition of the subspecialty of neuroanaesthesia.

References

(1) Jefferson G. Sir William Macewen's contributions to neurosurgery and its sequels. In: *Sir Geoffrey Jefferson, Selected Papers*. Springfield, Il: Chas C. Thomas, 1960; 132–49.

(2) Bowman AK. *The life and teaching of Sir William Macewen*. London: William Hodge & Co, 1942; 94–8.

(3) Macewen W. The introduction of tubes into the larynx through the mouth instead of tracheotomy and laryngotomy. *Glasgow Med J* 1879; 9: 72–4; and 12; 218–21.

(4) Macewen W. Clinical observations on the introduction of tracheal tubes by the mouth instead of performing tracheotomy or laryngotomy. *Br Med J* 1880; 2: 122–4, (July 24), 163–265, (July 25).

(5) Watt OM. *Glasgow anaesthetics 1846–1946*. Clydebank: James Pender, 1962, 19.

(6) Rowbotham ES, Magill IW. Anaesthetics in the plastic surgery of the face and jaws. *Proc Roy Soc Med* 1921; 14: 17–27.

(7) Watt OM. *Glasgow Anaesthetics 1846–1946*. Clydebank: James Pender, 1962; 15.

(8) *Board of Managers Reports, Glasgow Royal Infirmary 1882–83*, Archives, University of Glasgow.

(9) Watt OM. *Glasgow Anaesthetics 1846–1946*. Clydebank: James Pender, 1962: 21.

(10) James CDT. Sir William Macewen and anaesthesia. *Anaesthesia* 1974; 29: 743–53.

(11) Macewen W. Introduction to a discussion on anaesthetics. *Glasgow Medical J* 1890; 34: 321–32.

(12) Miller JD. William Macewen: Master of Surgery. *Virginia Medical J* 1979; 106: 362–8.

(13) McNalty A. Sir Victor Horsley: His life and work. *Br Med J* 1957; 2: 911–20.

(14) Green JR. Sir Victor Horsley. A Centennial Recognition of his impact on neuroscience and on neurological surgery. *Barrow Neurol Instit Quat* 1987; 3: 2–16.

(15) Paget S. *Sir Victor Horsley, A study of his life and work*. London, Constable, 1919: 40–41.

(16) Frost E. Central nervous system effects of nitrous oxide. In: Eger EI, II, ed. *Nitrous Oxide N₂O*, New York: Elsevier, 1985; 157–76.

(17) Shapira M. Evolution of anesthesia for neurosurgery. *New York State J Med* 1964; 64: 1301–5.

(18) Horsley V. On the technique of operations on the central nervous system. *Br Med J* 1906, 2: 411–23.

(19) Horsley V. Brain surgery. *Br Med J* 1886, 2: 670–5.

(20) Lyons JB. *Citizen surgeon*. London: Peter Downay, 1966.

(21) Paget S. *Sir Victor Horsley. A study of his life and work*. London: Constable, 1919: 184.

(22) Horsley V. On the technique of operations on the central nervous system. Address in Surgery, Toronto, *Lancet* 1906; ii: 484.

(23) Mennell Z. Anaesthesia in intracranial surgery. *Am J Surg* 1924; 38 (Anesth Suppl): 44.

(24) Behrend CM. Fedor Krause und die Anfänge der Neurochirurgie in Deutschland. *Deutsche Med Wochenshcrift* 1957; 82: 519–20.

(25) Jefferson G. Fedor Krause und die neurologische Chirurgie Fedor Krause Gedächtnisvorlesung in: Jefferson AA, et al eds. *Acta Neurochirurgica* Vienna: Springer-Verlag, 1960, 9: 661–4.

(26) Krause F. *Surgery of the brain and spinal cord based on personal experiences*. Trans, H Haubold, M Thorek. New York: Rebman & Co, 1912, Vol 1; 137–8.

(27) Braun H. Uber die Lokalanästhesie im Krankenhaus nebst Bemerkung ü die Technik der örtlichen Anästhesierung. *Beitr z. Klin Chir* 1909; 62: 641–85.

(28) Krause F. *Surgery of the brain and spinal cord based on personal experiences*. Trans, H Haubold, M Thorek. New York: Rebman & Co, 1912; Vol 3: 957–8.

(29) Bier A. Versuche über cocainisirung des Rückenmarkes. *Deutsche Zeitschrift für Chirurgie*, 1899; 51: 361–9.

(30) Fulton JF. *Harvey Cushing: A Biography*. Oxford: Blackwell, 1946; 69–70.
(31) Beecher HK. The first anesthesia records (Codman Cushing). *Surg Gynec Obstet* 1940; **71**: 689–93.
(32) Shepherd DAE. Harvey Cushing and Anaesthesia. *Can Anaesth Soc J* 1965; **12**: 431–42.
(33) Fulton JF. *Harvey Cushing: A Biography*. Oxford: Blackwell, 1946; 95.
(34) Cushing HW. Concerning a definite regulatory mechanism of the vasomotor center which controls blood pressure during cerebral compression. *Bull Johns Hopkins Hosp* 1901; **12**: 290–6.
(35) Cushing HW. On the avoidance of shock in major amputations by cocainization of large nerve trunks preliminary to their division. With observations on blood pressure changes in surgical cases. *Ann Surg* 1902; **36**: 321–45.
(36) Cushing HW. On routine determinations of arterial tension in operating room and clinic. *Boston Med Surg J* 1903; **148**: 250–6.
(37) The Division of Surgery of the Medical School of Harvard University—*Report of Research Work, 1903–04, Bulletin 11*, March 1904, 1–41.
(38) Fulton JF. *Harvey Cushing: A Biography*. Oxford: Blackwell, 1946; 115–6.
(39) Cushing HW. Some principles of cerebral surgery. *JAMA* 1909; **52**: 184–92.
(40) Halsted WS. *Surgical Papers*. Baltimore: Johns Hopkins Press, 1924; 167–78.
(41) Fulton JF. *Harvey Cushing: A Biography*. Oxford: Blackwell, 1946; 578.

25.2   Sir Victor Horsley (1857–1916) and anaesthesia

IAN D. CONACHER
Freeman Hospital, Newcastle upon Tyne, UK

At the 1906 Annual General Meeting of the *British Medical Association*, held in Toronto, Canada, the Address in Surgery was given by Sir Victor Horsley. It was entitled, 'On the Technique of Operations on the Central Nervous System', and was the dissertation of a man at the pinnacle of his career—a Knight of the Realm and a fellow of the Royal Society, with a brilliant academic record and an exceptional wealth of surgical experience on which to draw upon. The address included much of the pioneering work on operations in the central nervous system.

It is just over a century since Horsley conducted the first successful surgical removal of a spinal cord tumour, here in London, at the National Hospital, Queen Square. It is therefore appropriate to consider how this man of influence came to reach the conclusions on the conduct of anaesthesia that are so prominently promulgated in that section of his historic address which begins with the words, 'The all important question of anaesthesia must next be considered.' (1).

These words, uttered by probably the most eminent surgeon of his generation, are perhaps remarkable from our point of view because the prevailing attitude—and it sometimes seems if little has changed—was to pressurize novices into rushing the induction of anaesthesia and to be contemptuous of accurate and sophisticated systems for the delivery of volatile anaesthetic agents (2). Bear in mind that the anaesthetic climate in the United Kingdom was in a state of flux. In particular, there was much debate about chloroform. At this time Horsley, Waller, Sir Charles Sherrington, and Doctors McCardie and Dudley Buxton were members of an investigative committee, set up under the auspices of the British Medical Association in 1901, and which was to give its final and definitive report in 1910.

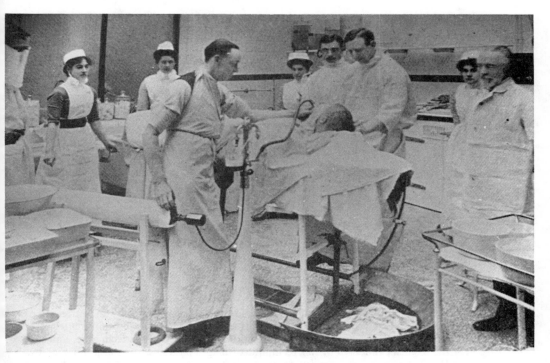

Figure 1   The Operating Theatre, Queen's Square, London 1906. Sir Victor Horsley, observed by Kocher of Berne, prepares to operate on a patient anaesthetized by Dr Powell.

Agents and techniques

Horsley's preference was always general anaesthesia. His requirements of an agent was that it produce hypnosis, analgesia and 'the convenience of influencing the blood pressure at will'. Morphine, used in the early days of neurosurgery by Horsley as an adjuvant to chloroform anaesthesia, was no longer favoured for, as we are informed by Buxton (3), Horsley was one of the first to note the detrimental effect this drug had on those whose respiratory centres are involved in a pathological process.

Recognizing, as a general rule, that chloroform was the more dangerous agent, particularly in context, because of its paralysing effect on the respiratory centre, Horsley expounded on its use.

Accompanying the text is this picture (Fig. 1). To the right of the patient's head stands Horsley. The distinguished looking, bearded gentleman is Professor Theodor Kocher of Berne, one of Europe's foremost surgeons of the day, and himself an authority on anaesthesia, who had an ether mask design attributed to him (4). The anaesthetist is a Dr Powell, one of two professional anaesthetists mentioned and to whom Horsley ascribes some of his experience; the other was Dudley Buxton.

The anaesthetic system shown in use in Fig. 1 is worthy of closer study. The inhaler is the model designed by Vernon Harcourt with whom Horsley was working closely at the time on Chloroform Committee projects. It was regarded as an accurate device and supplied up to a 2% concentration in air. Certainty of the patient receiving the accurate dose was achieved by ensuring a good seal at the face mask with wet towels. In addition, a facility for providing the patient with oxygen was arranged by plumbing in a cylinder to the system.

The text is accompanied by a stylized illustration, (Fig. 2), in which the degree of pain stimulation from the various tissue layers being dissected is plotted alongside the recommended concentration of chloroform. A peak is reached during induction, and a second peak at the

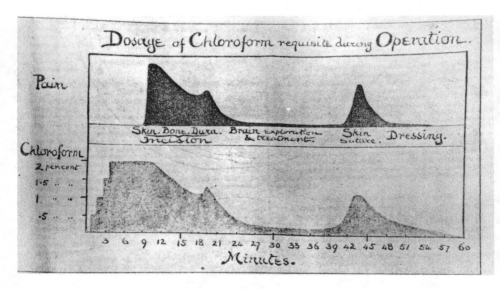

Figure 2   Horsley's stylized illustration of a chloroform anaesthetic for neurosurgery.

late stage of surgery to cover skin suture and avoid precipitating vomiting. In between the concentration is cut right down as the least sensitive parts, including the brain matter, are operated upon. What this picture hides is an additional flexibility to the technique, and the reason for the oxygen cylinder. For this technique of neuroanaesthesia was accompanied by another of Horsley's algorithmic concepts—one to deal with haemorrhage. So successful was this that Horsley came to regard operative bleeding as a problem with a simple solution.

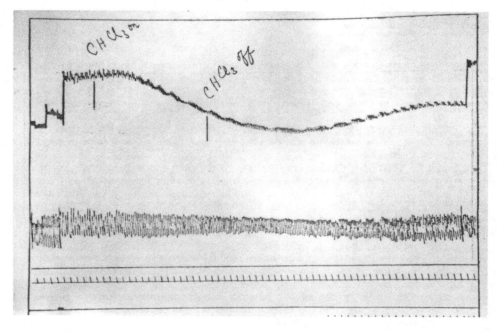

Figure 3   The effect of the introduction of chloroform on the carotid artery pressure of a dog anaesthetized with ether.

As it has been put:

> *'if it were capillary hot water stopped it, if it were venous then oxygen stopped it, and if it were arterial the judicious use of chloroform would suffice to lower the blood pressure and so put an end to the haemorrhage.'* (5)

The complex physiological changes brought about by such simple adjustments were not hidden from Horsley for like virtually all his statements there was backing from evidence obtained in clinical practice, and from meticulous animal experimentation. This calculated use of the hypotensive effect of an anaesthetic must be one of the earliest times, if not the first, that deliberate hypotension was systematically employed. Fig. 3, also from the Toronto lecture, is a kymograph recorded from a dog anaesthetized with ether. The time marks are 2 second intervals, the lower trace is of respiration, the upper of blood pressure recorded from a carotid artery. The effect of the deliberate introduction of chloroform is clearly demonstrated and recorded.

Biographical

Biographical accounts of Horsley, recognizing his greatness, describe him as belligerent, intolerant, and outspoken. One of those to see him in his worst light, initially at any rate, was the budding medical star, the American Harvey Cushing. Their first encounter, in July, 1900, is described in Fulton's biography of Cushing (6):

> *'He found Horsley living in seemingly great confusion: dictating letters during breakfast to a male secretary; patting dogs between letters; and operating like a wildman. H. C. gave him a reprint of his paper on the Gasserian ganglion, whereupon Horsley said he would show him how to do a case. They drove off next morning in Horsley's cab, after sterilising the instruments in H.'s house and, packing them in a towel, went to a well-appointed West End mansion. He dashed upstairs, had his patient under ether in five minutes and was operating fifteen minutes after he entered the house; made a great hole in the woman's skull, pushed up the temporal lobe—blood everywhere, gauze packed into the middle fossa, the ganglion cut, the wound closed, and he was out of the house less than an hour after he entered it. This experience settled H. C.'s decision to leave London for he felt that the refinements of neurological surgery could not be learned from Horsley.'*

This extraordinary description of Horsley is possibly distorted. It is based on Cushing's recollection of an occasion many years earlier and transcribed by one of his students. It is at variance with that of Ernest Sachs (7), another American witness of Horsley's technique. However, it is all too evident from the description how the gentle, painstaking, fastidious Cushing, who was to make these very traits tenets of neurosurgery, was so put off by the Englishman at his most cavalier. He came to admire Horsley, even to like him but, although they met on other occasions, I do not think he ever saw Horsley operate again.

Like Cushing, Horsley had developed an interest in anaesthesia early in his medical career. For Cushing it was something of a baptism of fire, for even as a medical student he felt responsible for the death of a man to whom he administered ether (8). For Horsley it was an academic interest. Newly qualified, the workings of the brain had begun to fascinate him and he embarked on some experimentation—initially on himself.

The first of two published biographies of Sir Victor Horsley, that by his friend Stephen Paget, informs that in the year 1881 Horsley was anaesthetized 'about fifty times in all.' Ether, chloroform, and nitrous oxide were all tried. Some times he administered to himself, and on others contemporaries anaesthetized him (9). The gradual, sequential decline in both cerebral and subtentorial function under the influence of these various agents intrigued him. Little of his results were ever formally published but there is one amazing report in the journal *Brain* in 1883/4 (10). Entitled, somewhat low-key, 'Note on the Patellar Knee-Jerk', it has in its preamble a description of the different effects each of these three anaesthetic agents has on tendon reflexes. By quoting what is essentially the methodology in the paper it is possible to gauge just how dangerous these experiments on his own brain were:

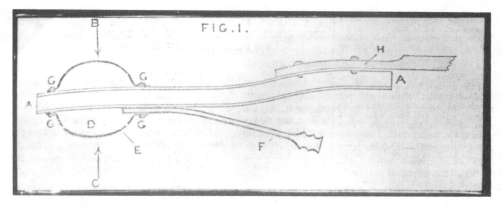

Figure 4   Diagram of Horsley's device for recording vocal cord movement in an anaesthetized dog.

'*To avoid the possibility of error in stating the depth of narcosis, only the results (fifteen in number) made on myself is here stated, but the facts were verified by observations made on other subjects.*

In all cases the anaesthesia produced was complete; after the usual symptoms attending the commencement of the administration of the pure gas were fully marked, absolute unconsciousness followed in from 90 to 120 seconds.

The anaesthesia was pushed until rigidity and sometimes cyanosis resulted. The recovery of consciousness was very frequently attended with considerable muscular spasm and semi-coordinated convulsive struggles and excitement.'

There followed that period of his most brilliant research work when he was Professor Superintendent of the Brown Institution. This complex was part of the University of London. It was here that Horsley did his animal experimentation, including some specifically anaesthetic orientated studies—most notably those on the effect of ether on the larynx. These were published with Dr F. Semon (later Sir Felix Semon) in the *British Medical Journal* in 1886. The two papers detail study results on more than 20 animals of various species (11).

In the second of these papers there is an interesting illustration (Fig. 4). The first impression is that it seems to be of a prototype cuffed endotracheal tube. Sadly, serendipity did not operate. Although it is of a structure designed for the airway it is, in fact, his recording device for one of the experiments detailed in these papers. The tube was inserted through a tracheotomy in an anaesthetized dog, with the cuff lying between the vocal cords. Any excursions of these were picked up by an air-filled cuff and transmitted to a recording tambour via the conduit that looks so much like the pilot tubing of a modern endotracheal tube.

Horsley was to move in great and influential circles and his counsel was to be sought on many issues. Before the Royal Commission of 1907, inquiring into vivisection, his defence for protagonists hinged on several pillars, of which a particularly pertinent one is this:

'*I wish to draw the attention of the Commissioners to the fact that the risk of death from anaesthesia has always been justly looked upon as a great reproach; and I have to express my personal opinion that it is purely a matter of knowledge of the dose required, and that, as regards the education of students in anaesthetising patients, no one ought to be allowed to render a human being unconscious before he has had practice on animals.*' (9)

Some of the evidence is presented in a way that would make a historian cringe or even make the subject of this study turn in his grave in far off Mesopotamia where he died in 1916 while serving the British Forces. However, the facts speak well for themselves and I suggest that the specialty of anaesthesia may owe this extraordinary Englishman a significant amount of recognition.

It is difficult to measure, let alone quantify what his contribution was. There is that foolhardy self experimentation, motivated out of academic interest but which must have given him a sympathy for the patient undergoing a stormy anaesthetic induction few of us can ever hope to gain. There is the animal research from which stemmed observations of practice which are still relevant today. There are his surgical techniques which have been left to posterity and there are his far-sighted views on the teaching of anaesthesia.

Principally, probably his legacy, is the attitude of mind that he engendered. His own intimate experience made him develop a respect for anaesthesia. Here was a branch of medicine of such import that it could not be left to the unsupervised junior doctor or nurse, or delegated to unqualified personnel, or hurried. He respected the views of those who shared an interest in the subject and, when eminent and of influence gave them (whether they be chemists, physiologists or clinicians) the kind of patronage a fledgling specialty could benefit from. He probably recognized that surgery and anaesthesia are an immutable partnership and would have welcomed a climate in which specialists of each enjoy equal professional status.

Conclusion

Sir Victor Horsley may not always have agreed with his fellow surgeons but he would not have disapproved of his views being shared with practitioners of the science and art of anaesthesia.

Acknowledgment

The author is grateful to Mr David Essenhigh, FRCS, Consultant Urologist, Freeman Hospital, Newcastle upon Tyne, England, for alerting me to Horsley's experiments in anaesthesia, and to the current Editor of the *British Medical Journal* for allowing reproduction of the illustrations.

References

(1) Horsley V. On the technique of operations on the central nervous system. *Br Med J* 1906, ii: 411–23.
(2) Macnalty A. Sir Victor Horsley: his life and work. *Br Med J* 1957, ii: 911–16.
(3) Buxton D. In *Anaesthetics: Their uses and administration*, 6th Ed. London: H. K. Lewis & Co., 1920: 335.
(4) Bryn Thomas K. In *The development of anaesthetic apparatus*, 1st Ed. Oxford: Blackwell Scientific, 1975: 252.
(5) Jefferson G. Sir Victor Horsley, 1857–1916. *Br Med J* 1957, i: 903–10.
(6) Fulton JF. In *Harvey Cushing*, 1st Ed. Illinois: Charles C. Thomas, 1946: 163.
(7) Sachs E. Reminiscences of an American student. *Br Med J* 1957; 916–7.
(8) Hirsch NP, Smith GB. Harvey Cushing: his contribution to anesthesia. *Anesth Analg* 1986; **65**: 288–93.
(9) Paget S. In *Sir Victor Horsley*, 1st Ed. London: Constable & Co. 1919: 40/187.
(10) Horsley V. Note on the patellar knee-jerk. *Brain* 1883/4; **4**: 369–71.
(11) Semon F, Horsley V. On an apparently peripheral and differential action of ether upon the laryngeal muscles. *Br Med J* 1886: 445–7.

25.3   Harvey Cushing (1869–1939) and
                    his mysterious paper on intracranial hypertension

MAURICE S. ALBIN
University of Texas Health Science Center, San Antonio, Texas, USA

One of the most seminal papers in the neurosciences literature appeared in the September, 1901, issue of the *Bulletin of the Johns Hopkins Hospital* by Harvey Cushing, entitled

'Concerning a Definite Regulatory Mechanism of the Vaso-Motor Centre Which Controls Blood Pressure During Cerebral Compression.' (1). Fundamental concepts of intracranial compliance, cerebrovascular dynamics, and brainstem ischaemia are delineated by this paper which also impacts importantly on the anaesthetic management of the patient with intracranial hypertension. In a sense, this article represents the first wave of a flood of important contributions made by Cushing that both changed the face and set the tone of modern neurosurgery and also influenced anaesthesia. Yet, the circumstances surrounding the publication of this paper are baffling, mysterious, and possibly gives us an inner glimpse of an individual who appears to have been vulnerable, immature and slightly desperate—a stark contrast to the poised, disciplined and autocratic image that we generally associate with Cushing.

The publication

Let us first examine some aspects of the paper itself and then the background of Cushing's activity during the time this paper was being formulated.

The details of the paper

The first page of the paper contains the first footnote:

'*Reprinted from the* Archives Italiennes de Biologie *for 1901,'*

yet a review of this Journal during 1901 reveals that Cushing did not have anything published there or in any other Italian Journal. The second footnote on the first page contains the notation:

'*I am deeply indebted to Professor Mosso in Turin and to Professor Kronecker in Berne for extending to me the privileges of their laboratories while carrying out these observations.'*

Cushing certainly did spend time in the laboratories of these two academicians, and more will be said about this later on in this presentation.

Another striking feature of this Cushing *magnum opus* lies in the paucity of references concerning work previously done in this area. In fact, there are no bibliographical references cited in the length and breadth of this paper, despite the reasonable assumption that Cushing was certainly familiar with the findings of Naunyn and Schreiber (1881) (2) and Spencer and Horsley (1892) (3) to name but a few scientists who had contributed significantly to some of the concepts described by Cushing.

Parallel publication

One is fascinated to find that hardly a year later, in 1902, Cushing publishes a much more complete paper (4) giving full credit to the many individuals preceding him who had worked in the field. The names listed (Fig. 1), are among the greats in physiology, pathology, and surgery.

Interestingly enough, a companion piece to the 1901 paper was also published by Cushing in 1902, this time appearing in the German medical journal, *Mittheilungen aus den Grenzgebieten der Medizin und Chirugie* (5), of which Bernard Naunyn was the Editor. This German version was personally submitted by Professor Theodor Kocher of Berne, Switzerland, (Fig. 2), the great surgeon who sponsored Cushing, arranged for him to work in the physiology laboratory of Professor Kronecker, and who assigned Cushing his project concerning brain compression. Cushing drew the wrath of Naunyn who appendixed a note at the end of Cushing's paper (Bemerkung zu obigen Aufsatz—Remarks on the above essay) stating that Cushing had not discovered anything new, had not cited the paper by Naunyn and Schreiber in 1881, but that the article was being published out of deference to Kocher (6)! Cushing responded to this oversight by including the name of Naunyn in his 1902 American paper (4). Thus, in a period of a little more than one year, Harvey Cushing published three papers using nearly the same experimental data.

THE

AMERICAN JOURNAL

OF THE MEDICAL SCIENCES.

SEPTEMBER, 1902.

SOME EXPERIMENTAL AND CLINICAL OBSERVATIONS CON-
CERNING STATES OF INCREASED INTRACRANIAL
TENSION.[1]

THE MÜTTER LECTURE FOR 1901.

BY HARVEY CUSHING, M.D.,

ASSOCIATE IN SURGERY, JOHNS HOPKINS UNIVERSITY.

GENTLEMEN: It is my privilege to bring before the College this
evening, as the Mütter lecture, some of the results of a series of experimental observations which relate chiefly to the intracranial circulation
as it is influenced by local pathological processes—a subject which,
from a bibliographical standpoint, is prominently associated, among
others, with the names of Haller and of Astley Cooper, of Fluorens
and Majendie, of Key and Retzius, of Leyden, of Althan, of Kussmaul
and of François Franck, of Naunyn, Mosso, von Bergmann, of Horsley
and Adamkiewicz, of Leonard Hill, and, more recently, of Kocher.

My personal introduction to the subject was due to the interest of
Professor Kocher, of Bern, and the investigations as originally undertaken at his suggestion had for their primary objective point the determination whether during an increase in intracranial tension the capillaries and smaller bloodvessels of the brain were dilated from venous
stasis, or, on the other hand, whether a condition of capillary anæmia
was brought about by such a state.

This question, naturally one of fundamental importance for the proper
explanation of the phenomena attending states of cerebral compression,

---

[1] This paper, in substance, was presented before the College of Physicians of Philadelphia,
on December 3, 1901. Its experimental basis will appear in Naunyn and Mikulicz's Mitteilun-
gen aus den Grenzgebieten der Medizin und Chirurgie, 1902, No. 9. under the title "Physiologische und anatomische Beobachtungen über den Einfluss von Hirnkompression auf den
intracraniellen Kreislauf und über einige hiermit verwandte Erscheinungen."

VOL. 124, NO. 3.—SEPTEMBER, 1902.

Figure 1   First page of September, 1902, paper from the American Journal of Medical Sciences.

Cushing's European tour

What was the chronology of events leading to the 1901 paper? Cushing reached Berne on
31 October, 1900, and was asked by Professor Kocher to look at the question of the blood
pressure and respiratory responses to intracranial hypertension working in the laboratory of
Professor Kronecker (Fig. 3). The latter also gave Cushing a project concerning neuromuscular
contractility relating to ionic concentrations in the frog's leg preparation which was published

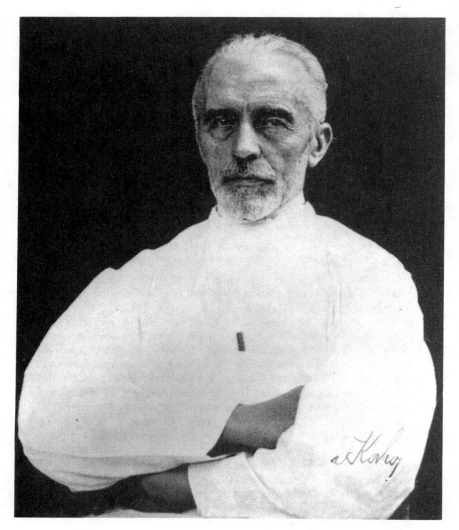

Figure 2   Photograph of Theodor Kocher, Professor of Surgery, University of Berne.

in the *American Journal of Physiology* in 1901 (7). Cushing partitioned his time between his laboratory work and visits to Professor Kocher's clinic.

By the middle of March, 1901, his experimental work had gone so well that he made plans for a 'Grand Tour' of northern Italy, leaving Berne on 20 March, 1901, and spending nearly a month in Turin working in the laboratory of the physiologist, Professor Angelo Mosso, where Cushing repeated and elaborated on some of his work done in Kronecker's laboratory. Cushing was helped by Mosso in developing new physiological recording techniques which Mosso asked him to write up and send in for publication. Cushing left Turin on 31 April, 1901, and visited Florence, Pisa, Bologna, Padua, and Venice. On 10 May, 1901, Harvey Cushing visited The Ospidale di San Matteo where he saw the sphygmomanometer developed by Riva-Rocci used routinely in this hospital (8), sketched it, was given a model of the inflatable cuff (by Dr Orlandi) and returned to Berne the next day. Cushing published his famous paper on blood pressure determinations in the operating room and clinic in 1903 (9).

Back in Berne, Cushing spent his time completing his experimental studies and also attended Kocher's clinics. On 3 June, 1901, he defended his intracerebral pressure experiments before

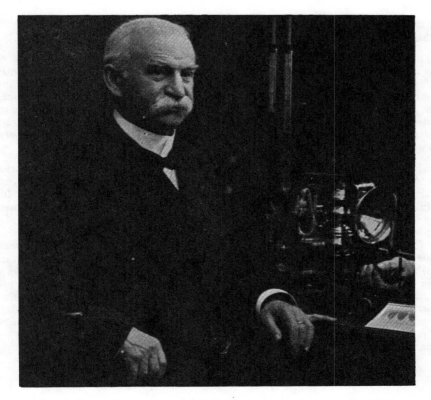

Figure 3   Photograph of Hugo Kronecker, Professor of Physiology, University of Berne.

a group of Professors of the Medical Faculty, and, on 13 June, 1901, he finished his manuscript (which was translated by the physiologist—philosopher Leon Asher), and delivered it to Kocher who submitted it to Bernard Naunyn.

Cushing left Berne on 27 June, 1901, the day Professor Mosso wrote informing him that he had presented Cushing's work at the Academy of Sciences of Turin, but could not get it published until November. In the same letter Mosso suggested that he would like to present Cushing's paper at the Fifth International Congress of Physiology whose meeting would take place in Turin, 17–20 September, 1901, with publication taking place in November, 1901.

Cushing spent most of July, 1901, visiting Sherrington in Liverpool and then McRae in Glasgow, returning to the United States on 23 August, 1901.

A need to establish priority

One can only speculate when the 'mysterious' manuscript was sent for publication in the September, 1901, issue of the *Johns Hopkins Hospital Bulletin* (1). We know that Kocher read it after Cushing returned from Turin on 11 May, 1901 and said 'Your paper from Mosso is clear, short and convincing—has all the characteristics of a truly valuable and lasting contribution to our knowledge.' (6) Is it possible that after hearing Kocher's laudatory comments, he might have had some gnawing doubts about the format of Mosso's presentation of the paper? After all, he *did* work in Mosso's laboratory, and while examining some of Mosso's patients, he formulated the concept of cerebral perfusion pressure by which the blood pressure increases as intracranial hypertension advances. Could it be that Cushing was concerned with Mosso's motives? That in the event of publication, he would not be the senior author or even that Mosso might publish the article without Cushing's name on it at all?

The last paragraph of this paper (1) superbly describes the conclusions from the experimental data that has stood the test of time:

> *'As a result of these experiments a simple and definite law may be established, namely, that an increase of intracranial tension occasions a rise of blood pressure which tends to find a level slightly above that of the pressure exerted against the medulla. It is thus seen that there exists a regulatory mechanism on the part of the vaso-motor centre which, with great accuracy, enables the blood pressure to remain at a point just sufficient to prevent the persistence of an anemic condition of the bulb, demonstrating that the rise is a conservative act and not one such as is consequent upon a more reflex sensory irritation.'*

Thus, we can envisage an individual, threatened by the potential loss of scientific priority for an 'Arbeit' that most justifiably belonged to him, responding in a panic mode by sending his manuscript to the *Johns Hopkins Hospital Bulletin* for immediate publication. In all probability the manuscript was mailed to Baltimore a short time after Kocher complimented him on the 'Mosso Report', and his doubts were confirmed after reading the 27 July, 1901, Mosso letter.

The footnote proclaiming that the paper was reprinted from the '*Archives Italiennes de Biologie* for 1901' is most difficult to explain. Did Cushing believe that his paper (sent in by Mosso) would somehow turn up in this journal, or perhaps Cushing had confused the journal with the proceedings of the Fifth International Congress of Physiology that had a November, 1901, publishing date, and would appear there? The simultaneous submission of two similar manuscripts to two different journals was certainly known to Kocher and most probably by Naunyn, which certainly did not help the reputation of the scientific neophyte, Harvey Cushing, in his early interactions with the European scientists.

In partial defence of his actions, Cushing writes to Arnold C. Klebs:

> *'. . . As a matter of fact, when I wrote that paper in Kronecker's laboratory I had very little chance to study the literature; if I had, I'd probably never have done the work.'* (6)

Conclusion

These events give us a momentary inner glimpse of an individual succumbing to the frustrating fear of lack of recognition and responding inappropriately. Is it possible that this early fall from grace served as a goad to reinforce his overwhelming drive to achieve scientific greatness?

References

(1) Cushing H. Concerning a definite regulatory mechanism of the vaso-motor centre which controls blood pressure during cerebral compression. *Johns Hopkins Hosp Bull* 1901; **12**: 290–2.

(2) Naunyn VB, Schrieber J. Aus der medizinischen Klinik in Konegsberg i Pr Uber Gehirndrucke. *Arch Exp Pathol Pharmacol* 1881; **14**: 1–112.

(3) Spencer W, Horsley V. On the changes produced in the circulation and respiration by increase of the intracranial pressure or tension. *Phil Trans Roy Soc Lond* 1892; **182**: 201–54.

(4) Cushing H. Some experimental and clinical observation concerning states of increased intracranial tension. The Mutter Lecture for 1901. *Am J Med Sci* 1902; **124**: 375–400.

(5) Cushing H. Physiologische und anatomische Beobachtungen uber den Einfluss von Hirnkompression auf den intracraiellen Kreislauf und uber einige hiermit verwandte Ercheinungen. *Mittheilungen aus den Grenzgebieten der Medizin und Chirurgie* 1902; **9**: 773–808.

(6) Fulton JF. *Harvey Cushing, A Biography*. Springfield, Ill: Charles C. Thomas, 1946: 754.

(7) Cushing H. Concerning the poisonous effect of pure sodium chloride solutions upon the nerve–muscle preparation. *Am J Physiol* 1901; **6**: 77–90.

(8) Thomson EH. *Harvey Cushing, surgeon, author, artist.* New York: Neal Watson Academic Publications, 1950: 347.

(9) Cushing H. On routine determinations of arterial tension in operating room and clinic. *Boston Med Surg J* 1903; **148**: 250–6.

25.4   Amussat (1796–1856) and Senn (1844–1908).
                             The holy duo of venous air embolism

MAURICE S. ALBIN and DAVID ROBINSON
University of Texas Health Sciences Center, San Antonio, Texas, USA

'. . . *Believing that it is in good practice to prepare for war in time of peace, I intend on this occasion to call your attention to one of the most dreaded and, I may add, one of the most uncontrollable courses of sudden death; I allude to air-embolism.*' (Senn, N. *An experimental and clinical study of air-embolism,* 1885) (1).

It has become firmly entrenched in the psyche of the anaesthetist that venous air embolism (VAE) only occurs in the sitting position, and then only in cases involving neurosurgical procedures. Reports of VAE developing in non-neurosurgical procedures (during hysterectomy, hip surgery, caesarean sections, exploratory laparotomies, to name but a few) are met with surprise and almost disbelief by many practitioners of anaesthesia and surgery (2). Yet a historical review indicates that the pathophysiological basis of VAE was firmly established in the 19th century and concepts of prevention and treatment already extant (3,4). In fact, our knowledge of the factors relating to VAE starts in the 17th century with the work of the Tuscan scientist Francisco Redi noting that he could cause death in a large variety of animals (dogs, horses, foxes, and sheep) by blowing air into their veins. The chronology of experiments on VAE during the 17th, 18th, and early 19th centuries were essentially physiological studies dealing with the artificial injection or insufflation of air. These scientists (including Brow–1749, Haller–1757, Morgani–1760, Tissot–1784, Bichat–1800 and Nysten–1811) did not consider spontaneous air aspiration and the problems of surgery.

The clinical problem and its evaluation

François Magendie crossed the experimental line and moved into the clinical realm with his paper of 1821 (5). Magendie described a case where the surgeon Bauchene was operating on a young locksmith for a tumour on the clavicle (on Bastille Day, 1818). After Bauchene mobilized the clavicle, he heard a hissing sound, the patient lost consciousness and died 15 minutes later. The autopsy showed a huge tear in external jugular vein. Magendie understood the physio-pathology involved and even thought that air could be aspirated from the right heart via a cannula. From 1821 on, till the end of the 19th century, numerous surgeons in France, Germany, Austria, Great Britain, and the United States published a considerable number of reports concerning VAE, its symptomatology, physiopathology, and treatment. These included eminences such as Dupuytren, Velpeau, Larrey, Roux, Malgaigne, Mott, Stevens, J. C. Warren, Von Wattmann, and the great Virchow (1,4).

Besides those mentioned above, four individuals stand apart because of their great contributions to our understanding of VAE, and these are John Rose Cormack, (Edinburgh) (6),

John E. Erichsen, (London) (7), Jean Zulema Amussat, (Paris) (4), and Nicolas Senn, (Milwaukee) (1).

Cormack presented his prize thesis, 'On the Presence of Air in the Organs of Circulation' to the medical faculty of the University of Edinburgh in 1837, described previous work done by the French, discussed the problem of air entering the body during vein dissection and its treatment. Interestingly, he describes some animal experiments by James Young Simpson who assisted him in the laboratory.

Erichsen read his paper 'On the proximate cause of death after spontaneous introduction of Air into the Veins, with some Remarks on the treatment of the accident' (24 pages), at the 13th meeting of the British Association for the Advancement of Science, and this was published in 1844 in the *Edinburgh Medical and Surgical Journal*. He describes carefully organized animal experiments, the findings of right heart dilatation and pulmonary blood vessel plugging, the peculiar sound heard when air enters the right heart, the use of ligatures to repair the tear in the veins, placing the patient in a recumbent position, and maintaining blood flow to heart and central nervous system as part of the treatment of VAE.

The work of Amussat and Senn

While the papers of Cormack and Ericksen stand out as important additions to our knowledge of VAE, the works of Amussat and Senn are unusually cogent, complete in their conception and modern in their understanding of the mechanisms involved and the treatment modalities used. For these reasons we have dubbed Amussat and Senn the 'holy duo' of venous air embolism. They also begin and end the 19th century, and anticipate the modern concepts concerning VAE that developed in the 1960s and 1970s.

Jean Zulema Amussat (Fig. 1) of Paris published his memorable 255 page book in French on VAE in 1839. The title (translated) is 'Research on the Accidental Introduction of Air into the Veins,' and it is subtitled, 'When Air is introduced through an injured vein, might it cause sudden death?' (4). Prior to this book on VAE, Amussat had published extensively on genito-urinary problems and vascular disease. As a fascinating side-note, this same Amussat invented a double-valved nasal ether inhaler popularized by Cloquet in 1847.

Amussat's book is a treasure-trove of information concerning the early history of VAE, and he gives a chronology (complete with references) at the end of the book starting with Francisco Redi in 1667, ending with Bouley's work in 1839. This tome consists of four parts, the first concerning his own animal experiments and the second describing observations made by other investigators on VAE in both humans and animals. In the third section he tries to explain the phenomenon and mechanism of action of VAE, and in part four he discusses practical inferences learned from the problems concerning VAE.

Part one consists of three chapters in which animal experiments (dogs, rabbits, sheep, and horses) are carried out under the conditions of spontaneous introduction of air into the veins (chapter 1), when air is delivered forcibly into the veins (chapter 2), and (chapter 3) experimental research into methods aimed to attenuate or treat the effects of VAE.

Amussat concludes and notes that the introduction of air produces a peculiar bruit, that the intensity of the phenomena is proportional to the size of the opening of the vein, the volume of air aspirated, its proximity to the heart and the force of aspiration, that autopsy immediately after death constantly reveals a distended right heart, ballooned with air mixed with blood, while the left side of the heart is almost empty, that the cause of death can be attributed to the interruption of the pulmonary circulation; that the *vertical position favours the introduction of air*, and that it is possible to aspirate almost all the air from the heart using a tube located in the right heart and attached to a glass syringe for aspiration!

Part two is fascinating, since Amussat collects the experiences of more than 35 surgeons who published clinical case reports involving VAE, many of whom did autopsy examinations soon after death. In some of the cases, air was also found in the coronary sinuses and on the arterial side of the circulation. Amussat notes that the incidence of VAE was not appreciated because autopsies were either not performed or else not done carefully.

Autopsy finding in man and animals are discussed in part three and Amussat emphasizes the constancy of findings relating to the highly distended right atrium, the relative lack of

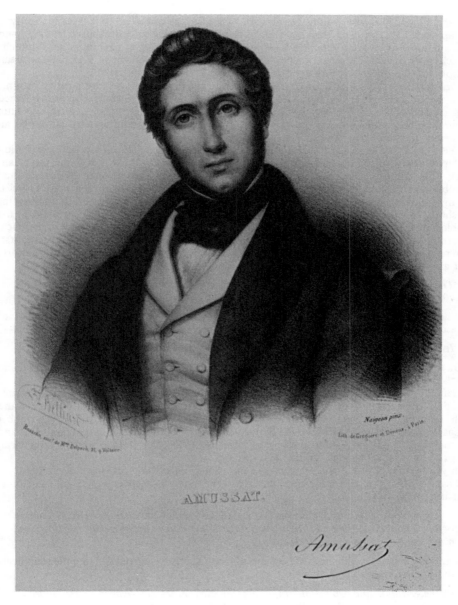

Figure 1   Engraving of Amussat at approximately 35 years of age.

fullness of the left side of the heart, the 'bellows' effect during inspiration, which is capable of entraining air through an open vein, the fact that some of the venous complexes form sinuses *that remain open*, and that the more forceful the inspiration the more marked the aspiration of air.

In part four, Amussat insists that experimental animal surgery is critical in investigating surgical problems, and points out the great amount of information gained in experimental research concerning VAE. He indicates the need for careful dissection near the jugular, auxiliary and subclavian vein complexes and that one can ligate, compress or insert sutures in these veins if tears occur. If air continues to enter, Amussat advises one to place a flexible cannula into the right atrium, and aspirate the air with a glass syringe connected to it. Finally, Amussat has appended a short chapter about sudden death after parturition attributed to VAE, and cites a number of authors who have described these cases—shades of contemporary thinking! Especially so, in light of the recent report by Malinow (8) and co-workers on VAE and caesarean section and the review by Robinson and Albin on VAE in obstetrics! (9).

Nicholas Senn (1844–1908) of Chicago brings up the tail end of the 19th century with his definitive, sophisticated, 116 page, 1885, article on air embolism (1). Senn was an accomplished surgeon and educator. He was involved in numerous pioneering clinical and experimental research in abdominal surgery, contributed to military medicine and was the author of an important textbook on the principles of surgery (10).

There are 17 major headings in his study including a section on 'Intra-Arterial Insufflation of Air.' Because of space limitations we will address only the salient features of this important work. Like Amussat, Senn generates a well defined historical view of VAE, well supported by bibliographical references. Similarly, Senn includes numerous animal experiments carried out in his laboratory on a wide variety of animals. Early in the paper Senn notes that the veins (in sheep) in close proximity to the heart were at a negative pressure. He then looks at the problem of aspiration of air into the superior longitudinal sinus (SLS) and describes the clinical report by Volkmann and the experimental work by Genzmer (one of Volkmann's assistants), who replicated this in the animal. Senn's experimental work on VAE and the SLS shows clearly that air was entrained when the head was elevated and he states:

> *'The force of gravitation constitutes the most important factor in determining the admission of air into an open sinus of the dura mater; . . . '*

When VAE occurred, Senn noted the loud churning or splashing sounds that could be heard on ascultation. To prevent air from entering this sinus he recommends:

> *'It is of the greatest importance to keep the head at a level with the heart . . . '*

Direct preventive measures involved continuous irrigation of the operative field and prophylactic ligation of the sinus.

Senn thought that the immediate cause of death after intravenous injection of air in animals was due to mechanical overdistension of the right ventricle, acute cerebral ischaemia and asphyxia from obstruction to the pulmonary circulation. He reviews and analyses a large number of cases (more than 120) in which the major veins were involved (including the internal and external jugular, auxiliary, subscapular, subclavian, facial, anterior thoracic, superficial cervical, femoral, internal saphenous, uterine and diploic).

In yet another clear-cut series of experiments, Senn successfully turned to direct puncture and aspiration of the right ventricle to remove the air-blood mixture causing right ventricular over-distension. He stated:

> *'Aspiration of the right ventricle for venous air-embolism when done early enough (before a fatal dose of air has been forced into the pulmonary artery), must be considered in the light of a life-saving operation.)*

Similarly, Senn experimented with a pliable Nelaton catheter introduced into the right heart via the jugular vein and concluded:

> *'Catheterization and aspiration of the right auricle for air-embolism compare favorably with puncture and aspiration of the right ventricle as a life-saving procedure, but the former operation is more dangerous on account of the tendency to the formation of a thrombus within or around the catheter.'*

Senn placed great importance on the role of the gravitational gradient in VAE and prophetically states:

> *'Statistics tend to show that the accidental admission of air into the veins was more frequent before anesthetics were used, a fact that the patients were then usually placed in a sitting or semi-recumbent position during the operation, positions favorable to the return of venous blood from the cervical region.'*

The quintessence of Senn's approach to the problem of VAE lies in his statement that:

'The timely removal of the air is the only rational treatment in all cases where simpler measures have proved inadequate in preventing a fatal termination.'

Summary

In spite of the historical, experimental, and clinical wisdom shown by these two innovative scientists, who published their findings more than a hundred years ago (1,4), and in spite of present day accurate methods for diagnosing and techniques of treating VAE, we still find many physicians reluctant to accept the possibility of venous air embolism occurring in procedures other than neurosurgical cases in the sitting position.

References

(1) Senn N. An experimental and clinical study of air-embolism. *Ann Surg* 1885; 2: 197–313.
(2) Albin MS, Babinski MF, Gilbert TS. Venous air-embolism is not restricted to neurosurgery! *Anesthesiology* 1983; 59: 151.
(3) Lesky E. Notes on the history of air-embolism. *Ger Med Monthly* 1961; 6: 159–161.
(4) Amussat JZ. *Recherches sur l'introduction accidentelle de l'air dans les veines*. Paris: Germer Baillière, 1839: 255.
(5) Magendie F. Sur l'entrée accidentelle de l'air dans les veines. *J Physiol Exp Paris* 1821; 1: 190–6.
(6) Cormack JR. *On the presence of air in the organs of circulation* (thesis). Edinburgh: John Carfae and Son, 1837: 56.
(7) Erichsen JE. On the proximate cause of death after spontaneous introduction of aire into the veins, with some remarks on the treatment of the accident. *Edinburgh Med Surg J* 1844; 61: 1–24.
(8) Malinow AM, Naulty JS, Hunt Co, Datta S, *et al*. Precordial ultrasonic monitoring during cesarean delivery. *Anesthesiology* 1987; 66: 816–9.
(9) Robinson D, Albin MS. Parturition and venous air-embolism. *Obstetric Anesthesia Digest*, April 1987, 38–40.
(10) Senn N, Senn EJ, Friend E. *Principles of surgery*. 4th Ed. Philadelphia: Davis, 1909.

25.5

Heinrich Braun (1862–1934).
A German pioneer in anaesthesia

WOLFGANG RÖSE
Medical Academy, Magdeburg, German Democratic Republic

The 125th anniversary of the birthday of the distinguished German surgeon Heinrich Braun (Fig. 1) offers an opportunity to remember some of his remarkable contributions to the development of anaesthesia at the end of the 19th and in the beginning of the 20th century.

Braun's first experiences in anaesthesia occurred a century ago in 1887, when he was completing his medical studies in Leipzig. As a medical student he had to administer anaesthetics in the surgical clinic of Thiersch and he recalls in his autobiography that:

'Thiersch praised me, because I was able to chloroform the patient in such a way, that the surgeon could perform a long operation while he was talking to him.' (1)

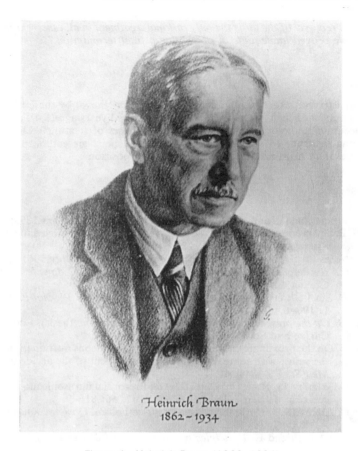

Figure 1   Heinrich Braun (1862-1934).

For the following 40 years of his professional life Braun, who mainly worked as a surgeon, was permanently interested in anaesthesia. Beside numerous outstanding achievements in surgery he enriched the new medical specialty anaesthesia with three important contributions—the introduction of adrenaline as a vasoconstricting agent with local anaesthetics and support for its use in cardiac resuscitation, the publication of the first German textbook on local anaesthesia, and improvements for the practice of inhalation anaesthesia.

The introduction into clinical practice of adrenaline as vasoconstrictor with local anaesthetics

Heinrich Braun became acquainted with the problems of local anaesthesia from 1888 onwards when he came under the influence of the surgeon Oberst in Halle and read Schleich's monograph 'Painfree operations', which had been published in 1894. In 1895 he started experimenting with infiltration techniques. One of the limiting factors to widespread use of local anaesthesia was the toxicity of cocaine, the agent then used. To minimize the side effects of cocaine Braun applied local hypothermia as well as a tourniquet to stop the venous return of the local anaesthetic. In 1900 he became aware of a pharmacological possibility of producing local vasoconstriction by employing an extract of animal suprarenal glands. He obtained the substance, mixed it with cocaine and injected the mixture into his forearm and produced:

'local anaesthesia with previously unknown intensity and duration.' (1)

This was the beginning of a series of experiments which were published in *Archiv für klinische Chirurgie* (2) with the title 'The influence of tissue vitality on local and general poisoning of local anaesthetics and the importance of adrenaline for local anaesthesia'.

This classic paper describes the results of numerous experiments on himself, investigations in animals, and administrations to patients. The author compared the effects of applying a tourniquet, using hypothermia and using adrenaline without local anaesthesia (to investigate its specific vasoconstrictor effect). He wrote:

> *'A pure adrenaline solution with some saline for preventing oedema, does not alter tissue sensibility.'* (2)

In order to look for side-effects, he injected himself subcutaneously with doses up to 0.5 mg adrenaline in a 1 : 1000 dilution. After five minutes he felt palpitations in his chest and an increased heart rate for a minute and a half. A tenfold diluted solution (1 : 10 000 adrenaline) given in doses up to 1 mg was not followed by side effects. This 1 : 10 000 solution was later used in patients.

A vasoconstrictor effect could be demonstrated experimentally with adrenaline solutions in 1 : 100 000 and even in a 1 000 000 dilution.

The next step was to determine the influence of adrenaline on the local anaesthetic effect of cocaine using different concentrations of cocaine and adrenaline and comparing it with cocaine injections without vasocontrictors. Braun summarized his findings by stating:

> *'These investigations demonstrate without exception, that the addition of a very small dose of adrenaline, or an adrenaline-containing extract of the suprarenal glands, increases the local anaesthetic effect of cocaine enormously such that diluted cocaine solution is as effective or more effective than concentrated solutions without this addition. After injection into the tissues a diluted cocaine-adrenaline solution anaesthetises a bigger area than the infiltrated region and interrupts the conductance of nerve fibres, when it is injected in their neighbourhood. In addition the cocaine anaesthesia is prolonged many times.'* (2)

As a logical consequence Braun demonstrated in rabbit experiments that the animals were able to survive doses of cocaine which would otherwise have been lethal, if 10 minutes earlier a small amount of adrenaline was injected into the same area.

Adrenaline for resuscitation

Braun also discussed the resuscitative qualities of adrenaline, writing in 1903 he stated:

> *'Further experiences are to be collected in treating states of collapse by intravenous injection of suprarenal extracts and adrenaline; it should be tried especially in cases of cardiac arrest during anaesthesia. Gottlieb successfully resuscitated animal hearts, even after 5 minutes of cardiac standstill, using compression of the thorax or massage of the heart and injection of adrenal extract. Schäfer's apparently challenging proposal to inject the substance in such cases directly into the heart is perhaps not so risky as it seems to be.'* (2)

Publication of the textbook 'Local Anaesthesia, it's Scientific Basis and Practical Use'

The first edition of Heinrich Braun's textbook on local anaesthesia was published in 1905. This first manual of local anaesthesia gave detailed descriptions of techniques for every region of the body. Many of them were originated or modified by the author himself and had been personally used by him in numerous cases. Seven editions of this textbook, each of them up-dated, were printed during Heinrich Braun's lifetime. In the second edition of 1907 (3) detailed recommendations were given on spinal anaesthesia (called 'medullary anaesthesia') including descriptions of instruments (Fig. 2) and drugs. The first English translation of the textbook was published by Lea and Febiger in 1914.

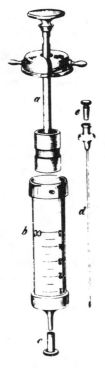

Figure 2   Injection device for
medullary anaesthesia (3)

Contributions to improved inhalation anaesthesia

The emphasis placed on Braun's fundamental discoveries in local and regional anaesthesia sometimes results in his contributions to general anaesthesia being overlooked. In 1901—two years before his famous article on adrenaline— he published a paper 'On combined anaesthesia and its rational use' describing the physical and clinical effects of ether and chloroform and the advantages of combined administration (4). He describes apparatus which made it possible to administer the inhalational anaesthetics in fairly precise doses, (Fig. 3) and a modification of this apparatus (Fig. 4) enabled the anaesthetic mixture to be insufflated by a tube into the pharyngeal cavity.

Almost 30 years later, having been closely engaged in hospital construction and organization in addition to his clinical work for more than two decades, he drew attention to the need to eliminate anaesthetic polluted air from the operating theatre to avoid inhalation by the staff and described a technique for doing so (5).

Summary

The surgeon Heinrich Braun contributed significantly both experimentally and in clinical practice to the early stages of the science of pain relief—anaesthesiology. His influence was apparent both in Germany and further afield.

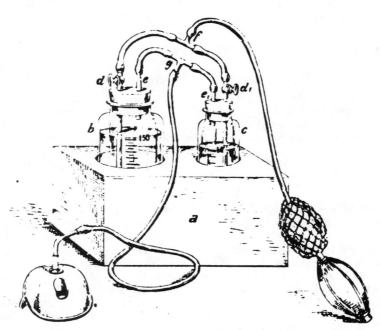

Figure 3   Apparatus for combined inhalation anaesthesia with ether and chloroform (4)

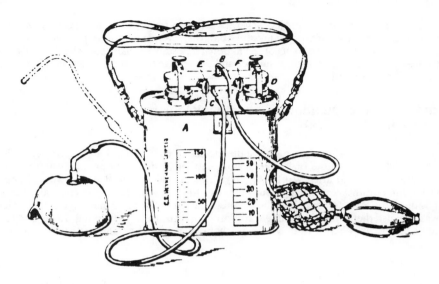

Figure 4   Portable device for inhalation anaesthesia by mask or insufflation tube (4)

References

(1) Braun H. Heinrich Braun. In: Grote R. *Die Medizin der Gegenwart in Selbstdarstellungen* Leipzig: Meiner, 1925: 1-34.
(2) Braun H. Über den Einfluß der Vitalität der Gewebe auf die örtlichen und allgemeinen Giftwirkungen localanästhesirender Mittel und über die Bedeutung des Adrenalins für die Localanästhesie. *Arch klin Chir* 1903; **69**: 541-91.
(3) Braun H. *Die Lokalanästhesie, ihre wissenschaftlichen Grundlagen und praktische Anwendung*, 2nd Ed. Leipzig: JA Barth, 1907.
(4) Braun H. Ueber Mischnarkosen und deren rationelle Verwendung. *Arch klin Chir* 1901; **64**: 201-35.
(5) Braun H. Die Operationsanlagen. In: Gottstein A, ed. *handbücherei für das gesamte Krankenhauswesen*. Berlin: Springer, 1930: 1-45.

25.6   The women physician anaesthetists of San Francisco, 1897-1940. The legacy of Dr Mary E. Botsford (1865-1939)

SELMA HARRISON CALMES
Kern Medical Center, Bakersfield, California, USA

A unique situation existed in the world of anaesthesia in San Francisco between 1897 and 1940; the specialty was dominated by women physicians. This paper documents the large number of women who were professional physician anesthetists (the term used at that time in the United States rather than 'anesthesiologist') in San Francisco during this period and examines the reasons why this situation probably evolved.

Work on another historical project several years ago resulted in the discovery that there were a surprising number of women anesthesiologists, women who were publishing scientific papers and who were even presidents of the national and state specialty societies. This discovery led to a new project to determine the number and percentage of women physicians in anesthesia as it evolved as a specialty.

A study of the population of anesthesiologists in the USA 1920–1948

This was a population study based on the directories of the United States' specialty societies between 1920 (the date of the first directory of anesthetists publication) and 1948 (that of the first directory published after World War II) (1,2). The study revealed that women doctors were found in anesthesia practice about twice as often as were male physicians and twice as often as might be expected based on their representation in the physician population. Briefly, this was because there was a feminine tradition in anesthesia in the United States due to the heritage of nurse anesthetists and, consequently, women physician anesthetists were accepted

Table 1

California members of the American Association of Anesthetists in 1920

Botsford, Mary	Oldenbourg, Louise
Burrows, Robert	Palmer, Caroline
Kavanagh, Mary Francis	Rithwilm, Lorruli
Martin, Jean	Talman, George
Mosgrove, Anna	Veach, H. C.
Murphy, Mary	

Table 2

Rank order of states by number of anesthetists, by year

	Total MD anesthetists	Women MD anesthetists
1920	New York (41)	California (11)
	Ohio (18)	Illinois (4)
	California (17)	New York (4)
	Massachusetts (14)	Texas (2)
	Illinois (14)	Indiana (2)
1930	New York (303)	California (48)
	Ohio (192)	New York (14)
	California (161)	Illinois (11)
	Pennsylvania (101)	Ohio (8)
	Illinois (93)	Massachusetts (7)
1940	New York (357)	California (55)
	Ohio (216)	Illinois (27)
	California (161)	New York (26)
	New Jersey (96)	Massachusetts (15)
	Pennsylvania (94)	Ohio (12)
1948	New York (505)	California (54)
	California (219)	New York (42)
	Ohio (214)	Illinois (23)
	Massachusetts (157)	Massachusetts (19)
	Pennsylvania (133)	Ohio (14)

Table 3

Professional MD anesthetists, total and female, by year

	San Francisco	Los Angeles	New York City	Boston
1920	8(11)	3(6)	1(4)	1(1)
1930	27(42)	12(83)	1(14)	4(7)
1940	26(39)	12(74)	12(26)	4(15)
1948	18(40)	7(58)	29(420)	8(40)

( ) = Total number physician anesthetists

by the surgeons, who no doubt hoped that women doctors would combine the submissiveness of nurse anesthetists with the medical training that many now realized was necessary for safe anesthesia practice. Anesthesia was also poorly paid at that time, and thus was unattractive to many men, and women doctors had fewer practice options than did men.

While working on this population study, it was noted that there were a large number of women physician anesthetists in California. An example is the list of names of the Northern California members of the American Association of Anesthetists (AAA, the first national anesthesia society in the United States) in 1920 (Table 1).

The next step was to arrange the States in rank order by the largest total number of members and by female members, by year, (Table 2). Although New York always had the greatest number of members, California always had the most female members. The number of female members in four major cities were then tabulated (Table 3). The largest number of women in anesthesia practice in San Francisco is striking.

Why had this fascinating situation happened? California always had many more women medical graduates than other states after 1876, when the first woman graduated from a state medical school (3), but, for many years, there was only one hospital to which women physicians could go to to receive the increasingly important hospital training. This was the Children's Hospital of San Francisco, founded in 1875 by three women physicians (4). The Children's Hospital of San Francisco was one of nine hospitals formed by women doctors in 19th century America to provide training that was not often available to women physicians at other medical institutions. The other women's hospitals, and 17 women's medical colleges, were located in the East and Mid-West (5), so there were many more opportunities for medical women in those areas.

Dr Mary E. Botsford

As California's women medical graduates were 'funnelled' through the Children's Hospital because they had no other place to go, they saw Dr Mary Botsford (1865–1939) at work. Dr Botsford was probably the first woman physician anesthetist in America, and she was almost certainly the first Californian who specialized in anesthesia*. An 1896 graduate of the Medical Department of the University of California (now the University of California at San Francisco, UCSF), she decided in 1897 to devote her practice to anesthesia after seeing how sick patients became after anesthesia and surgery. For the first two years, she did not earn any income from her anesthesia practice and supported herself by doing general medicine in the afternoons (6).

A charismatic, energetic leader, she trained at least 46 women in this specialty and then sent them out to hospitals in surrounding areas and other parts of California. Some of these were the women who were on the list of Northern California AAA members in 1920 as a cross check with the State of California Medical Directory volumes for the period shown. They were all graduates of California medical schools who interned at the Children's Hospital and trained with Dr Botsford. The women were very loyal to her, and she literally controlled anesthesia in the state for nearly 20 years. This was much resented by the men. Because of the many women she trained, the major Bay Area hospitals did not have nurse anesthesia, in contrast to most other hospitals in the United States, until after the Botsford generation of trainees was gone.

*This statement is made after extensive reading in the California medical journal and early anesthetic journals.

She did a considerable amount of scientific research, some of it with Arthur Guedel and Chauncey Leake, and she wrote many scientific papers, a number of which are of special interest (7–9). She also had a number of medicopolitical 'firsts'. She led the effort to get a section on anesthesia in the State medical association and was the first president of that group (10). The present state society of anesthesia evolved from that organization, so she can be said to have been its first president. She was responsible for the passage of a state law, the first in the United States, requiring that anesthesia be taught in medical schools. She was also the first faculty member in anesthesia at UCSF, and she was the first full professor of anesthesia at that institution. She was the third female president of the Associated Anesthetists of the United States and Canada in 1930 (11,12,13).

Botsford's legacy is gone now; the percentage of women members in the present American Society of Anesthesiologists, is the same in San Francisco as nationally. The women physicians who provided anesthesia in the San Francisco area in the period 1897 to 1940 were all of the same generation. They died out when the 'funnelling' of all women medical graduates through a single hospital ended during World War II, when hospitals started taking women physicians for hospital training positions because they were unable to get men, and, when subsequently, more men began to enter anesthesia after World War II as the specialty became more technical and better paid.

What we can learn from this unique situation in San Francisco during that time is that, given the opportunity (for example, the manpower needs of a developing specialty, the chance to organize as the result of the 'funnelling' of all women medical graduates through a single institution, and a charismatic leader like Mary Botsford, women physicians became leaders at a time when their total numbers were very small. Analysis of this situation also in San Francisco makes it clear how women physicians were constrained in other specialties and in other geographic areas.

References

(1) *Directory of the American Association of Anesthetists* 1920.*
(2) *Directory of Anesthetists* 1930, 1940 and 1948 (International Anesthesia Research Society, Cleveland), in the Wood Library-Museum, Chicago, Il.*
(3) Brown A. The history of the development of women in medicine in California. *California and Western Medicine* 1925; **23**: 8–9.
(4) *Anonymous. The story of Children's Hospital.* n.d. pamphlet. Archives and Special Collections on the History of Women in Medicine, Medical College of Pennsylvania, Philadelphia.
(5) Walsh MR. *Doctors wanted: No women need apply. Sexual barriers in the medical profession 1835–1975.* New Haven: Yale University Press, 1977; 180, 221.
(6) Doyle HM. *A child went forth: the autobiography of Dr Helen McKnight Doyle* New York: Gotham House, 1935: 307–8.
(7) Leake CD, Guedel AE, Botsford ME. The stimulating effect of carbon dioxide inhalations in dementia praecox catatonia. *Calif West Med* 1929; **31**: 20–3.
(8) Botsford ME. The use of sodium isoamylethyl barbiturate in children. *Anesth Analg* 1931; **10**: 221–3, and
    Botsford ME. Preoperative medication. *Calif West Med* 1931; **34**: 35–6.
(9) Botsford ME. Minimum standards for anesthesia service. *Anesth Analg* 1932; **11**: 11–5.
(10) Minutes of the First meeting, Section on anesthesiology, Medical Society, State of California, Yosemite, 15 May, 1922. Archives of the California Society of Anesthesiologists, San Mateo, California.
(11) McMechan F. Editorial. *Am J Surg* 1922; **36** Anesth Supp: 123.
(12) McMechan F. More honors richly deserved. *Am J Surg* 1924; **38** Anesth Supp: 89.
(13) Anonymous. Mary E. Botsford 1865–1939. *In Memoriam, University of California*. Berkeley, CA: University of California, 1939: 8–9.

*This analysis was presented at the annual meeting of the American Association for the History of Medicine in San Francisco 6 May, 1984. The paper is available from the author.

25.7   Georg Perthes (1869–1927). A pioneer of
                  local anaesthesia by blocking peripheral nerves
                        with the use of electrical stimulation

M. GOERIG, K. FILOS and H. BECK
University Hospital Hamburg, Federal German Republic

'It is a hard task to give freshness to the old and authority to the new. But still, it is true that it is upon the old that we must build the new.'

R. Matas (1)

Regional nerve block of the upper and lower limb may provide the safest form of anaesthesia for many surgical procedures when administered properly. Nevertheless this advantageous technique is not so often used, as the success of this anaesthesia depends on accurate placement of the local anaesthetic solution in close proximity to nerve trunks. The desired paraesthesias elicited by the physician and reported by the patient must be interpreted correctly by both. This requires an anaesthetist trained in this technique and a patient, who is capable of the appropriate responses. This is not often the case. On one hand, the anaesthetist may not have

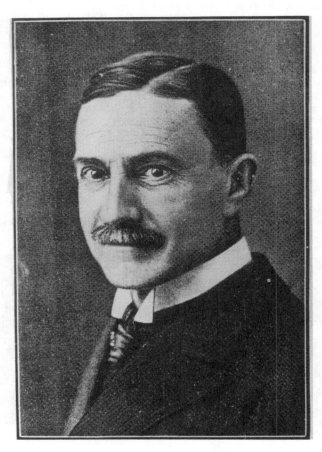

Figure 1   Georg Perthes (1869–1927)

had an opportunity during his training to develop expertise in this technique and, on the other hand, the patient, even when alert and cooperative, may misinterpret the paraesthesias due to his age, disorientation or sedation. If communication is impossible the incidence of unsatisfactory anaesthesia will be high and the administration of supplemental inhalation or intravenous anaesthesia will be necessary. These difficulties may be overcome by objective technique which is now successfully used worldwide—the use of the nerve stimulator. This highly sophisticated technique was first mentioned exactly 75 years ago when the German surgeon Georg Perthes published his article, 'Conduction Anaesthesia with the Help of Electrical Simulation' in the *Münchener Medizinische Wochenschrift* (2).

Born in Moers, Rheinland, on 17 January, 1869, Perthes (Fig. 1) studied medicine at the Universities of Freiburg, Berlin and Bonn (Fig. 2). From 1892 he became an assistant surgeon to the well known Friedrich von Trendelenburg, who was highly respected for his operation techniques, and, who in 1871, designed a tracheal tampon cannula with the first inflatable cuff (3,4,5).

Animal and self experimentation by Georg Perthes

Perthes had great influence on the development of the techniques of regional block anaesthesia (conduction anaesthesia) and then started to look for further improvements by locating peripheral nerves by means of electricity. For this purpose, he designed a special injection nickel needle as a stimulating electrode for use with weak electric currents. This was insulated with lacquer—the tip being uncovered. Using an induction coil the physician was able to operate the machine (Fig. 2) by foot-contact. To control the efficiency and extent of the anaesthesia produced by the anaesthetic solution, he employed the so called 'strong current' of the internal coil, which was connected with a 'faradic brush'. The intensity of the wanted faradic current could be determined by changing the internal metal-block. The moistened cotton-covered indifferent electrode was positioned 'best under the patient's seat' (2). Tests in the laboratory using the sciatic nerve of anaesthetized dogs, enabled him to produce fasciculations in the muscles innervated by that nerve. The nearer the tip of the needle to the trunk of the nerve, the greater the effect. Later, he directly stimulated the peroneal nerve of patients, whose lower limbs had to be amputated. A trial with his own ulnar nerve showed clearly, that the desired effects—

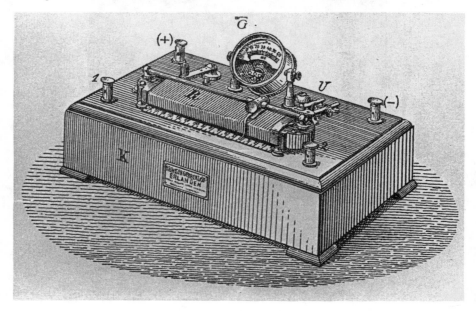

Figure 2   Potentiometer, similar to the model, used by Georg Perthes

producing typical fasciculations and paraesthesia—could be obtained by using minimal current, without producing any pain. This was enough evidence to start a clinical trial (2).

Clinical trials

Having given a detailed description of his apparatus in his article Perthes presents his results in 22 patients who were undergoing different surgical procedures, 15 on the lower limbs and seven on the upper limb. Ages ranged between 16 and 74 years and several of these patients would be classified today as 'high risk patients'. The operations included extended surgical procedures and reconstructive orthopaedic operations, amputations of the foot, tuberculosis of the foot joint, club foot, abscesses of the knee joint, complicated dislocations, an amputation of the upper arm for a malignant sarcoma and reposition of a bleeding dislocation of the elbow joint etc. To anaesthetize the sciatic nerve, he used the dorsal approach, which was first described by Läwen (6) and later modified by Jassenetzky-Woini (7). He was completely successful with electrically conducted anaesthetic procedures for the lower limb, but with the remaining cases he was not satisfied, due to an insufficient anaesthesia. His initial inexperience with this new technique is mentioned as a possible cause. In another case, after the obturator nerve was located by the same method, typical muscular fibrillations of the adductor-muscles could be produced by the electrical stimulation—a sign of proper nerve location and 8 ml of procaine 3% was injected. Unfortunately, he did not succeed in anaesthetizing the crural nerve at the same time, so that he quoted this case as a failure.

All 7 peripheral nerve blocks of the brachial plexus by the supraclavicular method, which had been described some months before by D. Kulenkampff (8) were performed satisfactorily.

The dosages of the local anaesthetic procaine (novocain) used by him for this new anaesthetic technique ranged between 0.45 g to 0.9 g. Generally 30 ml of procaine was injected, when typical muscle contractions had been produced. Initially, the nerve blocks were carried out with a 2% solution but as a result of his increased experience, he later employed a 3% solution to obtain a rapid and more intensive effect with longer duration of nerve blockade. The onset

Zentralblatt für Chirurgie

herausgegeben von

K. GARRÈ,   F. KÖNIG,   E. RICHTER,

in Bonn,   in Berlin,   in Breslau.

37. Jahrgang.

VERLAG von JOHANN AMBROSIUS BARTH in LEIPZIG.

Nr. 31.   Sonnabend, den 30. Juli   1910.

13) Perthes (Leipzig). Abgemessener Druck zur schmerzlosen Erzeugung künstlicher Blutleere.

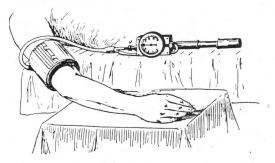

Figure 3   The 'Kompressor'.

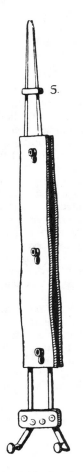

of anaesthesia was observed between the 3rd and the 30th minute and lasted for more than 90 minutes, with a maximum of 150 minutes. He described the effects of total sensory blockade with only partial muscle relaxation in some cases but in other patients complete relaxation of the muscles was observed.

Perthes did not observe any toxic reactions in his patients. The different onset times he explained by him as to whether the injection was made directly into the substance of the nerve ('endoneural') or was distributed around the nerve trunk, so that the trunk was bathed in the anaesthetic solution ('perineural').

He produced optimal bloodless surgical conditions, by using his 'Kompressor'—his own invention which he described in 1904 (9). This device was applied as a cuff to the limb being operated upon (Fig. 3) and before the pressure cuff was inflated, the blood of the extremity was removed by wrapping the extremity with a bandage (9). Perthes usually added the newly discovered adrenalin (1903) to local anaesthetic solutions, thereby augmenting their effect (10), and he introduced less toxic but more potent anaesthetics, new techniques and new anatomical approaches, this improving effectiveness of local anaesthesia could be recorded (11–14). Georg Perthes also suggested the use of insulated forceps (Fig. 4) for locating peripheral nerves intraoperatively, for use especially when reconstructive nerve-surgery had to be performed (15). He recommended this method for the identification of motor and sensory nerves during an operation and specially for pain therapy when the sciatic nerve had to be blocked in cases of sciatica.

Most of his patients were premedicated one hour before conduction anaesthesia was started with a mixture of scopolamine and pantopon given intramuscularly. This pharmacological combination was described in 1911 by C. L. Leipoldt as 'the ideal pre-anaesthetic narcotic' (16). The prospect of patients being wide awake during surgical procedures was of great concern to Perthes. He therefore recommended preoperatively premedication on the ward to allay apprehension, minimize discomfort and produce a light sleep. These optimal conditions were provided for the reduction

Figure 4   A bipolar-electrode for electrical nerve stimulation intra-operatively, recommended by Perthes. (c. 1916).

of stress in both the pre- and intra-operative periods. It is not an exaggeration to regard Georg Perthes technique as a forerunner of a modern concept of premedication (3).

He strongly recommended this preliminary administration of drugs for sedation for patients, who had to be operated under local and conduction anaesthesia for three reasons: first, most of the patients were incapable of an adequate cooperation with the physician performing the conduction block due to the stress of operation, second, some of them became agitated during the local injection and were unable to make the appropriate responses, and third, other patients did not report paraesthesial, even in cases when the needle was in the correct position relative to the nerve trunk. It therefore appeared to him that a better method was to have objective control of the motor effect rather than rely on the subjective feelings of the patient. During all surgical operations the premedicated patients were able to give adequate responses, the twilight sleep did not minimize the success of anaesthesia performed.

Three of the patients undergoing surgical procedures of the lower limb were older than 70 years and, according to today's assessment, they would be classified as high-risk patients. Perthes especially recommended his technique for these patients, which he believed had a number of advantages over spinal anaesthesia which was widely used at that time. It seems however that

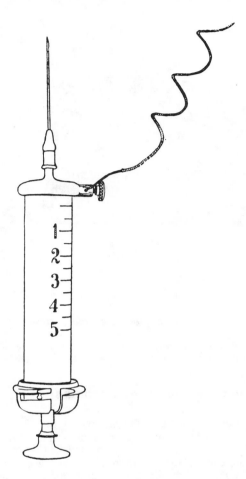

Figure 5   Hughson's—device for localisation of peripheral nerves by electrical stimulation (1922).

the electrical technique was not used a great deal practically although it was mentioned in all the leading textbooks at that time—for example, in the well known German textbook for local anaesthesia *Lehrbuch der Lokalanaesthesie für Studenten und Ärzte*, edited by Georg Hirschel 1913, and in Heinrich Braun's *Local Anaesthesia—Its Scientific Basis and Practical Use* (13). A similar device for localization of nerves by electrical stimulation (Fig. 5) is described in James Tayloe Gwathmey's second revised edition of *Anaesthesia* 1924 (18,19) but there is no reference to the original article of Georg Perthes which was published exactly 12 years before (2). In 1928, Kulenkampff in collaboration with Perkins published a review of brachial plexus anaesthesia techniques and drew attention to the advantages of employing the method of locating the plexus with Perthes' device (20).

It seemed that this modern technique was virtually forgotten. This may have been due to the cumbersome technique or Perthes' reported failures. In general, peripheral nerves were blocked after producing paraesthesia with the tip of the needle. This method has continued to be used in daily anaesthetic practice, although it is well known that post anaesthetic neurological sequelae are considerably increased and a high percentage of failed anaesthetic blocks occurs (14,18,20–24).

In 1962 Greenblatt and Denson reported on a 'Needle-Nerve-Stimulator-Locator: Nerve Blocks with a New Instrument for Locating Nerves' (21). The system was a transportable, transistored, nerve stimulator by which the use of electrical stimulation became practical and

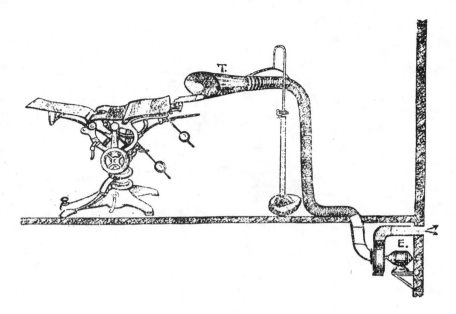

Figure 6   A suction pump for the operating theatre (1926).

widely applicable and another great impetus to its use in local anaesthesia (25–32). It is however certain that the original description was that in Georg Perthes article (2).

Atmospheric pollution by anaesthetic vapours

In one of the last articles published by Georg Perthes he is concerned with the various problems and toxic side effects of inhalational anaesthetics—especially of ether—to the staffs of the operation theatres (33). He therefore recommended and designed an electrical operating exhaust fan with an inlet close to the top of the operation table in the neighbourhood of the patients head (Fig. 6). Within five minutes the air of the operation-room could be totally changed. As a result of his efforts he describes an important improvement of efficiency of his staff (33).

Conclusion

Georg Perthes died of a heart failure at Arosa, Switzerland on 3 January, 1927, (34). His perfection of the methods of local and regional anaesthesia were steps forward in the evolution of the new specialty. Several of these developments sank into oblivion, as they were too impracticable, probably due to the cumbersome technique required at that time. Others achieved an immediate and lasting popularity. Many of his techniques were discarded to be rediscovered in due course and reapplied with excellent results. The successes and failures of Georg Perthes must be considered important to illustrate his highly developed understanding of the science of anaesthesiology.

References

(1) Matas R. Local and regional anaesthesia: a retrospect and prospect. *Am J Surg* 1934; **25**: 189–96 and **25**: 362–78.
(2) Perthes G. Ueber Leitungsanaesthesie unter Zuhilfenahme elektrischer Reizung. *München Med Wochenschr* 1912; **47**: 2543–8.

(3) Angerer K v. Zur Erinnerung an Georg Perthes. *München Med Wochenschr* 1927; **7**: 245–6.

(4) Jüngling. *Georg Perthes zum Gedächtniss*. Tübingen, 1927; 28–32.

(5) Makowsky L. Fünf Jahrhunderte Chirurgie in Tübingen. Stuttgart, *Verlag von Ferdinand Enke*, 1949: 85–90.

(6) Eulenburg A. Real-Encyclopädie der Gesamten Heilkunde. Vol. IV, Berlin-Wien; Urban & Schwarzenberg, 1908.

(7) Läwen A. Ueber Leitungsanaesthesie an der unteren Extremität, mit Bemerkungen über die Technik von Injektionen an den Nervus Ischiadicus bei der Behandlung der Ischias. *Zentralbl Chir* 1900; 252–69.

(8) Jassenetzki-Woino. Leitungsanaesthesie des N. Ischiadicus. *Zentralbl Chir* 1912; **30**: 1021.

(9) Kulenkampff D. Die Anaesthesierung des Plexus brachialis. *Zentralbl Chir* 1911; **40**: 1337–40.

(10) Perthes G. Abgemessener Druck zur schmerzlosen Erzeugung künstlicher Blutleere. *Zentralbl Chir* 1910; **31**.

(11) Braun H. Über den Einfluss der Vitalität der Gewebe auf die örtliche und allgemeine Giftwirkung lokalaaesthesirender Mittel- und über die Bedeutung des Adrenalins für Localanaesthesie. *Arch klin Chir* 1903; **69**: 64–82.

(12) Hirschel G. Die Anästhesierung des Plexus brachialis bei Operationen an der oberen Extremität. *München Med Wochenschr* 1911; **29**: 1555–6.

(13) Hirschel G. *Lehrbuch der Lokalanästhesie für Studierende und Ärzte*. Wiesbaden, Verlag von J F Bergmann, 1913: 124.

(14) Braun H. *Local Anesthesia—Its Scientific Basis and Practical Use* Ed. 3, Philadelphia, Lea & Febiger, 1914: 223–4 and 423–4.

(15) Härtel F. *Die Lokalanästhesie. zweite, neubearbeitete Auflage, Stuttgart*, Verlag von Ferdinand Enke, 1920: 62.

(16) Perthes G. Ausführung der Nervennaht. In: *Handbuch der Ärztlichen Erfahrungen im Weltkriege 1914–1918*. Herausgeg. v Schjerning, Otto v, Band II, Zweiter Teil. Leipzig, Verlag von Johann Ambrosius Barth, 1922: 270–8.

(17) Leipoldt L. Some remarks on pantopon anaesthesia. *Lancet* 1911; 369–71.

(18) Little D, Stephen CR. Modern balanced anesthesia: A concept. *Anesthesiology* 1954; **15**: 246–61.

(19) Gwathmey JT. *Anesthesia* New York and London: The Macmillan Company, 1924, 481.

(20) Hughson. Localisation of cutaneous nerves by electrical stimulation, applied to nerve-block anesthesia. *Johns Hopkins Hosp Bull* 1922; **33**: 338–9.

(21) Kulenkampff D, Persky MA. Brachial plexus anaesthesia. *Ann Surg* 1928; **87**: 883–91.

(22) Greenblatt GM, Denson JS. Needle nerve stimulator-locator: nerve blocks with a new instrument for locating nerves. *Anesth Analg* 1962; **41**: 599–602.

(23) Wright BD. A new use for the block-aid monitor. *Anesthesiology* 1969; **30**: 236–37.

(24) Magora F *et al.* Obturator nerve block: An evaluation of technique *Br J Anaesth* 1969; **41**: 695–8.

(25) Chapman GM. Regional nerve block with the aid of a nerve stimulator. *Anaesthesia* 1972; **27**: 185–93.

(26) Montgommery SJ *et al.* The use of the nerve stimulator with standard unsheathed needles in nerve blockade. *Anesth Analg* 1973; **52**: 827–32.

(27) Yasuda I, *et al.* Supraclavicular brachial plexus block using a nerve stimulator and an insulated needle. *Br J Anaesth* 1980; **52**: 409–11.

(28) Raj P. Der Einsatz des Nervenstimulators für periphere Nervenblockaden. Klinische Anaesthesie—*Current Reviews, Graz*: Akademische Druck-und Verlagsanstalt, 1982: 1–7.

(29) Berry FR, Bridenbaugh LD. The upper extremity: somatic blockade. In: Cousins MJ, Bridenbaugh PO, eds. *Neural blockade in clinical anaesthesia and management of pain*. Philadelphia-Toronto: Lippincott Co, 1984: 296–319.

(30) Postel J, März P. Elektrische Nervenlokalistion und Kathetertechnik. *Regional-Anaesthesie* 1984: **7**: 104–8.

(31) Winnie AP. Plexus anesthesia. In: Hakanosson Lennart, ed. *Perivascular techniques of brachial plexus block*. Edinburgh-London-Melbourne and New York: Churchill Livingstone, 1984: 210–20.

(32) Raj P. Adjuvant techniques in regional anaesthesia. In: Raj P, ed. *Handbook of regional anaesthesia*. Edinburgh-London-Melbourne and New York: Churchill-Livingstone, 1985: 249–58.

(33) Perthes G. Schutz der am Operationstisch Beschäftigten vor Schädigung durch die Narkosegase. *Zentralbl Chir* 1925; **16**: 853–5.

(34) University-Archives of Tübingen, Department of Surgery, *personal communication*, (No. 859 AZ 572/Perthes).

25.8   Mark Lidwell (1873–1968) and his anaesthetic machine

CHRISTINE BALL
Alfred Hospital, Prahan, Victoria, Australia

Mark Lidwell was born in England in 1873 and emigrated to Australia with his parents in 1896. He studied medicine at Melbourne University and graduated with Honours in 1902. He subsequently gained a Doctorate in Medicine in 1905. After holding various hospital appointments he moved to New South Wales where he took up general practice in Beecroft, a small rural area. He later moved to Strathfield where he gave up general practice to become a specialist physician (1).

In 1913 he joined the staff of the Royal Prince Alfred in Sydney as Honorary Assistant Physician. The same year he was also appointed the first tutor in anaesthetics at the hospital and the first lecturer in anaesthetics of the Faculty of Medicine. He became an Honorary Physician in 1926 and was admitted as a Foundation Fellow to the Royal Australian College of Physicians.

In 1930 the Royal Prince Alfred established a department of Anaesthetics and appointed Mark Lidwell as Honorary Director. He held this position until 1934. He was subsequently also made a Foundation Fellow of the Faculty of Anaesthetists, Royal Australasian College of Surgeons.

In 1921 he delivered a paper entitled 'Some Modern Methods of Anaesthesia' which was subsequently published in the *Melbourne Journal of Anaesthesia* (2). In it he stated:

> *'The anaesthetist should next consider what he really is. He is in fact a necessary evil. He does not cure the patient but only dulls the patient's senses so that the surgeon can do his work. He is to the surgeon what the vice is to the mechanic . . .'*

The Lidwell machine and his techniques

The paper went on to describe his anaesthetic techniques and the machine he designed in 1913 for 'mechanical,' or insufflation anaesthesia.

> *'I have found that after the anaesthesia has been even there has been considerably less postoperative vomiting. An absolutely even anaesthesia is only to be obtained by mechanical means . . . Mechanical anaesthesia has other advantages. It reduces abdominal movements to a minimum, or if the surgeon is working in the region of the head and neck, the anaesthetist can remain out of the way.'*

Lidwell had two preferred methods of induction. The first was the use of 25% solution of oil of bitter orange in spirit sprinkled on the mask to eliminate the smell of the ether. The second involved the administration of ethyl chloride prior to the introduction of ether.

Anaesthesia was then maintained using the Lidwell machine and insufflation anaesthesia via an intrapharyngeal, oral artificial airway was used with a tube passed into it from the machine. A towel was draped over the patients face in order to maintain anaesthetic depth. Nasal catheters were used for the pharyngeal method and a Belfast linen catheter for the intratracheal. This was passed under direct vision using a Chevalier Jackson laryngoscope.

The Lidwell machine itself was a portable machine weighing 7 kg and easily packed into two small handbags. The machine involved compressed air being delivered to an ether vaporizer (1,3). An ether/air control device allowed varying concentrations of ether vapour to be delivered. The ether vaporizer could be immersed in a warm water bath to prevent cooling. Lidwell was opposed to direct heating of the ether as he claimed it had no benefit and was theoretically wrong.

From the vaporizer the ether/air mixture went through a trap bottle, then to a crude mercury pressure blow off valve and subsequently to the patient. The ether temperature was measured. The Lidwell machine was manufactured by Eliot Bros. of Sydney. Subsequently the Anaesthesia and Portable Machine Company devised a machine which was functionally the same. However, in conflict with Lidwell's beliefs, it contained an electric lamp heater for the ether making it a potentially dangerous piece of equipment.

The Lidwell machine was used for over 30 years for endotracheal and endopharyngeal insufflation anaesthesia. Dr Lidwell retired from active staff in 1938 but served in various capacities throughout World War II. He died in 1968 at the age of 95.

References

(1) Hotten MT. Obituary—Dr Mark Lidwell *Official J Roy Prince Albert Hosp* 1968; Sydney.
(2) Lidwell M. Some modern methods of general anaesthesia. *Melbourne J Anaesth* 11 June, 1921; 482–85.
(3) Catalogue of the Geoffrey Kaye Museum.

25.9 Sir Francis Shipway (1875–1968). Anaesthetist by Royal Appointment

PETER A. COE
Guys Hospital, London, UK

Francis Edward Shipway was born on 6 December, 1875, at Chiswick. He was educated at Christ's College, Cambridge, graduating BA in 1897 and MA in 1901. He completed his medical training at St Thomas's Hospital, London, graduating MB, BCh, in 1902, and held residency posts at St Thomas's in obstetrics and casualty. After this he undertook post-graduate training in Vienna and obtained a doctorate in 1907. His interests had become focused on anaesthesia and he returned to London to take up a post in anaesthesia at the Royal Victoria Hospital For Children in 1908, before accepting a post at Guy's Hospital which he held until his retirement in 1935.

Shipway and the evolution of anaesthetic apparatus

Shipway was one of the first anaesthetists to appreciate the importance of temperature regulation during anaesthesia, (1,2), condemning the old 'rag and bottle' methods of anaesthesia where patients were forced to inhale through a cold hoar-frost as ether evaporated on the mask, and feeling that this contributed to patient cooling during surgery.

Dissatisfaction with these methods led him to look for ways to administer vapours. *The technique of intra-tracheal insufflation* had been described by Samuel Meltzer and John Auer in 1909 whilst they were working at the Rockefeller Institute. They discovered that a curarized animal could be kept alive by continuous insufflation of the trachea, with or without rhythmic respiratory movements. The technique for use in man was introduced into the United Kingdom by the Liverpool surgeon Kelly although the patients were not curarized. Kelly described his own apparatus in 1912 (3). He used a narrow bore (22 FG) intra-tracheal catheter passed by direct laryngoscopy to the carina. Continuous insufflation of anaesthetic vapours resulted in a mean airway pressure of 10–33 mmHg being applied to the airway, and a state of continuous positive pressure breathing resulted. This resulted in anaesthesia and oxygenation; occasional deflation of the lungs allowed carbon dioxide removal.

Shipway purchased a Kelly's machine in 1912 and subsequently modified it in 1914 (4). The modified machine consisted of an ether chamber through which air was insufflated, the mixture then passed through a humidifying chamber then into a warming vessel before reaching the intratracheal catheter. A mercury pressure limiting valve was included, as well as a tap to allow periodic deflation of the lungs, and a thermometer to measure the temperature of the outgoing gases. The main improvement over Kelly's machine was a longer delivery tube into the ether vaporizer which gave a higher ether output. The apparatus could be driven by a foot pump of by a 1/16 H.P. electric pump. The equipment was made by Messrs Mayer and Meltzer of Great Portland Street, London, and special intubation catheters were available as well as a Shipway Laryngoscope which he described as being modified from Hill's pattern.

Warm ether

Shipway, with the help of the physiologist M. S. Pembrey, next designed a much simpler apparatus, the warm ether/chloroform intra-tracheal apparatus, introduced in 1916 (5). This consisted of a hand bellows, a glass ether bottle, a Dudley-Buxton's modified Junker's chloroform bottle and a vacuum flask, used as a warming device, (Fig. 1). Air was insufflated by the bellows into either or both vaporizer bottles depending on the position of the selector control.

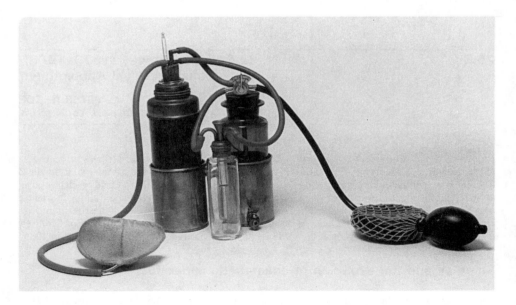

Figure 1   Shipway's warm ether apparatus 1916.

These bottles stood in metal pans containing water at about 75 degrees F. which provided latent heat of vaporization. Then the vapour laden air passed into the vacuum flask which contained water at about 120 degrees F, passing down a metal 'U'-tube to pick up heat before passing to the patient via a narrow bore delivery tube.

Research at the time by Shipway and Pembrey measuring the airway temperature showed that a range of temperature of 48.2–86.9 °F could be expected with open drop methods and 87.8–93.2 °F for their warm ether technique (2). Shipway claimed many benefits from the warm ether technique including:- fewer post-operative respiratory complications, protection against airway soiling, suitability for head and neck surgery and for thoracic surgery when the pleura was open, and the production of relaxation during abdominal surgery or where bowel obstruction would lead to risk of aspiration.

Shipways apparatus marked the end of the open drop methods in major centres and he subsequently developed the apparatus into a less cumbersome device described later in 1916 (6). This sturdy machine consisted of a central ether reservoir, dropping liquid into a central vaporizing chamber where it mixed with the insufflated air. The vaporizing chamber was surrounded by a hot water jacket, the temperature of which would be maintained at a recorded 110–120 °F. The air/ether mixture was insufflated to the patient who had the benefit of an overpressure valve and a tap to allow periodic deflation of the lungs. It was powered by foot bellows or an electric pump. This was the anaesthetic apparatus used during the first trans-auricular mitral valvotomy (7) performed at the London hospital on 6 May, 1925. The patient breathed spontaneously and the airway pressure varied from 8–20 mmHg according to the degree of deflation of the left lung required. The operation was successful and the patient lived another 7 years.

The use of warmed ether became very popular at this time and Shipway's colleague from Guy's Hospital, Geoffrey Marshall, used this apparatus on the Flanders battlefront (8).

This period saw the introduction of nitrous oxide in combination with oxygen in modern anaesthetic practice. In 1920 Shipway designed his own nitrous oxide/ oxygen/ ether outfit (Fig. 2) which was in some ways superior to machines designed by H. E. G. Boyle from St Bartholomew's (9), and his Guy's colleague, G. Marshall (10,11). It consisted of two nitrous oxide

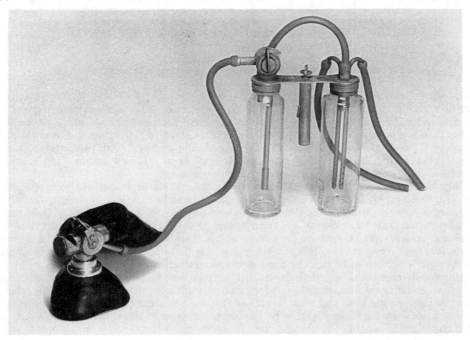

Figure 2   Shipway's nitrous oxide:oxygen:ether apparatus 1920.

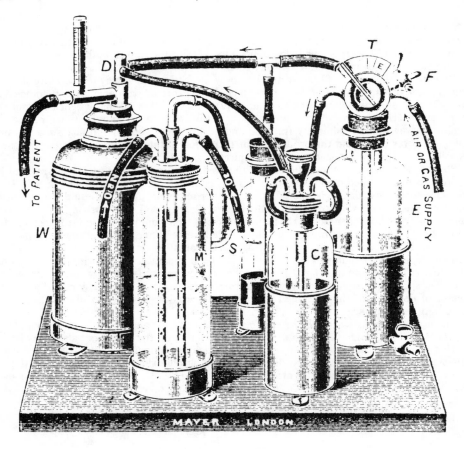

Figure 3   Shipway's nitrous oxide:oxygen:ether:chloroform apparatus 1922.

cylinders and one oxygen cylinder, both having reducing valves with long levers to control gas flow via the cylinder needle valves. A spirit lamp hung on the nitrous valve to prevent freezing as the cylinder cooled. The gases passed through a water-sight bottle, into a glass ether bottle then into a three way rebreathing valve with a Cattlin bag. In contrast Boyle's initial machine did not have reducing valves and delivered the gas into the tail of the rebreathing bag. However Boyle had published details of his machine in 1917 and his name has become identified with British continuous flow anaesthetic machines.

Shipway designed a further nitrous oxide/ oxygen/ether /chloroform insufflation apparatus in 1922, based on his 1916 warm ether intratracheal apparatus (12) (Fig. 3). This system also included a water-sight bottle for nitrous oxide and oxygen, the outlet of which could then either pass into the ether or chloroform vaporizers or go straight into the patient via the vacuum flask warming device. This system considered of five glass bottles in metal pans. The system must have been very cumbersome and it is not suprising that the more simple Boyle's machine of the 1920's became to be used by most British anaesthetists.

Shipway designed other equipment including, his own wire frame mask which had bilateral side tubes enabling the anaesthetist to give warmed vapour to one side and oxygen to the other, or to be used during head and neck surgery so that the anaesthetic tubing could pass to the opposite side from the surgery. One of his last inventions prior to his retirement was an airway with an inflatable cuff to be used during intra-nasal surgery when the cuff on this oral airway could be inflated to protect the airway from soiling. A detachable airway cap enabled the anaesthetist to distance himself from the surgery (13,14). Shipway was interested in resuscitation techniques and designed an intra-cardiac needle which was later modified by Langton Hewer to the pattern with which we are now familiar (15,16,17).

Research achievements

Bromethol. The 1920s were marked by the introduction of many new agents and techniques. Shipway pioneered the use of bromethol (Avertin) (18), which was given rectally, and provided basal narcosis which could be supplemented by local techniques, nitrous oxide, or ether. Bromethol spared the patient an inhalational induction and was popular for the nervous or thyrotoxic patient. His own series of 1600 administrations showed that the agent was safe if used in accordance with the established principles of the day.

Ethyl chloride was a popular agent for short procedures, and his series of 15 000 administrations in the dental chair was reported as not having resulted in a single fatality (19). As children often found the pungency of ethyl chloride unacceptable, Shipway recommended dropping a little eau de Cologne onto the facemask to disguise the smell (20).

Anaesthetic gases. In his later clinical years he began work to find a replacement for nitrous oxide, experimenting with ethylene, propylene and acetylene but this work was eclipsed by the discovery of cyclopropane in the USA by Waters in the early 1930's.

Divinyl ether. He had more success with his work with C. Langton Hewer and C. F. Hadfield, when this trio were the first to use divinyl ether in Britain (21). The findings of the first clinical study were that it was a potent agent with a wide margin of safety, and notable for lack of airway irritation, but it was inflammable and belonged to a group of agents characterized by the potential for hepatotoxicity, and so they advised that its maximum administration be limited to 90 minutes duration.

Professional achievements

Shipway was President of the Anaesthetic Section of the Royal Society of Medicine in 1926, and presided over the 1932 centenary meeting of the British Medical Association. Other honours included Honorary Membership of the Association of Anaesthetists of Great Britain and Ireland and Honorary Fellowship of the Faculty of Anaesthetists, Royal College of Surgeons of England in 1949.

He anaesthetized King George the Fifth twice in 1928 for rib resection, the surgery being performed by Sir Hugh Rigby. The surgery was protracted but despite this it is recorded that the King was not troubled by anaesthetic sequelae, a tribute to Shipway's skill. For his services he was appointed Knight Commander of the Royal Victorian Order in 1929 (22,23,24,25,26).

He was one of the founders of the Guy's Anaesthetic Committee, initially Secretary he became Chairman in 1919. Whilst serving on the committee he established the use of anaesthetic records in the operating theatre, organized the upgrading and maintenance of anaesthetic apparatus and improved the professional standing of anaesthetists in the hospital.

Conclusion

Sir Francis was an anaesthetic autocrat and would cancel patients on his lists if he thought it was in their best interests to avoid surgery. This lead to personality clashes with hospital staff. His idea of more relaxation was regarded by one senior surgeon as 'less rigidity'! After retiring in 1935, Sir Francis lived until 1968, witnessing the establishment of the speciality of anaesthesia in the National Health Service and the appointment of one of his junior anaesthetists from Guy's Hospital—Sir Robert Macintosh—as first professor of anaesthetics in Europe.

References

(1) Shipway FE, Pembrey MS. The influence of anaesthetics on the body temperature. *Proc Roy Soc Med* (Anaesth. Sec.) 1916; **9**: 3.

(2) Pembrey MS, Shipway FE. The importance of temperature in relation to anaesthesia. *Guy's Hospital Reports* 1914; **69**: 223–34.

(3) Kelly RE. Intratracheal anaesthesia. *Br J Surg* 1911; **i**: 90–5.

(4) Shipway FE. Apparatus for intratracheal anaesthesia. *Lancet* 1914; **ii**: 104.

(5) Shipway FE. The advantages of warm anaesthetic vapours and an apparatus for their administration. *Lancet* 1916; **i**: 70–4.

(6) Shipway FE. New apparatus for the intratracheal insufflation of ether. *Lancet* 1916; **ii**: 236.

(7) Ellis RH. The first trans auricular mitral valvotomy. *Anaesthesia* 1975; **30**: 374–90.

(8) Editorial. The war "warm ether". *Br Med J* 1916 **ii**: 268.

(9) Boyle HEG. Nitrous oxide-oxygen-ether outfit. *Proc Roy Soc Med* (Anaesth. Sec.) 1917; **11**: 30.

(10) Marshall G. Two types of portable Gas- oxygen- Apparatus. *Proc Roy Soc Med* (Anaesth. Sec.) 1920; **13**: 16–9.

(11) Shipway FE. Apparatus for nitrous oxide, oxygen and ether. *Proc Roy Soc Med* (Anaesth. Sec.) 1920; **13**: 19–20.

(12) Shipway FE. A combined anaesthetic apparatus. *Lancet* 1922; **i**: 490.

(13) Shipway FE. Airway for intranasal operations. *Br Med J* 1935; **i**: 767.

(14) Stanley-Sykes W. In: Ellis R, ed. *Essays on the first one hundred years of anaesthesia*, Vol 3. Edinburgh: Churchill-Livingstone 1982: 106–7.

(15) Shipway FE. Anaesthesia and resuscitation. *Br Med J* 1931; **ii**: 1135–6.

(16) Langton-Hewer C. *Recent advances in anaesthesia and analgesia*. Vol 3. London: Churchill, 1939: 200.

(17) Shipway FE. Recovery after stoppage of heart. *Br Med J* 1935; **i**: 326.

(18) Shipway FE. Rectal narcosis. *Guy's Hosp Gaz* 1931; **45**: 2–5.

(19) Shipway FE. General anaesthesia in dental operations. *Br Med J* 1927; **i**: 468.

(20) Shipway FE. Ethyl chloride for dentistry. *Br Med J* 1919; **ii**: 90.

(21) Shipway FE, Hadfield CF, Langton Hewer C. Use of vinesthene. *Lancet* 1935; **i**: 82.

(22) Seed RF. Anaesthesia at Guy's past and present. *Guy's Hosp Gaz* (Guy's Hospital 250th anniversary edition) 1976; 154–7.

(23) Obituary notice, Sir Francis Shipway. *Guy's Hosp Gaz* 1969; **83**: 55–6.

(24) Obituary notice, Sir Francis Shipway. *Anaesthesia* 1969; **24**: 296–7.

(25) Obituary notice, Sir Francis Shipway. *Br Med J* 1969; **iv**: 649.

(26) Black A, Black C. *Who was Who 1961–1970*. London: Black, 1972.

25.10   Dennis Emerson Jackson (1878–1980)

JOHN B. STETSON

Rush Presbyterian–St Luke's Medical Center, Chicago, Illinois, USA

Prefatory note

When my abstract was submitted the writer did not know Professor Lucien Morris would be on the programme with the same topic (Paper 25.11). As we have not collaborated, there may be some redundancy; hopefully this will be minimal as this biography will report many other

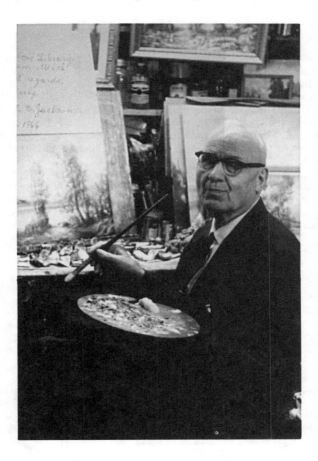

Figure 1   Dennis Emerson Jackson at age 88.

contributions of an extremely dynamic investigator, teacher, pharmacologist, text-book writer, journal editor, medical instrument maker, and theorist who gave us closed circuit carbon dioxide techniques, positive pressure intrathecal ventilation, and trichlorethylene anaesthesia. He had a wonderful sense of humour, was an amateur (actually a semi-professional) artist, violin maker, and a very poor business man.

Early years and education

Dennis Emerson Jackson (Fig. 1) was born September 3, 1878, on a homestead in southern Indiana. His father was a Civil War veteran. He was orphaned as a boy and he and his brother were raised on a farm by his maternal grandfather. There, in 1889, he witnessed his first anaesthetic; his younger brother received chloroform after injuring his shoulder. Twenty six years later he published his first paper on anaesthetics. In 1906 his appendix (normal) was removed. In addition to nausea from ether, his arms were paralysed for a year, (one wonders about shoulder braces).

In 1899, he began teaching in a one room school. Somehow, he managed to obtain teaching certificates each year. In 1903 he entered Indiana University (IU) to, in effect, have a high school as well as college education. Malaria, yellow fever, and other epidemics passed through; the hearty survived. He received his AB in 1905 and ended his one room school teaching career.

Postgraduate studies and research

That summer he was a graduate student at the University of Chicago. In June his handwriting was neat and he had given a dog ether by artificial 'respiration'. By July his handwriting was hurried, but he had learned that 80:20 $N_2O:O_2$ was safe for complete anaesthesia at 1¼ atmospheres and how to make ethylene.

Then back to IU to be an Assistant in Pharmacology and earn an AM in 1906. He married in 1906 and spent the 1906 year at the University of Chicago as a Fellow (resulting in his first publication, with S. A. Matthews, 'The action of magnesium sulphate upon the heart and the antagonistic action of some other drugs' (1). By 1908 he had his PhD from IU and was an Assistant Professor.

Washington University (WU) in St Louis was expanding and in, 1910, he joined them as an Associate in Pharmacology. His commuting did not stop as he also attended Rush Medical College in Chicago. In November of 1910 his daughter Helen was born, a month premature, by Caesarean section. The nitrous oxide anaesthetic, administered by Dr Isabella Herb, produced maternal cyanosis; some 20 odd years later, Helen learned anaesthetic techniques from

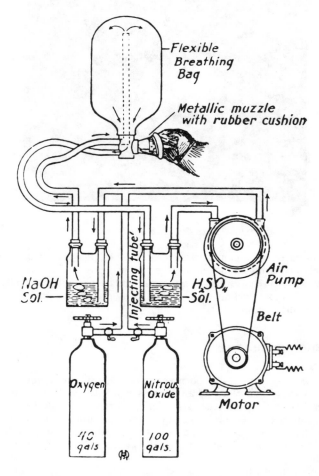

Figure 2   Schematic of closed nitrous oxide:oxygen anaesthesia machine shown with dog mask (this type of machine was used on human patients). Jackson's original machine contained valves and traps which were removed when found necessary (Inter J Orthodontia 1916; 2: 544–62).

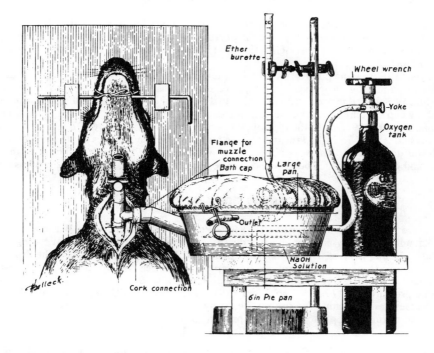

Figure 3   *Closed ether anaesthesia as taught to the medical students. The tube on the cephalad end of the tracheal 'T' tube could be attached to a tambour for recording respiratory movement (from: Jackson DE,* Experimental pharmacology. *St Louis: CV Mosby, 1917.)*

Dr Herb. In 1912 DEJ saw:-

> *'boy about ten years old anaesthetized with nitrous oxide . . . soon became very cyanotic, gasped, struggled and finally lay as if he were dead . . . some better and cheaper method of giving the gas should be available.'*

The 50¢ cost for 'gas' was the cost of many meals to the indigent out-patients. In 1913 he received his MD from Rush in Chicago. As a student he also was full time faculty at WU in St. Louis, wrote two monumental papers on the pharmacology of vanadium (2) (3) and another on the pulmonary action of the adrenal glands (4), published other papers, designed equipment, and had time to drink beer.

Early work on carbon dioxide absorption at University of Washington St Louis

By 1914 DEJ was settled in at WU (St Louis). He had thought out what he needed to build a carbon dioxide absorption anaesthesia machine, had organized a machine shop next to his laboratory, and in 1915 went to a plumbing shop to buy the pieces for the machine. The machine used liquid sodium hydroxide to absorb carbon dioxide, sulphuric acid solution to pick up excess moisture, a pump to circulate the gases, and had valves. A patent for a 'Process for the production and maintenance of general analgesia and anaesthesia' was filed 19 August, 1915, and patent 1 202 391 granted 24 October, 1916. Within a short time the machine was simplified and the valves removed (Fig. 2) (5). DEJ now had his narcotics stamp, and was ready to practise. His machine was used on the patients of Drs (?Otto) Henry Schwarz and Willard Bartlett.

At this time the *Journal of Laboratory and Clinical Medicine* was founded in 1915 DEJ was a founding Associate Editor (for pharmacology). He wrote the keynote paper, 'A new method for the production of general analgesia and anaesthesia with a description of the apparatus used, (6) (1915; **1**:1–12). The Silver Anniversary issue of this journal was dedicated to DEJ (the only member of the original Editorial Board alive) and he was still an active member of the Board!

The year 1917 saw the publication of DEJ's text-book laboratory manual (7). The students learned to administer closed system oxygen:ether, with carbon dioxide absorption, to their dogs (Fig. 3). Soldered pie-pans held the liquid hydroxide solution for carbon dioxide absorption. A bathing cap stretched over the pie-pan rim acted as a reservoir bag! The second edition did not follow until 1939. Due to the type of contract he signed with Mosby, DEJ made no profit from his books and Mosby had the right to use his illustrations and plates in other publications, which was done. As for his own opinion of his work, he told Dr Theodore Striker he did not understand why another such book would ever be published; everything was already in his book.

Washington DC. Arsphenamine and anaesthesia

Trials were in progress in 1918 when DEJ left Washington University for Washington, DC. Arsphenamine was new and some 'early deaths' were reported with its use. Working at the US Public Health Service, DEJ found slow injection of an alkaline solution of the drugs was not deleterious to his dog preparation, but rapid injection caused up to a 100% increase in pulmonary artery pressure (made worse by adrenaline resuscitation) with a 25–50% fall in systemic pressure (8) *J Pharm Exp Therap* 1918; **12**:221–42). DEJ designed and fabricated a new anaesthesia machine for use by the Army, but it was refused because its use would necessitate training people to use it, as opposed to 'pouring' ether.

The University of Cincinnati and continuing interest in anaesthesia

From Washington, DC, DEJ moved to the University of Cincinnati where he became professor and head of the department of pharmacology (later also the Edward Wendland Professor of Materia Medica and Therapeutics). In 1923 he hosted an 'Anesthesia Week,' probably the first national anaesthesia post-graduate course. Dr Francis H. McMechan, the father of professional anaesthesia in the United States aided in obtaining supplies and equipment. Physicians came from as far as Texas and Colorado, a long train trip. They heard 'rumours' of Arno Luckhardt's experiments with ethylene (probably from Dr Frances E. Haines). The Scroll of Recognition was presented to DEJ in 1923 by the National Anesthesia Research Society (the parent of the International Anesthesia Research Society). He was the keynote speaker at the first national Congress of Anesthetists in the United States and in 1925 was appointed Honorary President of the NARS.

A question of priority

Work with different anaesthesia machines continued and DEJ, ever the poor business man, had troubles with his patents (contested by Clark, Teter, and Heidbrink). In correspondence (1921) with the patent office he described a circle system with soda-lime canister between the mask and rebreathing bag with a description of how nitrogen wash-out is performed when the anaesthetic is begun through to closing the system and replacing metabolic oxygen. He knew, and reported, that the soda lime would act as a bacterial trap. A circle system with a canister to hold 'one and one-half to two pounds of soda lime' was described with Thomason in 1927 (8) and nitrogen wash-out was discussed. The authors reported over 200 administrations of ethylene with the machine. This reference was listed by Dr Brian Sword in his 1930 article (9) as though it was one of DEJ's 1915, '16, or '17 articles. Sword worked with Richard von Foregger, the equipment manufacturer, in developing his machine (9). Sword's machine was marketed, DEJ's was not. Sword generally receives credit for introducing circle absorption, DEJ's achievement is generally forgotten. Von Foregger did not forget DEJ's early work however; in 1940 he wrote DEJ about his original 1915 machine and later funded a reconstruction of a duplicate. Drs Ralph Waters and E. A. Rovenstine also seemed confused with their DEJ references. Waters, in 1924 (10) notes 'Mann' as co-author, missed DEJ's 1915 report, lists two 1916 articles (the circulating pump machine and dog-pie pan absorber), but describes a box plethysmograph system not reported by DEJ until 1928 (11). (An investigation of certain respiratory phenomena, *J Pharm Exp Ther* 1928; 33:263–4) (a unit comparable to an 'iron lung' was also described in this report and it was noted it had been used on humans). Waters repeated the same 'errors' in 1926 (12) and 1936 (13) (but his 1947 Centennial review article in *Anesthesiology* (14) carried the correct 1915 DEJ citation (6). Dr Rovenstine (15) in 1936 listed the 1915 citation (6) in 1936, then described the 1928 experiment (11). He wrote,

> *'Waters observed the work done in Jackson's laboratory and was convinced the principle should be developed clinically . . .'*

In fact Waters *wrote* to DEJ 29 September, 1920, (incorrectly addressing it to Washington University, but it was forwarded) but did not visit. They corresponded, but Waters did not attend the 1923 Anesthesia Week in Cincinnati. In December, 1935, DEJ wrote:-

> *'By a queer coincidence my daughter (who is a medical graduate) went to Wisconsin last summer to study the closed system of anaesthesia with Dr. Waters. I suppose this was another version of casting bread upon the Waters.'*

Artificial respiration

DEJ practised intratracheal ventilation as well as the box negative pressure system. The paper 'The use of artificial respiration in man: Report of a case' was refused by the JAMA in 1930 but published locally in the *J Med Cincinnati* (16). A 24 French catheter was used with leak of excess volume. The ventilator was made (and marketed) by the Max Wocher Company of Cincinnati. An eighteen year old man suffered ventilatory arrest when ether was administered for a planned cerebral decompression. The patient was resuscitated, DEJ brought his machine from the laboratory, attached it to the intrathecal catheter and adjusted the volume by chest excursion and stethoscope monitoring. The patient lived for twenty two hours, then the heart 'failed.' At autopsy there was a cerebral abscess 'containing four to six ounces of pus.' The head nurse objected to the treatment '. . . because the large number of persons who came to watch the patient created a bad mess for her to clean up.' The Max Wocher Company marketed many other laboratory devices designed by DEJ. In 1942 he received princely royalties of $191.97 from Wocher.

Trichloroethylene

DEJ believed that tic douloureux was caused by orbital muscle spasms pinching a nerve (17) and used trichloroethylene as an analgesic for treatment. In October of 1933 he presented his paper 'A study of analgesia and anaesthesia with special reference to such substances as, trichloroethylene and vinesthene, together with apparatus for their administration' at the International Anesthesia Research Society Congress and was published a year later (18) in *Anesthesia and Analgesia*. An apparatus the same as the one illustrated in the article was reconstructed after DEJ's death from pieces found in boxes containing a seventy-five year accumulation of spare parts is in the Wood Library-Museum. 'Clinical experiences with the use of trichloroethylene in the production of over 300 analgesias and anesthesias' was published in 1935 (19). The senior author of this report, Dr Cecil Striker (later a renowned diabetes specialist) told his son Theodore (now Chief of Anesthesiology, Cincinnati Children's Hospital), that based on this experience he was a better anesthesiologist than Ted (Theodore) could ever hope to be (personal communication from Ted Striker). Signs of depth, including rapid respiration, were delineated. Unfortunately, the Council on Pharmacy and Therapeutics of the American Medical Association found trichloroethylene wanting. It was lost to the profession until World War II when the late Mr C. Chalmers' (of Muswell Hill) letter reached Dr Charles Hadfield and Dr C. Langton Hewer who carefully investigated the drug and delineated its strengths and weaknesses (20).

Jackson as student and academic

Jackson had many pharmacological interests. He felt the nasal mucosal vessels responded in a manner akin to the pulmonary vasculature and arranged apparatus to measure the dog's intra-nasal volume and the changes wrought by different drugs.

DEJ had pictures of the medical students and learned their names (which he never forgot—he recognized students at their fortieth reunions) before they entered his classroom. He could tell if anybody was missing and always spotted a wool-gatherer and asked that person a question. As the answer progressed, he would say, 'yes, yes' in an encouraging manner with a twinkle in his eye, then at the end, depending upon the answer he might say, 'yes, that was absolutely wrong.' Once a student cribbed his answer from a text hidden in his lap. DEJ complimented him on his concise answer, but noted (without seeing the book) that he had read the wrong chapter and directed him to the page containing the correct answer.

DEJ was made Emeritus in 1948, but continued to work in his laboratory. In 1955 he published 'A special method for recording the actions of the heart: the cairivibograph and the vibogram' (21). The device amplifies and records changes in airway air movement that reflect changes in heart size.

When not making medical gadgets, he made violins with a cantilever bridge. He enjoyed oil painting and exhibited at physicians' art shows. In 1954 he received a Special Plaque from the American Society of Anesthesiologists, Inc. (ASA) and in 1958 he was 'saluted' in *Anesthesia and Analgesia* (the writer probably did not know he had been honoured in the same journal over a third of a century earlier). The year 1963 was marked by receiving both the ASA's Distinguished Service Award and the Citation of Merit of the Academy of Anesthesiology. He joined Harold Griffith, Philip Woodbridge, and Ralph Knight in 1968 at the American Society of Anesthesiologists, Inc. headquarters for a Distinguished Visitors Program. The following year, the University of Cincinnati's Sesquicentennial Year, he was awarded an Honorary Doctor of Science Degree.

His last medical publication was an editorial essay, 'What causes cancer?' (22). Two thirds of a century after his first publication, he was still 'pitching' (bowling). His thesis was cellular escape from nervous system control, perhaps caused by viral damage. His centennial, 1978, was marked by hundreds of letters, cards, and telegrams. As the oldest living member, he continued to receive his membership card from the fraternity Sigma Xi until death interrupted his magnificent life on 24 March, 1980.

Acknowledgments

This biography would not have been possible without the kind assistance of DEJ's son, Charles. I also wish to thank Drs Charles Aring, William Dornette, Benjamin Felson, J. 'Tom' Martin, Carl Minning, Lucien Morris, 'Ted' Striker, Mrs. Harry Shirkey and staff at the University of Cincinnati who have rendered generous assistance and suggestions.

References

(1) Matthews SA, Jackson DE. The action of magnesium sulphate upon the heart and the antagonistic action of some other drugs. *Am J Physiol* 1907; **19**: 5–13.
(2) Jackson DE. The pharmacological action of vanadium. *J Pharmacol Exp Ther* 1911–12; **3**: 477–514.
(3) Jackson DE. The pulmonary action of vanadium together with a study of the peripheral reactions of the metal. *J Pharmacol Exp Ther* 1912–13; **4**: 1–20.
(4) Jackson DE. The pulmonary action of the adrenal glands. *J Pharmacol Exp Ther* 19; **4**: 59–74.
(5) Jackson DE. An experimental investigation of the pharmacological action of nitrous oxide. *Int J Orthodontia* 1916; **2**: 544–62.
(6) Jackson DE. A new method for the production of general analgesia and anaesthesia with a description of the apparatus used. *J Lab Clin Med* 1915; **1**: 1–12.

(7) Jackson DE. *Experimental pharmacology*. St Louis: Mosby, 1917.
(8) Thomason H, Jackson DE. Carbon dioxide filtration method for general analgesia and anaesthesia. *Anesth Analg* 1927; **6**: 181–3.
(9) Sword BC. A closed circuit method of administration of gas anaesthesia. *Anesth Analg* 1930; **9**: 198–202.
(10) Waters RM. Clinical scope and utility of carbon dioxide filtration in inhalation anaesthesia. *Curr Res Anesth* 1924; **3**: 20–2.
(11) Jackson DE. An investigation of certain respiratory phenomena. *J Pharmacol Exp Ther* 1928; **33**: 263–4.
(12) Waters RM. Advantages and techniques of carbon dioxide filtration with inhalation anaesthesia. *Anesth Analg* 1926; **5**: 160–2.
(13) Waters RM. Carbon dioxide absorption technic in anaesthesia. *Ann Surg* 1936; **103**: 38–45.
(14) Waters RM. Absorption of carbon dioxide from anaesthetic atmospheres. Historical aspects. *Anesthesiology* 1947; **8**: 339–47.
(15) Rovenstine EA. Carbon dioxide absorption method for inhalation anaesthesia. *Am J Surg* 1936; **34**: 456–62.
(16) Jackson DE. The use of artificial respiration in man; Report of a case. *J Med Cincinnati* 1930; **11**: 515–9.
(17) Jackson DE. The treatment of tic doloreux. *J Med Cincinnati* 1934; **15**: 127–9.
(18) Jackson DE. A study of analgesia and anesthesia with special reference to such substances as trichlorethylene and vinesthene (divinyl ester) together with apparatus for their administration. *Anesth Analg* 1934; **13**: 198–203.
(19) Striker C, Goldblatt S, Warm IS, Jackson DE. Clinical experience with the use of trichlorethylene in the production of over 300 analgesias and anesthesias. *Anesth Analg* 1935; **14**: 68–71.
(20) Hewer CL, Hadfield CF. Trichlorethylene as an inhalation anaesthetic. *Br Med J* 1941; 1 924–7.
(21) Jackson DE. A special method for recording the actions of the heart: The cairivibograph and vibogram. *Anesthesiology* 1955; **16**: 536–43.
(22) Jackson DE. What causes cancer? *Cincinnati Med J* 1974; **55**: 130–1.

25.11   D. E. Jackson 1878–1980: A perspective

LUCIEN E. MORRIS
Seattle, Washington, USA

In the early 1920s several prominent basic scientists were strongly supportive in the founding of the National Anaesthesia Research Society which three years later became the International Anaesthesia Research Society (IARS) as it is known today. Their participation is readily identified through the inclusion of their names on the editorial masthead of the publication, *Current Researches in Anesthesia and Analgesia* which was started in 1922 as the official journal of the National Society. Individually and collectively these basic scientists participated in the birth and nurture of anaesthesiology as a fledgling clinical speciality in the United States of America. Foremost among this group was Dennis Emerson Jackson, PhD, MD who was then Professor of Pharmacology at the University of Cincinnati Medical College.

The 1923 course in anaesthesia

In 1923 Jackson organized at Cincinnati for the benefit of early specialist physicians, a course of laboratory demonstrations teaching applicable basic principles of physiology and pharmacology pertinent to the clinical practice of anaesthesia. About twenty-five clinicians from all over the country attended the week long course. They were stimulated by his enthusiastic teaching and most appreciative of his effort to improve and update their education with respect to developing knowledge and understanding of the pharmacological action of drugs used in or related to the practice of anaesthesia. As a mark of appreciation, Professor Jackson was at the next annual meeting presented with the Society 'Scroll of Recognition' and subsequently was made honorary president of the first congress of the IARS. In subsequent years the Society Scroll of Recognition was presented to Allen W. Rowe, Professor of Pharmacology at Boston University, and to Professors Yandell Henderson and Howard W. Haggard, both of the Laboratory of Applied Physiology at Yale University.

Jackson as teacher

Professor Jackson was undoubtedly a stimulating teacher of Pharmacology. His teaching of medical students was reinforced through their extensive laboratory participation. His remarkable text book on *Experimental Pharmacology*, published in 1917 (1) and revised in 1939, is replete with detailed descriptions of novel devices which reflect the imaginative approach of a practical mechanician able to turn ordinary household items into functional laboratory apparatus. Several of his ideas were of importance to the field of anaesthesia and especially to the development of carbon dioxide absorption in the closed system.

The closed system

Jackson took basic concepts which had already been developed by those scientists studying respiratory metabolism and applied them in the design of apparatus for the economical and physiological administration of anaesthetic gases and vapours in a closed system. On the basis of his laboratory experience he recommended use of the system for clinical anaesthesia (2). Although Jackson was not the first to try closed system rebreathing of anaesthetics the introduction of his ingenious equipment into basic laboratory teaching in two major medical schools, and his several subsequent revisions in design, attracted attention and interest to a logical concept and method. Indeed, after his initial paper (2) Dr Jackson produced in the next several years no less than five papers which described various design modifications of apparatus he made for the closed system absorption of carbon dioxide during anaesthesia. Two of these designs were also included in the 1917 edition of the textbook *Experimental Pharmacology*. One apparatus as pictured in figure 116 of the 1917 textbook is of special interest because it clearly portrays a prototype of what later came to be known as a 'to and fro absorption system'. It is a device utilizing a modified deep baking pan into which respired gases were simply exhaled and again inhaled from the closed container. Oxygen and small measured amounts of liquid anaesthetic agent were added as needed. Carbon dioxide was removed from the gas mixture by exposure to liquid alkali retained in a pan at the bottom of the cake pan. Tidal volume was accommodated by a lady's flexible shower cap fastened over the top of the pan to make the system air tight.

There was not general acceptance of Jackson's devices for clinical usage probably because of understandable concern about the potential hazards of the liquid alkali, but also reflecting the common phenomena of inertia and resistance to change. In the second edition of *Experimental Pharmacology* (1939) it was pointed out that solid chunks of either sodim or potassium hydroxide or granular soda-lime would be easier and safer to use than strong alkaline solutions. In the revised textbook, the description of a 'to and fro' device for animal anaesthesia again used the modified cake pan and shower cap but also had an interposed chamber for holding soda lime with which a major part of each tidal volume would come in contact. This was after Waters' 1924 publication describing the use of soda lime for carbon dioxide absorption in a 'to and fro' system for clinical anaesthesia with ether (3) and subsequent to the introduction of cyclopropane in the early thirties for which the closed system was a virtual necessity.

After a slow beginning and many rebuffs, the idea of the closed carbon dioxide absorption system was ultimately supported and implemented by others. However, despite inherent merit of the closed system methods and improvement of equipment by subsequent modifications, general application of the method has seemed to wax and wane in parallel with the popularity of cyclopropane. Now used with newer anaesthetic agents by only a relatively few perceptive specialists it remains for a new generation of anaesthetists to rediscover the economic and environmental benefits and more importantly, the educational and clinical rewards of mastering the use of the truly closed absorption system.

Jackson's innovative idea had stimulated the development of clinically useful closed carbon dioxide absorption systems. In recognition of the significance of his contributions the American Society of Anesthesiologists in 1963 presented its Distinguished Service Award to Dr Jackson. Dr Jackson maintained an interest in anaesthesia throughout his professional career. In 1933 he introduced trichlorethylene as an anaesthetic, which by a curious twist could not be used in the carbon dioxide absorption system.

Biographical

Dennis Jackson was a self sufficient individual innovator and original thinker. He was born 3 September, 1878, in Ridgeport, Indiana as the elder son of school teachers, Theophilus Job Jackson and Ellen Pickard Jackson. Orphaned when Dennis was eight years of age, the boys were brought up by maiden aunts and an uncle on a southern Indiana farm. Dennis demonstrated early both mechanical ability and a penchant for making useful things out of scrap. He did well in schoool, read voraciously and was a winner in spelling contests, but by his own account had only one year of high school (4). He did not like farm work and turned to teaching for several years in the traditional multiple grade one room school house in order to earn money to further his own education, originally intending to become a teacher of Latin. He was able to enroll at Indiana University by passing an entrance examination. He made up his high school course lacks and earned three degrees at Indiana (AB in 1905, AM in 1906 and PhD in 1908). During his undergraduate years, he took a course from Professor William Moenkhaus who taught physiology in the Department of Zoology. With the start of a new medical school at Indiana University, Professor Moenkhaus became head of the new medical Department of Physiology and Jackson was first his assistant, then instructor and, after earning the PhD, was appointed assistant Professor and assumed the obligation of teaching courses in pharmacology. Two years later he was appointed Assistant in Pharmacology at Washington University in St Louis where he remained for eight years and rose to Associate Professor before moving to the University of Cincinnati as Professor and Chairman of Pharmacology. In addition to organizing programs for teaching pharmacology, Dr. Jackson commuted frequently to Chicago to complete his own medical education at Rush Medical College. It was his empathy for indigent patients observed in the Chicago clinics which motivated him to seek a cheaper and better method for providing benefits of analgesia and anaesthesia for clinical use.

The latter years. A personal association

Dennis Jackson lived for more than 100 full years and throughout his life maintained a continuing interest in science, people, teaching, and the use of shop tools. Author, landscape artist, editor, educator, enthusiastic gadgeteer, medical historian, physician, professor, researcher, teacher and violin maker are all useful descriptions of his many talents and activities.

The writer had a particular interest in Dennis Jackson because he and his wife were long time family friends of his parents. Dr Jackson and his father were both ex-Hoosiers who became faculty colleagues at Washington University in St Louis. Each was among the pioneer group in new off-shoots from Physiology, Jackson in Pharmacology, the writers' father in Biochemistry, and each subsequently became head of an independent department in his chosen discipline.

Although Dr Jackson had seen the writer as a child, our acquaintance was largely limited to the last decade of his life and the occasions of visits to his home in Cincinnati two or more times each year. Prior to that time meetings had only been occasional. In his nineties he was still vigorous and an avid reader; there were always open current journals of anaesthesiology or pharmacology on the coffee table in front of his couch. He was still asking searching critical questions; a stimulating and interesting man because he did not seem to lose interest in the world around him and its puzzlements. These visits were much enjoyed because of mutual interests and friends and his sense of humour. After he left Cincinnati and went to live with his son in Virginia the writer visited him twice. Once was in the hospital on Christmas Day in his 101st year just after he had had a pacemaker implant and the second three months later, a year before his death. He came to the door to let his visitors in, was pleased to have visitors who wanted to see him, but for the first time, he did not know the reason for a special interest in him. The writer was privileged to know him and proud of his accomplishments and contributions to the specialty of anaesthesiology.

References

(1) Jackson DE. *Experimental pharmacology*. St Louis: CV. Mosby Company, 1917.
(2) Jackson DE. A new method for the production of general analgesia and anaesthesia with a description of the apparatus used. *J Lab Clin Med* 1915; **1**: 1–12.
(3) Waters RM. Clinical scope and utility of carbon dioxide filtration in inhalation anesthesia. *Can Res Anesth* 1924; **3**: 20.
(4) Jackson DE. *Handwritten autobiographical notes*, 1973.

25.12   Mathew Kasner Moss (1879–1945)

ROD WESTHORPE
Geoffrey Kaye Museum of Anaesthetic History. Royal Australasian College of Surgeons, Melbourne, Australia

---

Mathew Kasner Moss was born in 1879 and graduated in medicine from Melbourne University Australia in 1902. After a few years of hospital and general practice in Echuca in Northern Victoria, he moved to Perth, Western Australia, and entered General Practice. In 1930 he was appointed Honorary Surgeon to Perth Hospital.

He was a keen sportsman and had the distinction of representing both Victoria and Western Australia in interstate rowing. He is distinguished also by serving twice (in 1933 and 1944) as President of the Western Australian Branch of the British Medical Association.

Although involved in many aspects of medical practice, his prime interest was in anaesthesia. He eventually embarked on a specialist anaesthetist practice; however, only a few weeks later, he died, at the age of 66.

In the practice of anaesthesia, he was renowned as an innovator and inventor, particularly in relation to endotracheal anaesthesia and the development of vaporizers.

Endotracheal anaesthesia

He was responsible, together with Gilbert Troup, for introducing endotracheal anaesthesia to Western Australia in the 1920's. In association with this he designed a laryngoscope, which could be inserted from the side of the mouth for use in patients with short necks and prominent teeth.

Vaporizer

An inventor of some note he is best remembered for his Vaporizer, one of the earliest attempts at vaporizer design in Australia. It was designed in 1917 and consisted of two metal cannisters, one for chloroform and one for ether. Air was pumped from a foot bellows to pass via simple screw valves into one or both chambers. The ether cannister was warmed by a variable power DC heating coil and had provision for the insertion of a thermometer. Normally, the indication for increased heating power was the condensation of water droplets on the metal lid of the cannister. Air from the bellows was made to bubble through the liquid ether or chloroform via numerous small holes on the bottom of the gas inlet tube placed near the base of the cannister.

The mixture and amount of ether and chloroform vapour in the gas delivered to the patient was controlled by the needle valves, and the resultant mixture was then allowed to pass through a warmed vacuum flask before reaching the patient.

Despite the elegance of his device, Kasner Moss eventually discarded it in favour of his modification of Lidwill's apparatus in which he used a large glass jar as the vaporizer, floating a layer of ether on top of a volume of water in which a heating element was immersed.

He realized that warming of the air and vapour at a distance from the patient was of little value and he attempted to devise a heating system closer to the intratracheal catheter, but with little success.

Summary

Although none of Kasner Moss's devices or methods remain in use today, he stands out in the history of anaesthesia in Australia as an innovator, and is remembered for his worthy contribution to the practice of medicine in general.

25.13   A perspective—E. I. McKesson (1881–1935)

LUCIEN E. MORRIS
Seattle, Washington, USA

The activities and controversial ideas of Elmer Isaac McKesson made his hometown, Toledo, Ohio well known to those who practised the specialty of anaesthesia during the second, third and fourth decades of this century. He was for a time, of international prominence—largely because of his advocacy of nitrous oxide as the sole anaesthetic agent by techniques in which hypoxia was almost certainly a factor. McKesson died in 1935 so that the writer's knowledge of him is a reflected view from contacts with several of his students and colleagues (especially Fred Clement and Ken McCarthy) and more importantly from his writing in which he set down his ideas and described his techniques and the equipment for which he became famous. (1) Unfortunately the McKesson name is so closely associated with hypoxic techniques in the use of nitrous oxide that many of his fundamental concepts and other contributions have not received the full recognition that an objective evaluation would seem to warrant. McKesson evidently believed that the action of other anaesthetics when deep enough for relaxation depended upon depletion of oxygen available to the patient. This gave him the support to proceed with nitrous oxide in mixtures with oxygen percentages that are now viewed as hypoxic.

The purpose of this paper is to review the major contributions of McKesson and to consider why McKesson is today, in fact, not as well known an historic figure as he might be. For this evaluation, it is useful to know something of the man himself.

Biography

Elmer Isaac McKesson was born in Walkerton, Indiana in 1881 and brought up in that semi-rural environment. He graduated from high school in Walkerton, went on to a teachers college and then to North-western University and the University of Chicago after which he returned to Walkerton to serve two years as teacher and principal of the high school.

He next entered Rush Medical College in Chicago from which he graduated MD in 1906 and then went on to Toledo, Ohio for an internship at The Toledo Hospital. Following his internship, McKesson began private practice in the relatively neglected field of anaesthesia.

He recognized the important relationships between anaesthesia and various aspects of physics, chemistry and physiology in all of which he had more than ordinary interest, partly because of his background as a high school teacher. Because of his educational interests he also became associated with the Toledo Medical College, (a proprietary school which existed from 1882 until 1914) at which he served as Faculty Secretary and as Associate Professor of Physiology until that school became defunct in 1914.

After the closure of the Toledo Medical College, McKesson turned his attention towards the postgraduate education of physicians and dentists interested in the practical aspects of anaesthesia. For these postgraduate efforts, he co-opted the help of basic scientists including Professor Dennis Jackson of Cincinnati, the pharmacologist who had, in 1915, described a closed system for anaesthesia in which carbon dioxide was absorbed by liquid alkali and in which respired gases were circulated by an electric fan to reduce both resistance and dead space of the apparatus.

McKesson's scientific philosophy

McKesson was actually an inventive genius with mechanical skills and was well versed in physics. He also had a good understanding of the then current knowledge of physiology, especially of respiration and circulation. This combination of abilities and interests provided him with a perspective about some aspects of anaesthesia which was well beyond that of the average physician of that time. He was well acquainted with Haldane's concepts of respiration and used this knowledge to develop equipment and techniques for 'fractional rebreathing' which was an advance and may have been a major factor in the success of his nitrous oxide techniques as he applied them.

He identified physical factors related to the administration of inhalation agents and devised appliances for successful application of these principles. The first McKesson apparatus for anaesthesia was developed by 1910 and made available to the rest of the world through the Toledo Technical Appliance Company, of which he was president. His business interests were successful and he became a well liked and popular figure in the community.

His charisma was legendary and is reflected in the professional leadership and many organizational positions he enjoyed.

His writings about clinical anaesthesia, McKesson touch on many fundamental concepts the physiological basis for which are as valid today as then. Anaesthesiologists accept and apply many of his ideas today although most do not realize that he was the first, or among the first, to clearly enunciate them. The breadth of his clinical teaching contributions is impressive. A selected partial list of McKesson teachings reveals the scope of his interests and the depth of his understanding of problems and solutions as applied to general anaesthesia:

1. He taught that anaesthetics including nitrous oxide are cardiovascular depressants.

2. He pointed out that the signs of the anaesthesia levels are largely muscular (and so with use of modern intravenous muscle relaxants, many signs of anaesthesia depth have been eliminated.

3. He emphasized the importance of the presence and character of respiration as useful physiological information. He considered the sigh under nitrous oxide to be an important indication that all was well.

4. He emphasized the importance of mouth to mouth insufflation for resuscitation of infants.

5. He moved toward effective resuscitation in anaesthesia by incorporating in his equipment a means of exerting positive pressure to ventilate a patient who reached the point of apnoea

or respiratory difficulty. He taught that positive pressure is useful for maintaining the airway and reestablish ventilation in cases of apnoea. (The life support technique of artificial ventilation by manual compression of the anaesthetic bag was apparently not generally practiced prior to McKesson.) Positive pressure was also recommended to combat dilution from air leaks and to improve an obstructed airway giving the patient a better chance to breathe spontaneously. He pointed out also, that it was necessary to use positive pressure with an open pleura.

6. He was very much concerned with the size of the tidal volume and total amount of ventilation, and the relationship of dead space in the patient to those respiratory parameters. The equipment made for fractional rebreathing provided means for rebreathing any desired measured volume of each exhalation (2). This was a logical development combining useful features of both total rebreathing and continuous flow. Control over ventilation through the respiratory stimulant effect of carbon dioxide was achieved without the frank asphyxia which occurred with total rebreathing. The markedly increased ventilation effected by retained carbon dioxide provided an increased alveolar turnover which in turn brought nitrous oxide more rapidly to maximum effect as well as delivering more oxygen to the alveoli.

7. He was acutely aware that with respect to any given respired concentration of anaesthetic, the development of a corresponding maximum level of anaesthesia was a function of time (today we would talk about the fraction of alveolar concentration over the fraction of inspired concentration (FA/FI) as plotted against time);

8. He pointed out that in mountain sickness, vomiting is related to hypoxia and suggested that the same correlation might be true in anaesthesia.

9. He pointed out that the oxygen need in patients differed according to the biological variations and that indeed the nitrous oxide requirement was also different and he cited the anaemia patient who might need only 30–40% nitrous oxide with the balance oxygen (so he was not so committed to the use of 100% nitrous oxide as many of us have been led to believe).

10. He tried the closed carbon dioxide absorption technique after Jackson had introduced it and discarded it because he could not maintain the depth of anaesthesia in a closed system without adding nitrous oxide (so he knew there was a loss of anaesthetic effect and may have been aware of the need to keep adding anaesthetic because of the redistribution of the anaesthetic agent to the other tissues.)

11. McKesson was one of the early physicians to use blood pressure apparatus during anaesthesia and to chart his observations. He drew heavily upon his recorded observations as a basis for many of his papers and presentations. Some direct quotations from McKesson's writing are illuminating:

> *'It is my rule when in doubt to try more oxygen. This is best accomplished by pressing quickly, but gently, the direct oxygen button to give a small puff of pure oxygen. When this little puff of oxygen, which reaches the brain in 5 to 6 seconds, gives its momentary effect, one learns at once whether the oxygen percentage in the mixture should be increased or decreased . . .'* (2)

He wrote this in 1915 and he is saying that he did not want his patients to depend upon a lack of oxygen to drive respiration. It was 1928 that Corneille Heymann actually described the hypoxic mechanism through the carotid and aortic bodies for which he was later awarded the Nobel Prize. In 1915 McKesson did not know the mechanism but he knew a practical fact that demonstration of the existence of an hypoxic drive which could be abolished by a single breath of 100% oxygen, was a useful thing to be viewed as a warning in anaesthesia:

> *'Until 1910 rebreathing had always been accomplished as Wells, Clover, Hewitt or Gatch had practiced it—by allowing the patient to breathe to and fro for a certain time into a bag of anaesthetic vapors which was larger than the patient's tidal respiration. This is total rebreathing since the whole breath is stored and rebreathed. In 1910 I devised a fractional method of rebreathing and constructed a special bag for that purpose. . . . on inhalation the bag is first emptied and the remainder of the inhalation comes from the fresh supply. . .'* (2)

'Circulatory depression has occupied the attention of the best medical minds . . . The tendency has been . . . to prevent the development of shock . . . It is not always possible to avoid the loss of blood. Even small blood losses may be sufficient to . . . (cause) . . . depression . . . That the loss of fluid in the blood vessels occurs by general dilatation including arterioles, capillaries and venules is beyond question. The rational treatment, therefore would be to . . . make up for such dilatation by the intravenous administration of some solution which will readily leave the vessels as the patient reacts. Physiologic saline . . . does meet the requirements . . . it is my practice to see that enough saline is administered intravenously to elevate the systolic blood pressure to within ten percent of its normal reading.' (3)

'Standing orders for definite doses of morphine are not practical. Some (patients) get too much and others do not get enough. . . . morphine, before and after operations, (should be) regulated not by standing order, but by the physiologic effect. Less standardizations and more individualization of treatment is needed.' (3)

So in retrospect it appears that McKesson was teaching and practicing a great deal of what we understand to be important today.

Conclusion

It is hoped that in this brief presentation, it has been possible to impart some understanding of the scope of McKesson's interests and observations and the importance of his ideas to the practice of current anaesthetists and to their background of information. In fact however, McKesson's influence other than the indirect and subtle ways already discussed is not really recognized today. McKesson had turned his real educational interests toward postgraduate short courses to benefit dentists and a few physicians, in which the purpose was all too often interpreted as being the learning of a technique rather than of basic principles in which he was also versed. And so it is that McKesson's apparent influence on modern anaesthesia is much diminished and less credit is given to his contributions than might seem appropriate.

A quotation from a letter of Ralph Waters is revealing:

'The tendency has been for people to credit him with mechanical inventions and disregard his one extremely important contribution to anaesthesia; namely, the introduction of graphic recording of the condition of patients. As far as I know, he deserves the credit for starting this type of thing, and it is the one thing for which he should be remembered. Apparatus is a fleeting thing, changing in style as do automobiles, but fundamentals like methods of record keeping will last forever.' (4)

References

(1) McCarthy KC, ed. *Some papers on "Nitrous oxide—oxygen anesthesia by Elmer Isaac McKesson, M.D."* Conjure House, Division of Business News Publishing Co., 1953.

(2) McKesson EI. *Am J Surg* (Anesth Suppl) 1915: 29–51

(3) McKesson EI. Presidential address, National Anesthesia Research Society. *Curr Res Anesth Analg* 1923; **2**: 43.

(4) Waters RM. Letter to Geoffrey Kaye, May 5, 1937.

25.14	Ralph M. Waters (1883–1979).* To teach doctors . . . a scientific basis for practice of anaesthesia

LUCIEN E. MORRIS
Seattle, Washington, USA

An historic event occurred sixty years ago when Ralph Milton Waters, after more than 10 years in a practice limited to clinical anaesthesia, accepted an academic appointment on the medical faculty at the Univeristy of Wisconsin. It was his stated purpose to establish a programme to train doctors to go out and teach other doctors a scientific basis and professional approach to the practice of clinical anaesthesia. By 1928 resident physicians were appointed to the first truly academic programme for the post-graduate training of physicians in the speciality of anaesthesia. The cooperation of basic science colleagues was enlisted so that physicians in training might benefit. The basic science foundations for anaesthesia were explored and joint efforts in research were initiated, especially in physiology and pharmacology, where residents in training were assigned for research time. An innovative clinical teaching programme began, including morbidity and mortality conferences (M & M), and literature review. In less than a decade the programme for postgraduate training in anaesthesia at Madison, Wisconsin became a focal point of interest in the medical world. Visitors came to be stimulated by new ideas, to learn about the organization of Dr Waters' teaching and then returned home to emulate the model.

The first full time Professor of Anaesthesia

Waters was the first full time Professor of Anaesthesia. His personal dynamics attracted a steady flow of graduate physicians into a previously neglected area. In 20 years there were a total of 60 residents appointed, who by spending up to a year or two or more in the Wisconsin environment were introduced to academic anaesthesia and received a major influence on their professional lives. Each physician in this postgraduate programme was exposed to a contagious enthusiasm and as a result went forth with a mission to share the perspectives and knowledge absorbed.

The heritage

Two-thirds of Waters' residents devoted at least a part of their subsequent years to teaching. Twenty of these have served as a chairman or director of a teaching programme in a medical school. It was due largely to the momentum of these efforts that anaesthesiology ultimately became established as a separate autonomous academic department in most American medical schools.

Although he made numerous momentous and individually noteworthy contributions to the organizational, administrative, and practical aspects in the development of anaesthesiology, Waters will be remembered most for effectiveness as a medical educator and for his personal dynamics whereby others were infused with his projected enthusiasm and motivation. From Waters' students and subsequently through the teaching by their students a major influence has been exerted on the speciality of anaesthesiology. In North American medical schools well over a hundred individual chairmen, and throughout the world hundreds of academicians and literally thousands of clinical anaesthesiologists, have been of the Waters professional lineage.

* This poster presentation displayed an outline of the highlights in Waters career and the honours he received, selected photographs of Wisconsin staff and the aqua-alumni, the 'Waters Tree', and a listing of United States Medical Schools at which chairmen of Anaesthesiology have been of the Waters' lineage.

Conclusion

The current professional position of anaesthesiology owes much to the vision of Ralph Waters and the contributions of successive generations of his students. What the future holds depends upon the extent to which we live up to the standards and responsibilities of our heritage.

25.15   'My dear dogfish' — A correspondence between
Ralph M. Waters (1887–1979) and Geoffrey Kaye (1903–1986)

GWEN WILSON[1] and LUCIEN E. MORRIS[2]
[1]Australian Society of Anaesthetists, New South Wales, Australia,
and [2]Washington, Seattle, USA

This presentation is intended to call attention to and provide a brief glimpse of an important historical correspondence between Geoffrey Kaye of Melbourne, Victoria and Ralph M. Waters of Madison, Wisconsin. Their acquaintance began on the occasion of Kaye's first visit to Madison in 1930 during the economic depression. The letters* reveal not only a mutual abiding interest and concern for anaesthesia related problems but also a deepening friendship which ultimately spanned nearly fifty years.

The men

The participants themselves are of major interest, with personalities quite unalike, each was a major contributor to the growth and development of our specialty, each the recipient of accolades and a legend in his own right. The fact that they became friends and carried on a voluminous correspondence for nearly half a century provides a file of historic importance because of the topics and issues covered by their exchanges.

Geoffrey Kaye (1903–1986) (Fig. 1) was born in Melbourne, Australia, and had his schooling in England during World War I. He graduated in Medicine from the University of Melbourne in 1926 and by 1927–28 was specializing in anaesthetics and showing an interest in research.

In 1929 he met F. H. McMechan, organizer of anaesthesia societies and congresses and editor of the journal *Current Researches in Anaesthesia and Analgesia*. Kaye had planned to undertake a tour in 1930 to visit various centres in Germany and England. McMechan persuaded him to include North America in his trip so that he would attend the annual Congress of Anaesthetists, and, further, made specific arrangements for Kaye to visit and observe prominent anaesthetists in their places of work. So it was through an introduction from Frank McMechan that Geoffrey Kaye became one of the first in a long procession of international visitors to see the new and exciting programme for post-graduate study of anaesthesia at the University of Wisconsin, which became the model for teaching doctors the scientific basis of clinical anaesthesia practice.

---

*We acknowledge with gratitude the kindness of Darwin D. Waters in giving us access to a major part of this historically valuable collection of correspondence.

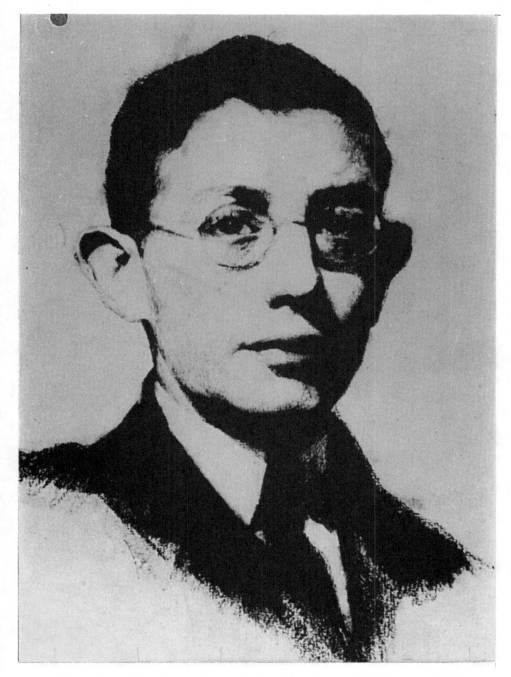

Figure 1   Geoffrey Kaye, as he was in the 1930s from a sketch by Norma Bull.

Ralph Waters (1883–1979) (Fig. 2) was born and educated in Ohio, USA. He graduated in 1912 from the School of Medicine, Western Reserve University in Cleveland. After more than 10 years of practice in clinical anaesthesia, he went in 1927 to the new Medical School Hospital of the University of Wisconsin at Madison as head of a new academic enterprise in anaesthesia.

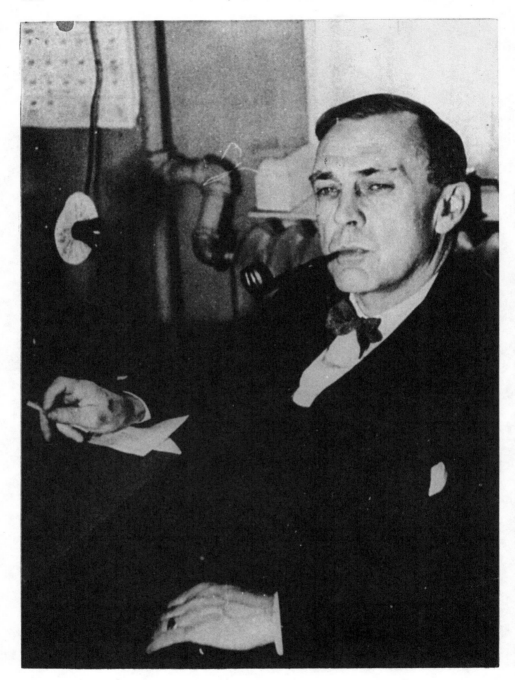

Figure 2   Ralph M. Waters and companion pipe at his office desk in the Wisconsin General Hospital.

Although 20 years older than Kaye he had limited his practice to the specialty of anaesthesia only a little over 10 years longer than Kaye. Nonetheless even though he had been in Madison for only three and a half years when Kaye visited in October, 1930, Waters held a unique position as a professorial head of a training programme in a medical school and was already recognized as a leader and driving force for change in anaesthesia education for all physicians.'

The dogfish

Kaye made a second visit to Madison in 1938 and in a description of the department subsequently written he indicated clearly that the department reflected the personality and activity of Waters himself. He further characterized Waters' relationship to others by a parable which we quote here as reported by Gillespie (1).

> *'There was once a dealer of Grimsby in England who used to store live cod in tanks until they could be sold to advantage on the London market. Having plenty of food, and no work to get it, the cod became so lethargic that the Billingsgate fishmongers complained that their flesh was quite insipid. So the dealer placed a live dogfish in each tank. The dogfish chased the cod around and gave them an interest in life so that they arrived in London in excellent condition.'*

The lethargy which afflicted the cod is parallelled in our work by *laissez-faire* and self satisfaction. The dogfish is the symbol of Ralph Waters. Geoffrey Kaye during his 12 years as the first Secretary of the Australian Society of Anaesthetists was something of a dogfish himself.

The letters

The letters, often six to eight pages long, reflect not only changing anaesthesia interests but also broad aspects of the world scene including social, geographic, economic, literary and political topics as well as personal concerns and frustrations. They contain detailed summaries of subjects heard at meetings and congresses attended with their frank critiques and evaluations of worth. The descriptive literary skills of Kaye paint vivid pictures of both Australian medical practice and geography as he travelled to various sections of the country in conjunction with his secretarial and organizational duties for anaesthesia. There are also case reports and vignettes describing observed incidents and experiences, as well as occasionally a visitor's impression of the foibles and practices of then prominent clinical anaesthetists.

In the audience attending this symposium are individuals perhaps better fitted to appreciation of the contents of these letters than any in the years to come for there are those here who were a part of the struggle, and part of the singular circumstances which made anaesthesia what it is today. For those who are younger, the letters will be a source of wonderment for the discussions centre upon techniques, concepts and principles ignored, forgotten, or absolutely taken for granted by later generations of anaesthetists. Many of the questions debated and the arguments pro and con are fundamental to understanding of origins of practices in present day anaesthetic services.

> *'Is excess of oxygen a good thing or a bad thing? Even in the pink patient does anaesthesia interfere with utilization of oxygen by tissues and cells?'*

> *'Can intubation really be satisfactorily performed under nitrous oxide alone? How many of our patients should be intubated? What size endotracheal tube should be used?'*

> *'Why was a higher incidence of post-operation pneumonia observed in Madison, Wisconsin than in Melbourne, Victoria? How prevalent is massive collapse of the lung?'*

> *'What effect did the differences between American and Australian surgeons have on the development of the specialty?'*

> *'Was certification of anaesthetists as specialists desirable or not?'*

The correspondence begins politely and formally, gradually relaxing to become completely open and sharing. The salutations of 'Dear Dr Waters' and 'Dear Dr Kaye' gave way only after several years to 'Dear Waters' and 'Dear Kaye'; eventually after his second visit to Madison in 1938, Kaye's greeting became rather regularly 'My Dear Dogfish'.

The following selected excerpts from the first decade may provide useful insight into the potential value of the file.

8 June, 1931

Dear Dr. Kaye:

Dr. Seevers, of the Pharmacology Department, has been . . . investigating the physiologic principles back in spinal anesthesia. . . . I think we can say, at the present time, that no case of spinal anesthesia need die as an immediate result of the anesthetic effect, provided proper artificial respiration is maintained.

Sincerely,
RMW

17 February, 1932

Dear Dr. Kaye:

. . . (We are reviewing) . . . about fifteen hundred cases of spinal anesthesia from the standpoint of post-anesthetic complications. The incidence is surprisingly and alarmingly high to me. . . . The trend (of this and other reports) . . . is that pulmonary complications are quite as frequent following spinal anesthesia as following the worst of the older types of ether administrations. . . . technique and management of spinal anesthesia cases is quite as important as that of inhalation anesthesia . . .

Sincerely,
RMW

3 April, 1932

Dear Dr. Waters:

Your letter of February 17th was delightful and calls for a prompt reply.

. . . Your remark as to the high incidence of post-operative complications after spinal anaesthesia is interesting, and I must ask my colleagues as to local impressions (I fear that local 'records' will be rather to seek). Myself, I do too few spinals to have data of any value . . .

Ever sincerely,
GK

28 February, 1932

Dear Dr. Waters:

One would never forgive oneself if one 'took a chance' . . . and things went agley. . . . it is a terrible thing to jeopardize a human life. For this reason, it is hard to teach students. Suppose I have a sick patient; how dare I entrust him to a student even though a student is entitled to learn to anaesthetize the very sick before he graduates? Again, I know that the student proposes to settle in . . . a locality where, if any anaesthetics be available at all, chloroform would be the only one. . . . Am I then to place a patients life in some jeopardy by giving him chloroform . . . purely that the student shall be taught . . .? I wish I knew the answer to all these questions; meanwhile, they are an obstacle in the path of hospital teaching.

Ever sincerely yours,
GK

12 April, 1932

My dear Dr. Kaye:

. . . (you ask) what we do in regard to teaching methods that we feel to be a disadvantage to one's own patients in order that students may have the experience . . . of open drop administration of ether. I used to sacrifice patient comfort . . . (for student experience but)

. . . I seldom do it now . . . (except for) occasional drop ether induction for tonsillectomy. I have come to the conclusion that if one gets the basic sciences, . . . the real physiology of respiration and circulation into their heads, the students will devise for themselves the mechanical means of conducting good anesthesia. I have had one or two students go out in small towns and rather surprise me at their ingenuity . . . one of them did . . . (use chloroform which in northern Wisconsin is) . . . as extensively used as it is in Australia. The modern youngster who comes from the basic science laboratories and who has not been taught open methods of anesthesia can be made to understand the rather simple technique of carbon dioxide absorption and can handle it somewhat easier than he can open methods. It is the fellow who has learned open (or other) methods first who finds it difficult to comprehend absorption technique.

Yours,
RMW

30 May, 1932

My Dear Dr. Waters:

. . . I am very interested in your views as to teaching of correct physiological principles to students (as against teaching open drop technique). . . . It . . . (is) . . . a standpoint so different from that held amongst us that I have to pause a while before making any comment. I never regarded myself as prejudiced, but I am not so sure now. My first reaction to something utterly different from my own and my colleague's practice is of a defensive character, revealing more prejudice than I knew I possessed.

Accept my best wishes
GK

4 October, 1932

Dear Kaye:

. . . Your slighting discussion of record systems interests me. We have long since come to the conclusion that our record system is rotten also. We get a great deal on paper here and file it away in the record rooms, but when we get it out, it is hopeless. A year ago, Tovell suggested the use of a punch card system like that used in business offices. We have spent the past six or eight months trying to get installed such a system here . . .

Yours,
RMW

20 November, 1933

Dear Kaye:

Our conclusion . . . was . . . that the preliminary investigation (of Cyclopropane) involving 450 cases justified a further careful study of the drug over a years period.

Yours,
RMW

4 September, 1934

Dear Kaye:

. . . We have an entirely new staff aside from Rovenstine since the first of the year, three of them new since the first of July. This means that both he and I can not be away at the same time. Doctor Schmidt will occupy our place on the program in Boston. We now have, in addition to Doctor Rovenstine, four excellent fellows who promise to do very superior work during the next four years. If they do not it will probably be my fault and not theirs. Breaking them into the routine of operating room technic, etc. however, is occupying most of the time now and very little investigative work is going on.

With very kindest regards, I am sincerely

RMW

15 October, 1934

Dear Waters:

. . . Our hospital has initiated post-graduate classes in practical anaesthesia, free to any who wish to attend. The response speaks well for the widening interest in the specialty . . . it means however, a good deal of work for the anaesthetic staff. . . . endotracheal gas anaesthesia . . . is becoming more an everyday procedure . . . (we are now trying) to establish as routine hospital services the methods which, a year or so ago, (were) the 'stunts' generally reserved for private practice.

Ever sincerely yours,
GK

1 May, 1935

Dear Kaye:

. . . There seem to be two of your letters unanswered. Perhaps . . . (because we have spent a lot of time) in the operating room. Rovenstine . . . left the first of January to try to start a similar organization at New York University Medical School. . . . I have stretched a point in letting another of the men on the service here help him out until January 1, 1936, thus our own service is deprived of experienced help.

. . . An electrocardiographic study of our one hundred cases with records taken before, every few minutes during, and ten hours after operation. This will be presented in Atlantic City by Dr. Kurtz, the hospital cardiologist. . . . The most startling (thing) being that very few cases indeed escape . . . change during anesthesia and operation to be worthy of note. Whether these changes are of great significance or not is difficult to tell, and whether they are due to agent, technique, or operative procedure is also difficult to be sure.

The total cases of cyclopropane up to date are I believe, in the neighborhood of four thousand. . . . for the years 1933 and 1934 the absorption technic constituted about 74% of our work . . .

. . . were you to come to the states again in the next few years, you will find anesthesia on a different basis than when you were here before. . . . On the whole the attitude decidedly favors professional anesthesia in most places. . . . There is a constant increasing interest on the part of medical societies and schools . . . (In our report) . . . a great deal of ether . . . was for tonsillectomies . . . in children and was given by open drop solely for training of senior students. Much of our work is influenced by teaching. . . . when it makes no difference (to patient care) . . . we often modify technic for teaching purposes.

With kindest regards and best wishes, I am sincerely,
RMW

8 January, 1936

Dear Kaye:

. . . I believe there is real progress being made for anesthesia in intrapleural work. . . . One of the . . . contributions . . . is what we call 'controlled respiration'. . . . That is the overventilation of a patient with the closed system so as to reduce the carbon dioxide content of the blood and tissue sufficiently to 'take the respirations away from' the patient. . . ., my impression is that much more physiologic conditions can be maintained . . . We have utilized such controlled respiration over periods as long as 2½ hours with the pleural cavity wide open. This of course, is always done with the closed endotracheal airway and practically always done with cyclopropane as the agent, although I have used a similar technic in upper abdominal work with ether anesthesia. When one thus controls the respiration himself, he can omit exchange for periods of time when the slightest movement of the lung would be an embarrassment to the surgeon. I think I can see the look of horror on your face after reading the above, nevertheless, I should like the opportunity of demonstrating it to you. There are many intriguing angles to such a technic.

Sincerely,
RMW

6 May, 1936

Dear Waters:

. . . I was very interested in your apnoeic stunt with CO_2 absorption. No, I have not the feelings of horror you impute to me. I can see that the apnoeia is got in a physiologic way and I shall be interested to try it.

. . . I admit that I have been too casual about absorption methods in the past . . . now to take them more seriously. I would like to see you at work again and intend to do so at the earliest opportunity.

Sincerely yours,
GK

11 January, 1937

Dear Waters:

. . . On the technical side, I have little to report except a growing call for endotracheal gas anaesthesia and (my) determined dislike for spinals in cases for which inhalational methods will do as well. . . . The new year brings some interesting little problems if I can find energy to work them out. . . . They have made me Lecturer in Anaesthesia at the University. The job, under the present curriculum, gives little scope for serious instruction but I hope to improve matters by degrees . . .

Cyclopropane has moved slowly in Australia, though Troup of Perth and Daly of Sydney have made a beginning. The rest of us are awaiting the results of your electrocardiographic studies. Ethylene has given such good results that our men are hesitant to change unless and until they appear to be able to do so safely.

Sincerely yours,
GK

5 May, 1937

My dear Kaye:

. . . The work here on cyclopropane has progressed very slowly. . . . (Dr. Meek) has, with the help of the various men on . . . (anesthesia service) . . . made a real contribution in a comparative study of cyclopropane, ether, and chloroform as to their cardiac effects as mirrored by the electrocardiograph. . . . Briefly, I think he has verified Levy that chloroform sensitizes to the effects of adrenalin and that deep cyclopropane may do likewise on occasion.

With kindest personal regards, I am sincerely,
RMW

28 July, 1937

Dear Waters:

Dr. Meek's work on cyclopropane seems to be 'the goods' and should do much to explain the cardiotoxic properties of this gas . . . The sudden and rather alarming cardiac syncopes reported with cyclopropane are thus brought into line with our old friend, 'primary cardiac inhibition' under chloroform. The name of Embley is taken as covering just about the last word on chloroform in Australia. . . . his (explanation of a) vagal overflow mechanics for chloroform syncope . . . when the anus is dilated, the prepuce clamped, or similar 'reflexigenous area' disturbed under light chloroform anesthesia . . . does not explain, however, deaths which occur in the induction phase before the patient is in any way interfered with . . . It has seemed to me that Levy's idea of ventricular fibrillation come nearer to explaining such incidents than could Embley's vagal irritability. . . . Dr. Meek would seem to have provided the connecting link, both in the case of chloroform and of cyclopropane. It seems a nice bit of research.

Ever sincerely,
GK

22 October, 1937

Dear Kaye:

. . . So far as I know, Dr. Meek has turned up nothing that would make one wish to question Embley's work. I hope you have not misunderstood Meek's work to prove that those difficulties are vagal in origin. It is much deeper than that and involves the irritability of . . . the ventricle itself, I think. Dr. Meek has not verified Levy's work in that he seems to find that really high concentrations of chloroform are essential to the ventricular fibrillation phenomenon. What probably happened in Levy's experiment was the effect of a single (breath of) high concentration after breath holding which he considered to have happened under light anesthesia. That, you remember, was John Snow's attitude.

. . . your statement that you will concentrate on undergraduates in the future, agrees with my own belief. I came here solely with the idea that . . . (for) . . . the future, it must start at the foundations and let the students know what anesthesia really means. The basic principle(s) of anesthesia must be translated from physiology and pharmacology to clinical medicine by a physician . . . the difficulty with getting . . . across to students . . . is in the correlation of their basic science training with the problems of clinical medicine and I do not hesitate to try to teach them the care of respiratory and circulatory emergencies in medicine whether or not they are related to definite problems of anesthesia. No one else on the clinical staff seems to serve this function and therefore I think it is up to the anesthetist. I am sure that such an attitude does no harm to anesthesia . . . and I think help is offered to the internist and the neurologist thereby.

With kindest personal regards, I am yours,

RMW

10 March, 1939

Dear Kaye:

. . . I should only like to leave with you the idea that . . . very slight mistakes in the construction of apparatus can result in very marked physiologic effects on occasion. The matter of the dead space in the mask is at present our chief worry. . . . particularly models for wee youngsters.

(There is) no need for selecting cases in which to use absorption technic provided the equipment is not at fault. There is no physiologic reason why the absorption technic should be less applicable to one patient than another. I can agree with you however, that if the absorption technic is giving poor satisfaction some other technic should be tried because the way the absorption technic is being used on this occasion is at fault and it may be impossible to find the fault. The absorption technic as such, if properly applied mechanically and chemically, is applicable in my estimation to anesthesia for all patients.

Sincerely,

RMW

23 March, 1939

My dear dogfish,

I am a rotten correspondent, but must plead pressure of many affairs.

. . . (After return) to Melbourne at the New Year I plunged straight into the university lecturing season and 'spoke my piece' on the requisite number of occasions, to the boredom of the students and the admiration of all beholders generally . . .

It has been an unusually important year from the teaching angle, in that Faculty had it in mind to wash out the university lectureship and to substitute three hospital lectureships . . . (fortunately) the Dean of the Faculty is against the proposal and it looks as though little more will be heard of it. . . . One of these days . . . there will be a Melbourne University Hospital with a proper Department of Anaesthesia. This is a goal for which we have to aim and, to aid in its realization, I mean to keep the teaching of anaesthesia as centralized as possible, and as closely in the University's hands as I can.

. . . (The new army midget anaesthesia) machine was delivered last week, and I sent the first one down to a public hospital . . . I thought the best test was not that given by a trained anaesthetist (who ought to be able to give a decent anaesthetic with two pickle bottles if necessary) but an untrained hospital resident . . . if the interns could use the apparatus, the army might too be able to do so . . .

I had just got over the fuss and bother with the army machine when they decided to hold a meeting of the Australian Society of Anaesthetists in Melbourne in April. That gives me a fortnight to work up a programme . . .

. . . Troup is the first of the interstate men to reach Melbourne. He arrived today, dined with me this evening, and then went on to a Congress of the Royal Australian College of Physicians . . . He (Troup) is a splendid chap and I hope that he will be president of the Australian Society of Anaesthetists for the coming year . . . at any rate, he deserves it.

. . . I have been, I fear, permanently 'grounded' as an airman; more stringent regulations have come into force, and, unless I can find someway of circumventing the regulations regarding visual efficiency, I may not be allowed to handle a 'stick' again in Australia. Renton's mother died and he got pretty run down and went away for a holiday, so that I have to do his work for him . . .

Finally, as a last straw, my cat has got diarrhoea and is trying to ruin my carpets. It has an unholy proficiency in escaping from confinements, reaching my study and there expressing its feelings on the matter.

The political horizon can only be described as lousy. . . . I think the world is mad. . . . I trust that my gloom is due rather to the cat's diarrhoea than to the true picturing of world events.

Ever sincerely,
GK

27 April, 1939

Dear Kaye:

. . . Your delightful letter was most gratefully received.

. . . You're a sly old owl—a littler bird than an owl has told me that ground was broken the other day for the new Melbourne University Hospital and I know you will have a real place to work and a real department before you know it.*

Your program for the meetings looks inviting. I agree with your estimate of Troup.

. . . A special outfit for one method (technic) or one drug, means you have to decide ahead of time what you are going to do in a given case. This I do not admit is right. One should be free to change at a moments notice both technic and agent at all times. So you see, eventually your modified army model is the only solution or else a single operating suite in which to work. Preferably the latter, of course.

Now as to the cat. I'm for her hook, line, and sinker. If one had cats enough about the house and they all had diarrhea, one wouldn't care whether the world went to war or not. Would one? Mean time, I'm interested in what Seevers can find out for us as to the effects of excess and the opposite of carbon dioxide in the body, the same for oxygen, a new way of contacting a closed breathing unit with the respiratory tract, possibly a new chemical absorber for soda lime and all the rest of the things we ought to know and do but have never known or done.

My best to the cat.

Yours,
RMW

The serial exchange of letters between these two men may be one of the most important collections of documents in the history of modern anaesthesia. They illustrate quite vividly the evolution of anaesthesia to become a recognized specialty. The struggles to gain recognition for anaesthesia were quite different in the USA and Australia, and these letters provide information that for anyone undertaking the future task of analysing world development of the specialty will be essential to the understanding of the early problems.

---

*The University of Melbourne does not yet have a professorial department of anaesthetics, so Kaye's hopes have still not been realized nearly fifty years later.

Reference

(1) Gillespie Noel A. Ralph Milton Waters: a brief biography. *Br J Anaesth* 1949; **21**: 197–214.

25.16   The contribution of two Brazilian physiologists to the
introduction of carbon dioxide absorption into clinical anaesthesia
An acknowledgment by Ralph M. Waters (1883–1979)

CARLOS PARSLOE
Hospital Samaritano, São Paulo, Brazil

On 22 October, 1923, Ralph Waters presented a paper during the Second Annual Congress of the National Anesthesia Research Society in joint meeting with the Interstate, Midwestern and Chicago Anesthetists at the Auditorium Hotel in Chicago. Its title was 'Clinical scope and utility of carbon dioxide filtration in inhalation anesthesia'. That paper, subsequently published (1), had all the prerequisites of a seminal paper: it was short, had one diagrammatic sketch of the carbon dioxide filtration technique and only 3 references.

The 1923 paper

Waters listed the practical results of the new technique under four headings, economy, convenience, welfare of patient and limitations. Under welfare of patients he stated: 'Body heat and moisture.

> *'Body heat and moisture are not lost. The use of filters has changed my attitude toward rebreathing. The principle of fractional rebreathing as held by McKesson, causing the patient to rebreathe approximately his excess tidal air over waking conditions seemed sound if one accepts Henderson's work on carbon dioxide. I believe now, however, that this benefit was not due to retained carbon dioxide, but to retained heat and moisture. This belief is supported by work published from a Rio de Janeiro laboratory some time ago inferring that Henderson's results in which he caused shock in dogs by means of induced hyperpnea, were due, not to excessive loss of carbon dioxide, but to loss of body heat and moisture. Attempts to duplicate Henderson's findings in Rio de Janeiro failed because of the warm, humid condition of the air in the Brazilian laboratory.' (1)*

The Henderson theory of shock

The concept of carbon dioxide filtration was diametrically opposed to the accepted physiological teaching of the time led by Yandell Henderson who introduced the theory that shock was caused by the loss of carbon dioxide from the body due to hyperventilation, a condition which had been called 'acapnia' by the Italian physiologist from Turin, Angelo Mosso. Rebreathing of expired air during inhalation anaesthesia had become an accepted practice since it conserved carbon dioxide, therefore supposedly preventing the appearance of shock. The regulation of breathing by carbon dioxide, as clearly shown by Haldane and co-workers in 1905 (2) lent impetus to Henderson's theory.

In 1906 Henderson at Yale University was attempting to record the volume curves of the heart. His laboratory possessed a 'minimum of apparatus, and in particular none for artificial respiration' (3). Here are the beginnings of the acapnic theory of shock as written by Henderson:

> 'In order to permit the placing of the cardiometer over the heart, it was necessary to open the thorax widely. Under these conditions the lungs collapse and it was necessary to blow air into them, so as to keep them distended, as well as to maintain respiration. To meet these requirements we had only a leaky hand bellows, and the janitor, who worked that implement for me, was compelled to keep up a rapid succession of pulmonary inflations; the lungs undergoing a considerable deflation between strokes. The overventilation was therefore tremendous—much greater than is possible before the chest is opened; and the animals quickly went into collapse and died. And the fact that was most striking was that the more energetic the janitor was with the bellows, the more rapidly the animals collapsed. Thus it appeared that an acute acapnia, simply from overventilation of the lungs, may cause failure on the circulation . . . From this beginning the use of rebreathing in connection with anesthesia made its way in a few years (between 1909 and 1919) into many surgical clinics and effected a notable decrease of anesthetic accidents and postoperative depression. It was a first step toward the control of the gaseous exchange that is the key to the control of respiration: a control that every capable anesthetist now maintains.' (3) [In 1905 Haldane, Priestley and Douglas] published their epoch-making studies on the part that carbon dioxide plays in the normal control of respiration as they demonstrated, the regulation of the volume of breathing by carbon dioxide is so precise that normal respiration maintains a nearly uniform concentration of carbon dioxide in the air of the lungs. So precise, indeed, is this regulation that even a slight decrease in the so-called "alveolar carbon dioxide" automatically induces a temporary decrease of even a cessation of respiration: the so-called apnea vera. . . . I undertook to extend this conception into the abnormal field, and in particular to analyse the problem of respiration under anesthesia. For this I was fortunately placed. It happened that, as my students then received no other instructions on experimental pharmacology, I had introduced as much of the subject as I could into my laboratory course in physiology. I believed—and I still believe—that no young doctor is really competent to administer anesthesia until he has been responsible—and has been duly rebuked—for causing a death under anesthesia: the death of a cat. . . . And in learning the importance of uniform anesthesia and how to administer it, those students afforded me opportunities to see a far larger number of deaths under anesthesia than (I am sure) any of my many friends among professional anesthetists have ever caused or witnessed. . . . Only yesterday a little girl two years old caught her hand in a washing machine. Taken to the accident room of the hospital this scared and suffering child was anesthetized and passed into a fatal apnea . . . (The excuse of course is "status lymphaticus" or some other fault of the patient; the intern responsible had never killed a cat). . . .' (3)

On 6 December, 1909, Henderson addressed the John Hopkins' Hospital Society. The topic was 'Fatal apnea and the shock problem.' He wrote:

> 'I pointed out the importance of rapid induction of anesthesia, avoidance of anxiety and excitement, use of preliminary morphine (then rare), and prevention of overventilation by means of rebreathing. In concluding I reported that I had tried a new method of resuscitation upon dogs during apnea with strikingly successful results. It consists in administering air or oxygen containing 5 or 6% of CO_2 and starting the subject to breathing by one or two artificial respirations.' (3)

The concept of acapnia as a major factor in disturbed physiology was enlarged by Henderson to explain more than failure of circulation through failure of the 'venopressor mechanism'. Acapnia became considered one of the dangers of anaesthesia leading to apnoea and causing, as a consequence, anoxia; anoxia, in turn, who lead to acapnia. This concept and the expanded role of acapnia as the explanation of fatal apnoea during anaesthesia and of shock after laparotomy, was accepted throughout the 1910–1930 decades. With Haggard, Henderson introduced mixtures of carbon dioxide and oxygen in the treatment of asphyxia, to restore vitality and to prevent pulmonary complications after surgical operations, to resuscitate asphyxiated newborns and as a treatment for carbon monoxide poisoning. Inhalation of mixtures of carbon dioxide and oxygen were widely practised throughout the world in the prevention and relief of postoperative atelectasis.

Yandell Henderson, a well known professor of physiology at Yale and a pioneer American Respiratory Physiologist, had conceived and developed the acapnic theory of shock which became widely accepted. As a consequence, the use of 'closed' techniques to administer inhalation anaesthetics was widely practised. In those days a 'closed' technique meant a rebreathing bag with provision for admission of air or oxygen and deliberate rebreathing of exhaled carbon dioxide in order to prevent its loss from the body. The 'open' technique was considered dangerous for the ever present possibility of apnoea due to hyperventilation and consequent decreased alveolar carbon dioxide (4).

Ralph Waters, an unknown clinician from Sioux City, Iowa, in the United States, was proposing a radically different concept of 'closed' administration of inhalation anaesthesia. In his apparatus all gases and vapours were rebreathed except carbon dioxide, which was removed by soda-lime contained in the 'filter'. This concept challenged the accepted rebreathing techniques and indeed was a direct suggestion that Henderson's theory was wrong.

Waters's references

An analysis of the references in Waters's paper, that offered him support for this radical conceptual change is revealing. He first quoted Jackson's two original papers on carbon dioxide absorption during anaesthesia in animals, published in 1915 and 1916 (5)(6) which Waters simplified by the use of granular soda-lime and extended into clinical practice. The second consisted of two papers by Henderson's and co-workers on acapnia and shock, published in 1915 and 1917 which supported rebreathing of carbon dioxide during inhalation anaesthesia (7,8). But it was the third reference that gave Waters the physiological basis to use carbon dioxide filtration. It was entitled 'The nature of surgical shock and Henderson's theory of acapnia' and was published in 1918 (9) by two Brazilian brothers, both physiologists, Alvaro and Miguel Ozorio de Almeida, who, during the summer of 1912 in their laboratory in Rio de Janeiro, Brazil, had repeated Henderson's hyperventilation experiments in dogs with negative results.

The Brazilian paper

The Ozorio Almeida brothers employed respiratory rates of 200 per minute during several hours with closed and bilaterally open thoracies in dogs. No state of shock developed in their animals and those which did not have an open chest were able to recover and walk at the end of the experiment—apnoea persisting only a few minutes. The brothers reasoned that all determinants of the state of shock as described by Henderson had not been taken into account and some factor must have escaped his observation (10).

They argued further that, *a priori*, taking into consideration physical factors, hyperventilation would lead to cooling of the animal. Such cooling theoretically would be a function of 5 factors, the temperature of inspired air, its degree of humidity, the quantity of air passing into the lungs per minute, the quantity of heat capable of being produced by the animal in unit of time as a defence against cooling and the mass of the animal—that is, the quantity of heat produced (proportional to the dog's mass) that was accumulated (10). Cooling of the dogs would lead to coma, death occurring when the central temperature reached a sufficiently low degree. Close examination of Henderson's and their own experimental protocol led them to single out 'climate' as the different factor in the two instances (10). Their initial experiments had been performed in January (summer in Brazil) when the temperature of the air in Rio de Janeiro:

'frequently ranges from 32 to 34°C (89.6 to 93.2F) during the day and its percentage of humidity is always very high. . . . In our experiments there was evident formation of acapnia without the slightest change of the internal temperature of the animal, and, moreover the state of shock did not occur.' (9)

They argued further that, *a priori*, taking into consideration physical factors, hyperventilation would lead to cooling of the animal. Such cooling theoretically would be a function of five factors, the temperature of inspired air, its degree of humidity, the quantity of air passing into the lungs per minute, the quantity of heat capable of being produced by the animal in unit of time as a defence against cooling and the mass of the animal—that is, the quantity of heat produced (proportional to the dog's mass) that was accumulated (10). Cooling of the dogs would lead to coma, death occuring when the central temperature reached a sufficiently low degree. Close examination of Henderson's and their own experimental protocol led them to single out 'climate' as the different factor in the two instances (10). Their initial experiments had been performed in January (summer in Brazil) when the temperature of the air in Rio de Janeiro:

> *'frequently ranges from 32 to 34°C (89.6 to 93.2F) during the day and its percentage of humidity is always very high. . . . In our experiments there was evident formation of acapnia without the slightest change of the internal temperature of the animal, and, moreover the state of shock did not occur.'* (9)

After those initial negative results they proceeded to hyperventilate dogs with artificially produced cold air (18°C (64.4F) with 30 to 40% relative humidity) resembling the ambient conditions existing in the North American laboratory. Under those experimental conditions their animals became hypothermic, developed a state of coma and died.

They concluded that dogs hyperventilated with the warm and humid summer air of Rio de Janeiro lost carbon dioxide but did not lose heat and water vapour. Whereas dogs hyperventilated with cold, dry air, lost body heat and moisture along with carbon dioxide. Therefore, the cause of shock could not be acapnia as suggested by Henderson, which existed on both sets of experiments, but rather the loss—of heat and water which occurred only in the ambient conditions of the New Haven laboratory or artificially produced in Rio de Janeiro. They further explained Henderson's failure to cause 'shock' when mechanical dead space was added, by stating that it was not due to preservation of carbon dioxide but by the avoidance of heat and water loss.

> *'The air exhaled from the lungs, charged with humidity and at high temperature, was reinjected at each new compression of the bellows thus avoiding cooling of the experimental animal.'* (10)

The results and conclusions of this work, published in 1913 in French (10), did not come to the attention of English speaking physiologists. With the growing importance of the shock problem during World War I they decided to publish in 1918 a résumé of their work in English in the *Journal of the American Medical Association* (9). This was the paper that caught the attention of Ralph Waters. The main conclusions were:

> *'1. Excessive and prolonged artificial respiration produces coma and death only when it is made with air having a sufficiently low temperature and humidity. 2. If the temperature and humidity of the air are sufficiently raised, the respiration may be prolonged indefinitely without obtaining this result. 3. Since the conditions described in the preceding paragraph produce strong acapnia, it is clear that this state has no relation to coma. 4. It was the coma resulting from the internal cooling of the animal that Henderson confused with a state of shock. 5. The continuous failure of Henderson to obtain what he thought was shock, when respiration was made with air already once breathed, proves that under such conditions it is impossible to obtain the internal cooling of the animal because expired air is saturated with moisture and has a relatively high temperature.'* (9)

Waters's application of the Brazilian results

It is a tribute to Ralph Waters's capacity for critical analysis that, knowing nothing about those two physiologists working in faraway Brazil, he was sufficiently wise to accept their correct interpretation of the results of the hyperventilation experiments. Thus, on the basis of work in animals, Waters introduced into clinical anaesthesia a technique which provided absorption of expired carbon dioxide. It was obvious that carbon dioxide filtration during anaesthesia did not cause shock in his patients. In 1927 Waters wrote:

'We have for several years used a technique in which a filter for carbon dioxide is interposed between the mask and a rebreathing bag, allowing complete rebreathing of anesthetic mixtures with the addition only of enough oxygen to supply metabolic needs. When using this technique, rebreathing of some 200 cc of each inspiration takes place, this much being contained in the mask and filter between the soda lime and the face. We have long noticed that this technique gave us quite an ideal respiratory rate and volume in the average case.' (11)

Was this statement his lenient way of not antagonizing the proponents of rebreathing? In only two instances Ralph Waters made reference to Yandell Henderson's theory. In 1927 he wrote:

'Fortunately, and unfortunately, the researches in carbon dioxide of the New Haven school of physiologists have entered the literature of anaesthesia in the past decade: fortunately, because these researches are brilliant and have taught us many facts of the greatest importance; unfortunately, because the facts have been made use of by practical anaesthetists in some quarters to make easy their work without sufficient investigation as to what by-effects may accompany the altered physiology which their method induce.' (11)

And on 23 June, 1937, he read a paper at a meeting of the Canadian Medical Association, Section of Anaesthesia, in Ottawa and stated:

'Henderson deduced from his experiments that surgical shock results from low carbon dioxide in the blood and tissues; that low carbon dioxide in the blood and tissues is a usual accompaniment of anaesthesia; and that hyperventilation of the lungs by the use of carbon dioxide and oxygen mixtures should prevent post-operative pulmonary atelectasis. All three of these deductions are fallacious.' (12)

The controversy between fractional rebreathing and carbon dioxide absorption in inhalation anaesthesia ended with the statement which appeared in *Fundamentals of Anesthesia* (13) clearly reflecting Waters's thinking:

'Carbon dioxide is a waste product, do not hinder its excretion without a purpose in doing so. Depletion of carbon dioxide does not *cause shock.'*

It is interesting to conjecture: 1. If the brothers Álvaro and Miguel Ozorio de Almeida had not published their work in English, would Ralph Waters have introduced carbon dioxide filtration into clinical anaesthesia? Certainly at the time no work, published in English, challenged Henderson's theory and it made sense to use fractional rebreathing during inhalation anaesthesia. 2. Did Ralph Waters in 1923 realize the impact of his new technique on anaesthesia? Would he be surprised to find it still being used daily, 64 years later, all over the world and presently undergoing a period of renewed interest? Indeed, absorption of carbon dioxide is the only true universal anaesthesia system—the level of alveolar carbon dioxide being independent of fresh gas flow and an inverse function of the degree of alveolar ventilation, which is indirectly under the control of the anaesthesiologist.

Conclusion

In the introduction of carbon dioxide absorption into clinical anaesthesia four professors played a major role. One was a pharmacologist, Jackson, and three were physiologists, Henderson and the brothers Ozorio de Almeida. But it was a clinician, Ralph Waters, who developed the physiological concept of anaesthesia. In his brain and hands the old 'closed' system lost its asphyxial or hypercapnic properties to become a normoxic and normocapnic technique. For the first time the rebreathing bag was used to rebreathe oxygen and anaesthetics but not carbon dioxide. Antiphysiological rebreathing had become physiological by the removal of carbon dioxide, an anathema at the time. Anaesthesia had entered its modern period. For as long as carbon dioxide absorption is used, the name of Ralph Waters will be remembered, but the acapnic theory of shock is only past history.

References

(1) Waters RM. Clinical scope and utility of carbon dioxide filtration in inhalation anesthesia. *Curr Res Anesth Analg* 1924; **3**: 20–2.
(2) Haldane JS, Priestley JG. *Respiration.* 2nd Ed. Oxford. Oxford University Press, 1935.
(3) Henderson Y. *Adventures in respiration. Modes of asphyxiation and methods of resuscitation.* Baltimore: Williams and Wilkins Co, 1938: 16–25.
(4) Gatch WD. The use of rebreathing in the administration of anesthetics. In: Gwathmey JT, ed. *Anesthesia.* New York: D. Appleton and Co, 1914: 100–16.
(5) Jackson DE. A new method for the production of general analgesia and anaesthesia with a description of the apparatus used. *J Lab Clin Med* 1915; **1**: 1–12.
(6) Jackson DE. An experimental investigation of the pharmacological action of nitrous oxide. *Intern J Orthodontia* 1916; **2**: 544–62.
(7) Henderson Y, Bryant J. Closed ether and a color sign. *JAMA* 1915; **65**: 1.
(8) Henderson Y, Haggard HW, Prince AL. Observations on Surgical Shock. *JAMA* 1917; **69**: 965.
(9) Osorio de Almeida A, Osorio de Almeida M. The nature of surgical shock and Henderson's theory of acapnia. *JAMA* 1918; **71**: 1710–1.*
(10) Ozorio de Almeida A, Ozorio de Almeida M. Véritable cause du coma produit par la respiration artificielle excessive et prolongée.*
(11) Waters RM. Carbon dioxide: its place in anaesthesia. *Can Med Assoc J* 1927; **17**: 1510–3.
(12) Waters RM. Carbon dioxide. *Can Med Assoc J* 1938; **38**: 240–3.
(13) Subcommittee on Anesthesia of Division of Medical Sciences, National Research Council. *Fundamentals of anesthesia, an outline.* 2nd Ed. Chicago: American Medical Association Press, 1944: 21.

*Reference 10 gives the correct spelling Ozorio whereas reference 9, the paper translated into English, gives an incorrect spelling with *s* instead of *z*.

25.17   Arno Benedict Luckhardt and the introduction of ethylene

JOHN B. STETSON
Rush Presbyterian—St Luke's Medical Center, Chicago, Illinois, USA

Luckhardt was born 26 August, 1885, in Chicago. His parents had emigrated from Germany to have their family in the 'New World'. Unfortunately, his father Gustav Adolph (a pharmacist)

died 21 February, 1887, of 'apoplexy'. His mother, Aurelia (Weber) supported her sons Albert Edmund and Hilmar Eric (ABL's baptismal names) by teaching and tutoring. Another son, Ernst, had died at age 2 of diphtheria. As the German school at which she taught was in a poor neighbourhood, in 1897, she sent her sons to board at Conception Abbey, a Benedictine Monastery in Missouri. ABL learned the classics, enjoyed what little free time he had, and later confided to his nephew he had had enough religion at Conception to last the rest of his life.

In 1903, he left Conception and matriculated at the University of Chicago:

> *'It was a hot day. I had waited a long time. Finally I got to a table where a woman asked me to fill out a card; I did, and wrote my name simply as "Luckhardt". . . . "We have to have more than that. What is your first name?" I had never like the name, Hilmar, so I hesitated. ". . . let me have your initials . . ." . . . I answered, "A" that being the first letter of the alphabet. "Fine . . . give me another," so I gave her "B". Later I expanded the initials to Arno, an old family name, and Benedict, the saintly man. . .'*

His mother did not approve; later he named his first born son Hilmar Francis to placate her (1). He earned the BS in 1906, MS, 1908, PhD, 1911, and MD Rush Medical College (then an integral part of the University of Chicago) in 1912. He was Phi Beta Kappa and Sigma Xi.

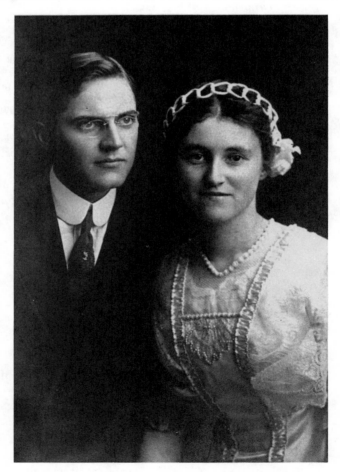

Figure 1   Arno B. Luckhardt and Luella La Bolle, 1912.

In 1908, he and friends started the University of Chicago Chapter of Gamma Alpha, a Graduate Scientific Fraternity. The students ate dinner together, then played cards. Dr William Crocker, a plant physiologist, often played whist with them. Dr Crocker and Mr Lee I. Knight, at the request of Wisconsin carnation growers, were studying the poisonous effects of illuminating gas on budding and flowering carnations. The gas was toxic to the flowers, 1:40 000 in air; ethylene, a component of the gas, was toxic at a concentration of 1:2 000 000 in air. ABL stored this information in his memory.

In graduation year (1912) he married Luella Catherine LaBolle of Somonauk, Illinois (Fig. 1). The local newspaper devoted a great deal of space to Ms LaBolle; of ABL it was noted:

> 'The groom is a Professor in the University of Chicago, but so far as I know, he has always acted the part of a gentleman.' (2)

Actually, at that time, ABL was an instructor (asst. prof. 1914, assoc. prof. 1920, prof. 1923, chairman 1941). ABL's older brother Albert Edmund married Luella's sister, Ruby, forming a very close family.

ABL did a very short stint of family practice (perhaps to earn money) after graduation, but the rest of his career was at the University of Chicago in the physiology department. For recreation, he did play one game of golf (25 September, 1911). He wore a stiff white collar, a white bow tie, and a pince-nez with a gold chain going around his left ear (2). His hobbies were horticulture, a rock garden, medical history (and the associated rare books), the life of Dr William Beaumont, and during the summer, Wabigama Country Club in northern Michigan.

ABL, the famous Dr A. J. Carlson ('Ajax'), and some associates had a joint vacation area (W. C.C.). His children (Hilmar Francis—later music faculty, University of Wisconsin, Paul Gregory—later a geologist and Mary Aurelia Miesse—still alive) went there for 'fifty summers' where their father had them tend vegetable and flower gardens. The men did not shave while at W. C.C.. ABL picked up guests at the train station with whiskers, red 'long johns' showing, in a red model 'T' Ford with 'WABIGAMA COUNTRY CLUB' painted on the side and milkweed hanging from all corners.

Ethylene

At the University of Chicago ABL spent long hours in the laboratory. In 1918, an associate, R. C. Thompson, generated ethylene, and the gas was tried on frogs and white rats. Unlike carnations, castor bean plants, and flowering sweet peas, they were not affected. The ethylene was increased, and at 90% ethylene, 10% oxygen, the frogs and rats 'seemed to go to sleep.'

Animal experiments

World War I slowed down ABL's investigation of ethylene. In 1922, J. Bailey Carter, a student (who after medical qualification became an internist and ultimately a Professor at Rush Medical College), carried on the research with ABL. Frogs, mice, rats, guinea pigs, kittens, and dogs were studied. Carter did comparative quantitative studies of ethylene-oxygen versus nitrous oxide-oxygen (3). Dogs were anaesthetized with a closed carbon dioxide absorption system as developed by Dennis Jackson (4).

Human experiments

The investigators were now ready for human trials. On Sunday, 21 January, 1923, ABL '. . . as a dutiful husband, took the family to church,' but he did not note if he attended the service as, 'then went to the physiological laboratory, where I met Carter' (3). Using a Clark gas apparatus, ABL anaesthetized Carter (Carter was anaesthetized first as he was not married—personal communication from Mrs J. B. Carter). Carter then anaesthetized ABL. During the animal experiments the ethylene had been laboriously made by the interaction of absolute alcohol and phosphoric acid (under the direction of Professor Fred C. Koch) to produce a pure product (5). ABL and Carter used 'Calorene' as sold for welding (99% ethylene, 1% unknown) on each other! ABL knew if he could persuade Dr A. J. Carlson ('Ajax'), the head of the department, to join the experiment, he would 'volunteer' others.

In the trials, the subject raised his arm from a reclining position while taking the ethylene and the falling of the arm was the end point. ABL felt he knew Ajax's preferences so he gave him ethylene 'straight' (ethylene is gaseous dehydrated ethyl alcohol). Ajax's arm hit the wall with a loud crack and ABL did not know if he should call a surgeon or a mason. After a minute or two Ajax awoke and claimed he was 'analyzing his experiences' but not asleep. A second trial was made and a pin put through his toe (personal communication, Mrs Carter). Ajax then 'volunteered' J. Blumenstock, A. C. Siedan, N. Kleitmann, and K. Phillips. All had eaten and they smoked and lit matches in the tiny room (Sunday is obviously a good day for dangerous experiments). On 28 January, ABL and Carter anaesthetized each other for ten minutes and C. Johnson, T. Boyd, and G. Turner for five minutes each. On 4 February, ABL was anaesthetized by Carter while the surgeons Dallas B. Phemister and Eugene Cary watched. The surgeons were then anaesthetized and Carter 'kept under' for fifteen minutes (again, all had consumed large breakfasts).

Isabella C. Herb, Professor of Anaesthesiology at Rush, reminisced:

> *'One day during commencement exercises, a voice behind me, in a sort of stage whisper, said, "Dr. Herb, I wish that you would come over to the laboratory of physiology. I want to demonstrate the anesthetic property of a gas I have been investigating." I turned around to see who the speaker was, as I did not recognize the voice, and was surprised to see the earnest, almost pathetically eager face of a young man whom I had seen occupying a seat in the college a few years before.'* (6)

Dr Herb was ill for two weeks, then on Sunday, 11 March, 1923, she and anaesthesiologists, Mary Lyons and Frances Haines attended a demonstration with eight other surgeons and physicians.

Clinical trials

Three days later ABL stood by at Presbyterian Hospital as Herb (Fig. 2) administered ethylene to a young man while Dr Arthur Dean Bevan removed sebaceous tumours from his scalp (shades of Crawford Long!). By 1 October, 1923, a thousand ethylene:oxygen anaesthetics had been administered at Presbyterian Hospital to patients aged from 3 to 88 years. No premedication was employed, but Herb administered 90% ethylene and 10% oxygen.

Gastrectomies were performed under ethylene:oxygen anaesthesia (the patients were wasted from their disease). When necessary ether was added, but in reading the articles the impression is gained that there was an attempt to do everything with ethylene:oxygen alone to prove its values. In a bit over a year ABL was author or co-author of a half dozen articles and the chapter on ethylene anaesthesia in the second edition of James Taylor Gwathmey's text (*Anesthesia*, N.Y: Macmillan, 1924).

Carter and ABL were offered $2 000 000 by a group of patent lawyers, but refused because of professional ethics. They gave the drug to the public gratis, then discovered: 'What one gives for nothing is worth just that much' (3). Although many people quickly adopted ethylene (one of the best early papers was by John S. Lundy of the Mayo Clinic who had been Herb's student, but never gave less than 20% oxygen (7)), there were many who were critical of the drug (a generation later curare received the same treatment).

The explosion hazard was cited (clinically useful ranges of dosing are *not* explosive). Although ether explosions and fires were not reported, ethylene ones received wide news coverage. Some said thyroid patients receiving iodine therapy would iodinate the molecule after inhalation. ABL studied halogenated ethylenes and demonstrated their lack of clinical effect and the types of toxic symptoms that would appear if they were present (4).

Nitrous oxide manufacturers were against ethylene (as could be expected) and charged three times as much for it as for nitrous oxide. The worst misadventure was an untried manufacturing system that left carbon monoxide as a contaminant. Several patients died. Reading 'between the lines' of some of ABL's later published talks, one gained the impression comments were

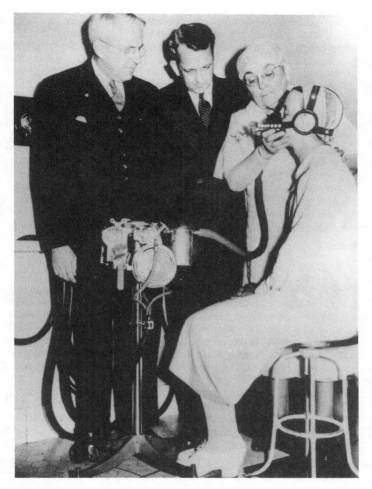

Figure 2   Arno B. Luckhardt, J. Bailey Carter, and Isabella C. Herb posing with a McKesson gas machine. Presbyterian Hospital, Chicago. Date unknown.

made to him suggesting that if he had patented ethylene, he could have controlled the quality of the product. He was also criticized for being a 'guinea pig'. ('What would become of your family if anything happened to you?') Poor ABL; guilt for being great.

In 1928, ABL received the Scroll of Recognition from the International Anesthesia Research Society (6) and in 1933 he was Honorary President of this society (8). In his Presidential address he noted a report of one death per 332 721 ethylene administrations and another report of a million administrations without an explosion: ethylene was safe. ABL said his reward for his discovery was letters from grateful patients.

Luckhardt's other interests

In the mid-1930s cyclopropane came into use and interest in ethylene waned except among those anaesthesiologists who were adept in its employment and did not seek relaxation (excellent for thyroids, mastectomy, and other superficial operations). As ABL pointed out, he had 'blundered into this field solely because of idle curiosity of the pharmacological action of . . .' ethylene. He had many other interests.

In his handwritten résumé forms on file at the University of Chicago, he placed his parathyroid and secretion research ahead of ethylene in importance.

ABL was sympathetic to the problems of dentists and delineated the physiological effects of adrenaline-procaine solutions (9). He was a charter member (1930) of the Council on Dental Therapeutics of the American Dental Association and served on the Council until 1948. He was President of the American Physiological Society, 1932–1934 as well as President of the Federation of American Societies for Experimental Biology and Medicine in 1934. As a Rockefeller fellow, he visited Germany in 1924–25.

His interest in medical history has been noted. He collaborated with James Henry Breasted in the interpretation of the Edwin Smith surgical papyrus (2 vols. Chicago, University of Chicago Press, 1930). His extensive collection of Beaumontiana was given to the Beaumont Museum at Prairie Du Chien, Wisconsin. When lecturing to the medical students about gastric physiology, he would have a gastric tube in place so the students could sample his digestive juices to confirm Beaumont's discoveries.

The title of his 1930 talk, 'Historical High Lights and Shadows in the Discovery of General Anesthesia' (10), is a reflection of his feelings about the ether controversy. He was frank to admit his hero worship of Edmund Andrews who introduced nitrous oxide:oxygen mixtures (11).

Conclusion

ABL retired in 1950, but continued to consult for a pharmaceutical company. Several years later he had a CVA, but his mind remained bright. In November, 1957, he was invited to Florida to receive an Honorary Membership in the American Dental Association. As he had never been to Florida and had not been feeling well, he looked forward to the trip and Florida sun. Two days after this honour (6 November) he died. He is said to have choked on a piece of lobster (personal communication from Mary Luckhardt Miesse); perhaps as a residual of his CVA he had a poor cough reflex. His extensive library, at the suggestion of Logan Clendening was sold so that others could enjoy the rare volumes and his estate receive the funds. His bookplate, a bespectacled jackass in mortar board and academic gown with the seal of the University of Chicago is well known among medical bibliophiles.

A memorial service was held 15 March, 1958. He was justly described as *Scientist*, *Teacher* and *Friend*. It was revealed that after retirement (although his income was minimal) he presented a substantial cheque to the new Chairman of the Department of Physiology with the statement:

> '*Someday a student is going to come to you who is hungry or in trouble. Use this and say nothing about where it came from. If you need more let me know.*'

The funds were used. Love goes both ways and shortly thereafter five of his former pupils anonymously established a fund to supplement his retirement pay. Other admirers established the Arno B. Luckhardt Fund to provide fellowships for students in Physiology. He was a giant in intellect, ability, humour, and kindness. An example was a comment to a graduate student:

> '_____, *you put your name on this; I'm a Professor and have no place to go, but you are young and it may help you rise.*'

He was as great as his ideals, Beaumont and Andrews, and very worth copying as a role model.

Acknowledgment

Mr Robert Luckhardt, son of Dr Albert Luckhardt, was of invaluable assistance in providing Luckhardt family information.

References

(1) Bing FC. With Professor A. B. Luckhardt, on the trail of Dr. William Beaumont. *Fed Proc* 1977; **37**: 2506–9.

(2) University of Chicago School of Medicine. Dr. Luckhardt retires. *Bull Alumni Assoc* 1950; **7**: 1 & 9.

(3) Luckhardt AB. An adventure in research. *J Ohio State Dental Soc* 1944; **18**: 71–9.

(4) Kistler GH, Luckhardt AB. The pharmacology of some ethylene–halogen compounds. *Anesth Analg* 1929; **8**: 65–74.

(5) Luckhardt AB, Carter JB. The physiologic effects of ethylene. A new gas anesthetic. *JAMA* 1923; **80**: 765–70.

(6) Luckhardt AB. Sundry remarks on ethylene–oxygen anesthesia. *Anesth Analg* 1928; **7**: 12–6.

(7) Lundy JS. The comparative value of ethylene as an anesthetic. *JAMA* 1924; **83**: 350–5.

(8) Luckhardt AB. Biological reactions to ethylene anesthesia: A résumé. *Anesth Analg* 1934; **13**: 102–4.

(9) Pickering PP, McCooey CJ, Steinmeyer HP, Luckhardt AB. Possible cardiovascular changes in local anesthesia. *J Am Dent Assoc* 1939; **26**: 1823–8.

(10) Luckhardt AB. Historical high lights and shadows in the discovery of general anesthesia. *Anesth Analg* 1930; **9**: 241–53.

(11) Luckhardt AB. Edmund Andrews, M.D. and his "oxygen mixtures". *Anesth Analg* 1940; **19**: 2–11.

25.18	The life and work of Sir Ivan Whiteside Magill, KCVO

K. G. LEE
Westminster Hospital, London, UK

Ivan Whiteside Magill was born at No 4 Barnhill Terrace (now known as 10 Curran Road), Larne, Co. Antrim, N. Ireland, on 23 July, 1888. Ivan was one of five children of Samuel Magill, a prominent businessman, councillor, Presbyterian and Freemason of Larne, and Sara Magill (née Whiteside). Thus he could boast no family medical background (1). He was educated at Larne Grammar School from 1900 to 1906, and showing prowess as a sportsman, he graduated MB ChB BAO from Queen's University, Belfast, in 1913. Having received little formal training in anaesthetics, and having given some sixty general anaesthetics as an undergraduate (2), he qualified with a certificate that he had 'received practical instruction in the administration of anaesthetics, and had personally administered an anaesthetic.'

Immediately after qualification, Magill came to England; after a short period in general practice in Leicester, he took resident posts in Liverpool, first at Stanley Hospital, then at Walton Hospital. He showed a predilection for surgery, rather than anaesthetics at the time (3).

The Great War broke out in August, 1914, and in 1915 Magill took a temporary Commission in the Royal Army Medical Corps, serving as Captain in the RAMC during the remainder of the War, particularly with the Irish Guards at the Battle of Loos, and in a field hospital near Rouen.

He married Edith Robinson (daughter of Thomas Robinson of Banbridge, Co. Down) in 1916. She was a physician who later worked as a school doctor with the London County Council. They were to have no children.

The Sidcup story

At the end of hostilities, Magill was posted to the Barnet War Hospital (now Barnet General Hospital), where he gave occasional anaesthetics, before moving to the Queen's Hospital for

Facial and Jaw Injuries (now Queen Mary's Hospital), Sidcup, Kent. Also posted to Sidcup at that time was another RAMC officer, Stanley Rowbotham. Together, they began to work in the new field of facial plastic surgery, made necessary by four years of war, under Major, later Sir Harold, Gillies. With little anaesthetic experience between them and no precedent in this hazardous branch of anaesthetics, Magill and Rowbotham were offered the option of anaesthetics, and their pioneering partnership started (4).

They realized that success lay in control of the airway during facial and jaw surgery. Intratracheal insufflation was available, and Magill and Rowbotham began to work with this. Next, they added a second, pharyngeal tube to allow expiratory gas to escape; this enabled them to pack the throat and separate the airway from the surgical field. To-and-fro breathing through a single rubber endotracheal tube was then perfected, culminating in Magill's description of endotracheal anaesthesia and blind nasal intubation in 1928 (5).

Apparatus

In parallel with the development of these techniques Magill also experimented with, designed and developed the necessary apparatus for them. His first publication was the description and illustration of forceps for placement of the insufflation catheter under direct vision in 1920 (6)—apparatus which has remained in the anaesthetist's armamentarium, although no longer used for its original purpose. He designed a range of rubber endotracheal tubes, both for oral and nasal use, together with appropriate curved metal connectors.

He developed portable, table-top apparatus for the delivery of anaesthetic gases (the anaesthetist in those days was often itinerant, taking his own apparatus with him). His first apparatus was for the delivery of warm ether in air by insufflation (1921); the second was for giving ether, nitrous oxide and oxygen (1923); the third was a combination of the first two (1927), while the fourth was an improved version of the third, incorporating dry gas flowmeters and a sparklet attachment for provision of carbon dioxide (1932) (7). This was the first apparatus to include a wide-bore fresh gas outlet (1.4 in (3.5 cm)), for attachment of a rebreathing bag and wide-bore breathing system. Neither the fourth apparatus nor the Magill attachment were described in the literature.

Magill also devised an intermittent flow apparatus for nitrous oxide and oxygen, as well as modifications of Chevalier Jackson's laryngoscope. He examined the problem of airway control in paediatric facial surgery; unable to find small rubber tubes of sufficient rigidity, he devised reinforced and armoured tubes (which he termed 'surgeon-proof tubes'). With these tubes he used a Y-connector, with fresh gas being delivered by fine-bore tube into the side limb, effectively giving 'T-piece' anaesthesia, predating Ayre's description in 1937 by several years (8,9).

Thoracic anaesthesia

After the Armistice, Magill and Rowbotham were employed at Sidcup on a part-time basis and each took several other posts in London Hospitals as well. An American plastic surgeon, one J. Eastman Sheehan, failed to persuade Magill and Rowbotham to emigrate and work for him in the USA (4).

Magill joined the staff of the 'Brompton Hospital for Consumption' in 1923, and was appointed 'Chloroformist to the Westminster Hospital' in 1924. Here he turned his mind particularly to anaesthesia for thoracic surgery, which consisted almost invariably of surgery for pulmonary tuberculosis at that time, with its problem of copious purulent lung secretions. He again developed new techniques, together with the necessary apparatus. Several centres were experimenting with anaesthesia for thoracic surgery at the time, culminating in techniques for giving one-lung anaesthesia.

Initially, Magill advocated that thoracoplasty be done under local anaesthesia together with light nitrous oxide and oxygen by mask, retaining the cough reflex; at first he considered intubation contraindicated, as it necessitated anaesthesia deep enough to obtund the cough reflex, so preventing clearance of secretions. Next he tried endotracheal intubation with intermittent tracheal suction, and devised a simple T-connector for the tube with a removable seal, facilitating suction. Magill then worked on bronchus blockade, using a balloon-tipped rubber suction catheter through an endotracheal tube, introduced using his own design of tracheoscope. This, however, proved difficult to use in practice. At the same time he developed further the idea of endobronchial intubation (already introduced in the USA) by producing tubes for more reliable introduction under direct vision using an intubating bronchoscope lying within the tube. By this means one-lung anaesthesia became a routine possibility (10). These advances were, of course, themselves improved upon by subsequent workers.

Other innovations

Magill was responsible for introducing some new agents into anaesthesia in the United Kingdom (UK). He brought back Nembutal (pentobarbitone) from the USA in 1931, and used it intravenously for basal anaesthesia. He tried a number of other new agents of the time; he described cyclopropane as a 'Godsend' in thoracic work, and Lundy's concept of 'Balanced anaesthesia' appealed to him (11). He later brought Arfonad (trimetaphan) back from the USA, describing the first few cases using it in the UK in 1953. This again demonstrated Magill's willingness to change his practice in the light of new advances (in 1934 he had stated:

> *'It appears to me unreasonable to expect the anaesthetist to stop bleeding by lowering the blood pressure, as can quite easily be done with chloroform.'*) (11)

The Diploma in Anaesthetics

Magill's other interest was in the status of anaesthesia as a speciality in its own right, and he realized the necessity of a diploma entailing appropriate training, experience and study. As Secretary of the Section of Anaesthetics of the Royal Society of Medicine (the only anaesthetic forum at the time in the UK) he was the first to suggest a Diploma in Anaesthetics, on the 6 November, 1931 (12). He was told by the Secretary of the Society that this was outside the scope of the Society, under its charter as an academic body. However, several members of the Section met and decided to form an independent body with this aim in mind. The Association of Anaesthetists was constituted on the 1 July, 1932, to concern itself with the political rather than scientific aspects of anaesthesia.

The first examination for the Diploma in Anaesthetics was held on 8 November, 1935. Magill was on the Board of Examiners, having worked to set up the venture; he did not, however, enjoy examining, and his standards were too high, so his fellow examiners soon persuaded him to retire from the Board. He was made President of the Anaesthetic Section of the Royal Society of Medicine in 1937.

Retirement

Magill remained in London throughout the Second World War; his house in Wimpole Street was bombed and destroyed in 1941—luckily there was no-one in the house at the time. He was adviser to the Emergency Medical Service and the Forces, and also to the Ministry of Health during the foundation of the National Health Service, ensuring the status of anaesthesia in the Service. He retired from his Health Service posts in 1955, but continued to work in London, giving his last anaesthetic at the age of 84. Fiercely independent, after his wife's death in 1973 he lived a secluded life in central London, near the Royal Society of Medicine, still attending meetings of the Anaesthetic Section until shortly before his death.

Royal anaesthetics

Magill anaesthetized several members of the Royal Family during his career, as well as many foreign dignitaries. He anaesthetized the Dowager Duchess of Gloucester in 1937—she had taken a full breakfast and, not surprisingly, vomited. He attended Princess Margaret's appendicectomy in 1955, and later attended the Duke of Windsor, Prince Charles and Princess Anne. (He did not anaesthetize King George VI.) In recognition of his services, he was invested Commander of the Royal Victorian Order in 1946, and Knighted KCVO by the Queen in 1960.

Honours

Many honours were also bestowed on Magill by the medical world in respect of his pioneering work. He was awarded the Henry Hill Hickman medal of the Royal Society of Medicine in 1938, and the medal of the Ulster Medical Society in 1939. In 1945, Queen's University, Belfast, awarded him an honorary Doctorate of Science; Queen's had accepted his wife's MD thesis in 1920, but had rejected his own (based on endotracheal anaesthesia) on the grounds that it was unlikely to be of much value. Magill was later awarded the John Snow medal in 1958, and the medals of the Canadian Anaesthetists Society in 1963 and the American Association of Plastic Surgeons in 1965. He was made Honorary Fellow of the Royal Society of Medicine in 1956, and of the Faculty of Anaesthetists and the Association of Anaesthetists in 1958. Magill delivered a number of lectures after his retirement, giving a fascinating insight into the advances in anaesthesia during his career; these include the Frederick Hewitt Lecture of 1965, and the paper he presented as the first recipient of the Ralph Waters award in 1966 (13,14).

Conclusion

In summary, Sir Ivan Magill was a world doyen of anaesthesia. He was an innovator and pioneer—often using his manual dexterity in making prototype devices in his own home, while developing techniques now taken for granted. Throughout his career he retained a progressive outlook, able to change his opinion and practice in the light of new developments. He maintained the physical fitness he acquired as a school and university sportsman. Although he disliked formal teaching, he taught by demonstration and example, setting a standard in anaesthetic care.

He was a visionary at a time when anaesthesia was rapidly advancing, setting the foundation of anaesthetic training, postgraduate examination and the present-day status of the specialty.

Sir Ivan Magill died on 25 November, 1986, in his 99th year. He had been a legend in his own lifetime.

References

(1) Page R. The Barnhill lad who became a consultant to Royalty. *Larne Times* 1987: January 22nd.
(2) Magill IW. Anaesthesia: The Magill story. In: Gillies H, Millard DR, eds. *The principles and art of plastic surgery*. Vol. I. Boston and Toronto: Little, Brown and Co.
(3) Rowbotham S, Ivan Magill. *Br J Anaesth* 1951; **23**: 49–55.
(4) Condon HA, Gilchrist E, Stanley Rowbotham. *Anaesthesia* 1986; **41**: 46–52.
(5) Magill IW. Endotracheal anaesthesia. *Proc Roy Soc Med* 1929; **22**: 83–7. (Also reproduced in *Anaesthesia* 1978; **33**: 580–6.)
(6) Magill IW. Forceps for intratracheal anaesthesia. *Br Med J* 1920; **2**: 670.
(7) Bryn Thomas K. *The development of anaesthetic apparatus*. Oxford: Blackwell. 1975.
(8) Gordon Jones RG. A short history of anaesthesia for hare-lip and cleft palate repair. *Br J Anaesth* 1971; **43**: 796–802.
(9) Ayre P. Anaesthesia for intracranial operation. *Lancet* 1937; **i**: 561–3.
(10) Mushin WW, Rendell-Baker L. *The principles of thoracic anaesthesia*. Oxford: Blackwell. 1953.
(11) Magill IW. Modern views on anaesthesia. *Newcastle Med J* 1934; **14**: 67–78.
(12) *Minutes of the meetings of the Council of the Section of Anaesthetics of the Royal Society of Medicine*. Meeting of Friday November 6th, 1931. Pages 300–1.
(13) Magill IW. An appraisal of progress in anaesthetics. *Ann Roy Coll Surg* 1966; **38**: 154–65.

(14) Magill IW. The heritages of the past are the privileges of the future. *Anesthesiology* 1967; **28**: 202–8.

25.19

Sir Ivan Whiteside Magill (1888–1986)
and tracheal intubation

W. K. PALLISTER
The Middlesex Hospital, London, UK

Ivan Whiteside Magill (Fig. 1) was born at Larne, Northern Ireland, on 23 July, 1888. He died on 25 November, 1986, in Bristol at the home of his nephew Dr Campbell Laird, aged 98—or as Ivan himself would have said 'in my 99th year!'. At a meeting held at the Royal Society of Medicine on 9 June, 1978, to mark his 90th birthday, Dr Bryn Thomas chronicled his contributions to anaesthesia, and pointed out 'That when Sir Ivan was born, anaesthesia itself was but 42 years old'. This account, in his own words compiled from tape recordings, galley proofs and his own lecture typescripts covers a period two-thirds as old as anaesthesia:

> 'Now I will go back to the time when I was a student in the year 1910, and when I went first to see an operation in the theatre, I was struck by the fact that anybody who was qualified as a doctor was expected to be able to given an anaesthetic for any operation—whatever it may be. In other words—there was no training!
>
> I was launched into the medical profession, and qualified as a doctor, on the certificate to say that I had received instruction in anaesthesia—and had personally administered one anaesthetic. That gives you an idea of the training that existed in those days. In fact my experience as a student made me quite frightened of it, because I could see that when I was qualified I would have to undertake this onerous task for which I was not really adequately trained.
>
> However, the War came along (the first war) and, at the end of the war, by chance, I was posted to a hospital on the outside of London, and I had to give some minor anaesthetics there. And there was a demand for an anaesthetist at the Queen's Hospital, Sidcup. Well, I was offered the job, and I said "Alright". The reason that I took this job was not because I knew anything about anaesthetics, but my wife was living in London at the time, and I knew that this hospital for facial and jaw injuries was at Sidcup. And I had seen that name on the back of a bus. So I said "Right—I'll take the job".
>
> I went to Sidcup, with my scant knowledge of anaesthetics—and I got to this hospital and I said "What kind of Hospital is this?" And they said "Oh, this is a facial hospital" I said "What do you do—do you give anaesthetics with a Junker, or something?" Anyway, I very soon learnt what I was up against. There was something like 600 beds of wounded soldiers—all of whom had been wounded in the face and jaws.
>
> Now anaesthesia at that time was limited to a Shipway Apparatus—which was a development of the original Junker—having an Ether bottle as well—and it was activated by hand bellows—or by an oxygen cylinder. We used a Hewitt's airway—or any oral airway—or sometimes a small tube slipped into the pharynx—but the difficulty of maintaining the airway through an operation which lasted some four hours—and sometimes entailed the entry of blood into the pharynx, was a tremendous job (1).
>
> At the time I joined Queen's Hospital, Ether inhalation was in vogue. The slot in a Philips pharyngeal airway was fitted with an angle piece, made from a 303 cartridge case. Ether was blown into an attached funnel through a Shipway apparatus. This funnel magnified the patient's breath sounds, which enabled the anaesthetist to introduce his

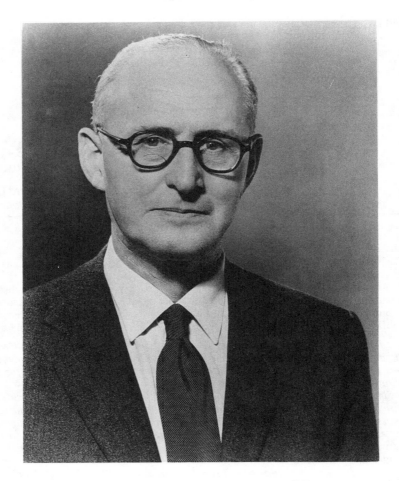

Figure 1   Sir Ivan Whiteside Magill, KCVO

*ether, and follow his patient's breathing well away from the surgical field. It did not
however, allow for access to the patient's airway, and as any pharnygeal tube is an easy
prey to obstruction, it could cause a severe—and even fatal strain—on the patient. A
bone graft case is recalled, in which the pharyngeal airway obstinately persisted in partial
obstruction during the entire procedure. Although the patient was at no time in acute
distress, at the end of 4 hours he was so exhausted that he died (2).*

*Well I was joined there by my old friend, Stanley Rowbotham, and between us we
worked out that the whole essence of success in anaesthesia in these cases was control
of the larynx. Well, we knew that Elsberg in America had devised the endotracheal
technique, it was devised of course before I went to this hospital in 1919, and we began
to use endotracheal insufflation.*

*Now when I say insufflation, I mean insufflation. We used an air pump driven by
an electrical device, a motor, which drew in air, to which ether was added—drop by
drop. And this was true insufflation—in other words, you blew in enough air so that
if there was any blood in the pharynx, it was blown out. And also was blown out the
ether exhalations—which were not so very good for the surgeon. Anyway—that was
quite a relevation—insufflation anaesthesia was quite something. And people came to
observe the plastic surgery—which was a development at that time; and they very soon
got wise to the fact that plastic surgery was done with the assistance of the anaesthetist*

who made the job possible. Now when I say insufflation, I want you to understand that there was one tube—a catheter—pumping air into the trachea. I used to demonstrate to the spectators how safe it was. I took a jug of water at the end of the operation, and poured it into the patient's mouth to show that respiration was completely under control.

However, as I've said—with bleeding into the mouth, the surgeon was covered with a spray of blood, and Gillies, who was the surgeon at that time, he said "Maggi—you seem to get this anaesthetic into the patient alright, don't you think you could devise some method of getting it out, so that I am not anaesthetised?" So we got to work on that. And we used, first of all a Hewitt's airway, and a pack—and then we eventually used a tube through the nose—a piece of rubber tubing of indifferent quality, and were able to pack the throat. Well, now, after that we discovered that with operations inside the mouth, it was a constructive idea if the anaesthetic could be given through the nose (1).

The difficulty of expiration in endotrachel anaesthesia was solved somewhat dramatically in 1922. A soldier with an extensive jaw deformity had had a tracheal catheter passed through the nose, but owing to the deformity and contracture of the lower jaw, expiration became laboured. Attempts to find a free channel by means of rubber tubes were quite unsuccessful, until one of these tubes accidentally entered the trachea along with the catheter. The relief which followed, left no doubt as to the value of two tubes (2).

So Rowbotham and I developed what we called the "Two tube method of Anaesthesia", that is to say we insufflated through a catheter into the trachea in the manner I have described to you, but in addition we passed a second tube into the trachea to deal with expiration. In that way, the pharynx could be packed, and the surgeon protected from the exhalations—and the sprayed blood.

Well I've told you how we started off with the insufflation technique using ether. Well, I found that to use nitrous oxide and oxygen, which came into popularity at the end of the first war (the Americans used it on their casualties) by the insufflation technique, was not a practical procedure, because—first of all it was grossly expensive (it cost 8 shillings (40p) a gallon in those days). Secondly you had got a patient who was dark— and not breathing very well, and it was not a very satisfactory method. (1) Eventually McKesson came over to this country and he demonstrated the use of gas and oxygen without any adjunct whatsoever and he demonstrated with his machine, that you could give an anaesthetic for any facial operation.

I think it was Professor Macintosh, who described the saturation technique as "You convert an A1 individual into a C3 individual, as regards his physical condition, by three bouts of asphyxia". Zebulon Mennell, when he saw this demonstration by McKesson, said "The signs of secondary saturation are the signs of impending death!"

At first we'd pass the catheter with a stilette in it through the nose—Rowbotham used a stilette to puncture the catheter, and lift it into the trachea. I myself thought it would be better not to injure the catheter—and I devised a pair of forceps, which I believe still exists in some museums.

Well now—I've told you my early experiences of insufflation—but then there came a time when I was faced with a problem that really was quite something. I was faced in private practice with a patient who had been in Switzerland, and received some very nasty injuries in the neighbourhood of the eye, and she had, this lady of about 24, she had had about 7 anaesthetics. Now when Gillies was called upon to do some plastic surgery this lady said "I want it to be fully understood that I am not having ether or chloroform. I have had them before—and unless there can be a guarantee that I do not have those anaesthetics—then—I shall not have the operation." Well I was a poor man at that time, and I didn't want to lose my practice. So I began to figure out "What have we got?"

This operation will take one hour, or an hour and a half. I said "I think there's only one anaesthetic that I think is available for this job and that's nitrous oxide and oxygen. Now I thought "How am I going to do that?" Insufflation is no good. I said the only way to do this is with a wide bore tube and a bag. And I made a rubber tube with a ⅜ths of an inch bore, and I made a strong angle piece—and I anaesthetised this patient after a preliminary of omnopon and scopolamine. I anaesthetised her with pure nitrous oxide and oxygen, after the manner that was done in those days when you saturated *the patient with nitrous oxide—then you saturated them with oxygen—and when you had done that once or twice—then you were able to deal with the patient.*

That was the origin of the wide bore tube for to and fro breathing. And that patient, at the end of operation sat up and said "I don't mind having that again". At the same time it was also the origin of the device that is sometimes known as the Magill attachment—I've never written it up in any way—but I'd like to tell you about it because when I used it first there was a bag attached to the machine and this bag was covered by a net which did not come into play unless the bag was sufficiently inflated. The tension on the bag was balanced exactly by the tension on the expiratory valve, and I believe that in some outlying places, they still use that piece of equipment at the present time.

And that was the origin of the wide bore tube. Then the problem arose, how was I going to get these tubes? The kind of rubber tubing we had in hospitals, that was drainage tubing, had not got the necessary consistency. So I went to a rubber shop in Tottenham Court Road, they sold footballs, they sold coils of rubber tubing. I came to an arrangement with the man who sold these coils (because rubber is a thing subject to the ravages of time—when it's fresh out of the extruder it's very soft, and then it gradually gains a certain amount of consistency) that he would give me the tail ends of the coils when he had finished with them. And for quite a long time I got my pieces of rubber tubing from this man. His place was destroyed one night by Hitler, with a bomb.

Manufacturers were completely disinterested in anaesthetic apparatus at that time. Then Charles King came into the picture. I said "Well Charles, these things are in demand I find that when I deposit these tubes around hospitals they are stolen. And he was interested. So he got busy with the rubber companies. He produced miles of tubing— and he had two girls in the back of the shop with soldering irons, finishing them off. We discarded miles of these tubes! Now, of course, you know that rubber tubes have been made by various manufacturers. To me, rubber tubes, when of the right consistency, have nothing to beat them; but I did say in America in 1952, that I felt certain that with the development of the plastic elements, eventually a tube would be devised which would be completely clear, and would have all the qualities that one associates with a good rubber tube. I believe that that day has already arrived. (1)

For blind intubation, free nasal breathing should be determined before induction. Cylindrical gum elastic catheters up to 23 French Gauge can usually be passed through the nose without causing injury. It is inadvisable, in my opinion, to use a larger tube than this, or any other hard material, if trauma and bleeding are to be avoided. Commercial rubber tubing is the most satisfactory material. It is firm enough to maintain its patency, and sufficiently resilient to pass over mucous membranes without causing injury.

The tube should be cut obliquely, sterilised and lubricated. It is then passed along the floor of the nose, close to the septum. The course of the tube should be visualised as is that of the needle in regional anaesthesia. When a point is reached at which the respiratory sounds are heard at maximum intensity, the tube will usually enter the glottis, if pushed on, during inspiration. In the case of failure, before resorting to speculum, or forceps, rotation of the tube to one side or the other will frequently bring its end into the desired position. The importance of dexterity in intubation is now obvious. Some of the chief difficulties which arise may be traced to a faulty position of the patient's head. Hyperextension, as adopted by some surgeons for bronchoscopy is not only unnecessary, but actually increases the difficulty of intubation. The head should have the same relation to the neck and trunk in the recumbent, as in the erect position. A pillow may therefore have to be placed below the occiput. The correct position on the table is that in which the cervical vertebrae are in normal relation to the dorsal vertebrae, and are not extended. The head itself is slightly extended on the Atlas, so that the mandible is approximately at right angles to the table. These, in fact are the relative positions of the air passages instinctively adopted by a man as he scents the air, or drinks a pint. When a mesial section is taken through the head and neck in this position, it is clear that the course of the air passage from nostril to glottis is a curve. Introduced through the nose, a rubber tube with a similar curve can be made to follow that course quite naturally, and will enter the glottis in a large percentage of cases, in preference to the oesophagus.

Intubation can be carried out through the mouth, or through the nose, according to the site of operation. When the oral route is selected, I prefer to pass the tube by direct vision with the aid of a speculum, which should have a wide slot at the side. A self contained battery in the handle is a convenient means of illumination.

The commonest question I have had to answer is "How do you know the tube is in the trachea?" It seems to me that when a tube 26 cms long is passed through the nose in its entirety, the presence or absence of free ingress, and egress of air through the lumen is sufficient evidence of its position. (2)

In 1935 I was invited to Paris to the International Congress of Plastic Surgeons; there I demonstrated on a cadaver that the trick of blind nasal intubation depended purely upon anatomy. Later at the request of one of the French surgeons, I agreed to give an intratracheal anaesthetic. At this hospital the anaesthetist was, as often as not, a porter with a chloroform bottle. The surgeons were used to much coughing, struggling, and other respiratory commotion. The intra-tracheal tube went in easily, and the patient was breathing so quietly that one of the French doctors whispered "Il ne respire plus, Il est mort?" "Procedez, s'il vous plait" I answered with amusement "Ca marche tres bien!" (3).

In private practice in the 1920s–1930s the general practitioner considered that the patient was his in the first instance, and they all resented that anybody outside should be called in to give an anaesthetic. Most anaesthetists in those days were General Practitioners. He would say "what are you going to give 'ether or chloroform—or what'?" I said "well something quite simple!" You see, I got a bit foxy, about that time, because I had already discovered that if you had control of the patient's larynx, you could get away with light anaesthesia without saturating the patient with ether to the deepest possible depth. So I anaesthetised the patient with a mask and an ether drop bottle, and when I got the attention of the General Practitioner turned away, and looking at something else, perhaps the clock, "what is the time?" I used to intubate the patient blindly through the nose with a rubber tube, and I continued to give the anaesthetic with a Schimmelbusch mask and a drop bottle and at the end of the operation I removed the mask—and the tube, you see, inside the Gamgee pad. So you see he never saw the tube!' (1)

References

(1) 'Reminiscences' Sir Ivan Magill. Address to the Department of Anaesthesia. The Middlesex Hospital, London W1. Jan 24th 1974.
(2) Magill IW. Technique in endotracheal anaesthesia. *Br Med J* 1930; **1**: 817–9.
(3) The Magill story: Chapter 3, 57–70. In: Gillies H, Millard R Jr, eds. *The Principles and Art of Plastic Surgery* Vol. 1. Boston and Toronto: Little, Brown and Company.

25.20   Philip Dudley Woodbridge (1895–1978). A Renaissance man

JOHN B. STETSON

Rush Presbyterian—St Lukes Medical Center, Chicago, Illinois, USA

Philip Dudley Woodbridge (Fig. 1) was born on 11 November, 1895, in Brookline, Massachusetts, the second of three children. His family tree included many physicians and

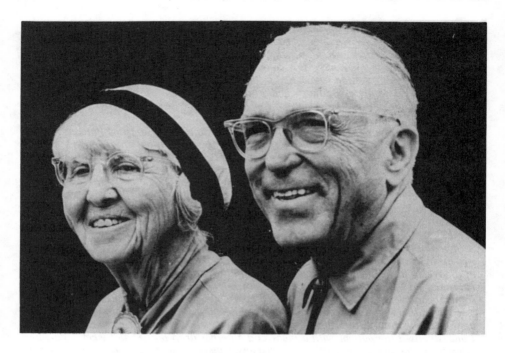

Figure 1   Philip D. Woodbridge and his wife Marion, 1964.

the founders of Woodbridge, Connecticut and Woodbridge, New Jersey. Woodbridge Hall at Yale was named for a family member. His father, a Professor at the Massachusetts Institute of Technology (MIT) pioneered modern concepts of heating and ventilation and designed the systems for the US House of Congress. His father also pushed through Congress a bill to outlaw using the mails for lotteries. PDW was raised in the Congregational Church and later characterized himself as being a perfectionist and Puritan as a youth. He was drawn to the study of medicine by a talk given by Dr Wilfred Grenfell, 'The Laborador Doctor'. His beloved brother acquired tuberculosis in Laborador and died while an MIT student.

Always a diligent student, PDW graduated from Phillips Academy, Andover, Massachusetts in 1913 and from Harvard (*cum laude*) in 1917. At Harvard he studied English literature, the classics, and music. He then entered Harvard Medical School and graduated MD in 1921. World War I was in progress and he was drafted for three months. He was 'impressed with folly of war and brainwashing of drill.' He played the viola for eight years in the Harvard Symphony Orchestra. Later he played for twelve years in the MacDowell Club Orchestra with Arthur Fiedler as conductor. Although he came from a well established family, his father was a cardiac invalid and retired about the time PDW entered college. He lived 'on a shoestring'—a 5¢ bowl of soup and crackers constituted many of his meals.

Anaesthesia Internship (1921—1923) was at Hartford Hospital. He also trained for four months at Boston Consumptives' Hospital and four months in the Contagious Disease section of Boston City Hospital.

Anaesthesia training

In 1924 he started general practice in Connecticut, married Marion Crane Maercklein, and took two weeks of anaesthesia training with Dr Brian C. Sword. He then;

'*Soon found I knew more about anaesthesia than anyone except three between Boston and New York City.*'

In 1927 he became John Lundy's First Assistant at the Mayo Clinic and remained a year 'learning local anaesthesia.' His son, Dudley Hooker, was born in 1928 in Rochester, Minnesota. The family (PDW, wife, infant, and dog) returned to Boston via automobile through Canada so Phil could visit Canadian anaesthetists and learn more about endotracheal intubation. PDW noted later in life that he performed the first endotracheal intubation done at the Mayo Clinic.

At the Lahey Clinic

Joining the staff at the Lahey Clinic, Boston, (1928), he remained until 1940. He was Head of the Department 1938–1940. He was knowledgeable, a hard worker, an active investigator, a good teacher, indefatigable in advancing and promoting the specialty, scrupulously fair, and, unbending.

Spinal anaesthesia was used for all operations below the diaphragm. At times, a sedated patient would moan during a high exploration. Before a gallery of visiting surgeons, a patient moaned; Dr Lahey turn to PDW and said, 'Under these circumstances we give the patient a barbiturate, don't we, doctor?', PDW stood up and said, 'We do not, it is not physiologic,' then sat down. On another day, the same thing occurred to another anaesthesiologist. He bustled to the foot of the table (saphenous vein infusions were used) and injected saline. Dr Lahey was mollified and all went well. Later Phil scolded his colleague for being deceptive; to PDW the end did not justify the means.

The staff members had desks grouped together (face to face) in one room. At the end of the day they would do their paper work, prepare reports, and so on. PDW would say nothing, but the next day a colleague might find a note from Phil concerning some duty or assignment. When his old co-workers related these stories it was always with a laugh and a final comment that he was always 'exceeding fair' and honest.

In personal habits, he was careful with his diet so he would remain thin and wiry, wore woven shoes so his feet could 'breathe,' and discarded the undershirt (vest) before Clark Gable made this popular in the film, 'It Happened One Night' with Claudette Colbert.

Automobiles

If he had a passion, it was convertible automobiles with air-cooled engines. Friends date his activities by his vehicle. When Franklin air-cooled engined cars were no longer available, he switched to an Oldsmobile Hydramatic drive. After World War II he obtained a VW convertible with an air-cooled engine. Unfortunately, VWs are too small for American touring. He returned from a European trip in 1964 with a Citroen convertible with adjustable-height suspension (good in snow and to reach the Mt Toby Quaker Meetinghouse while it was under construction). Finally, he switched to Saabs because they have front wheel drive. He installed direction signals on his cars in the 1930s and removed hood (bonnet) ornaments as 'deadly.'

Resident training

While at the Lahey Clinic PDW organized a resident training programme (as he also later did at Temple University and Reading Hospital). The instruction sheets he prepared for the trainees stressed compassion and understanding. He was a founding member of the American Board of Anesthesiology (1938), received diploma number nine, and was President, 1945–1946. He also helped found the 'Travel Club.'

Scientific papers

During the twelve years he was at the Lahey Clinic, he published 26 scientific articles, helped develop the Connell flow meters and anaesthetic machine (technologically so far ahead of its time that the market for the machine was limited), the Horton intercoupler to reduce the incidence of static sparking, and a non-collapsing endotracheal tube (important in the days of enormous colloid goitres). He wrote that he was the first person in the United States to use acetylene as a general anaesthetic (date not given). Acetylene is mentioned in a 1933 article (1).

The 26 articles reflect development of the specialty prior to World War II. Eight articles are on progress, choice of method and economics, four each on regional blocks and spinal anaesthesia, three about the value of carbon dioxide absorption techniques, two each on cyclopropane, evaluation of surgical (anaesthetic) risk, and prevention of static sparking (explosions), and one a description of his non-collapsing endotracheal tube. Six of the articles were published in the *New England Journal of Medicine*, six in the *Surgical Clinics of North America*, and three each in *Anesthesia and Analgesia* and *The American Journal of Surgery*. Often, articles in two different journals would be similar (again, a reflection of the era). The two articles on preventing static sparks appeared in the *Journal of the American Medical Association* (1939).

The articles were concise, well organized, scientific, and directed toward improved patient care. His articles on therapeutic nerve blocks (such as alcohol for tic) were prescient of the modern pain clinic as well as a reflection of then current medical problems (spinal for treatment of ileus).

His reviews of closed system anaesthesia, to-and-fro and circle, demonstrated the economy of the system (9¢ an hour for soda-line, 15¢ an hour for oxygen), stressed the conservation of body heat, and reduction of explosion hazard by reducing gases and vapours in the operating room.

He was a pioneer in popularizing spinal anaesthesia, first with procaine, then with metycaine which he helped to introduce, finally with hyperbaric pontocaine.

He advocated administration of intravenous amytal and ephedrine just prior to spinal block for sedation and preservation of a safe blood pressure.

His 1936 surgical risk scale (2) is a preview of the later ASA Physical Status scale. He noted:

> *"A history of the patient's activities and symptoms is far more valuable than the physical examination . . .".*

His contributions concerning explosions were classic. He surveyed active anaesthesiologists and found the incidence of explosions per 100 000 administrations (ether, 1.73 ± 0.31; ethylene 2.44 ± 0.86; cyclopropane 3.85 ± 1.22). He then enlisted the aid of Professor Warren Horton of MIT and developed a high resistance intercoupler so patient, table, anaesthesiologist, and machine all had the same potential and any sparking would be outside the danger zone (area of gas leak at the mask). The introduction of cyclopropane was championed by Woodbridge. His knowledge of carbon dioxide absorption techniques allowed him to use the gas properly.

Later career and interests

As an extremely intelligent person, he knew he was not meeting all of his personal problems. He left the Lahey Clinic (1940) and worked on the staff of the Grace-New Haven Hospital in 1941 while he underwent psychoanalysis at Yale. In 1966, he wrote of this experience '. . . emerged a changed and changing person.'

Philadelphia

He then went to Temple University (1942) where he was Professor and Chief of Anesthesia. At Temple he started a residency training programme but wrote no important articles. In Philadelphia he alternated between the Presbyterian Church (good sermons, 'gorgeous' music) and the Quakers. As the Quaker spirit matched his, he soon joined them. Outside the hospital he worked on the American Peace Terms Committee.

Reading, Pennsylvania

He was unable to make satisfactory business arrangements at Philadelphia so he left in 1945 to head the department at Reading (Pennsylvania) Hospital. He again started a residency programme and wrote an article and a chapter detailing anaesthetic techniques for otolaryngological surgery.

Greenfield, Massachusetts

Business arrangements were again poor and in 1950 he returned to New England and entered the private practice of anesthesiology in Greenfield, Massachusetts. In Greenfield, his house was on a 36 acre wooded ridge overlooking the Connecticut River Valley. His exercise was cutting trees to preserve his view and for firewood. He became Clerk and Recording Clerk of Quaker Meetings (when he reported he was an agnostic he was told the Quakers had a place for him). He belonged to the American Civil Liberties Union, United World Federalists, the Fellowship of Reconciliation and took part in peace and civil rights marches. He played the piano and violin as well as the viola and performed in the area's symphony orchestra and string quartets.

Papers

His pen began to flow again and he wrote important anaesthesia papers as well as letters and articles about mankind's danger of nuclear self-destruction. One of his first medical achievements after moving to the freedom of private practice in Greenfield was development of the concept of compressed gas tank pin indexing (3). Industry accepted his suggestion; like so many of his contributions, this important safety feature does not bear his name. The medical articles in Greenfield included a review of operative risk for a medical cyclopedia, a chapter on ethylene for a comprehensive review text, and a general review for an American Medical Association text (PDW was active in the Anesthesia Section of the AMA, when this organization was important to the specialty). He espoused the use of chlorpromazine in a manner that is still being copied with droperidol. The 1955 meeting of the American Society of Anesthesiologists was held in Boston. PDW was Chairman of the General Activities Meeting and wrote the information booklet.

In 1957 he published, '*Changing concepts concerning depth of anesthesia*' (4). He divided the elements of 'anaesthesia' into sensory (afferent), motor (efferent), undesirable reflexes, and mental (sleep). He turned to Professor Herbert M. Howe who gave PDW the Greek *nothria* as a better word than anaesthesia. Woodbridge seems to have developed his ideas without knowledge of Professor T. Cecil Gray's concepts concerning 'The Disintegrative Action of the Central Nervous System' (5). Nothria did not become a popular word. When PDW was Chairman of the Section on Anesthesiology of the American Medical Association (1963), he presented a talk entitled *The Components of General Anesthesia*, (6). It is roughly the same as his 1957 paper, but nothria is not mentioned (nor is the 1957 paper listed in his references!).

One of his most interesting papers was published in 1961. Entitled *A technique for staying out of trouble while using cyclopropane*, (7) PDW delineated an ingenious method of maintaining a non-explosive mix of cyclopropane, ethylene, and oxygen. Following induction and a three to four minute cyclopropane wash-in, nitrogen wash-out, flows are adjusted so cyclopropane plus ethylene totaled 1000 ml/minute. To this is added 333 ml/min. of oxygen (25% oxygen). Metabolic oxygen is added to this mixture (about 300ml/minute). For light narcosis 100 ml/min. of cyclopropane plus 900 ml/min of ethylene is employed. For medium narcosis, the ratio is 200 to 800. These combinations are non-flammable. If nitrous oxide is used to replace ethylene, the mixtures become flammable! What a shame, Phil worked out this wonderful system at the beginning of the era of non-flammable anaesthetic vapours.

'Retirement'

By 1966, Phil was three-quarters retired (age 71) and withholding a portion of his federal income taxes as witness to his protest of the Vietnam war. His hobbies continued as well as interests in photography, sailing, speed-reading, accurate use of language, reform of the calendar and of English spelling, man's lack of interest in hygiene (cigarettes, obesity), and 'organized religion's frequent cruelty thru (sic) the ages.' At age 73 he retired. In 1968 he was invited to the headquarters of the American Society of Anesthesiologists to be honoured in its Distinguished Visitor Program.

Several years later, while driving, he had a pain in his chest, a feeling of imminent death, but managed to pull off the road and stop. He awoke in a hospital on oxygen therapy. The electrocardiogram did not reveal a myocardial infarction. John Severinghaus 'guessed a pulmonary embolism' and recommended aspirin which PDW probably took for the rest of his life.

His first wife had died (1970) and PDW had married Ruth Fraser, a Quaker friend, a 'very intelligent peace activist.' He continued to play in the local symphony and remained fairly active.

He died 11 December, 1978, ten years after 'retiring,' the passing of a unique, humane scholar and a Renaissance Man.

Acknowledgments

The author is indebted to Mr Dudley Hooker Woodbridge, Drs Morris Nicholson, Leo Hand, Alan Sessler, and John Severinghaus. Their kind assistance made it possible to prepare this limited account of some of PDW's many contributions.

References

(1) Woodbridge PD. Better gas anaesthesia. The carbon dioxide absorption method. *N Engl J Med* 1933; **208**: 632–40.
(2) Woodbridge PD. Preoperative estimation of the anaesthetic and surgical risk. *Am J Surg* 1936; **34**: 410–8.
(3) Woodbridge PD. A pin index system for gas bottles. *ASA Newsletter* March 1952; **16** (iii): 8.
(4) Woodbridge PD. Changing concepts concerning depth of anaesthesia. *Anesthesiology* 1957; **18**: 536–50.
(5) Gray TC. Disintegration of the nervous system. Joseph Clover Lecture. *Ann Roy Coll Surg Engl* 1954; **15**: 402–19.
(6) Woodbridge PD. The components of general anaesthesia. A plea for blocking the sensory pathways. *JAMA* 1963; **186**: 641–5.
(7) Woodbridge PD. A technique for staying out of trouble while using cyclopropane. *Anesth Analg* 1961; **40**: 32–41.

25.21   The contribution of Harold Randall Griffith
                                                    (1896–1985) to anaesthesia

DEIDRE M. M. GILLIES and J. EARL WYNANDS
Queen Elizabeth Hospital of Montreal, Quebec, Canada

The name of Harold Randall Griffith is best known for his courageous introduction of neuromuscular blockade into the practice of anaesthesia. This all-important step took place on 23 January, 1942, at the Homeopathic Hospital of Montreal (now the Queen Elizabeth Hospital of Montreal), when a 20-year-old plumber undergoing appendicectomy was given a total dose of 5 cc of Intocostrin (extract of unauthenticated curare, Squibb) for a one-hour operation. This was after about a year of cogitation regarding the pros and cons of using this drug, which had been supplied to him by Dr Lewis Wright of E. R. Squibb and Sons. Others had also received the drug for trial but their results, following animal experimentation, had been somewhat disastrous and it had been rejected as much too dangerous for clinical use.

Over the next six months curare was given by Dr Griffith to a further 24 patients and in July, 1942, the classic paper, 'The use of curare in general anaesthesia' was published in *Anesthesiology* (1).

This epic change in anaesthetic practice could not have occurred so quickly or so simply in the present climate of 'informed' consent and endless testing and re-testing for safety, in all situations, that is required by governments. Dr Griffith's guidelines to his first use of arrow poison were, that there was a need for better muscular relaxation during certain surgical procedures, that, if the patient stops breathing, 'I know how to ventilate him by squeezing the bag', and the fact that Dr Bennett in Nebraska has been giving curare to soften the effects of ECT therapy without serious problems (2).

It is appropriate at this point to quote, from the original anaesthetic record, the description by Dr Griffith of this first use of curare:

> '*REMARKS*
> *Intocostrin, Squibb (Curare) 3.5 cc given intravenously in 1-1/2 min. as operation started—no appreciable effect on pulse or respiration. After 5 min. another 1.5 cc of intocostrin given. Apparently complete relaxation of abdominal muscles resulted and continued for 20 minutes, during which time cyclopropane was lightened. At the end of this period muscle tone returned, probably from wearing off of curare effect. Cyclopropane was then increased in concentration and anaesthesia continued in the usual way. There was no demonstrable change in pulse, B.P. or respiration.*'

With the advent of this new tool, which revolutionized the practice of anaesthesia, surgical progress has known no bounds.

Dr Griffith's many contributions to the development of anaesthesia

This was not the first occasion when Dr Harold, as he was known to all his many trainees, grasped and refined a new concept or recognized the possible advantages of new drugs. Griffith's interest in anaesthesia developed while he was a medical student and even at that time he developed an acute awareness of the subtleties essential for safe anaesthetic practice. He wrote his first paper entitled 'Some practical observations on general anaesthesia' in 1922 when he was still a medical student at McGill. The sample anaesthetic records in this prize-winning essay outshine those kept by many of our colleagues today (3).

Ethylene

All the anaesthetic agents that were available at that time were used by him but he did develop a preference for intratracheal ethylene (4) over nitrous oxide and used this drug for about ten years—the only anaesthetist in Montreal to do so.

Cyclopropane

In October, 1933, a visit by Dr Griffith to Dr Waters in Madison, Wisconsin, revealed a new gaseous agent that appeared to be far superior to ethylene. This was cyclopropane—also explosive but much more potent. Its anaesthetic properties had been proved in animals by Lucas and Henderson in Toronto but, when offered for trial to the anaesthetists of that city, there had been reluctance to accept it, and thus Ralph Waters was the pioneer user of the new agent. Griffith became the first to use cyclopropane in Canada, on 30 October, 1933 (5), and he continued to use it until he retired in 1966. In fact, at the age of 89 years he wrote an essay on his favourite anaesthetic agent (6) to celebrate more than 50 years since its first use.

The use of this new agent, which was very expensive (at 50 cents a gallon), necessitated a change in the technique of administration to a closed system with carbon dioxide absorption. Griffith quickly accepted this major change and worked on improvements. Aids used to maintain a tight system were an inflatable balloon on the endotracheal tube and the use of the Leech pharyngeal bulb gasway.

Thoracic surgery was in its infancy in the early thirties and was only contemplated for patients with severe abscess-producing pulmonary diseases. Operation was usually followed by contamination of the 'good lung' and a high mortality rate. To reduce the possibility of this Dr Waters (7) suggested the use of a cuffed endotracheal tube inserted into either the right or left main bronchus, and Dr Harold was quick to understand the significance of this approach. He, in turn, offered to Dr E. Archibald, a Montreal thoracic surgeon, the idea of a bronchial blocker (8).

Recovery and intensive care

Since Griffith was also the Medical Superintendent of the hospital he was quick to adopt innovative ideas about areas of specialized patient care and in 1943 opened the first Post-Operative Recovery Room in Canada (9). This was thought to be a waste of money by many at that time—but would any anaesthetist today feel safe without such a facility?

In time and with increasingly more complicated medical and surgical undertakings, it seemed appropriate to start an Intensive Care Unit in 1961 at the Queen Elizabeth Hospital. There was only one other such unit in Canada at that time. This was followed by a unit designed for the special care and monitoring of the acute cardiac patient.

Teaching and research

Although Griffith had had no formal training in anaesthesia he realized the need for this if it was to progress as a specialty. He discovered later in life that he had a talent for imbuing students with his wisdom and pragmatism. Thus, he developed an Anaesthesia Training Programme for the Armed services during World War II. This developed into a three-year diploma course and is now the specialist training programme at McGill University.

As Chairman of the Department of Anaesthesia at McGill, he felt that teaching had to be supplemented by research and he persuaded Sir Henry Dale and the Wellcome Trust to support a research professorship. Sir Gordon Robson set up the Department of Research in Anaesthesia which is now directed by Professor K. Krnjevic. However, this was an independent department within the University and has not become what Griffith envisaged. This is now being rectified by the setting up of an endowed chair which will bear his name, and which will be an integral part of the Department of Anaesthesia at McGill.

National and international organizations

The importance of sharing knowledge and experience amongst colleagues was an early interest of Griffith's and he became involved in the organization of associations of anaesthesia, at first locally then nationally. He became President, Canadian Anaesthetists' Society (1943–46), and later, Founder President of the international World Federation of Societies of Anesthesiologists.

Scientific articles and a conclusion

He produced many papers on many different subjects, all written in clear concise language. In 1963, on the 21st anniversary of the first successful anaesthetic use of curare, a volume of his writings was produced by his colleagues and entitled, 'The Boundless Realm of Anesthesiology' (3). In this and in other papers published thereafter he leaves us many words of wise advice and these remain, today, the essence of the safe practice of anaesthesia.

His favourite dictum was the motto of the Canadian Anaesthetists' Society—chosen by his friend and predecessor in the McGill Department of Anaesthesia, Dr Wesley Bourne:

'KATHEUDONDAS PARATEROUMEN'
(We watch closely those who sleep)

References

(1) Griffith HR, Johnson GE. The use of curare in general anaesthesia. *Anesthesiology* 1942; **3**: 418–20.
(2) Bennett AE. Curare: A preventive in traumatic convulsive shock therapy. *Am J Psych* 1941; **97**: 1040.
(3) *The boundless realm of anaesthesiology: A collection of the works of Harold Randall Griffith.* 1963.
(4) Griffith HR. Intratracheal ethylene–oxygen anaesthesia. *Can Med Assoc J* 1929; **21**: 294–6.
(5) Griffith HR. Cyclopropane anaesthesia: a clinical record of 350 administrations. *Can Med Assoc J* 1934; **31**: 157–60.
(6) Griffith HR. *Personal communication*, 1985.
(7) Gale JW, Waters RM. Closed endobronchial anesthesia in thoracic surgery. *J Thorac Surg* 1932; **1**: 432–7.
(8) Archibald E. A consideration of the dangers of lobectomy. *J Thorac Surg* 1935; **4**: 335–51.
(9) Griffith HR, MacMillan M. A post-operative recovery room and blood bank. *Can Hosp* 1946; **23**: 38–40.

References

PART VII
SPECIAL PRESENTATIONS

Chapter 26
POSTERS

The subject matter of the majority of the posters have been included in previous chapters indicated by the cross references.

26.1 The history of the faculty of anaesthetists of the Royal College of Surgeons of England.
Aileen K. Adams and **Richard S. Atkinson**
(See *Chapter* 8. *Paper* 8.1.)

26.2 Memorabilia of Sir Ivan Magill, KVO.
D. J. Wilkinson and **Audrey Eccles**
(See also *Chapter* 25. *Papers* 25.18 & 25.19.)

26.3 Finding the real Crawford Long. Discovery of an historical photograph.
M.A. Albin
(See *Chapter* 24. *Paper* 24.1.)

26.4 To keep the Ether Dome a show place.
M. Tverskoy
(See *Chapter* 6. *Paper* 6.5.)

26.5 John Snow's Monograph "On the inhalation of the vapour of ether".
A. Matsuki
(See *Chapter* 24. *Paper* 24.2.)

26.6 To teach doctors—a scientific basis for the practice of anaesthesia.
L. E. Morris
(See *Chapter* 25. *Paper* 25.14.)

26.7 Classic papers from the *British Journal of Anaesthesia*.
P. A. Coe and **A. P. Adams**

26.8 Whose were these?
P. Frost
(A presentation of minor pieces of anaesthetic equipment designed by anaesthetists and bearing their names with historical notes on the persons concerned.

Chapter 27
VIDEO AND FILM PRESENTATIONS

27.1 Video recordings of eminent anaesthetists.
The Wood Library of the American Society of Anesthesiologists

27.2 Historic films on anaesthesia.
H. Essex-Lopresti

27.3 Historic films from the ICI Archives.
Imperial Chemical Industries Limited

List of registrants

R. Acland
9 Tole Street, Ponsonby, Auckland, New
Zealand

C. K. Adam
6 Sillerhole Road, Leven, Fife, Scotland
KY8 5NA

A. K. Adams
Dean, Faculty of Anaesthetists,
Royal College of Surgeons, 35–43 Lincoln's
Inn Fields, London, England

C. N. Adams
West Suffolk Hospital
Hardwick Lane, Bury St Edmunds, Suffolk
IP33 2QZ

M. Adt
Deutsches Herzzentrum Berlin,
Augustenburger Platz 1, 1000 Berlin 65,
W. Germany

A. A. Al-Mazrooa
King Abdulaziz University Hos,
PO Box 6615 Jeddah, Saudi Arabia

M. S. Albin
7703 Floyd Curl Drive, San Antonio, Texas
78284, USA

L. G. Allan
Windmill Cottage, 64 Watchet Lane, Holmer
Green, Bucks, England

R. S. Atkinson
75 High Cliff Drive, Leigh on Sea, Essex
SS9 1DQ, England

N. Azzopardi
11 Preca Street, Lija, Malta

S. M. Baguneid
King Khaled Eye Hospital,
PO Box 7191, Riyadh 11462, Saudi Arabia

R. Bailey
PO Box 360, Roseville,
NSW 2069, Australia

B. Baker
Otago University, Dunedin, New Zealand

C. Ball
19 Mason Avenue, Elwood 3184, Victoria
3184, Australia

B. J. Bamforth
University of Wisconsin, Madison W1,
53705 USA

A. Bardeen-Henschell
412N Lake Road, Oconomowoc WI 53066,
USA

Dr P. J. F. Baskett
Frenchay Hospital, Bristol BS16 1LE,
England

G. S. Bause
Yale University School Medicine,
Department of Anesthesiology
333 Cedar Street, PO Box 3333, New Haven,
Connecticut, USA

J. Beinart
Wellcome Unit for History of Medicine,
45–47 Banbury Road, Oxford OX2 6PE,
England

Dr R. Bell
42 Stonegate Drive, Ancaster L9G 3R7,
Canada

N. A. Bergman
3181 SW Sam Jackson Park Road, Portland, Oregon, 97201, USA

A. M. Betcher
Orthopaedic Institute, Bernard Aronson Plaza, 301 East 17th Street, New York NY 10003, USA

K. J. Betten
6072 Old Post Road, Kalamazoo, Michigan 49009, USA

R. Binning
19 Nizells Avenue, Hove BN3 1PL, England

K. J. Bird
Royal Berkshire Hospital, London Road, Reading, Berks, England

T. E. Black
3010 Provincial, Ann Arbor, Michigan 48104, USA

C. Blogg
Radcliffe Infirmary, Woodstock Road, Oxford OX2 6HE, England

R. Bodman
409 Admiralty Place, Prince Street, Dartmouth, Nova Scotia, Canada B2Y 4L3

J. Bottome
3533 South Alameda, PO Box 6530, Corpus Christi, Texas, USA

T. B. Boulton
Royal Berkshire Hospital, Reading RG1 5AN, Berks, England

J. B. Bowes
Cottles, Publow, Pensford, Bristol BS18 4JA

L. Brandt
Mainz University Hospital, D-6500 Mainz, German Federal Republic.

P. P. Bricknell
48 Boxwood Drive, Hershey PA 17033, Republic of South Africa

W. Brodzinski
4337 N.E. 22nd Avenue, Fort Lauderdale, Florida 33308, USA

A. M. Broennle
Children's Hospital, 34th Street, Civic Center Boulevard, Philadelphia, USA

D. A. R. Brown
1 Ady Street, Hunters Hill, NSW 2110, Australia

Dr M. W. Brown
6 Le Bourgage, Alderney, Channel Islands

R. C. Bryan-Brown
6431 Fannin, 5.020 MSMB, Houston, Texas 77030, USA

B. A. Burgess
7 Clevedale, Downend, Bristol BS16 2SQ, England

J. W. Burleson
Dekalb General Hospital, Decatur, Georgia, USA

M. Burrows
2 The Westwoods, Noctorum Road, Birkenhead, Merseyside, England

J. Burton
Rusty Stack, Bulkington Road, Wolvey, Nr Hinckley, Leics, England

R. Calverley
UCSD Medical Center H-770, 225 Dickinson Street, San Diego, CA 92103, USA

K. Chambers
94 Topsham Road, Exeter EX2 4RR, England

C. Chevalier-Thewissen
Rue Basse 2, 1180 Brussells, Belgium

J. A. Clarke
22 Copse Hill, Wimbledon, London SW20 0HG, England

W. G. Clayton
93 Whitefield Road, Stockton Heath, Warrington WA4 6ND, England

A. R. Clifford
42 Strickland Avenue, Glen Waverley, Melbourne, Australia

D. Coates
Bristol Royal Infirmary, Bristol BS2 8HW,
England

P. Coe
Guy's Hospital, London SE1, England

D. I. Conacher
44 Moorside South, Newcastle upon Tyne
NE4 9BB, England

E. Conner
5704 Apache Road, Louisville, Kentucky
40207, USA

I. Corall
Kings College Hospital, London SE5 9RS,
England

J. Corbett
42 Glenburnie Road, Mitcham, Melbourne
3132, Australia

T. G. Costello
16 Evans Road, Kew, Victoria 3101,
Australia

J. Couper
Medical University of S.A., Box 205, PO
Medunsa, South Africa

J. Cowan
13 Calais Court, Nepean, Ontario K2E 7E1,
Canada

R. Cowie
16 Kooyongkoot Road, Hawthorn, Victoria
3122, Australia

M. C. Crocker
795 Oak Street, Winnipeg, Manitoba
R3M 3RZ, Canada

K. Cvachovek
UL. 8 Listopadu 22, 169 00 Praha 6,
Czechoslovakia

S. Dalal
38 Partridge Road, St. Albans, Herts
AL3 6HH, England

J. Daniel
2 The Spinney, Hartlepool, Cleveland
TS26 0AW, England

R. W. E. Daniel
312 Buncombe Street, Raleigh, North
Carolina 27609, USA

H. Davenport
Northwick Park Hospital, Harrow, Middx,
England

J. J. de Lange
Free University Hospital, PO Box 7057,
Amsterdam, Holland

P. Debenham
206–600 Royal Avenue, New Westminster,
British Columbia V3M 1J3, Canada

D. Devchand
21 Forest Oak Close, Cyn Coed, Cardiff
CF2 6QN, Wales

S. Dhamee
8700 W. Wisconsin Avenue, Milwaukee,
Wisconsin 53226, USA

P. Dinnick
Brook Cottage Hospital, Empshott Green,
Liss, Hants GU33 6HU, England

F. Dorman
Hillingdon Hospital, Field Heath Road,
Uxbridge, Middx, England

D. Duda
Mainz University Hospital, D-6500 Mainz,
Federal German Republic

P. Duncan
16 Simpson Crescent, Saskatoon, Sask 57H
3C6, Canada

B. Duncum
26 St Edmunds Terrace, London NW8 7QB,
England

M. I. Edwards
Veterans Administration Center,
Philadelphia, Pennsylvania 19104, USA

M. El Gindi
Inz University Hospital, D-6500 Mainz,
Federal German Republic

R. H. Ellis
Linden House, 45 Eglington Road,
Chingford, London E4 7AS, England

S. Eriksen
Haderslev Sygerhus, Haderslev, DK 6100
Denmark

P. Fancourt-Smith
Vancouver General Hospital, 855 West 12th
Avenue, Vancouver BC, V5Z 1M9,
Canada

R. Fink
RN-10 University of Washington, Seattle,
Washington 98195, USA

Dr G. Flowers
13762 Northwood Road NW, Seattle,
Washington 98177, USA

A. Fortuna
Hospital Santo Antonio, Av Bernadino de
Campos 47, Santon SP 11100, Brazil

C. Foster
Glebe Farm, Sternfield, Near Saxmundham,
Suffolk, England

J. Freeman
Centre Hospitalier, Universitaire Vaudois,
CH-1011 Lausanne, Switzerland

E. Frost
Albert Einstein College of Medicine, Bronx
N.Y., 10461, USA

P. Frost
Glan Clwyd Hospital, Bodelwyddan, Nr
Rhyl, Clwyd, Wales

S. Garner
70 Latimer Road, Cropston, Leicester LE7
7GN, England

A. Gazder
124 Market Street, Sunbury PA 17801,
USA

L. Gemmell
Hafdd-y-Gynfawr, Glyn Ceriog,
Nr Llangollen, Clwyd, Wales

G. Gerson
2 Princes Crescent, Hove, BN3 4GS,
England

D. Gibb
St Vincent's Hospital, Victoria Street,
Darlinghurst NSW 2010, Australia

E. Gibbs
83 Church Street, Great Burstead, Billericay,
Essex CM11 2TS, England

D. M. M. Gillies
Queen Elizabeth Hospital, 2100 Marlowe
Avenue, Montreal, Quebec H4A 3L6

M. Goerig
2 Hamburg 20, Martinistrasse 52, Federal
German Republic

D. Goldstein
3824 Chandelle Lane, Port Arthur, Texas
77642, USA

T. Gordh
J. O. Wallins Vag 6, 17164 Solna, Sweden

E. Hackner
514 Hillcrest Road, Beverly Hills, CA 90210,
USA

P. Hall
7 Waterdale Road, Ivanhoe, Victoria 3079,
Australia

G. Hall Davies
Park House, 463 Birmingham Road,
Bordesley, Redditch, Worcs. B97 6RL,
England

W. K. Hamilton
University of California, San Francisco,
California 94143, USA

G. W. Hamlin
1 Grange Park Close, Leeds LS8 3BU,
England

H. B. Hannah
Queen Elizabeth Military Hospital, Stadium
Road, Woolwich, London SE18, England

O. Haxholdt
Vilvordehoj 11, Charlottenlund, DK 2920,
Denmark

I. Hayter
4875 Connaught Drive, Vancouver, British
Columbia V6J 4E4, Canada

U. Hintzenstern
Anderlohrstrasse 4, D-8520, Erlangen, Federal German Republic

Anthony Holland
Montreal General Hospital, 1650 Cedar Avenue, Montreal, Quebec H36 1A4, Canada

J. Horton
9 Orchard Close, Wenvoe, Gwent CF5 6BW, Wales

I. Houghton
BMH, BFPO 17, Federal German Republic

G. Housam
2053 James Street, Burlington, Ontario L7R 1H4, Canada

D. D. C. Howat
Flat 10, 40 Wimpole Street, London W1M 7AF, England

Hsu
675 Worcester Road, Wellesley Hills, MA 02181, USA

R. Hughes
Wellcome Research Laboratories, Beckenham, Kent BR3 3BS, England

R. G. Humble
University of Alberta, 12407-39 Ave, Edmonton, Alberta T6J 0N1, Canada

G. Huston
147 Annandale Road, Pasadena, California 91105-1405, USA

A. Hyman
622 W.168 Street, New York City, 10032, USA

M. T. Inman
Moorholme, Dousland, Yelverton, Devon PL20 6LY, England

A. T. J. Jasser
Faculty of Medicine, University of Aleppo, PO Box 3126 Aleppo, Syria

Sir A. Jephcott
21 Brilliant Street, St Heliers, Auckland 5, New Zealand

B. Jones
43 Bro Emrys, Talybont, Bangor, Gwynedd, North Wales LL57 3YT

H. M. Jones
Royal Gwent Hospital, Newport, Gwent, Wales

D. Joseph
Univesity of Sydney, 2006 Australia

M. B. Kamath
167 Sutton Passeys Crescent, Wollaton Park, Nottingham NG8 1EA, England

L. Kaufman
941 Finchley Road, London NW11 7PE, England

M. Kus
Copernicus Medical School, Kopernika 17, Krakow 31–501, Poland

K. Lech
Silesian Medical Academy, Katowice Ul Medykow 14, 40–752, Poland

J. A. Lee
73 Kings Road, Westcliff on Sea, Essex SS0 8PH, England

K. G. Lee
Westminster Hospital, London, England

Z. Lett
Caritas Medical Centre, 111 Wing Hong Street, Shamshuipo, Kowloon, Hong Kong

O. Lippman
S & W Foundation Roskildevej 14, Albertslund, DK-2620-Denmark

W. G. G. Loyn
Llechwedd, Banc-Y-Darren, Aberystwyth SY23 3LJ, Wales

P. Lye
Glan Clwyd Hospital, Odelwyddan, Rhyl, Clwyd LL18 5UJ, Wales

A. MacDonald
28 Newlands Road, Glasgow G43 2JD, Scotland

T. MacDonald
6/33 Elamang Avenue, Kirribilli, New South Wales 2061, Australia

J. A. MacDougall
20 Queen Square, Saint John, N.B. Canada E2L 1R7

J. Mainzer
1720 Louisiana NE 401, Albuquerque, New Mexico 87110, USA

R. Maltby
Foothills Hospital, 1403-29 Street NW, Calgary, Alberta T2N 2T9

R. Mansfield
Cherry Tree Cottage, Henley Hill, Surrey GU27 3HG, England

J. Marcy
220 N. Dithridge Street, Pittsburgh PA, 15213, USA

E. Mathews
54 Selly Wick Road, Selly Park, Birmingham B29 7JB, England

A. Matsuki
5 Zaifu-Cho, Hirosake, Aormori-Ken, Japan

M. Mauve
Veldweg 32, Laren NH, 1251 HD, Holland

C. McLaren
12 Broadacres, Broad Town, Wotton Bassett, Wilts, England

I. McLellan
Groby Road Hospital, Leicester, England

R. Mirakhur
Royal Victoria Hospital, Belfast BT12 6BA, Northern Ireland

L. Morris
15670 Point Monroe Drive NE, Bainbridge Island, Washington 98110, USA

P. Morris
29 Norris Road, Sale, Manchester M33 3GR, England

W. W. Mushin
30 Bettws-Y-Coed Road, Cardiff CF2 6PL, Wales

N. Naqvi
Bolton General Hospital, Minerva Road, Farnworth, Bolton, England

N. Newton
Guy's Hospital, St Thomas Street, London SE1 9RT, England

J. Nunn
Northwick Park Hospital, Harrow, Middx HA1 3UJ, England

C. H. Osborne
32 St Anns Way, Leeds LS4 2SQ, England

B. Owen
Ysbyty Glan Clwyd, Bodelwyddan, Nr Rhyl, Clwyd LL18 5UJ, Wales

A. Owies
Royal Melbourne Hospital, 7 Power Avenue, Hawthorn, Victoria 3122, Australia

W. K. Pallister
8 Upper Wimpole Street, London W1, England

S. Panjratan
Blacktown Hospital, Blacktown, N.S.W., Australia

C. Parsloe
Hospital Samaritano, Rua Conselheiro Brotero, 1486, 01232 S. Paulo SP, Brasil

P. Patel
221 Foxmeadow Drive, Winnipeg, Manitoba R3P 1T4, Canada

R. Patterson
143 Greenfield Avenue, Los Angeles CA, 90049, USA

S. V. Pavan
8 Mirrabooka Avenue, Homebush, New South Wales 2140, Australia

J. Pender
26311 Esperanza Drive, Los Altos Hills, CA
94022, USA

B. Philpott
12 Kingswood Firs, Grayshott, Hindhead
GU26 6EU, England

S. Pokrzywnicki
Editor, Polish Journal Anaesthesia,
Pl. Konstyttucji 3M, 78 Warsaw Pl 00-647,
Poland

R. W. N. Ramsden
42 Repton Drive, Newcastle, Staffs
STT5 3JF, England

H. Reinhold
247 Av. Winston Churchill, Bte. 8, B-1180,
Bruxelles, Belgium

L. Rendell-Baker
11201 Benton St, Loma Linda, California
92357, USA

J. Restall
Cambridge Military Hospital, Aldershot,
Hants GU11 2AN, England

D. L. Rice
Children's Hospital, National Medical
Centre, 111 Michigan Avenue,
Washington DC 20010, USA

J. G. Roberts
Flinders Medical Centre, Bedford Park,
South Australia 5042, Australia

Z. Rondio
National Research Institute, of Mother and
Child, Ul. Kasprzaka 17A, Warsaw

N. Rose
Worcester Royal Infirmary, Castle Street,
Worcester WR1 3AS, England

M. Rosen
45 Hollybush Road, Cardiff CF2 6SZ, Wales

M. K. R. Roy
General Hospital, Hartlepool, Cleveland
TS24 9AH, England

H. Ruben
Skodsborg Strandvej 260, 2942 Skodsborg,
Denmark

M. Rucklidge
Royal Lancaster Infirmary, Lancaster,
England

W. Runciman
6 Birkdale Crescent, Mt. Osmond SA 5064,
Australia

J. Ruphreht
Erasmus University, Azr Dijkzigt,
Rotterdam, Netherlands

G. B. Rushman
26 Tyrrone Road, Thorpe Bay, Essex
SS1 3HF, England

M. V. Ryssen
Dobbins, Castle Lane, Bramber, Nr
Steyning, W. Sussex BN4 3FB, England

W. Sabiniewicz
Apartment 12, 13 Av. De. L'Yser, 1040
Brussells, Belgium

T. Savege
The London Hospital, Whitechapel, London
E1 1BB, England

E. Schwarz
39 Belvoir Road, St Andrews, Bristol
BS6 5DQ, England

R. W. Schwarz
Inst. fur Anaesthesiologie,
Maximiliansplatz 1, D-8520 Erlangen,
Federal German Republic

W. Scott
Church Farm Cottage, Astwick, Stotfold,
Hitchin, Herts SG5 4BH, England

W. E. Scott
Church Farm Cottage, Astwick, Stotfold,
Hitchin, Herts, England

O. Secher
Blegdamsvej 9, 2100 Copenhagen 0,
DK-2100, Denmark

R. Seed
Riyadh Military Hospital, E230 Armed Forces Hospital, PO Box 7897 Riyadh 11159, Saudi Arabia

J. W. Severinghaus
UCSF, 1386 Hse, UCSF San Francisco CA, 94143, USA

R. N. Shah
2 Lime Crescent, Sandal, Wakefield WF2 6RY, Yorks, England

Z. P. Shah
4 Russellcroft Road, Welwyn Garden City, AL8 6QT, England

S. M. Shnider
University of California, 513 Parnassus Avenue, San Francisco 94143, USA

P. H. Simmons
Garden House, 3 Queens Road, Barnet EN5 4DH, England

I. Smith
8 North Deeside Road, Bieldside, Aberdeen AB1 9AJ, Scotland

T. Smith
5 Parkside Road, Reading RG3 2DA, Berks, England

W. D. Smith
11 Moorland Drive, Leeds, Yorks LS17 6JP, England

G. W. Snipes
2962 Las Palmas Court, Riverside, California 92506, USA

D. Soban
Borsetova 23, 61000 Ljublijana, Yugoslavia

L. Soper
217 Canyon Drive, Las Vegas, NV 89107, USA

D. Soucek
5847 Broadview Road, Cleveland, Ohio, 44134, USA

D. Spears
32 Roxwell Road, Chelmsford, Essex CM1 2NB, England

J. R. Spears
32 Roxwell Road, Chelmsford, Essex CM1 2NB, England

R. S. Srivastava
35 St Georges Avenue, South Shields, Tyne and Wear, England

J. E. Steinhaus
1365 Clifton Road, Atlanta GA 30322, USA

R. S. Stephen
15801 Harris Ridge Ct, Chesterfield MO 63017, USA

J. B. Stetson
Rush Medical College, St Luke's Medical Center, 1753 W. Congress Parkway, Chicago 60612, USA

P. Stow
6 Harrow Road, Knockholt, Sevenoaks, Kent TN14 7JT, England

M. S. M. Takrouri
Faculty of Medicine, Jordan University, Amman, Jordan

T. N. Taylor
60 Wood Vale, London N10 3DN, England

C. M. P. Theunissen
Medical Centre de Klokkenberg, Galderseweg 81, 4836 Ae Breda, Holland

T. A. Thomas
Bristol Maternity Hospital, Southwell Street, Bristol BS2 8EG, England

P. W. Thompson
2 Lakeside Drive, Cardiff CF2 6DF, Wales

S. Tirer
V. A. Medical Center, Woodlands University, Philadelphia, PA 19107, USA

D. Toren
3117 South 30th Street, Lincoln, Nebraska 68502, USA

K. Underwood
The White House, 2 St Martin's Road,
 Scarborough, N. Yorks. YO11 1QJ,
 England

R. M. Valkenburg
Groene Hilledyk 315, Rotterdam 3075, EA,
 Holland

J. Van Berkel
Diamant 5, Berkel en Rodenrijs, 2651 SH,
 Holland

J. Van Kleef
46 Park Leeuwenberghlaan, Leidschenden
 2267 BP, Holland

M. Van Wishe
Sanderij 8, Delden 7491 GX, Holland

L. D. Vandam
75 Francis Street, Boston, Massachusetts
 02115, USA

R. Vaughan
17 Ash Tree Close, Radyr, Cardiff CF4 8RY,
 Wales

D. Vermeulen-Cranch
Nijeenburg 82, Buitenveldert, Amsterdam
 1081 GG, Holland

I. R. Verner
67 Harley Street, London W1N 1DE,
 England

J. B. R. Walker
23 Weir Close, Mainstone, Plymouth, Devon
 PL6 8SD, England

C. Ward
Royal Infirmary, Huddersfield HD3 3EA,
 Yorks, England

B. Welsh
14 Tankerville Terrace, Smond, Newcastle
 on Tyne NE2 3AH, England

R. Westhorpe
Royal Children's Hospital, Parkville,
 Melbourne 3052, Australia

Dr D. Wilkinson
St Bartholomew's Hospital, London
 EC1A 7BE, England

J. Williams
231 Macquarie Street, Sydney, NSW 2000,
 Australia

V. Williams
8 Abbotts Close, Macclesfield, SK10 3PB,
 England

M. Wilmotte
24 Rue Curie, Seraing, B4100, Belgium

G. Wilson
74 Mitchell Parade, Mollymook, NSW
 Australia 2539, Australia

J. D. Wolff
Hoge Duin Daalseweg 13, 2061 AD
 Bloemendaal, Holland

C. Woollam
105A Newmarket Road, Norwich NR2 2HT,
 England

G. Wyant
University Hospital, Saskatoon,
 Saskatchewan S7N 0X0, Canada

D. Zuck
Chase Farm Hospital, Enfield, Middx,
 England

(NB: page numbers in italics refer to illustrations and diagrams)